Acute Rheumatic Fever
and
Chronic Rheumatic Heart Disease

Acute Rheumatic Fever
and
Chronic Rheumatic Heart Disease

SECOND EDITION

Editor

IB Vijayalakshmi

MBBS MD DM (Card) DSc FICC FIAMS FIAEFCSI FICP FCSI FAMS FISH FRCP (London)

Professor Emeritus of Pediatric Cardiology
Former Professor and HOD
Department of Pediatric Cardiology
Super Specialty Hospital [Pradhan Mantri Swasthya Suraksha Yojana (PMSSY)]
Bangalore Medical College and Research Institute
Former Head, Pediatric Cardiology
Sri Jayadeva Institute of Cardiovascular Sciences and Research
Bengaluru, Karnataka, India
President Elect of Indian Academy of Echocardiography

Foreword
George Cherian

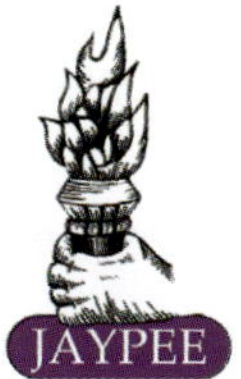

JAYPEE BROTHERS MEDICAL PUBLISHERS

The Health Sciences Publisher

New Delhi | London

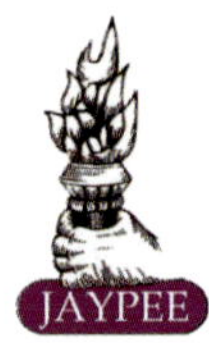 **Jaypee Brothers Medical Publishers (P) Ltd**

Headquarters
EMCA House
23/23-B, Ansari Road, Daryaganj
New Delhi 110 002, India
Landline: +91-11-23272143, +91-11-23272703
+91-11-23282021, +91-11-23245672
E-mail: jaypee@jaypeebrothers.com

Corporate Office
Jaypee Brothers Medical Publishers (P) Ltd.
4838/24, Ansari Road, Daryaganj
New Delhi 110 002, India
Phone: +91-11-43574357
Fax: +91-11-43574314
E-mail: jaypee@jaypeebrothers.com

Overseas Office
JP Medical Ltd.
83, Victoria Street, London
SW1H 0HW (UK)
Phone: +44-20 3170 8910
Fax: +44(0)20 3008 6180
E-mail: info@jpmedpub.com

Website: www.jaypeebrothers.com
Website: www.jaypeedigital.com

Inquiries for bulk sales may be solicited at: jaypee@jaypeebrothers.com

Acute Rheumatic Fever and Chronic Rheumatic Heart Disease / IB Vijayalakshmi

First Edition: 2011

Second Edition: **2023**

ISBN: 978-93-5465-878-5

Printed at: Samrat Offset Pvt. Ltd.

Dedicated To

All our patients of acute rheumatic fever,
chronic rheumatic heart disease and
thousands of rheumatic heart disease
patients in the past,
who taught the lessons to
the clinicians all over the world
and also dedicated to doyen of cardiology
late Dr S Padmavati who inspired many like me
and late Dr Chitra Narsimhan dedicated and devoted associate.

Contributors

Arati Dave Lalchandani MD (Med) DM (Card) FCSI FAPVIS
Board of Governors
AIIMS, Gorakhpur
Former Principal and Dean
GSVM Medical College
Kanpur, Uttar Pradesh, India

AS Chandrasekhara Rao MD DM (Card) FISE FICA FIAMS
FIMSA FICP FICC FACC FCSI
Consultant Cardiologist
Former Professor and Head
Department of Cardiology
Sri Jayadeva Institute of Cardiovascular
Sciences and Research
Bengaluru, Karnataka, India

Asha Moorthy MD DM FICP FCCP FIMSA FIACM FICC
Professor and Head
Department of Cardiology
Sri Ramachandra University and Saveetha University
(Emeritus)
Sri Ramaswamy Memorial Institute
Chennai, Tamil Nadu, India

Bo Remenyi MBBS FRACP PhD FCSANZ
Pediatric Cardiologist
Royal Children's Hospital
Research Fellow
Division of Child Health
Menzies School of Health Research
Darwin, Australia

Chandrakant B Patil MD (Med) DM (Card) Fellowships-WHO
Fellow in Interventional Cardiology (USA) Fellow of Cardiological
Society of India Fellow of Indian College of Cardiology Fellow of
Indian Academy of Echocardiography Fellow of IMA AMS
Visiting Faculty
Department of Cardiology
Manipal Hospital, Bengaluru
Cardiologist
Sri Shankara Cancer Hospital and Research Centre
Bengaluru, Karnataka, India
Member: Association of Physicians of India
Member: IMA

Late Chitra Narasimhan MD FICPC
Assistant Professor
Department of Clinical Pediatric Cardiology
Sri Jayadeva Institute of Cardiovascular Sciences and Research
Bengaluru, Karnataka, India

IB Vijayalakshmi MD DM (Card) DSc FICC FIAMS FIAE
FCSI FICP FCSI FAMS FISH FRCP (Lond)
Professor Emeritus of Pediatric Cardiology
Former HOD at
Sri Jayadeva Institute of Cardiovascular Sciences and Research
Bengaluru, Karnataka, India
President Elect of Indian Academy of Echocardiography

Jain T Kallarakkal MD DM FRCP
Senior Consultant
Department of Cardiology
Sree Narayana Institute of Medical Sciences
Kochi, Kerala, India

Monica Kher DNB (Gen Med) DNB (Card)
Cardiologist
Department of Cardiology
Aster Hospital
Doha, Qatar

Nicola Culliford-Semmens MBChB FRACP
Pediatric Cardiology Fellow
Department of Pediatric and Congenital Cardiology
Green Lane Pediatric and Congenital Cardiac Services
Starship Children's Health
Te Whatu Ora, Auckland, New Zealand

Nigel Wilson MBChB DCH MRCP FRACP FCSANZ
Pediatric Cardiologist
Department of Pediatric and Congenital Cardiology
Starship Children's Hospital
Honorary Clinical Associate Professor
Department of Pediatrics
University of Auckland
Auckland, New Zealand

Poonam Malhotra Kapoor MD DNB MNAMS FIACTA (Hony)
FTEE (Hony) FISCU (Hony)
Professor
Department of Cardiac Anesthesia and Critical Care
All India Institute of Medical Sciences (AIIMS)
New Delhi, India

Pradeep Vaideeswar MD
Professor
Department of Pathology (Cardiovascular and Thoracic Division)
Seth GS Medical College
Mumbai, Maharashtra, India

Prasanna Simha Mohan Rao MD
Professor and Head
Department of Cardiothoracic and Vascular Surgery
Sri Jayadeva Institute of Cardiovascular Sciences and Research
Bengaluru, Karnataka, India

Ramesh Arora MD DM (Card) FICC FCSI FIMSA FACC
Chief Cardiologist
Metro Hospitals and Heart Institute
Noida, Uttar Pradesh, India
Formerly Director
Professor and Head
Department of Cardiology
Maulana Azad Medical College and
Govind Ballabh Pant Hospital
New Delhi, India

Sarasa Bharati MD PhD FCCP FICP FEMSI FIAMS FICA FMMC
Director
Research, Training and Applications
Madras Institute of Orthopaedics and Traumatology (MIOT)
Hospitals
Chennai, Tamil Nadu, India

Saroja Bharati MD
Director
The Maurice Lev Congenital Heart and Conduction System
Center, The Heart Institute for Children
Advocate Hope Children's Hospital
Advocate Christ Medical Center
Oak Lawn, Illinois, USA
Professor of Pathology
Rush University Medical Center
Chicago, Illinois, USA
Clinical Professor of Pathology
Rosalind Franklin University of Medicine and Science
Chicago Medical School, North Chicago, Illinois
Visiting Professor of Pathology
University of Illinois Chicago
Illinois, USA

Shibba Takkar Chhabra DM (Card) FACC FCSI
Professor of Cardiology
Dayanand Medical College and Hospital
Unit Hero DMC Heart Institute
Ludhiana, Punjab, India

Sivasubramanian Ramakrishnan MD DM FACC
Professor of Cardiology
All India Institute of Medical Sciences
New Delhi, India
Editor-in-Chief
Annals of Pediatric Cardiology

Smita Mishra MD (Ped) FNB (Ped Card)
Head
Department of Pediatric Cardiology
Human Care Medical Charitable Trust (HCMCT)
Manipal Hospital
Dwarka, New Delhi, India

Sneha K Chunchanur MD (Microbio)
Assistant Professor
Department of Microbiology
Bangalore Medical College and Research Institute
Bengaluru, Karnataka, India

Late S Padmavati FRCP (Lond) FRCPE FAMS FACC FAHA FESC
DSc (Hon) PhD (Hon)
Former President
All India Heart Foundation
New Delhi, India

S Pruthvish MD (Community Med) DNB FISHWM FAMS
Director of Academics and Training
Sri Shankara Cancer Hospital and Research Centre
Former Professor and Head
Department of Community Medicine
MS Ramaiah Medical College
Bengaluru, Karnataka, India

Sudhayakumar N MD DM
Former Professor and Head
Department of Cardiology
Government Medical Colleges Kottayam and Kozhikode
Kerala, India

Usha Anand MD FPC
Associate Professor
Department of Pediatric Cardiology
Sri Jayadeva Institute of Cardiovascular Sciences and Research
Bengaluru, Karnataka, India

Foreword

I feel privileged to be asked to write a foreword to this book on *Acute Rheumatic Fever and Chronic Rheumatic Heart Disease*, edited by Professor IB Vijayalakshmi, one of India's leading Pediatric Cardiologists, who has herself contributed greatly to this field.

Rheumatic fever and rheumatic heart disease continue to be a major cause of mortality and morbidity even now in many parts of the globe and particularly so with poorer sections of societies. In 2005, it was estimated that the global burden of group A streptococcal diseases was still high with a prevalence of at least 20 million cases with around 3,00,000 new cases each year and as many deaths (Lancet Infect Dis, 5:685-94). Reappearance of rheumatic fever in parts of the Western world, points out the need for continued vigilance and attention to this problem. The WHO has brought out several technical reports and as recently as 2009 the American Heart Association has updated their scientific statement on the prevention of rheumatic fever and the diagnosis and treatment of acute streptococcal pharyngitis (Circulation, Vol: 119).

It is, therefore, right and proper that an updated book on *Acute Rheumatic Fever and Chronic Rheumatic Heart Disease* is being published from the Indian subcontinent. Most of the contribution in the newer sections like the role of echocardiography in the diagnosis of acute rheumatic carditis and nonsurgical treatment of rheumatic vascular heart disease has been given by the Indian workers.

Professor IB Vijayalakshmi, Professor Emeritus and former Head of Pediatric Cardiology at one of India's major institutions with the Sri Jayadeva Institute of Cardiovascular Sciences and Research is ideally placed to edit such a book. She has had a major interest in rheumatic fever and rheumatic heart disease and has made a notable contribution particularly in the area of echocardiographic criteria for the diagnosis of acute rheumatic carditis. She also has the distinction of being a member of the World Heart Federation Group for standardizing echocardiography in rheumatic heart disease. The book with a galaxy of distinguished contributors, I am sure will be a valuable reference resource for the years to come and this Second Edition upgraded the knowledge and advances till now, especially revised New Jones criteria that has included Echo as a major criteria to detect subclinical carditis that will change the epidemiological face of RF and RHD.

George Cherian MD DM FACC FAMS FRCP
Academic Head
Cardiology Division
Narayana Hrudayalaya Hospital, Bengaluru, Karnataka, India
Former Head, Cardiology Division
Christian Medical College, Vellore, Tamil Nadu, India
Former President, Cardiology Society of India

Preface

The purpose of this book is to describe the whole gamut of *Acute Rheumatic Fever (ARF) and Chronic Rheumatic Heart Disease (RHD)* and give the details of management by which the practitioners and the medical students can approach the diagnostic problem presented by children with this disease; through proper assessment and integration of the history, physical examination, investigations, especially the modern tool, the echocardiography and learn the prevention of the disease and its complications.

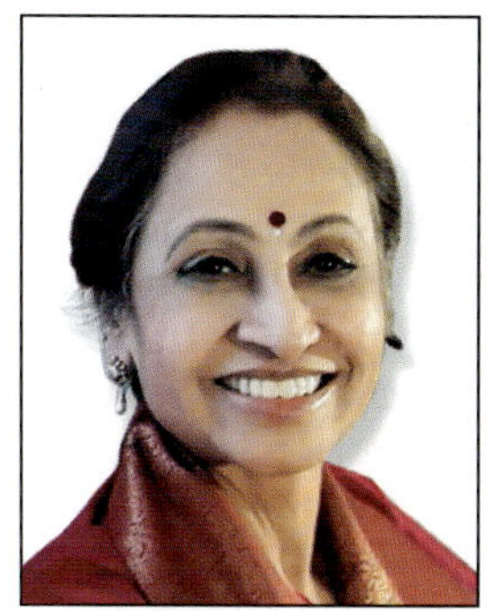

This monogram, in both its concept and design, is aimed at giving a comprehensive and complete knowledge about ARF and RHD to the pediatricians, physicians, cardiologists and all the medical students dealing with health problems in the socioeconomically poor community. I have not made an exhaustive or a complicated report. Instead, I have concentrated on the detailed description, practical successful approach to control the menace of ARF and RHD in the 21st century, which is the need of the hour.

The book begins with *Lessons Learnt from the History of Rheumatic Heart Disease, because* if I do not learn from the past, I cannot build the future. The doctors have learnt a lot from the pioneering work done by many great clinicians in the past. *Rheumatic Fever and Rheumatic Heart Disease: A 4-century Review with Special Reference to India* is written by a doyen, S Padmavati, who herself was in the forefront in the fight against this dreaded disease for decades. Notwithstanding the brilliant achievements of medical fraternity, ARF and RHD remains a major public health problem, throughout the developing countries of the world, that is to say, in most of the world's population. Therefore, the third chapter is *Epidemiology of Group A Streptococcal Infections, Rheumatic Fever, Rheumatic Heart Disease and Role of WHO*. Today, this disease is not seen much in the West. But, India is in the phase of epidemiological transition. On one hand there is a substantial burden due to RHD, on the other hand resources are scarce to treat and prevent the disease. Hence, the fourth chapter is, *Can We Change the Epidemiological Trend of Rheumatic Heart Disease in India?*

The ARF has not yet been completely eradicated, as prevention will be less than optimal until the pathogenesis of the disease has been totally elucidated. ARF is caused by a group A beta hemolytic streptococcal (GABHS). The process is triggered by an inadequate immunological response, both humoral and cellular, therefore, the *Etiopathogenesis and Management of Streptococcal Infection* is a very important and a basic chapter. The *Laboratory Diagnosis of Group A Beta Hemolytic Streptococcal Infections* is meant for educating all the practitioners about laboratory investigations and their usefulness. Saroja and Sarasa Bharati both pioneers in cardiac pathology have contributed *Etiopathogenesis and Pathology of Carditis in Rheumatic Fever*. *Pathology of Chronic Rheumatic Heart Disease* written by Pradeep Vaideeswar has brilliant photos of specimens by him, which will go a long way in the understanding of pathology of carditis in ARF and RHD.

Acute rheumatic fever is an acute, diffuse, nonsuppurative inflammatory disease that occurs in susceptible individuals as a late complication after an untreated *Streptococcus pharyngotonsillitis*. The infection itself sometimes being asymptomatic. The initial streptococcal pharyngotonsillitis is followed by latent period and then by the acute and chronic phases. There are four distinct phases characterizing the disease. The disease has the potential to involve the heart, joints, brain and subcutaneous and cutaneous tissues. Cardiac injury is the most important manifestation and it is the injuries to the heart which produce its clinical, social and economic impact. Hence, the third part consists of important chapters such as *Etiopathogenesis, Clinical Manifestation and Diagnosis of Acute Rheumatic Fever and Clinical Profile of Rheumatic Heart Disease* written by none other than a veteran teacher, AS Chandrasekhara Rao and Dr Sudhay Kumar. Probably, this is the first book on rheumatic fever, to dedicate one whole chapter to *Role of Echocardiography in Diagnosis of Carditis in Acute Rheumatic Fever* written personally by me because revision by American Heart Association (AHA) in 2015 has included ECHO as a major criteria in Jones criteria. The Vijaya's ECHO criteria given for diagnosis of carditis in ARF is very unique and will prove useful in future to the modern clinicians. The degree of cardiac involvement is quite variable, ranging from mild, asymptomatic valvulitis to severe carditis with significant acute mitral and/or aortic regurgitation resulting in heart failure. Many a times, subclinical valvulitis and indolent carditis is missed by best of the clinicians; more so because the auscultation is becoming the dying art among the younger clinicians, who fail to recognize the mild valvular lesions. Therefore, *Role of Echocardiography in Diagnosis of Carditis in ARF* and *Echocardiography and Transesophageal ECHO in Rheumatic Heart Disease* is added to this book and access to echocardiographic videos is given along with the book to assist the clinicians to improve their skill to detect the disease more accurately. It will certainly help in making an early and precise diagnosis of carditis and this modern modality, ECHO is now added as a major criteria to Jones criteria can certainly change the epidemiological face of ARF.

Both ARF and chronic RHD continue to pose serious concerns with regard to health, in many parts of the world and present a significant challenge for those involved in providing healthcare. In developed countries, although its incidence has been markedly reduced since the 1950s, ARF remains a risk because of its potential risk in many countries. There is consensus in some of the management strategies, but there are some issues in the management which are controversial. In some management strategies there is consensus and the guidelines are laid. But many of the treatment methods are old aged and not evidence based. Hence, there is confusion among the treating physicians. Therefore, the chapter *Diagnosis, Consensus and Controversies in the Management of Acute Rheumatic Fever* is useful to know the appropriate management and avoid mismanagement. *Medical Management of Rheumatic Heart Disease and Management during Pregnancy, Noncardiac Surgery and Infective Endocarditis* and How Important is *the Echocardiographic Screening for Rheumatic Heart Disease?* by Bogarka (Bo) Remenyi and Nigel Wilson is an added attraction to this book. This is aimed at making the clinicians to bring more children with RHD into the net of penicillin prophylaxis and prevent the further damage to the heart.

The 20th century was distinguished by the identification of GABHS pharyngitis as the cause of ARF and by the demonstration that the first attack of ARF and recurrence are preventable by the appropriate use of penicillin to treat and prevent these infections. *Prevention and Vaccine for Rheumatic Fever: How Far are We?* are extremely important and will go a long way in controlling ARF and RHD.

The disease is seen in its virgin condition undetected and untreated in many poor and backward areas. Therefore, chapters on *Natural History of Rheumatic Fever and Rheumatic Heart Disease* and *Cardiac Complications of Acute Rheumatic Fever* are added to caution the clinicians about the dreaded complications and to impress the importance of timely detection and management of consequences.

The repercussions of the disease involve patients of all ages, since the valvular sequelae can be carried throughout life. The children and adolescents, who are most frequently admitted to hospital with acute episodes, are the same group of patients who, after the fourth decade of life, form the largest group when analysis is focused on invasive intervention and death. Tremendous progress is made in interventional cardiology and cardiac surgery, the benefit of which should reach the patients of RHD in advance stage. Therefore, chapters on *Non-surgical Management of Rheumatic Heart Disease* written by most experienced, Ramesh Arora who has the highest number of papillary thyroid microcarcinomas (PTMCs) to her credit in the world. Juvenile rheumatic heart disease is peculiar to Indian subcontinent, hence, special emphasis is on *Transcatheter Treatment of Rheumatic Mitral Stenosis in Pediatric Age Group*. There is an all important chapter *Surgical Management of Rheumatic Heart Disease*, which contains care of native and prosthetic valve and anticoagulation. RHD, besides being considered the most frequent condition necessitating valvular surgery in adults, even the non-surgeons should know about the prosthetic valve complications. The economic impact must also be considered, not only with regard to the financial cost of clinical and surgical treatments but also relative to the loss of productivity as the result of disability acquired at an early age. The last but not least, the book ends with the positive note with the last chapter *Rheumatic Fever, Rheumatic Heart Disease Registry and Control Program*. This chapter consists of proforma and protocols for ARF control program to be conducted from the remotest place to nationwide. This special chapter is meant for motivating the youngsters to take up preventive and epidemiological projects rather than sit in the clinic and treat the terminal cases. If the morbidity and mortality due to ARF and RHD is reduced in the children and they lead hale and healthy life then the purpose of writing this book is fulfilled.

The book could not have been written without the help of many other individuals whose names do not appear in the list of contributors. I thank all my contributors for their efforts in contribution toward making this book possible. I am now able to include color illustrations throughout the book and give access to videos of ECHOs in ARF and RHD through QR code scanning. of ECHOs in patients with carditis and RHD. The influence of this is likely to be truly spectacular and special.

My grateful thanks to late Dr Chitra Narasimhan, who labored beyond the call of duty in her efforts to obtain all the chapters on time and to complete some of the chapters. I am also indebted to Usha Anand, who co-authored a chapter and made the corrections of the proofs a pleasurable task rather than a chore. I also express my thanks to my various colleagues who permitted me to use illustrations from various previous collaborative ventures. I have cited their contributions in the legends to the specific figures, hoping that I have not made any omissions. I hope that this book will be of some value to not only to those involved in the practice of cardiology but also to the medical students and clinicians practicing in the periphery. Most of all, I sincerely hope that the lessons learnt from this book will benefit the helpless patients and reduce the disease burden on patients and economical burden on the society.

My heart goes out to the children suffering from ARF and RHD. The present scenario of ARF and RHD in poor children is pathetic. It makes me feel sad and say:

"Dawn is nowhere in the sight,
yet I am waiting for the light"

But I am sure with determined effort at controlling the menace of ARF and with the proper understanding of the disease, utilizing ECHO criteria for early and precise diagnosis and appropriate preventive measures, I can definitely succeed in eradicating ARF from the surface of the globe. So my sincere prayer is:

"Oh God grant me the serenity to accept what
I cannot change (poor socioeconomical condition)
courage to change the things I can
(diagnostic criteria, bringing awareness)
the wisdom to know the difference"

I have the fond hope that this honest effort of mine, will go a long way in changing the epidemiological trend of ARF and eventually succeed in eradicating RHD worldwide and then we can say the RF licks the joints and bites the heart is a thing of past.

IB Vijayalakshmi

Video Content

Echocardiography for the diagnosis of carditis in acute rheumatic fever and chronic rheumatic heart disease.

- Dedication
- Revised Jones criteria, 2015.
- 6th revision of the Jones Criteria for the diagnosis of acute rheumatic fever in the era of Doppler echocardiography.
- Major changes in original Jones criteria.
- Clinical diagnosis of carditis.
- Echo can assess.
- Doppler findings in rheumatic valvulitis: Jones criteria, 2015.
- Doppler findings in valvulitis.
- Morphological findings on Echo in rheumatic valvulitis.
- M-mode Echo features.
- Thickened valve leads to reduced mobility.
- Parasternal long axis in 13-year-old RHD patient MV thickness is > 7 mm. (RHD: rheumatic heart disease; MV: mitral valve)
- Thickened mitral and aortic valve.
- Physiological mitral regurgitation.
- Physiological mitral regurgitation in PLX.
- Pathological MR with central jet. (MR: mitral regurgitation)
- Pathological MR. (MR: mitral regurgitation)
- Physiological versus pathological regurgitation.
- Trivial AR. (AR: aortic regurgitation)
- Beaded appearance (histopathology).
- Beaded appearance of mitral valve (histopathology comparing with Echo).
- Parasternal long axis shows beaded appearance.
- Nodular club like AML in RHD. (AML: anterior mitral leaflet; RHD: rheumatic heart disease)
- Vijaya's Echo score.
- How specific are Vijaya's Echo criteria?
- Results of auscultation versus Echo.
- Summary—revised Jones criteria: subclinical carditis.
- "Echo detectable" subclinical carditis, is it of clinical benefit? Yes
- Unless valve regurgitation is associated with other features.
- Thickened MV, AV, and beaded appearance. (AV: aortic valve; MV: mitral valve)

- Efficacy of Echo criteria.
- Parasternal long-axis view.
- Echo can differentiate functional MR from pathological. (MR: mitral regurgitation)
- Myxomatous MV with prolapse of scallops. (MV: mitral valve)
- Severe aortic cusp prolapse.
- Classical beaded appearance of MV in short axis. (MV: mitral valve)
- Severe mitral regurgitation.
- Severe MR in PLX and four-chamber view. (MR: mitral regurgitation)
- Torn chordae, flail MV with severe MR. (MR: mitral regurgitation; MV: mitral valve)
- Echo features of carditis.
- A 3-year-old boy with ARF. (ARF: acute rheumatic fever)
- Modified two-chamber view.
- Both mitral and aortic valves are thickened.
- Torn chordae tendineae with mitral regurgitation.
- Diagnostic of ARF with carditis. (ARF: acute rheumatic fever)
- Echo helps in decision making.
- A 3-year-old girl with ARF. (ARF: acute rheumatic fever)
- Chordal tear prolapse with severe MR in an 8-year-old boy.
- Apical four-chamber view.
- ALCAPA with MR. (ALCAPA: anomalous left coronary artery from pulmonary artery; MR: mitral regurgitation)
- ALCAPA confirmed with angiography. (ALCAPA: anomalous left coronary artery from pulmonary artery)
- Identify the features of pancarditis.
- Pancarditis.
- Case profile of patient with I° AV block. (AV: atrioventricular)
- Apical three-chamber view.
- Tear of chordae tendineae with MR. (MR: mitral regurgitation)
- Chordal tear with severe MR. (MR: mitral regurgitation)
- Tear of chordae tendineae.
- Torn chordae moving freely between LV and LA flail MV with severe MR. (LA: left atrium; LV: left ventricle; MR: mitral regurgitation; MV: mitral valve)
- Case profile.
- Short axis illustrating beaded appearance.
- Classical beaded appearance of MV and AV. (AV: aortic valve; MV: mitral valve)
- Clinical description.
- Modified two-chamber view shows moderate PE, severe MR, and MVP. (MR: mitral regurgitation; MVP: mitral valve prolapse; PE: pulmonary embolism)
- Pericardial effusion.
- Case profile.
- Apical four-chamber view.
- Apical five-chamber view.

- Echo PLX: severe MR and severe AR. (AR: aortic regurgitation; MR: mitral regurgitation)
- MVP with club-like thickened AML and PML. (AML: anterior mitral leaflet; MVP: mitral valve prolapse; PML: posterior mitral leaflet)
- How Echo is superior?
- Aortic valve showing active valvulitis.
- Nonrheumatic pathological MR and mild AR. (AR: aortic regurgitation; MR: mitral regurgitation)
- Gradient in abdominal aorta aortoarteritis.
- Case profile.
- Modified two-chamber view with severe MR. (MR: mitral regurgitation)
- Pericardial effusion, preserved LV function is rheumatic (LVEF—60%). (LV: left ventricle; LVEF: left ventricular ejection fraction)
- Is it recrudescence of rheumatic activity? Or SBE? (SBE: subacute bacterial endocarditis)
- Submitral aneurysm versus AML tear. (AML: anterior mitral leaflet)
- Carditis, AHA, 2015. (AHA: American Heart Association)
- Subclinical carditis.
- Subclinical carditis.
- Doubtful RF. (RF: rheumatic fever)
- What to do if diagnosis is not certain?
- Writing group statement.
- Rheumatic heart disease (RHD).
- Assessment of severity of mitral stenosis.
- M-mode in MS. (MS: mitral stenosis)
- Mitral valve area by planimetry.
- Commissural morphology.
- Valve morphology and subvalvular apparatus.
- Subvalvular stenosis.
- Submitral fusion.
- Grading of MS. (MS: mitral stenosis)
- Tips to measure MVOA. (MVOA: mitral valve orifice area)
- Limitation of planimetry.
- Pressure gradient.
- Evaluation of pulmonary hypertension.
- Data of percutaneous transvenous mitral commissurotomy (PTMC) in juvenile mitral stenosis (JMS), poster presented at Transcatheter Cardiovascular Therapeutics (TCT), Washington DC, 2002.
- Challenges of BMV in juvenile mitral stenosis. (BMV: balloon mitral valvuloplasty)
- BMV in juvenile MS. (BMV: balloon mitral valvuloplasty; MS: mitral stenosis)
- PTMC in juvenile MS (until 2016). (MS: mitral stenosis; PTMC: percutaneous transvenous mitral commissurotomy)
- Youngest child of MS. (MS: mitral stenosis)
- Mitral stenosis (MS), tricuspid stenosis (TS), and tricuspid regurgitation (TR) in a 3-year-old child.
- Shortest patient of MS to undergo BMV. (BMV: balloon mitral valvuloplasty; MS: mitral stenosis)

- A 12-year-old child with critical MS. (MS: mitral stenosis)
- Continuous wave (CW) cursor on tricuspid valve to demonstrate TS and TR. (TS: tricuspid stenosis; TR: tricuspid regurgitation)
- Juvenile MS/malignant MS. (MS: mitral stenosis)
- MVOA measurement by planimetry increased from 0.2 to 1.4 cm^2 after BMV. (BMV: balloon mitral valvuloplasty; MVOA: mitral valve orifice area)
- Post-BMV, the MVOA is better MV gradient reduced from 35/15 to 13/7 mm Hg. (BMV: balloon mitral valvuloplasty; MV: mitral valve; MVOA: mitral valve orifice area)
- Catheterization data of 12-year-old female of critical MS, height—130 cm.
- Post-BMV MR. (BMV: balloon mitral valvuloplasty; MR: mitral regurgitation)
- Post-BMV MR two jets in an 8-year-old girl. (BMV: balloon mitral valvuloplasty; MR: mitral regurgitation)
- Catheterization data of an 8-year-old female.
- Pre-BMV. (BMV: balloon mitral valvuloplasty)
- Post-BMV apparently good result.
- Do not miss the eccentric jet.
- Catheterization data.
- Restenosis.
- 16 Post-BMV, restenosis after 6 years. (BMV: balloon mitral valvuloplasty)
- Challenges of BMV in mitral restenosis. (BMV: balloon mitral valvuloplasty)
- Post-BMV restenosis.
- Post-BMV restenosis after 6 years.
- The eccentric MR with severe submitral fusion. (MR: mitral regurgitation)
- MVP, MS, and MR in an 8-year-old girl. (MR: mitral regurgitation; MS: mitral stenosis; MVP: mitral valve prolapse)
- Post-closed mitral commissurotomy and later BMV, RHD–MS, TS, severe TR, AS with AR. (AR: aortic regurgitation; AS: aortic stenosis; BMV: balloon mitral valvuloplasty; MS: mitral stenosis; RHD: rheumatic heart disease; TR: tricuspid regurgitation; TS: tricuspid stenosis)
- Commissural morphology.
- Valve morphology and subvalvular apparatus.
- Subvalvular stenosis.
- Submitral fusion has deformed the balloon.
- MS, MR, AS, AR, TS, TR, and AF with CCF. (AF: atrial fibrillation; AR: aortic regurgitation; AS: aortic stenosis; CCF: congestive cardiac failure; MS: mitral stenosis; MR: mitral regurgitation; TR: tricuspid regurgitation; TS: tricuspid stenosis)
- Giant RA with severe TR. (RA: right atrium; TR: tricuspid regurgitation)
- Giant LA needs plication. (LA: left atrium)
- BMV during pregnancy. (BMV: balloon mitral valvuloplasty)
- Safe PTMC in pregnancy. (PTMC: percutaneous transvenous mitral commissurotomy)
- Echo-guided balloon across MV into LV. (LV: left ventricle; MV: mitral valve)
- BMV during pregnancy. (BMV: balloon mitral valvuloplasty)
- Contraindications to BMV. (BMV: balloon mitral valvuloplasty)
- Transthoracic echocardiography (TTE) versus transesophageal echocardiography (TEE) for thrombus in left atrial appendage (LAA).

- LA body clot. (LA: left atrium)
- Spontaneous Echo contrast (SEC) on transesophageal echocardiography (TEE).
- Contraindications to BMV. (BMV: balloon mitral valvuloplasty)
- Periprocedural TEE and 4D Echo have gained great importance to assess paravalvular leak. (TEE: transesophageal echocardiography)
- Spontaneous Echo contrast with organized clot in LAA—relative contraindication. (LAA: left atrial appendage)
- TEE showing thrombus on interatrial septum—contraindication for BMV. (BMV: balloon mitral valvuloplasty; TEE: transesophageal echocardiography)
- Football in the heart.
- SBE prophylaxis. (SBE: subacute bacterial endocarditis)
- Echocardiographic assessment of aortic stenosis.
- Apical five-chamber view shows AS in a case of RHD with MS, MR, and TR. (AS: aortic stenosis; MR: mitral regurgitation; MS: mitral stenosis; RHD: rheumatic heart disease; TR: tricuspid regurgitation)
- Dextrocardia with severe AS and rheumatic MS. (AS: aortic stenosis; MS: mitral stenosis)
- Balloon dilatation of AS and MS. (AS: aortic stenosis; MS: mitral stenosis)
- Result of BMV. (BMV: balloon mitral valvuloplasty)
- May–Thurner syndrome.
- Assessment of aortic regurgitation.
- M-mode AML flutter in AR. (AML: anterior mitral leaflet; AR: aortic regurgitation)
- Aortic regurgitation.
- Color Doppler.
- Diastolic flow reversal in descending aorta.
- Echo of diastolic flow reversal in descending aorta.
- Vena contracta width.
- AR with vegetation on AV. (AR: aortic regurgitation; AV: aortic valve)
- EF: 10–15%, inoperable. (EF: ejection fraction)
- Grading of MR by vena contracta width. (MR: mitral regurgitation)
- Tricuspid stenosis and regurgitation.
- Missed diagnosis can be disastrous for the patient.
- The disease in AV and TV is likely to progress despite BMV. (AV: aortic valve; TV: tricuspid valve; BMV: balloon mitral valvuloplasty)
- Post-BMV the MVOA is better MV gradient reduced. (BMV: balloon mitral valvuloplasty; MV: mitral valve; MVOA: mitral valve orifice area)
- Summary.
- Conclusion.
- 2012 WHF criteria for echocardiographic diagnosis of RHD. (RHD: rheumatic heart disease; WHF: World Heart Federation)
- Borderline RHD. (RHD: rheumatic heart disease)
- Echocardiographic criteria for individuals aged >20 years.
- Congenital MV anomalies must be excluded. (MV: mitral valve)
- Criteria for pathological regurgitation.

- Test your skill—Case I.
- Parasternal long axis.
- Test your skill—Case II.
- What is the Echo score and what is the diagnosis?
- Test your skill—Case III.
- What do you see?
- Test your skill—Case IV.
- What is the diagnosis?
- Test your skill—Case VI. Is it pathological or physiological MR?
- What is your decision?
- Is MR physiological or pathological? (MR: mitral regurgitation)
- What is the impression?
- What is the decision?
- Echo prevents damage at three levels.
- Carry home message.
- Conquer the unconquered.
- Acknowledgement.
- All working together for a cause.

Contents

Lessons Learnt from History of Rheumatic Heart Diseases

IB Vijayalakshmi

> *"The glory of medicine is that it is constantly moving forward, that there is always more to learn. The ills of today do not cloud the horizon of tomorrow, but act as a spur to greater effort."*
>
> —**William James Mayo** (1861–1939)

■ INTRODUCTION

Hippocrates in 400 BC provided the first description of arthritis. Since then thousands of studies have contributed to the better understanding of the rheumatic fever (RF) and rheumatic heart disease (RHD). The earliest concept of RHD began as "articular rheumatism" in the 17th century. Guillaume de Baillou (France) is credited with the first description of "acute rheumatism" in the 17th century. Since then this disease has ravaged the world for the past 4 centuries, afflicting the children, adolescents, and young adults. It has been diagnosed and treated more effectively since the 20th century, thanks to the lessons learnt from centuries of experience of clinicians. Still it has remained as a burning problem in many developing countries, where the clinicians, society, and governments have not learnt lessons from the history. Therefore, the history of RF is of relevance to modern medicine, so that lessons learnt from the past experience can help to evolve appropriate preventive strategies in countries where the disease is still endemic.

The striking and progressive changes that were seen with poststreptococcal infections—acute arthritis, pericarditis, endocarditis, chorea, and myocarditis are quite distinct. The history of RF has taught us much about the pathophysiology and epidemiology of this autoimmune disease. It has also taught us the methods of prevention. However, in spite of much research the link between "the throat and the heart" remains elusive. Unless this is established full control of the disease may not be possible.

■ HISTORY IN THE 18TH CENTURY

"Rheumatism" was a routine complaint in the 18th century. RF was embedded in the diagnostic category of "rheumatism", a broadly defined group of illnesses characterized by fever, aches, and pains of the limbs and overall debility.[1]

Thomas Sydenham (England) separated "articular rheumatism" from gout and although he gave a masterly description of chorea, he did not recognize its rheumatic nature!

In April 1798, Mr TM was struck down with rheumatism while traveling in England. He was very familiar with the beginning stages of this illness, for he had been afflicted with rheumatism yearly since the age of 9. There was a preliminary period of fever and chills, which he and his

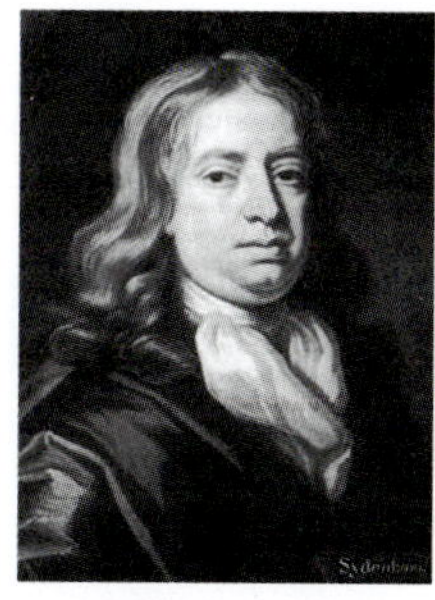

**THOMAS SYDENHAM
(1624–1689)**

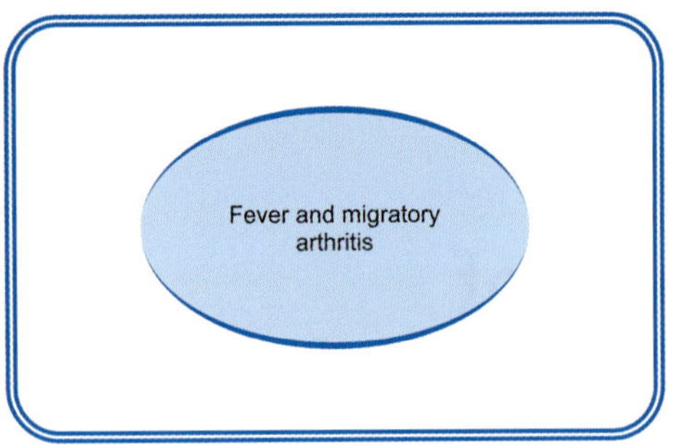

FIG. 1: Rheumatism in the 18th century.

family attributed to a needless exposure to dampness and cold weather, followed by considerable swelling, redness, and tenderness of his knees, ankles, and wrists. This arthritis had a peculiar twist: it moved from joint to joint, lasting in one spot for a few days or a week before moving to another location. His family put him to bed for several weeks and he recovered completely after each bout. Despite the considerable debility during the active stage of the disease, he had been left with no permanent handicap. Therefore, rheumatism in the 18th century consisted of only fever and migratory arthritis **(Fig. 1)**.

> Lesson learnt is arthritis in RF is characteristically flitting in nature and recovers completely without permanent handicap.

The clinicians, by the last years of the 18th century, appreciated cardiac involvement in ills also characterized by "rheumatism". Mr TM's tenth bout began in the accustomed way: knees and ankles red, swollen and tender, occurring after an unfortunate submersion into a cold spring pond. What set this episode apart from earlier ones was an "oppression in his chest" and the palpitation of his heart. After 3 weeks, these chest complaints led to extreme breathlessness and a feeling that he was "about to expire". So different was this addition to his regular rheumatic complaints that he traveled to London to consult a hospital based physician. There he met Dr William Charles Wells at St. Thomas's Hospital. Wells listened to the young man's story and quickly confirmed that Mr TM had what physicians in the late 18th century called "acute rheumatism". What was entirely new in Wells's experience was the history of "oppression in the chest", heart palpitations, and breathlessness. Wells confirmed that the heart was involved by palpating the pulse and feeling the heart bound against Mr TM's chest wall. Wells believed that he was seeing a new aspect of a

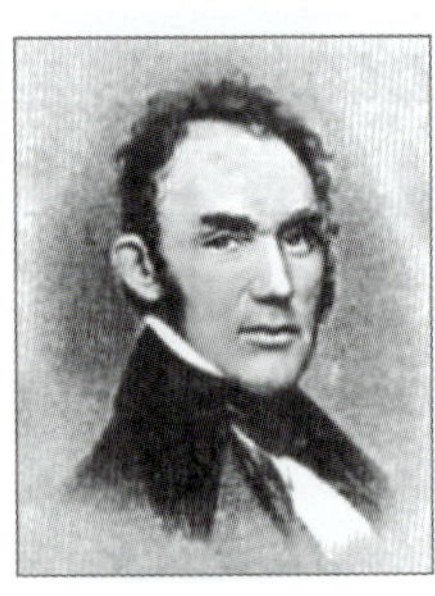

WILLIAM CHARLES WELLS (1757–1817)

common disease; he called it "rheumatism of the heart".[2] Mr TM, like most sufferers from acute rheumatism, survived even repeated attacks of this disease.

HISTORY IN THE 19TH CENTURY

In early 19th century, Wells called attention to the experience of David Dundas, sergeant surgeon to the king, who reported nine patients with heart disease and rheumatism in 1809. Most had suffered chest pains, anxiety, and increased pulse, ascites (fluid in the abdomen), pleural fluid, or peripheral edema following one or more attacks of acute rheumatism. Seven of the nine were under 22 years of age and seven died, usually after a period of several months. He autopsied six and found the heart enlarged in most; excess pericardial fluid surrounded one heart and in several others the pericardium adhered to the surface of the heart.[3]

When later Wells published Mr TM's history with 13 additional cases in 1812, he did not claim priority for his observation linking heart disease with rheumatism. Rather, he credited David Pitcairn, a prominent British physician, with the initial association in 1788. Pitcairn failed to publish his remarks on the subject, so Wells considered his paper to be serving the purpose of recording Pitcairn's idea, to which he added his own cases.

William Charles Wells, provided an early description of the new face of rheumatism. One of his case histories gave details of Miss AL, a 16-year-old girl who had been well until her current affliction. Her fatal illness began in early August 1806. Wells also remarked that Matthew Baillie, a Scottish pathologist, had made the initial autopsy investigation of a patient with rheumatism dying from heart disease.[4] Following Wells's lead some practitioners began looking for heart disease in cases of rheumatism. James Russell, a surgeon from Birmingham, provided an example from 1814. Seth Bassett, a 22-year-old wagoner, came to Russell with painful joints. Russell, aware of the writings of Baillie, Dundas, and Wells, took a special interest when Bassett developed chest pain, shortness of breath and a rapid pulse several weeks later. Russell confidently believed that Bassett had an inflamed heart.[5]

Following René Laennec's introduction of the stethoscope in 1816, practitioners' acquisition of auscultatory skills that correlated sounds at the bedside with structural changes at the autopsy table took decades. RF has not been a static disease which patients and physicians have viewed from different vantages over the past 2 centuries. Technology, thus, confirmed rheumatism's change in biological character. Bouillaud's use of the stethoscope followed Wells's observation by more than a quarter of a century and initial reports of cardiac involvement by nearly 50 years. This is not to argue that technology played no role. The stethoscope cemented cardiac damage to acute rheumatism in the minds of many practitioners by contributing fresh bedside evidence. And it extended the link between heart injury and rheumatism to include the many *asymptomatic* cases in which the injury was so mild that it went unnoticed by the patient. By mid-century, then, experience and technology were available to diagnose whether the pericardium or endocardium was involved in acute rheumatism. The stethoscope was not, of course, as helpful in determining myocardial damage, which was often silent. In 1821, René Laennec listed "gouty or rheumatic affections" as an occasional cause of pericarditis.[6]

William Potts Dewees, a physician from Philadelphia, described the case of AB, an 8-year-old girl. In mid-November, the young girl developed swelling and redness of her wrists and ankles shortly after a sore throat, chill, and cough; suddenly she was overwhelmed by a "great oppression" in her chest and shortness of breath so severe that she could not lie down; a week later she was dead.[7] Similar case reports increased over the next decade and a Parisian medical student, Joseph Irénée Itard, was able to sustain a 24-page thesis for graduation from medical school, entitled "Considérations sur le Rhumatisme de Coeur" in 1824.[8]

Initially, sounds emanating from the lungs received most attention. Only by the 1830s, did clinicians begin to sort out which abnormal heart sounds came from a particular chamber or valve of the heart.[9] Jean Baptiste Bouillaud, a Parisian clinician who had been a student of Laennec, applied this new instrument to rheumatic patients in 1837, greatly enhancing the ability to describe cardiac injury while the patient lived. Significantly, the stethoscope also permitted Bouillaud to discover patients with *asymptomatic* heart disease.[10]

Bouillaud and the Stethoscope

Most initial reports resulted from specific and striking complaints of patients, external inspection of chest and pulse, followed by confirmatory autopsies. The stethoscope changed this. While René Laennec's introduction of the stethoscope in 1816 has been well studied by historians, a great deal less is known about the reception by practitioners of this technological breakthrough. The acquisition of skills among practitioners that correlated sounds at the bedside with structural changes at the autopsy table took time. The best historical accounts demonstrate that the stethoscope received a slow but steady welcome from clinicians, especially among those physicians who had been trained in Paris.

Using a stethoscope, Jean Baptiste Bouillaud (1796–1881)[11] argued convincingly in 1836 that there was a "constant coincidence either of endocarditis or of pericarditis with acute articular rheumatism".[10]

Over the 19th century, rheumatic fever's biological changes and the progression of clinical thinking shifted emphasis from fever and joints to the heart. Individual cases showed that cardiac injury was part of rheumatism. Hospital studies showed that most debility and death resulted from heart disease. The "typical" case demonstrated that heart involvement was the most vital element in rheumatism from the point of view of prognosis **(Fig. 2)**.

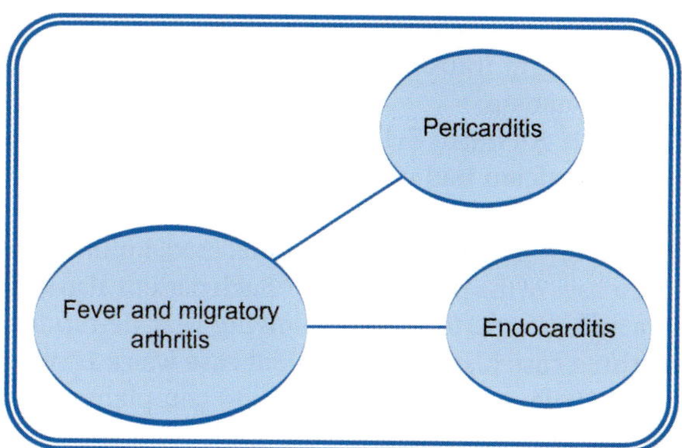

FIG. 2: Acute rheumatism in the 1830s.

Despite the growing association of heart disease with acute rheumatism, clinicians still gave central importance to fever and joint pains. These were the complaints that brought the patient to the practitioner. These were the criteria needed to make a diagnosis. These were the objects of therapy. But heart damage had joined fever and joint pains as an associated manifestation and *death resulted from heart disease.*

In September 1835, Bouillaud had been called to consult in the case of a 19-year-old boy who had been admitted to La Charité Hospital 2 weeks earlier. The boy's admitting physician asked Bouillaud's advice when the young man developed chest pain in addition to his joint complaints. On this initial visit, Bouillaud placed his hand on the chest and felt a "very distinct vibration which immediately led me to announce the existence of the bellows, file, or saw sound", which he confirmed when he applied his ear to the boy's chest. He interpreted his findings to mean that the boy had the valvular damage of endocarditis. He visited weekly, each time recording his cardiac findings. A month after his initial visit, he found the boy had improved. This time he examined his patient with a stethoscope and discovered that the abnormal heart sounds had largely disappeared. This and other experiences led Bouillaud to observe that "in auscultating the sounds of the heart in some individuals still laboring under, or convalescing from acute articular rheumatism, I was not a little surprised to hear a strong, full, saw or bellows sound ... such as I had often met in chronic or organic induration of the valves, with contractions of the orifices of the heart".[10]

In a short monograph devoted entirely to the subject, Bouillaud gave a systematic approach to examining the heart in patients with rheumatism. Like other members of the Paris School, the term often used by historians of medicine to describe extraordinarily creative hospital based medicine which grew out of educational and clinical innovations of the French Revolution, Bouillaud made extensive use of percussion and auscultation, and he followed unsuccessful cases to the autopsy room.[12] Hospital based, Bouillaud saw enough cases to estimate that nearly one half of people with acute rheumatism suffered from either pericarditis or endocarditis or both. Bouillaud's observation of the frequency of cardiac injury was another piece of evidence of the malignant transformation and increasing severity of acute rheumatism.

In 1838 Richard Bright (1789–1858), a prominent London physician had encountered so many patients with rheumatism, called attention in his Lumleian Lectures at the College of Physicians to the occasional association of chorea with diseases of the pericardium.[13] Each patient also suffered from acute rheumatism. The following year he reported in detail three case histories. The initial case was a 17-year-old boy who 12 days earlier "had begun to complain of general rheumatic symptoms; pains in the limbs, with puffiness and swelling of the wrists, and some other joints". 6 days later, he developed chorea: "his head was constantly thrown from one side of the bed to the other; his lips were closed, and opened with a smacking sound and when desired to put out his tongue it was protruded with all the forced grimace and difficulty observed in chorea". A rapid and irregular heartbeat "led to suspicions" that the heart was also affected. 16 days later, the boy died. At autopsy, Bright discovered that both the pericardium and the endocardium were involved. Careful dissection of the brain failed to yield any perceptible abnormalities.[14]

The New Face of Rheumatism

Rheumatism was a quite familiar health concern for patients and physicians at the end of the 18th century. Thomas Sydenham, who had turned his revolutionary zeal from Puritan causes to the many epidemic fevers plaguing his practice among London's poor, defined rheumatism in the late 17th century in a fashion that continued to serve practitioners a century later.

This disease happens at any time, but especially in autumn and chiefly affects such people in the prime of life. It is generally occasioned by exposing the body to the cold or immediately after having heated it by violent exercise or some other way. It begins: (1) with chillness and shivering, which are soon succeeded; (2) by heat, restlessness, thirst, and the other concomitants of a fever; (3) in a day or two and sometimes sooner, there arises an acute pain in some or other of the limbs, especially in the wrists, shoulders and knees; which, often shifting affects these parts alternatively, leaving a redness swelling in the part last affected; (4) in the beginning of the illness, the fever and the aforementioned symptoms do sometimes come together, but the fever goes off gradually whilst the pain continues and sometimes increases, occasioned by the derivation of the febrile matter to the limbs, which the frequent return of the fever, from the repulsion of the morbific matter by external remedies sufficiently shews.[15]

Cullen had appreciated that joint complaints separated into two distinct clusters: "acute rheumatism" in teenagers and young adults with short lived arthritis that left no permanent disability, and "chronic rheumatism" in older adults, in their 50s and 60s, with persistent joint complaints that often resulted in crippling arthritis. Ideas about RF evolved from what Cullen called "acute rheumatism", a term that others enlarged to "acute articular rheumatism", to place emphasis on the painful joints. In *First Lines of the Practice of Physic*, Cullen stated that rheumatism "seldom appears either in the very young or elderly persons, and most commonly occurs from the age of puberty to that of 35 years". He concurred with Sydenham that "the pains affect several joints, often at the very same time, but for the most part shifting this place and having abated one joint, become more violent in another".[16]

A New Outcome for Acute Rheumatism: Death

Beginning in the middle of the 18th century, physicians began to record a few who died from their bouts with rheumatism. These deaths contrasted sharply with the complete recovery that both patients and physicians anticipated with acute rheumatism. As with any new phenomenon, these deaths begged explanation. The precise reason for the deaths perplexed physicians because it was not at all clear why a temporary joint complaint should suddenly turn fatal. When this unusual event occurred, physicians would explain that the rheumatism had moved somehow from the joints to a vital organ. For example, Gerhard van Swieten, the great Viennese physician of the mid-18th century, noted in his *Commentaries upon Boerhaave's Aphorisms*, "while the rheumatism attacks only the joints, it is rarely fatal; but when it seizes the brains or lungs, it is highly dangerous, and sometimes occasions sudden death". Van Swieten gave only a cursory explanation of how rheumatism could move around the body. Early in his discussion, he claimed that "rheumatism derives its name from (the Greek word) to flow".[17] He had a vague notion that a misdirected rheumatic "poison" could flow from the joints to produce havoc elsewhere.

Sydenham and Cullen had spoken of diseased joints in a general way. Other observers sought to locate the site of disease more precisely within the joint itself. For example, William Balfour, a physician writing on the pathology of rheumatism early in the 19th century, claimed that the location of rheumatism was in the "cellular membrane" of the joints, by which he meant the connective tissue surrounding the joints. Balfour based his notion on his examination of living patients and not on dissection.[18]

Cullen, who was known for his meticulous classification of diseases, had struggled over where exactly to locate "acute rheumatism". It shared many characteristics with inflammation. Acute rheumatism produced swollen, painful joints that appeared to the examiner just like joints in other illnesses that were filled with pus or suppuration. In these latter conditions, the joints frequently were destroyed, leaving the patient crippled. In contrast, Cullen noted that the affected joints in rheumatism never contained pus and never were permanently damaged: "The acute rheumatism, though it has much of the nature of the other phlegmasiae (inflammation), differs from all these hitherto mentioned in that it is not liable to terminate in suppuration".[16] Acute rheumatism also differed from other forms of inflammation in that it moved from one joint to another without affecting the tissue in between.

The practitioners began to realize that the umbrella of "rheumatism" often covered many conditions that Sydenham and Cullen had never intended. Edward J Seymour, a physician at St. George's Hospital in London, noted that practitioners loosely used the term to cover many ills, both trivial and serious: growing pains in children, the limb pains that accompanied many febrile illnesses, the pains of nerves damaged by hemorrhage, debilitated constitutions, abuse of mercury, any pain stemming from muscles, bones, or joints, as well as the joint pain in rheumatism.[19]

William Charles Wells and "Rheumatism of the Heart"

Despite difficulty in defining acute rheumatism precisely, Wells had no trouble diagnosing acute rheumatism in Mr TM.[2] Wells recalled that two colleagues, David Pitcairn and Matthew Baillie, had mentioned similar cardiac difficulties in patients with acute rheumatism. After scouring the available medical literature, he could find only one or two additional references. Nevertheless, it is clear from accounts of patients suffering from acute rheumatism that practitioners were becoming aware of the cardiac connection before Wells. For example, van Swieten had reported that "sometimes, when the pain in the limbs ceases, there arises an anxiety in the breast, a palpitation of the heart, an intermitting pulse".[17] Despite this observation, van Swieten did not connect the rare involvement of the heart with the few patients he treated who died from rheumatism. Cullen, too, had called attention to the "full and hard pulse" that accompanied rheumatism on occasion.[16] In the first extensive statistical analysis of rheumatism, John Haygarth noted in 1805 that 55 out of 93 patients with acute rheumatism who had their pulse recorded had a heart rate > 96 bpm. Haygarth did not make the connection between heart damage and rheumatism, and an elevated pulse does not always mean heart disease (fever alone can raise the pulse). But, Haygarth's observation indicated that physicians were beginning to look at the heart when confronted with patients with rheumatism. Twelve of Haygarth's patients died. His detailed case histories indicate that three died with either severe chest pain or shortness of breath. While it is not possible to be certain of the exact anatomical cause of the deaths, it is likely that diseased hearts were responsible.[20]

> Lesson learnt was RF does not deform the joints but kills the patient due to involvement of heart. Hence "RF licks the joints but bites the heart".

Wells presented the experiences of nine of his patients, plus five from colleagues. Miss AL, the young woman who died

from cardiac complications, was Wells's fifth case. Eleven of these patients were teenagers, two were in their 20s and the oldest was 36. With fever and migrating arthritis, each clearly suffered from acute rheumatism. Like the cases of Mr TM and Miss AL, each had complaints explicitly related to the heart: chest pain, breathlessness, palpitations, irregular heartbeat, forcible or violent heartbeat or an enlarged heart. In each case, Wells or his colleagues confirmed cardiac involvement with examination of the pulse and inspection and palpation of the chest wall. Six patients died, a highly unusual outcome for acute rheumatism. The autopsies revealed that pericarditis, a collection of fluid resulting from an inflamed pericardium, was the cause of each of the deaths. One of the older patients had the additional finding of "excrescences" attached to the mitral heart valve, indicating injury to another of the heart's tissues, the endocardium. Of passing interest was Wells finding that one patient, Martha Clifton, also had "many of the tendons of the superficial muscles ... studded with numerous hard tumors", the first clear description of subcutaneous nodules, another ailment later associated commonly with acute rheumatism.

When Alfred Stillé discussed the death of a 23-year-old man from rheumatism, he stated to his listeners at the Pathological Society of Philadelphia in 1839 that examination of the heart in rheumatism had become routine.[21] In the same year that Bouillaud published, Henry Shuckburgh Roots (1785–1861) described a man he admitted to St. Thomas's Hospital in London who suffered from acute rheumatism and pericarditis, a diagnosis he made with the use of a stethoscope.[22]

There was a similar historical trail leading from rheumatism to chorea. Beginning in the 1830s, doctors began commenting on patients with rheumatism, some of them with heart disease in addition, who also suffered from uncontrollable movements or chorea. One early example came from Dr Yonge of Plymouth, England, in his 1840 description of Francis Hill, a 19-year-old boy who had suffered from rheumatism for 2 weeks before developing severe chest pains. What caught Dr Yonge's attention was: *irregular twitching of the muscles of the mouth and right side of the face; which is increased by speaking and occasions some hesitation: seemed unconscious of this till it was noticed, but says, on being asked whether it was habitual that it has come on during the previous week. (1 week later) Has walked from his lodgings but with great difficulty, from the very uncontrollable state of the voluntary muscles throughout the body: great difficulty in making himself understood; cannot remain for any time in one posture and although there is no spasm or violent action of the muscles, he is very unmanageable and gives his friends a great deal of trouble.... His gait is unsteady and tottering and he drags rather than lifts his feet. Francis worsened the next day and was hospitalized. The muscular agitation continues to increase; he occasionally strikes himself against objects, from inability to control or regulate movements. (His) articulation is almost unintelligible; the tongue is jerked out.... (Of note, one doctor heard a heart "bruit" on auscultation with a stethoscope, but Francis's violent movements prevented accurate description of the heart's injury).*

Over the next week, his chorea deteriorated. He died 11 days after entering the hospital. At autopsy, Dr Yonge concluded that the cause of death was the marked pericarditis (the cause of the chest pain) and endocarditis (which had produced the bruit, an extra sound heard when listening with a stethoscope that indicated disease). His brain appeared entirely normal. Chorea was the most dramatic punctuation of Francis's rheumatism, but it did not kill him.[23] Similar descriptions increased over the next decades until chorea joined heart injury as another new feature of rheumatism.

Bright suggested a linkage between acute rheumatism, heart disease, and chorea. This observation confronted him with a conundrum similar to the one that had faced Cullen and Wells: how to explain the connection between a minor, self-limited form of arthritis and a serious brain injury. Bright believed, although his postmortem dissections failed to demonstrate it, that rheumatic inflammation spread from the pericardium to the spinal cord then on to the brain, leading to chorea.[14]

Prompted by Bright's observation, Dr Yonge of Plymouth consulted Bright in 1840 about the case of Francis Hill, a 19-year-old gardener who struggled with his bout of rheumatism, endocarditis, and chorea.[23] Francis was so afflicted with his chorea that he could not walk, eat, or drink and required a straitjacket to prevent him from harming himself. After Francis's death, Yonge and Bright discovered that his mitral valve was seriously damaged; the spinal cord and brain, while carefully dissected, yielded no visible abnormalities.

Richard Bright thought his linkage of chorea with the now cardiac expanded acute rheumatism was a new observation. In its 19th century form, chorea overwhelmed the observer. Rheumatism had altered its biology again.

Acute Rheumatism Mutates again with Chorea

There was a comparable path leading from acute rheumatism to chorea, a dramatic movement disorder. In the middle third of the 19th century, chorea began to afflict some patients of acute rheumatism, another indication that rheumatism was changing its biological character. Again, it was Thomas Sydenham who gave chorea its classic description in 1686. This is a kind of convulsion, which attacks boys and girls from the 10th year to the time of puberty. It firstly shows itself by limping or unsteadiness in one of the legs, which the patient drags. The hand cannot be steady for a moment. It passes from one position to another by a convulsive movement; however, much the patient may strive to the contrary. Before he can raise a cup to his lips he makes as many gesticulations as a mountebank; since he does not move it in a straight line, but has his hand drawn aside by spasms, until by some good fortune he brings it at last to his mouth. He then gulps off at once, so suddenly and so greedily as to look as if he were trying to amuse the on lookers.[24] In Sydenham's practice, chorea and rheumatism did not occur together in the same patient.

> Lesson learnt is though chorea is part of rheumatism, it does not occur at the same time as joint pain.

PATIENTS AND DOCTORS

At mid-century, changing biology dictated a significant shift in the way practitioners approached patients with acute rheumatism. When confronted with patients with fever and joint pains, physicians routinely examined the heart, often with a stethoscope whether or not the person complained of chest pains. In addition, practitioners anticipated the possible onset of chorea. What was important was that physicians began to assign greater significance to heart damage. The rising prominence of the heart in rheumatism came from the growing clinical appreciation, backed up by autopsy reports that deaths from acute rheumatism resulted not from arthritis or fever but from injury done to the heart. Chorea, although seldom a cause of death and never accompanied with an autopsy finding, added complexity, misery, and certainly drama to acute rheumatism. While neither heart disease nor chorea occurred in every case of rheumatism, their presence was anticipated in the minds of practitioners **(Fig. 3)**.

The final third of the 19th century witnessed another shift in clinical thinking about RF. Individual case histories showed the considerable variability of the illness. Hospital based analysis demonstrated in a general way how RF affected populations. Neither approach was entirely helpful to the practitioner when confronted with sick patients and a mutating disease. What emerged in the 1880s was the concept of the "typical" case, which allowed for the necessary biological variability yet possessed common elements. Employing an epidemiological approach, which clustered elements from many cases, enabled physicians to make a certain diagnosis in a disease that was most uncertain in its

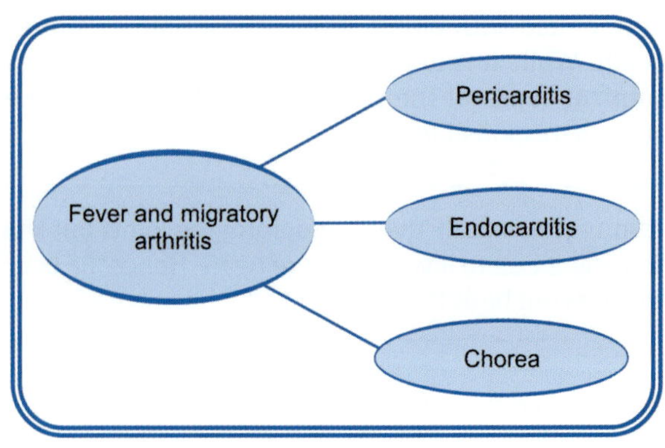

FIG. 3: Acute rheumatism in 1850.

presentation. Another advantage of this strategy was to follow patients over longer periods of time, demonstrating that RF was an illness of relapses and remissions, with increasing debility with each episode. Pioneering in this strategy was Walter Butler Cheadle, physician to the Hospital for Sick Children, Great Ormond Street, London.

> *Lesson learnt:* Along with arthritis and carditis, chorea also was part of acute rheumatism.

In mid-century, hospital-based physicians in Great Britain, with access to 100s of patients with the new biologically expanded rheumatism were able to analyze more carefully rheumatic fever's changing character. Using numbers and statistics, these physicians enumerated precisely how often heart injury and chorea joined fever and arthritis, what age groups were most vulnerable, what time of year rheumatism was most likely to attack and which therapies were most likely to succeed. Large hospital-based studies also noted that rheumatism was continuing to change: subcutaneous nodules sometimes appeared, erythematous rashes joined in some cases, tonsillitis had struck most victims. Significantly, these hospital-based reports recorded that heart disease gravely sickened patients.

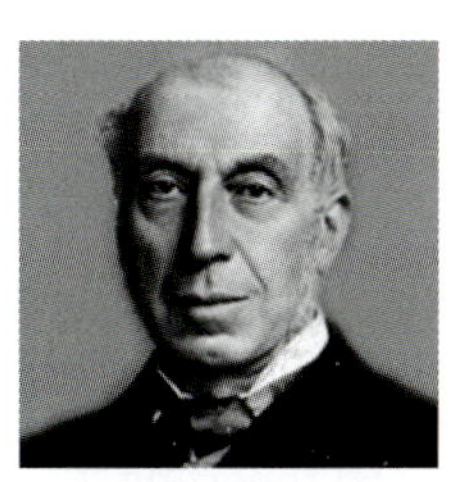

WALTER BUTLER CHEADLE (1835–1910)

From the mass of individual cases and hospital studies available, Cheadle identified rheumatic fever's common elements in 1886: fever, arthritis, pericarditis, endocarditis, pleurisy, tonsillitis, erythematous rashes, chorea, and nodules. This expanded list of symptoms alone signaled how far RF had traveled in a century. Over the course of this relapsing illness, Cheadle believed that most patients would suffer from most symptoms. Despite this expectation, Cheadle understood that not every patient experienced every possible complaint. He organized these symptoms, or "manifestations", into 10 common temporal sequences, or "series". For one example, in chart form he described the case of WS, aged 4.5 years, that Cheadle thought "typical" of many who suffered from RF.[25]

Cheadle's clinical organization of thinking about rheumatic fever provided practitioners with a helpful guide to diagnosis **(Fig. 4)**.

Indeed, no one has improved upon his general approach. Even T Duckett Jones's diagnostic criteria created in response to rheumatic fever's continuing biological evolution in the 20th century, which medical students began to memorize after 1944, were solidly based on Cheadle's efforts.

Social Setting of Acute Rheumatism

Practitioners in the 18th century, before the advent of heart disease and chorea, observed that people who succumbed to rheumatism often belonged to families who seemed to have a constitutional weakness that predisposed them to this disease. Several children in one house would have rheumatism at the same time; parents had suffered similarly when children themselves. In people so prone, rheumatism was thought to follow a chill brought on by exposure to cold and wet, reflecting the usual onset of the disease in fall, winter, or early spring. Physicians, thus, noted a social dimension to rheumatism. Not too infrequently, the victim, often poor and living in crowded circumstances, was

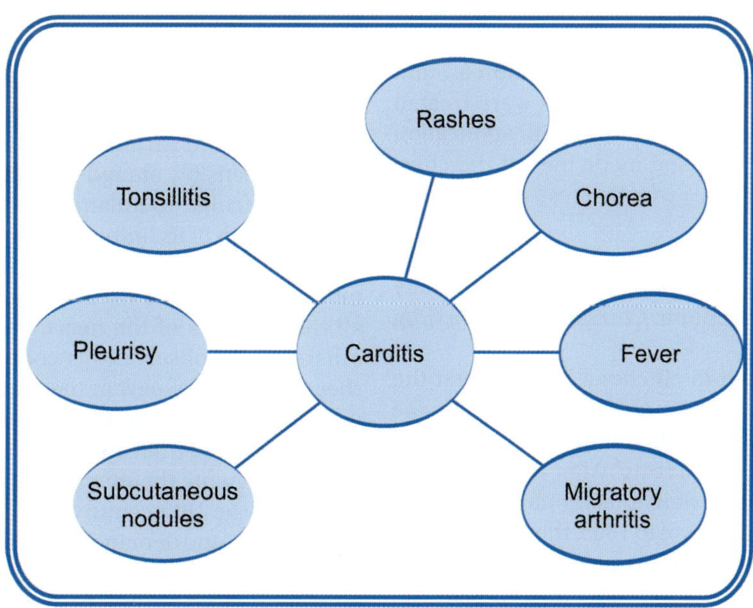

FIG. 4: Cheadle's rheumatic state (1889).

described as intemperate in drinking, eating, or sleeping. As such, physicians thought that rheumatism had seasonal, familial, and social dimensions.

THERAPY FOR RHEUMATISM IN THE EARLY 19TH CENTURY

Changing biology challenged therapeutics with its new injuries, but initially led to only a few fundamental changes. Until the end of the 18th century, doctors and patients addressed the complaints that brought patients to physicians like joint distress and fever. In addition, doctors worried about an underlying, but poorly defined, phlegmasiae, or inflammation. Bed rest, always a pillar in the care of any debilitating illness, formed the mainstay of treatment for acute rheumatism. Enforced rest, it was thought, prevented permanent damage to hurting joints. Physicians also directed attention to local and external care. Painful joints were frequently wrapped. Some doctors preferred linen; others flannel; still others a variety of plasters.[26] Opium became the prime drug for alleviating joint pain and after the march of acute rheumatism to the heart, for chest pain as well.[27] Reports from the first years of the 19th century indicated that opium was administered in doses large enough and frequent enough (often hourly) to relieve pain. Whether opium speeded the course of acute rheumatism or merely lessened troublesome symptoms was a debated point.[28]

Physicians at the end of the 18th century also treated acute rheumatism with depletive therapies commonly employed to lessen any form of inflammation: bleeding, purging, sweating, and local irritation. These measures continued during the first decades of the 19th century. Although he had altered how physicians thought about rheumatism, Bouillaud advocated these traditional treatments. Significantly, Bouillaud directed some of these customary remedies at heart injury, for example, cupping the chest wall over the heart in an effort to draw off inflammation around the heart. Pericarditis and endocarditis thus were treated both systemically with bleeding and locally with application of leeches or other locally applied medicines to the chest wall.[29] Physicians treated chorea with bed rest, restraint and occasionally sedatives.

Although Bouillaud supported substantial blood-letting, other physicians worried that such measures actually weakened their patients. In opium, Corrigan[30] found a drug that worked well.

Some physicians turned to cinchona bark to treat the fever of acute rheumatism. This use was prompted by the perceived similarities between rheumatism and malaria, i.e., high fever and a tendency to recur. After John Haygarth published his favorable experience using cinchona bark with 170 patients with rheumatism in 1805, the drug enjoyed several decades of popularity.[20] Many physicians combined standard therapies for inflammation with drugs for pain and fever.

Perceptions of physicians and patients that a variety of therapies worked quite well in acute rheumatism were enhanced by the nature of the disease to remit frequently on its own. In general, physicians stuck by traditionally favorite remedies and normally the patient recovered. When confronted with a patient who developed a serious case of chorea or heart disease, most physicians "threw the book" at the patient, hoping that one or all remedies would prevent death. The treatment of acute rheumatism was very much an open question in mid-century.

Through anatomical analysis of those who died from rheumatism, "acute rheumatism" became an inflammatory illness in most classification schemes. Yet it never comfortably fit into any nosological niche, largely because the joints and brains of victims, clearly diseased in life, appeared normal at autopsy. In a footnote, Baillie recorded that "Dr Pitcairn has observed this in several cases". Deformities of the heart valves were noted by Morgagni (Italy) in 1861, in autopsies of patients with history of articular rheumatism, just prior to Cheadle's reorganization of "clinical thinking".

Clinical Thinking

Repeatedly over the 19th century, rheumatic fever's changing biology forced physicians to sort out common and useful patterns in a disease that was becoming increasingly complex in its presentation. This sorting out occurred in distinct phases, clearly reflected in clinical reporting. Early in the century, practitioners, such as Wells and Yonge, wrote about individual cases that stressed elements peculiar to that patient. The focus centered on fever and the joint disease, but other manifestations, such as cardiac damage and chorea, were added to the picture in a supporting role.

As observations linking acute rheumatism and heart disease mounted, postmortem examinations showed that the pericardium was the main site of cardiac injury. An early exception was Dewees's findings at the autopsy of AB. He discovered that both pericardium and myocardium were involved: "Heart twice as large as usual and adhering by a thick coat of lymph to the pericardium... Two ounces of straw colored serum in pericardium. The texture of the heart was sensibly altered ... in the crispy semicartilaginous manner peculiar to inflamed muscles. I did not detect any inflammation of its lining membrane".[7]

Wells's earlier single description of endocardial injury indicated that acute rheumatism was capable of attacking all three tissues of the heart. Wells believed that his and others recent observations coupling heart injury to acute rheumatism were new at the end of the 18th century.[2] Is it possible that Pitcairn, Wells, Dundas, Dewees, and others simply observed what others had overlooked in the past? This is unlikely. Acute rheumatism was rarely a fatal disease until the end of the 18th century. Patients' new chest complaints were striking and demanded attention. Physicians confirmed with their usual examinations that the heart was behaving improperly and autopsies demonstrated definite cardiac injury. Careful physicians could not fail to miss either patient demands for alleviation of symptoms or the result of examination or autopsy. Even Haygarth, van Swieten, and Cullen who did not associate rheumatism with heart disease nevertheless did remark on these "unusual" symptoms. In the 18th century, patients with acute rheumatism were not discomforted except from their joint pains and fever and they did not die. A close look at the individual case reports from Wells and Dundas shows that these early patients were dramatically symptomatic.

What was likely was that acute rheumatism had changed its biological nature to include injury to the heart. Wells treated only nine patients with the new rheumatic heart complication in the span of 12 years and Dundas encountered a like number of patients over the course of 36 years. The observation that took Wells and Dundas years to repeat became a common place later in the 19th century. For example, a physician at St. Bartholomew's Hospital, PM Latham, tabulated that 13% of all patients admitted between 1836 and 1840 with the diagnosis of acute rheumatism suffered from pericarditis.[31] The proportion of patients with pericarditis as part of their rheumatism grew to 22% at Middlesex Hospital between 1853 and 1859[32] and 24% at Guy's Hospital between 1870 and 1872.[33] The prevalence of endocarditis in some hospitals was even higher.

History of Drugs in Acute Rheumatic Fever

Thomas Maclagan discovered in 1876 that salicin quickly lowered fever, eased joint pain and swelling and lessened chest pain by decreasing pericardial fluid.[34] It had no effect on chorea. Shortly, many salicylates with slightly varying chemical constituents became available, including aspirin, which formed a mainstay of therapy for RF in the early 20th century. Relief from joint illness, prolonged fever and chest pain brought excitement to doctors and patients alike; virtually overnight older therapies were cast aside. So effective was salicylate in alleviating distress that almost no physician critically analyzed its value to the injury that doctors feared most: endocarditis at the end of the 19th century and myocarditis in the 20th century. When these studies were carried out, some nearly a half century after the introduction of salicylate, the drug was found wanting in healing myocarditis, the heart injury then common. Here we see another consequence of the biological mutation of RF. We now know that salicylate effectively lowers fever, reduces joint pain and swelling, eliminates some of the pericardial inflammation that leads to the painful accumulation of fluid and probably (although doubt still exists) cuts some early endocardial inflammation. In other words, salicylate eased both the distresses that brought patients to doctors and the forms of heart disease that doctors most feared at the end of the 19th century. Salicylate did not influence myocarditis, which eventually led to the undeserved conclusion that it was ineffective in RF.[35]

Coburn "Activity" and Aspirin

The concept of rheumatic "activity", which combined clinical evaluation with laboratory confirmation, provided a novel way of assessing the value of aspirin. Helen Taussig, a pediatrician at Johns Hopkins who began her career studying RF before shifting her interests to congenital heart disease as RF waned, was among the first to suggest that aspirin speeded the return of the sedimentation rate to its normal value.[36] Alvin Coburn developed this idea.

Coburn argued that the treatment should be directed at "activity", not symptoms. In his view, physicians had erred in giving aspirin only as long as patients complained of fever, chest discomfort, or joint pain. Overt symptoms ended long before the cessation of "activity", measured by the sedimentation rate. Withdrawing aspirin too soon permitted ongoing cardiac damage. Coburn estimated that nearly 40% of patients relapsed when doctors and patients stopped aspirin at the point when fever and joint pain ended. Breaking new ground, Coburn proposed administering large doses of aspirin, up to 10 g a day, as soon as the diagnosis was made and continuing the drug until all signs of "activity" were extinguished for at least 2 weeks. This often meant that aspirin needed to be taken for months. To ensure that patients received sufficient aspirin, he advocated giving it intravenously at least at the beginning of therapy and measuring blood levels to make certain that the physician had not overshot or undershot his therapeutic mark.[37] When aspirin was used in this fashion, the patient experienced comfort from reduced fever and cessation of joint pain. In Coburn's hands, aspirin also dampened the effect of rheumatic carditis. None of his patients relapsed.

Coburn's advice to treat "activity" was heeded almost without question and continues to serve as one guidepost for therapy in RF. His innovation provided a rationale for length and efficacy of therapy. And most doctors accepted that the best and safest way of monitoring aspirin was with guidance from the serum level. Some early reports supported Coburn's findings.[38] Not all were convinced, however, that his high-dose regimen of aspirin effectively treated heart disease. From Coburn's Presbyterian Hospital came reports that colleagues could not improve outcomes with Coburn's more aggressive approach.[39] Some encountered serious overdosing despite careful monitoring of the serum aspirin levels.[40] Others could not verify that aspirin hurried the return of the sedimentation rate to normal values.[41] Still others argued that high-dose aspirin benefited only pericarditis.[42]

What seems likely is that Coburn's more precise use of aspirin and "activity" collided with rheumatic fever's biological evolution. Always effective for fever, joint complaints and pericardial fluid, salicylate, when first employed at the end of the 19th century, seemed more effective against heart disease simply because pericarditis was then more common. Aspirin was far less capable in treating the newer form of heart disease. Thus, as pericarditis waned, the perception waxed that aspirin was worthless in any form of heart injury. Nevertheless, when Coburn developed his aggressive high-dose aspirin treatment, RF injured the heart far less seriously than it had when Thomas Maclagan first used salicin 75 years earlier. This lessening of impairment may well have left the impression of the benefits of Coburn's treatment.

> Lessons learnt are the concept of "rheumatic activity" and remarkable improvement of the symptoms with Aspirin.

Radiation

A few physicians approached chronic myocardial inflammation with an entirely different therapeutic strategy. Beginning in the mid-1920s, Robert Levy, also at Presbyterian Hospital in New York, used radiation. His rationale was that X-ray killed inflammatory cells; in RF Aschoff bodies were sites of inflammation. Over a period of many years, Levy selected a small number of patients with evidence of myocarditis and gave them 4–25 radiation treatments for a total dose of about 1500 RAD, which in itself was capable of injuring the heart's muscle. Although Levy believed that his patients benefited from radiation, he was unable, of course, to obtain myocardial biopsies to verify his claims.[43] Never widely accepted, radiation nevertheless was assessed during World War II among naval personnel hospitalized with RF. Giving much lower doses, naval physicians could detect no benefit.[44]

Treatment for Congestive Heart Failure

Treating congestive heart failure with digitalis offered the hope of shortening the time a child spent in bed. Heart failure made the experience of RF even more desperate for victims. Shortness of breath, swollen legs, and greatly enlarged livers worsened the quality of life. Some of the earliest trials of digitalis pushed the dose to the point where toxic effects were evident on the electrocardiogram. In this fashion, children's heart disease actually worsened.[45] The narrow range between effective dose and overdose in children proved a difficult one to achieve, but when it was attained, victims of RHD benefited.[46]

Physicians at the House of the Good Samaritan worked out the details. The first line of therapy for congestive heart failure was restricting fluid intake and lowering dietary salt. If the child remained symptomatic, doctors added a mercurial or xanthine diuretic, both drugs with side effects in the 1940s. When these efforts were not enough, they added digitalis, carefully monitoring for ill effects. In this manner, most children showed signs of improvement.[47]

The concept of "activity", sulfonamide prophylaxis, and carefully monitored aspirin provided physicians with tools to combat RF. Without question, they improved the lot of victims of the disease. One cannot leave this conclusion without a parting, sympathetic remembrance for all those children who spent months or years in convalescent homes, some exposed to cold and the elements, in enforced bed rest, with few visits from parents and family. Some endured rigor producing fever for chorea. Others serious side effects from early sulfonamide or digitalis. A few overdosage of radiation and most had tonsils removed. Their travail is part of the history of RF.

■ HISTORY IN THE 20TH CENTURY

Moderating biology of RF in the 20th century is easy to spot. A close look at the central feature of RF carditis reveals the outline. Dramatic pericarditis and endocarditis of the late 19th century largely disappeared, replaced by myocarditis that was often clinically subtle and which might even smolder for decades with minimal perceived morbidity. In the last third of the 20th century, few, if any, streptococcal infections treated or not, injured the heart. There was diminishing of other symptoms. By the time that Jones published his diagnostic scheme in 1944, painful and migratory swollen joints had yielded to mildly sore joints without much swelling or arthralgia, melting away over the next decades to insignificant aches and pains. Chorea, once a major movement disorder with verbal and even psychiatric involvement, also disappeared, witnessed now, if at all, with only an occasional twitch. Subcutaneous nodules and erythema marginatum have also largely disappeared. In contrast to Cheadle, who anticipated that most patients would suffer from most symptoms at some point in their illness, for Jones the clinical problem was the difficulty of making a diagnosis in a disease of increasing rarity and diminishing severity. Most of his patients suffered from only one or two of rheumatic fever's many symptoms. To surmount these new hurdles, Jones separated the diverse complaints of RF into "major" manifestations and "minor" manifestations. The presence of only two "major" or one "major" and two or more "minor" manifestations was sufficient to make a diagnosis **(Table 1)**.

> *Lesson learnt:* Jones "major" and "minor" manifestations were helpful to make the diagnosis.

Molecular Biology

The prevention of rheumatic recurrences by antistreptococcal medication was confirmed in 1929 by Coburn and Moore. The relationship between GAS and RF was established only in 1931 by Collis (England) and Coburn (USA).[48] By 1935, variations in GAS resistance to phagocytosis of virulent, attenuated and avirulent strains were clearly confirmed and were summarized by Ward and Lyons.[49] They wrote, "the resistance to phagocytosis of the virulent variants appears to be associated with the presence of capsules on

TABLE 1: Jones criteria for the diagnosis of rheumatic fever (1944).	
Major manifestations	• Carditis • Arthralgia • Chorea • Subcutaneous nodules • Prior bout with rheumatic fever
Minor manifestations	• Fever • Arthritis • Abdominal pain • Chest pain • Rashes (erythema marginatum, among others) • Nosebleeds • Lung disease • Abnormal laboratory tests, such as elevated erythrocyte sedimentation rate, high white blood count

Source: Jones TD. The Diagnosis of Rheumatic Fever. J Am Med Assoc. 1944;126:481-4.

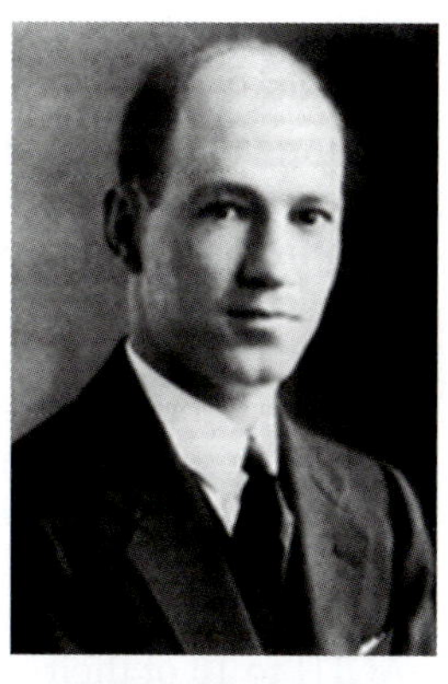

THOMAS DUCKETT JONES (1899–1954)

of the *Streptococcus* produced antibodies that "cross-reacted" with heart tissue. These antibodies, in theory, were the agents of cardiac injury.[53] Subsequent laboratory research demonstrated similar cross-reactivity between the *Streptococcus* and glycoprotein in heart valves, heart muscle, neurons in the caudate and subthalamic nuclei of the brain and joint tissues molecular evidence linking the *Streptococcus* to each part of the body attacked by RF. Different components of the *Streptococcus*, usually classified as M proteins, appeared responsible for antibodies targeting distinct tissues, accounting in theory for the variable symptomatic expression of RF in diverse people that has characterized so much of its history.

Epidemiologists in the 1930s did more than just provide evidence that streptococcal sore throats preceded RF. They recorded how prevalent the disease had become and as startling, and showed that its continuing biological evolution had started its march toward extinction. In an exhaustive study that summarized virtually all relevant epidemiological knowledge in 1930, John R Paul determined that approximately 840,000 or just <1% of Americans suffered significant and permanent heart damage from RF.[54] A decade later, Philip Hench estimated that the number had grown to 1 million, with an estimated 40,000 deaths each year.[55] Mortality did not tell the whole story. School health doctors in the United States and Britain calculated that between 1 and 2% of all school-age children had perceptible cardiac scars with varying degrees of handicap,[56] impediments that mandated special educational programs in most communities.[57]

Adrenocorticotropic Hormone and Cortisone

"A new era in the study and treatment of rheumatic diseases began on April 13, 1949", Benedict Massell precisely proclaimed, when Philip Hench and colleagues at the Mayo Clinic first gave patients cortisone and adrenocorticotropic hormone (ACTH).[58] Cortisone and ACTH hormones, known to physiologists for over a decade as "compound E" and "compound F", had not been available in sufficient amounts for human trials until 1948. The first patients to receive the hormones were victims of Addison's disease, who lacked normal levels of cortisone. Hench, who had edited annual critical surveys of literature dealing with rheumatological diseases since 1935, turned his attention to the potent anti-inflammatory characteristics of these compounds. Hench proposed their use, at much higher doses, in degenerative arthritis in adults and RF in children. His supposition was

the organisms.... No capsule can be demonstrated on the avirulent variant". The appearance of the colony depends to some extent on the length of incubation time. The younger colonies of 6–8 hours are of the mucoid type, being smooth, watery, and of regular contour. The prevention of first attacks of RF by the treatment of GAS Pharyngitis was done in 1949 by Massell and Wannamaker.[48] Later interest in RF waned, but curiosity about the *Streptococcus* and its fascinating biology continued strong. With Lancefield's discovery of the GAS surface M protein as a major virulence factor and the type specific protection afforded by its homologous M antibody,[50] the capsule was relegated to a secondary level of interest, especially because it appeared to be nonantigenic.[51,52]

However, to select GAS clones likely to be the most mouse virulent and to contain a large amount of M protein, Lancefield advised picking only the most highly mucoid colonies from the surface of a blood agar culture.

In the late 1950s, pathologists discovered that antibodies were attached to heart tissue removed during surgical repair of rheumatic heart valves. This provided molecular evidence that myocarditis smoldered long after the initial bout with RF and suggested that these antibodies mediated cardiac damage. In the early 1960s came proof that these antibodies were identical to *Streptococcus*-induced antibodies. In other words, a constituent

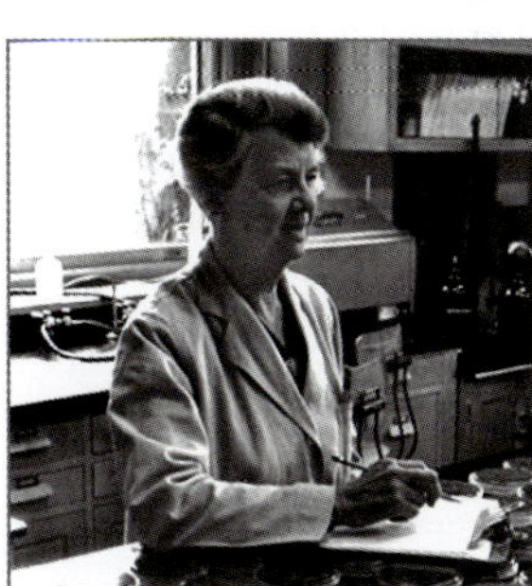

REBECCA CRAIGHILL LANCEFIELD (1895–1981)

that both drugs should lower fever, lessen the pain and swelling of arthritis and reverse the carditis all signs of inflammation in RF. Hench understood that giving pituitary ACTH resulted in patients' secreting higher than normal amounts of adrenal cortisone. In essence, giving either preparation resulted in increasing the level of cortisone available to lessen inflammation. At first, Hench treated just seven patients. He was impressed with the prompt response in abating symptoms and urged further study.[59]

Massell and physicians at the House of the Good Samaritan immediately accepted the task of exploring the effects of hormones and later in 1949 they administered ACTH to 10 of their sickest patients. Like many physicians who regularly treated those seriously ill with RF, Massell understood that aspirin had serious limitations, especially in healing carditis. His initial experience with hormones rendered him an ardent convert. He had good reason for his passion: even in these precariously ill patients fever vanished in a day, joint pain in 1–3 days, joint swelling in 2–3 days, pericarditis and congestive heart failure in <2 weeks. The sedimentation rate returned to normal in <1 month; nodules melted in <2 months. Large doses of ACTH had side effects: acne, stretch marks, headaches, and in a few cases psychiatric disturbances. More immediately, ACTH promoted fluid retention that initially worsened congestive heart failure. To Massell, the benefits of hormone were "striking" and far outweighed the complications, hitting a chord that was struck again and again throughout the medical profession.[58]

What followed was a cascade of reports from many hospitals that treated children with RF. For the most part they described experiences with a small number of patients, often just during the period when the drug was administered. In part, the small numbers were dictated by the epidemiological downswing of the disease: no hospital had enough patients, especially with life-threatening carditis, to conduct a study that would achieve statistical significance. There were other problems. What was the appropriate dose, for how long should treatment last, what signs should the clinician follow, how many side effects could be tolerated? Treatment with cortisone was often followed by a new phenomenon: a distressing "flare" or "rebound" of symptoms once medication was stopped. What did these new symptoms mean for the prognosis of the patient? Despite shortcomings, these early reports were uniformly enthusiastic, especially in the treatment of the sickest patients; those with pericarditis (fortunately now rare) and myocarditis complicated by congestive heart failure.[60]

Corticosteroid offered the hope of accomplishing what penicillin and aspirin could not: treating myocarditis. This potent anti-inflammatory steroid hormone ran headlong into rheumatic fever's changing biology and epidemiology. Fewer critically ill patients made drug trials more difficult. Fewer deaths and those occurring decades after initial illness made pathological evidence of success or failure nearly impossible. In some instances, steroids appeared to provide quick relief to myocarditis, but new problems swiftly

arose. Side effects were prompt and serious, preventing long-term use. Grave "rebound" occurred when the drug was withdrawn.[61] A careful multinational comparison between aspirin and steroids, carried out by the American Heart Association and the British Medical Research Council, demonstrated no superiority for hormones!

At Bellevue Hospital in New York City, physicians confirmed that hormones were strikingly effective in treating fever and arthritis and in improving the general "well-being" of the patient, for example, improving appetite. At issue, did hormone benefit the heart? In a discussion that bore striking resemblance to the debate on the value of salicylate 75 years earlier, the Bellevue doctors thought cortisone helped with pericarditis, perhaps aided myocarditis, but almost certainly did not prevent damage to heart valves.[62] Several groups concluded again from the perspective of their small numbers of patients that hormone produced no benefit to the heart but ladened the patient with serious side effects.[63]

Lesson learnt is cortisone has serious side effects and a distressing "flare" or "rebound" of symptoms once medication was stopped.

A clear mandate to remove the triggering *Streptococcus* with penicillin seemed the unavoidable conclusion to laboratory research. Here the dramatic moderating of streptococcal diseases in general and rheumatic fever in particular hindered efforts. Office-based research pointed to obstacles. Much streptococcal infection was now asymptomatic. Some streptococcal disease mimicked the common cold. Only a fraction of streptococcal illnesses produced the "classical" symptoms of sore throat with accompanying signs of fever, swollen lymph nodes, and exudative pharyngitis. In most office practice, only 1% of streptococcal throat infections progressed to cause RF and these few cases were far milder by every measure than cases of a generation earlier. With the simple office throat culture, physicians had the means of diagnosing streptococcal disease quickly and accurately, but determining which patients required culturing was problematic. With every epidemiological study pointing toward the marked reduction in the incidence of RF, some physicians in the 50s began to question whether close surveillance of the *Streptococcus* in the office setting was even necessary. Even parents of the children at greatest risk, those with prior episodes of RF, often neglected to take their offspring to the physician's office for monthly injections of penicillin. Most children did not suffer negative consequences.

■ PENICILLIN

Penicillin altered rheumatic fever's clinical landscape. Although Alexander Fleming had observed the bacteria killing nature of the penicillium mold in 1928,[64] penicillin

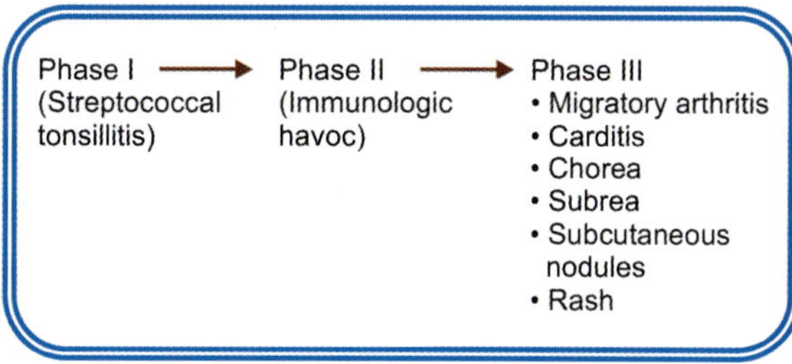

FIG. 5: Coburn's phases of rheumatic fever (1936).

largely remained for the next decade an effective laboratory tool for sorting out bacteria on blood agar plates. In the late 1930s, Howard Florey and Ernest Chain at Oxford revitalized Fleming's idea and systematically explored it. The older drugs like sulfonamide could prevent streptococci from multiplying but could not eliminate them from the pharynx. When physicians had stopped giving sulfonamide to patients, streptococci lingered in the throat to trigger RF. In sharp contrast, penicillin promptly killed all streptococci. The question was one of timing: would penicillin overcome the necessary delay between the acquisition of bacteria on the tonsils and the start of antibiotic? Older studies had implied that streptococci needed some time to initiate the rheumatic havoc (Coburn's Phase II) **(Fig. 5)** but the span of the therapeutic window of opportunity was uncertain.

A close look at one of the initial investigations reveals the power of their method. They enrolled over 1,600 recruits who suffered from sore throats severe enough to produce exudates of pus on their tonsils. Researchers cultured all for streptococci and tested all serially for antistreptolysin O. Randomly, they divided the recruits into a group that received penicillin and a control group that received no antibiotic, which was, of course, the prevailing approach in 1949 to the initial management of streptococcal tonsillitis. This random assignment eliminated a bias that had entered Caroline Bedell Thomas's earlier studies with sulfonamide when only those patients who were compliant received the drug.

Only two men in the penicillin group subsequently developed RF compared with 17 in the control group. Penicillin was clearly more effective than no treatment. A crucial benefit to this study was the calculation that 2% of patients with untreated streptococcal sore throats ultimately went on to develop RF, a prediction subsequently refined upward to 3%.[65]

Almost immediately, the treatment of streptococcal throat infections with penicillin became the recommendation of the American Heart Association. Because many physicians' offices did not have ready access to definitive culture techniques in the early 1950s, the AHA encouraged giving penicillin even in "suspected" cases.[66] With a similar study design, the Fort Francis Warren group determined that recruits benefited from penicillin even when the treatment began as long as 9 days after the start of throat symptoms.[67]

When long-acting benzathine penicillin became available, the Fort Francis Warren group demonstrated that a single injection eliminated streptococci from the throats of nearly 100% of sufferers.

Once the streptococci were gone, the threat of RF vanished.[68] So successful was long-acting penicillin that the navy began administering a single shot to all recruits in 1957.[69] Cementing the supremacy of penicillin over the more familiar sulfonamides, such as sulfadiazine, which doctors continued to use successfully in prophylaxis of recurrences, physicians at Fort Warren demonstrated once again that these drugs were unsuccessful in eliminating streptococci from throats and as such, had no role in the treatment of the preceding streptococcal infection.[70]

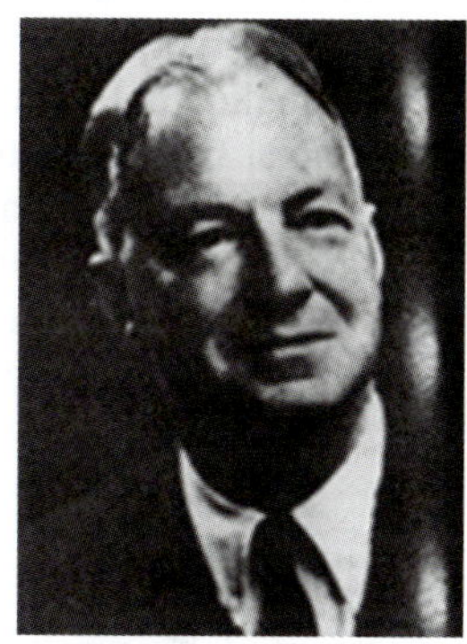

ALVIN F COBURN

Long-acting Injections of Penicillin for the Prevention of Rheumatic Fever

The people with the most at stake were those recovering from RF. Until now, the only measure of safety against relapse was the daily dosage of sulfonamide carried out for years. Would treatment with penicillin of subsequent streptococcal infections, instead of continuous prophylaxis, serve this population? At the House of the Good Samaritan, Benedict Massell too had a ready group of patients to study. Massell had taken over direction of much of the research at "Good Sam" after Duckett Jones became the medical director at the Helen Hay Whitney Foundation, which sponsored research in RF. Massell was able to culture throats thrice weekly of patients convalescing from RF. As soon as streptococci appeared (whether or not they produced symptoms in the child), he started penicillin. When he did so, only 6% of patients relapsed compared with nearly half of patients who served as controls. The lesson drawn was that penicillin used in this fashion was beneficial but not as effective as continuous prophylaxis with sulfadiazine, which, when followed, eliminated most relapses. In marked contrast to physicians at Fort Francis Warren, Massell studied only 46 patients.[71]

A natural consequence of the Fort Francis Warren investigations was to see whether penicillin would also be effective in a scheme of continuous prophylaxis. Initially, penicillin was available only in injectable form and as such was considerably less attractive for daily use than oral sulfadiazine. In the early 1950s, penicillin became available in oral tablets. Dosage was five times the intramuscular route and to be effective penicillin had to be given three or four times a day on an empty stomach, no mean task for parents to accomplish. Despite obstacles, penicillin proved highly efficacious. Its advantage over sulfadiazine was that physicians did not need to follow white blood counts looking for early signs of drug-induced toxicity.[72] The question arose whether patients and their families would be able to follow such a schedule for years. As a more palatable alternative, some doctors suggested, with initial clinical success, using oral penicillin intensively just 1 week each month.[73] For most physicians, the continuous daily prophylaxis with either sulfadiazine or penicillin was the safest recommendation for children who survived one bout of rheumatic fever.[74]

Long-acting penicillin, benzathine penicillin or "bicillin", changed the calculus of prophylaxis. Gene H Stollerman, who began a career devoted to streptococcal illness and RF at Irvington House, found in 1952 that a single monthly injection provided sufficient penicillin to prevent streptococcal infection. Its advantage, immediately appreciated by workers in the field, was that nurses, doctors, and parents could make certain that children received an adequate dose of the drug. Its disadvantage, also immediately appreciated by child recipients, was that the volume of penicillin required was sizable and its intramuscular injection painful.[75] Children balked so often that some physicians, including May Wilson, who was now working with a younger colleague, Wan Ngo Lim, at New York Hospital, offered oral penicillin coupled with frequent reminders from the office. Most doctors argued that monthly shots provided the most efficient means of prophylaxis.[76] In 1955, Stollerman formulated the general principles of prophylaxis: antibiotic for at least 5 years after the initial bout of RF, preferably penicillin, in monthly injections because it eliminated the difficulties of multiple daily dosing.[77] The recommendation extended even to children who did not suffer carditis as a major manifestation of RF, out of concern that a second or third bout might attack the heart.[78] Just how long to continue prophylaxis was a debated point. Clearly the risk of recurrence declined with time, especially after 20 years of age, but it never went away.[79] Despite this observation and the marked decline in RF, the American Heart Association in 1965 recommended prophylaxis for life.[80] Continuous penicillin posed theoretical problems. Would it lead to resistance of the group A β-hemolytic *Streptococcus*? Fortunately, that did not occur. Penicillin did result, however, in other resistant mouth flora, especially among nonhemolytic streptococci, that presented the worrisome possibility of untreatable bacterial endocarditis, always a concern for people with scarred heart valves.[81,82]

Penicillin and Public Health Programs

Prophylactic penicillin offered communities a cheap alternative to long hospital stays for convalescent care. Newton, Massachusetts, was among the first to act. After consulting with Duckett Jones and Benedict Massell, public health officials set up a program to identify those children who needed prophylaxis. First, Jones and Massell joined community leaders in public forums to educate physicians regarding the need to provide penicillin. Next, Jones and Massell asked Newton's doctors to cull their files for cases. Then public health officials sent questionnaires home with all 14,000 of the community's schoolchildren asking parents whether their child had ever received the diagnosis of RF. Responses revealed that 379 children had. The parents were directed to make an appointment with their physicians to confirm the memory and if correct, to seek penicillin tablets for continuous prophylaxis. Newton's doctors substantiated the parents' recollections for 214 of the children. If parents could not afford the price of penicillin, the Newton Health Department supplied it without cost. The program enjoyed considerable success. The questionnaire revealed that only 16% of children who needed prophylaxis had received the antibiotic before the start of the project. The program raised this to 80%. Of note, despite intensive physician and parent education that reached into every home and the availability of free penicillin, one-fifth of those in need did not receive the drug.[83]

> Lesson learnt is penicillin altered rheumatic fever's clinical landscape. Penicillin prophylaxis is the sheet anchor of prophylaxis.

Officials in Youngstown, Ohio, went further; they set out to prevent even first attacks of RF. Beginning in 1950, the same year that the Fort Francis Warren physicians reported the efficacy of treating the preceding bout of streptococcal sore throat, Youngstown public health officials went to work. A close look at their program illustrates the immensity of the project. It began with an intensive educational campaign public lectures, Parent-Teacher Association programs, radio shows, and newspaper articles that targeted, separately, physicians and nurses, school teachers and principals and parents, and children. The following year, officials put their program into gear. Any child with a sore throat was directed to report to the school nurse, who obtained a throat culture. The parent of an absent child received a phone call to determine whether the absence was due to tonsillitis. If so, the parent was urged to obtain a throat culture either at school or at a physician's office. Through both routes, nearly 900 cultures were obtained in 1951. Six percent of the cultures grew hemolytic streptococci. Both the parent and the child's physician received telephone notification of a positive culture with instruction for the child to seek medical attention. The following day, the school nurse once again called the parent to ask what action had been taken. Foolproof? Not at all. Despite these efforts, only half of the children received any penicillin; less than a third received a full course of the drug.[84] Community and state programs proliferated. In 1950 two states offered free antibiotics to needy patients; in 1958, the number grew to 29. These antibiotic programs joined the Crippled Children's Program public sector efforts which had grown to include all but one state in aiding "cardiac cripples".[85]

Lessons learnt: Intensive educational campaign like public lectures, radio shows, newspaper articles, awareness program for physicians, nurses' physicians, nurses, school teachers, principals, parents, and children needs to be done now in all the developing countries where RF is endemic.

The moderating nature of RF and hormonal therapies that carried serious side effects prompted physicians to rethink Duckett Jones's criteria for diagnosis. Initially revised in 1955 and again in 1965, the new guidelines called for more objective evidence before reaching a diagnosis. Recommending a lifetime punctuated with painful monthly injections placed an increased burden of proof upon frontline physicians. At mid-century, the challenge for the physician was the diagnosis, prevention, and treatment of an increasingly rare disease.

Inadequacy of Public Health Programs

The Biological Evolution of RF and Physician Error: Despite identification and treatment programs, children with RF still found their way to doctors' offices. Leaders in the field analyzed the reasons for these "preventable" cases. After talking with parents and children, physicians at Irvington House discovered that over 40% of bouts of RF were preceded by totally asymptomatic streptococcal illnesses, which had been detected only through rising antistreptolysin O titer in the blood.[86,87] Two-thirds of patients arriving with RF at the House of the Good Samaritan had not consulted a doctor for the preceding illness, largely due to the mild nature of the symptoms. The third who had attended a doctor received either an incorrect diagnosis or inadequate therapy.[88] A different, but no less distressing, story came from doctors at La Rabida Sanitarium in Chicago. Only one-third of patients with sore throats received a throat culture. Even more disturbing, only one-third of blood agar plates had been interpreted correctly by the physician as demonstrating the presence of hemolytic streptococci.[89] With these problems in mind, Benedict Massell advised parents and physicians: mothers should take a sick child's temperature four times a day. If the fever ever reached 101°, she should consult a physician. Unless the cause of the fever was clearly identified, a physician should obtain a throat culture. The appearance of any β-hemolytic colonies on the bacterial plate should dictate penicillin. Even these stringent guidelines, of course, did not detect totally asymptomatic cases or prevent physician error.[88]

Lesson learnt: Stringent RF Control Programs and Public Health Programs are very important.

Programs for prophylaxis of recurrences fared no better. Two-thirds of children discharged from Herrick House, a convalescent hospital 30 miles west of Chicago, were no longer taking penicillin at a follow-up visit. About half of the parents gave as a reason that they had stopped bringing their children to a doctor. The prescription had simply run out. As woeful, the other half selected doctors who did not understand the need for continuous prophylaxis. Some of these physicians stopped the penicillin because there was no evidence of heart disease, a sign, of course, of the measure's success and the need for its continuance.[89] A survey conducted by the US Public Health Service and the American College Health Association of over 500,000 first year students entering 137 colleges during a 5-years period in the late 1950s revealed the immensity of the problem. Only half of the adolescents in need of prophylaxis had ever been enrolled in a program; merely 12% arrived at college taking penicillin.[90] A similar poll of military recruits in 1960 revealed that only 7% of those in need received antibiotics.[91] One interpretation of this neglect was that RF had disappeared from the public mind as a health menace.

Sorting Out Therapy

The British Medical Research Council and the American Heart Association took up the responsibility of sorting out the appropriate therapy issue. The paucity of patients and the flush of excitement accompanying the dramatic first usage of cortisone were just two of the impediments to assessing the true worth of steroid hormones.[92] After the first enthusiasm for hormone waned, the need plainly emerged to establish its worth compared with aspirin, the flawed but nonetheless accepted treatment. Complicating matters still further was the question whether it made a therapeutic difference which hormone was used, ACTH, or cortisone. Early studies comparing hormones and aspirin could establish no obvious superiority, but these investigations, carried out in single hospitals, also suffered from lack of sufficient numbers of patients.[93-95] Even Benedict Massell, hormonal advocate, conceded in 1953 that the relative merit of competing drugs was an unresolved issue.[96]

In the hope of settling these therapeutic perplexities, the Medical Research Council of Great Britain and the American Heart Association collaborated in a carefully constructed, 12 hospital study. Its coordinators included many of the major leaders and institutions most closely involved with RF. Each of the over 500 patients had to meet Jones criteria for diagnosis, modified only to make it more rigorous by requiring observable swelling and limitation of motion of joints or arthritis, in place of Jones's original inclusion of simple joint pain or arthralgia. All patients received penicillin treatment for current streptococcal infection and were placed on penicillin prophylaxis. All endured the rigors of enforced bed rest. The patients were randomly assigned to one of three drug regimens: aspirin (at a dose somewhat lower than Coburn's suggested schedule), cortisone or ACTH. The duration of all three drugs was 6 weeks. Patients were kept in the hospital under observation during this period and for 3 weeks after stopping the drugs. Patients returned for clinic appointments monthly for 6 months and then every other month. The protocol thus seemed nearly perfect: the best investigators and institutions, rigorous diagnostic criteria, uniform administration of drugs, in hospital observation, close follow-up and conclusions subjected to demanding statistical tests. "Nearly" perfect in that detractors pointed out that there was not a group receiving no drug at all.

Sulfonamide and later penicillin brought similar enthusiasm. Shortly after Coburn singled out infection with the *Streptococcus* as the triggering event in RF (Coburn's Phase I), sulfonamide became available for treating bacterial infections, raising expectations that it was just the drug to combat the disease. Here rheumatic fever's unusual nature confounded early therapeutic attempts. Despite Coburn's well-articulated consensus that RF was not a widely disseminated infection, early studies treated symptomatic RF (Coburn's Phase III) with sulfonamide. The drug had no effect on heart, brain or joint symptoms and serious side effects actually worsened the patient's experience. When physicians correctly targeted the triggering sore throat for treatment, sulfonamide also came up short. It could not prevent Phase I from progressing to Phase II and III.[97] The first success with sulfonamide came in preventing relapses with daily doses of the drug administered throughout the year: in other words, not permitting infection to occur in the first place.[98] Newer sulfonamides produced fewer side effects and prevention was so attractive to the United States military that 100s of 1,000s of seamen received daily sulfonamide starting in 1944. Within months of this massive and very successful program, biological disaster struck: the *Streptococcus* became resistant to sulfonamide and diseases caused by resistant streptococci infected sailors. The US Navy had fewer cases of RF, but in the process it altered the germ.[99,100]

> Lessons learnt are sulfonamide had no effect on heart, brain, or joint symptoms, but had serious side effects which actually worsened the patient's experience. Still worse *Streptococcus* became resistant to sulfonamide. Therefore sulfonamides are not indicated in RF.

In 1959, Wilson[101] clearly demonstrated striking capsules formed in 3–6 hours, serum enriched broth cultures of GAS strains isolated from patients with virulent human infection. On properly prepared and preserved blood agar plates, the heavily encapsulated strains formed large, domed "mucoid" colonies and the size was measured by light microscopy using India ink preparations. Furthermore, the "matte" strains previously described by Ward and Lyons[49] and by Todd and Lancefield[102] were demonstrated to be initially "mucoid", but upon drying, they developed a roughened, "matte", collapsed (flat) surface. With use of phase contrast

microscopy, Wilson had also demonstrated virtually total resistance to phagocytosis of heavily encapsulated strains. In subsequent studies, resistance to "surface phagocytosis" of GAS strains by mouse and rat leukocytes was correlated with the degree of encapsulation or M protein content.[103]

This is not to argue that the history of RF can be reduced simply to an alteration of molecules. Rather, these molecular shifts set into motion biological and epidemiological changes that confronted patients and doctors with an ever changing health problem that demanded attention. To be sure, technologies, such as the autopsy, the stethoscope and electrocardiogram, the progression of medical thinking (individual case histories, large hospital-based studies, Cheadle's "typical" series, Coburn's "phases", and Jones's "major/minor" criteria), the organization of medical care into hospitals and various research strategies all helped to define and illuminate RF. If molecular biologists are correct in their singling out of M proteins as the ultimate culprit, the very nature of the disease lay beyond truly "curative" therapy until the cusp of the 21st century. This observation underscores the dilemma that patients and doctors have often faced in history: combating disease with the knowledge and tools at hand at a given moment, knowing full well that their efforts are not wholly adequate.

The complex bond between molecules, disease, epidemiology, and history continues. Insights about the M proteins suggested to Stollerman, an additional means for physicians to attack RF: a vaccine against M proteins, signaling an effort for humans to alter the molecular makeup of the *Streptococcus* and thus a chance to alter its history. The abrupt termination of an epidemic by such treatment was associated with the prompt disappearance of RF and simultaneously of the highly encapsulated strains belonging to the epidemic M types 1, 3, 5, 14, 19, and 24. After mass prophylaxis in military recruits resulted in the elimination of epidemic RF, persistent GAS carriage and sporadic pharyngitis were noted to occur relatively frequently without the reappearance of RF.[104,105] At about this time, two highly encapsulated strains that clearly caused RF (an M3 and an M5) were isolated by Alan Siegel from Chicago in two school children during their antecedent episodes of pharyngitis.[106] These virulent strains became the source of many subsequent studies of their virulence properties and of their potential for development of M protein vaccines. While studying these strains, Stollerman and Ekstedt[107] reported that encapsulation significantly shortened the chain length of GAS units, whereas, with loss of encapsulation or with growth in the presence of type specific anti-M antibody, their chain length was greatly elongated.

Variation of Virulence of Strains in a Single M Type

Four variants of a single M14 strain (M+ Capsule+, M+ Capsule_, M_ Capsule+ and M_ Capsule_) identified by Armine Wilson were used to study the innate host defense of germ-free mice[108] and of colostrum deprived piglets.[109]

Maximal virulence was demonstrated only in strains that were both M protein rich and heavily encapsulated.[110] Rothbard and Watson demonstrated that during convalescence from pharyngitis there is progressive loss of GAS strain virulence.[110,111]

By the 1960s, it became more evident that the high attack rate of RF noted in military epidemics did not apply to endemic GAS pharyngitis in schoolchildren.[112] GAS strains were more often cultured from clinically mild pharyngitis, as well from convalescent or asymptomatic carriers.[113] Though 20% of school children had positive throat cultures for GAS, the prevalence of RF abruptly declined. There was a difference in the virulence of GAS strains isolated from sporadic infections in schoolchildren from Chicago with that of the strains isolated from military epidemics.[114,115] Thus, it was proposed in 1969 that only certain heavily encapsulated strains were notorious for causing RF (rheumatogenic).[116] Further review of the existing literature[117,118] confirmed the limited M type association. After the standardization of an M typing system based on the nucleotide sequence encoding the N-terminus of the mature M protein, GAS reference laboratories widely adopted this sensitive method of M typing,[119] but identification of colony morphology as a marker of strain virulence was rarely noted.

> *Lesson learnt:* "Rheumatogenic" encapsulated strains of GAS are notorious for causing rheumatic fever.

The Return of Rheumatic Fever and Invasive GAS Disease

In the 1980s, focal epidemics of RF occurred in cohorts of children in several US states and Pennsylvania[120-123] and in some US military installations.[124,125] The M types of the strains causing these epidemics were eventually to be the same as the notorious rheumatogenic strains of the earlier World War II military epidemics.[126] The state of encapsulation of these strains was not reported originally and systematic studies of their virulence were not made.[127] Later, retrospective analysis of outbreaks of invasive GAS infection that followed revealed that mucoid colonies were often identified in some isolates from affected cohorts, notably, M types 3 and 18.[128]

Finally, a retrospective study of the colonial morphology of the GAS isolates recovered from patients with pharyngitis was made during several years of recurrent waves of acute RF.[129] For strains that had been carefully preserved at −70°C, there was a clear correlation between the outbreaks of acute RF and the prevalence of mucoid strains.[129] Identification of the genome of some of these strains revealed that a single virulent clone may have been responsible for the epidemics of RF reported from the Rocky Mountain States and elsewhere[130,131] and that a single genetically identified clone also caused an outbreak of invasive streptococcal disease among schoolchildren in Minnesota.[132]

Experimental Studies

By the mid-1970s, the adherence of GAS to pharyngeal cells was shown to be due to several fibronectin binding ligands, such as lipoteichoic acid[133,134] and the so-called F proteins,[135] rather than to M protein alone. The hyaluronate capsule's role was studied and it was demonstrated that it attaches to a hyaluronic acid binding protein, CD44, which is present on human epithelial cells[136-139] and which induces cytoskeletal rearrangements, resulting in disruption of intercellular junctions, thus allowing the microorganisms to remain extracellular as they penetrate the epithelium.

More recently, strains of M types 3 and 18 that were strongly associated with the reappearance of RF in the United States in the 1980s were shown to avidly aggregate type IV collagen.[140] Such aggregation was found to depend on the expression of both M protein and hyaluronate and was demonstrated in vivo (mouse skin) as well as in vitro.

Surgery for Rheumatic Fever

By 1970, surgically repairing or replacing heart valves had become routine on the surgical service, >20 years after the "revival" of valvular surgery in the late 40s.[141] These victims died, their weakened hearts worn out a decade before routine heart transplantation. Surviving RF meant that many victims could expect to lead fuller lives. Women of childbearing years were clear beneficiaries. By 1970, many women with the reluctant blessing of their obstetricians conceived and survived pregnancy.

In 1970, RF accounted for only 256 deaths in the United States, a startling decline from nearly 40,000 deaths in 1940.[142] Physicians who had trained at Boston's House of the God Samaritan, a hospital that specialized in the care of the sickest sufferers of RF and where many of the innovations of the 30s and 40s first saw light, remembered that some of the hospital's beds went empty during their training in the 50s.[143] Some of these same physicians remembered with persistent excitement their investigations into RF a decade earlier during World War II, because the disease, long in decline, briefly enjoyed an epidemiological encore in barrack[144] and ship[99] life that crowded recruits into tight living spaces. The stunning efficiency of sulfonamide and a few years later, penicillin in driving the nails into the coffin of a disease once so prevalent.[65] Unfortunately, same decline is not seen in developing countries with poor socioeconomical condition and overcrowding.

Antibiotics played a role, especially in prevention, but they were only a small part of the story. In fact, RF had been in decline for a half century before the discovery of penicillin.

In 1970, there were still vestiges of RF left visible for the newcomer to medicine. On rare occasions, a child came to the pediatric clinic with complaints so unusual that the question of RF arose. In such instances, the physicians would seek out of necessity the "gray-hairs", because the regular teachers, pediatric house officers, had no first-hand experience with the disease! The elders would enter into the examining room. If diagnosis was guessed correctly, great ceremony would be made in gathering together as many students and residents as possible for a demonstration and discussion of this fascinating disease! RHD brought laboratory scientists and clinicians together intellectually and physically. This disease ignited controversy even after its death in western countries. RF fascinates, because it is a disease that abounds with change. Historians anticipate that medical and public health ideas about a particular illness and how to prevent or treat it will change considerably over time, depending on the disease and on the social settings of patients and physicians. In this regard, RF does not disappoint.

By 1970, RF had almost disappeared in developed countries. For most families, the suffering it once produced took its place in the memory of an afflicted parent or grandparent! Its diminished nature properly dictated its lowered status. Physicians and medical students shifted interests elsewhere as well, for RF no longer produced serious health consequences in the west. It lingered a while in lectures, textbooks, and clinical lore and then was largely forgotten.

Floyd Denny, who participated in the initial trials of penicillin after World War II, remarked in 1986, "I am impressed that we have raised an entire generation of young physicians who have never seen a case of acute RF".[145] Only in the continued exaggerated concern over streptococcal sore throats, precautionary antibiotics before trips to dentists for those with suspicious heart murmurs and repeated and largely unnecessary, heart examinations looking for newly acquired heart disease during well child visits did patients and doctors still meet over the remnants of RF.

In 1980, echocardiography (ECHO) a modern tool was used to diagnose carditis. When ECHO is carried out in patients with acute RF diagnosed strictly, according to the Jones criterion, can avoid both overdiagnosis and underdiagnosis of carditis. A high incidence of carditis or subclinical carditis is detected by echocardiography when performed in patients with rheumatic chorea or arthralgia.[146] When I gave grand rounds at Fairview University, Minnesota and spoke on "Role of ECHO in precise and early diagnosis of carditis in ARF" Liz Bruanlin said, "This may be the only lecture you may hear on RF in the medical school, that too from the person who sees poor patients with RF everyday". I was surprised to see the enthusiasm among all the senior persons such as Ed Kaplan, Patricia Ferreri, Miller, and others. At the end of the lecture, there was a hot discussion. Ed Kaplan asked me, "With the application of ECHO for the diagnosis of carditis will there not be over diagnosis?" In reply, I asked him "If we over diagnose, at the most we end up giving penicillin injection for secondary prophylaxis, which is inexpensive. That is erring on the right side. If we do not use the ECHO and miss the diagnosis and the patient ends up with RHD, needing expensive balloon valvuloplasty or valve repair or replacement it is expensive and carries high morbidity and mortality. That is erring on the wrong side. If you have a choice, would you err on the right side or the

wrong side?". Ed Kaplan raised his arms and said, "You are disarming me". In a nutshell, the disease is eradicated in the US but the problem is huge in many developing countries like India. Hence, early and precise diagnosis of carditis in acute RF, though difficult, is very important in preventing serious consequences, morbidity, and mortality in young. Echocardiographic criteria are now very important in providing precise diagnosis of carditis or subclinical valvitis. These subclinical changes, detected only by ECHO, can persist and probably belong to a large group of patients who present later as RHD, without the past history of acute RF and prophylaxis. These echocardiographic criteria, therefore, should now be included as one of the major criteria in the Jones' system to permit diagnosis of carditis in the setting of acute RF.[147] ECHO can change the epidemiological face of RF in the 21st century.

■ SUMMARY

Rheumatic fever is an illness of skin, brain, heart, connective tissue, tonsils, joints, blood, and serum, all bound intimately to a member of the *Streptococcus* family of bacteria that causes several human diseases. Each component of the disease has its own history; together, as RF, they share a collective history. In addition, RF has been most responsive to the environment, especially living conditions and physical setting.

Rheumatic fever's researchers have also been its historians. Understandably, the disease which challenged physicians at the bedside, in the laboratory, or in the making of health policy has also stimulated historical reflection. These medical leaders have discussed some of the early descriptions and changing symptoms of the disease, analyzed the perplexing relation of the *Streptococcus* to RF, detailed some of the social dimensions of RF, addressed the value of therapies and provided thoughtful appraisals of rheumatic fever's disappearance. The history of RF is of relevance to modern medicine because it has taught us much about the pathophysiology and epidemiology of autoimmune disease and because RF is unique in the way that it has changed repeatedly over time. Lessons learnt from history are more important now in the developing countries where disease is still a burning problem. It is high time that the clinicians and policy makers in the developing countries learn the lessons from the history of RF and RHD.

■ STAGES IN HISTORY

There are three stages in the history of every medical discovery. When it is first announced, people say "*it is not true*", then a little later, when its truth has been borne in on them, so that it can no longer be denied, they say "*it is not important*". After that, if its importance becomes sufficiently obvious they say that anyhow "*it is not new*".

—**Sir James Mackenzine (1853–1925)**

ACKNOWLEDGMENT

We acknowledge the great contribution of all the pioneers and also the author English, Peter C who has recorded the events systematically and diligently in his book. We recommend reading this book of great interest and details. Rheumatic Fever in America and Britain. Copyright © 1999 by Peter C English. Reprinted by permission of Rutgers University Press.

REFERENCES

1. Swan J. The Entire Works of Dr Thomas Sydenham, Newly Made English from the Originals: Wherein the History of Acute and Chronic Diseases, and the Safest and Most Effectual Methods of Treating Them, are Faithfully, Clearly, and Accurately Delivered. London: Edward Cave at St John's Gate; 1749.

2. Wells WC. On Rheumatism of the Heart. Trans Soc Improv Med Chirurg Knowledge. 1812;3:373-424.

3. Dundas D. An Account of a Peculiar Disease of the Heart. Medico-Chirurgical Transact. 1809;1:37-46.

4. Baillie M. The Morbid Anatomy of Some of the Most Important Parts of the Human Body, 2nd edition. London: J Johnson G Nicol; 1797. pp. 44-6.

5. Russell J. Case of Rheumatism of the Heart, Successfully Treated. Edinburgh Med Surg J. 1814;10:18-21.

6. Laennec RTH. A Treatise on the Diseases of the Chest: In Which They are Described According to Their Anatomical Characters, and Their Diagnosis Established on a New Principle by Means of Acoustick Instruments. London: G Underwood; 1821. p. 266.

7. Dewees WP. A Case of Rheumatism with Metastasis, Producing Carditis, Pericarditis, Peripneumonia, and Pleuritis. Am J Med Sci. 1828;2:473-5, 22.

8. Stgerist HE. John Hopkins University bulletin of Institute of the history of Medicine. 1936;IV(10).

9. Davis AB. Medicine and its Technology: An Introduction to the History of Medical Instrumentation. Westport, Conn.: Greenwood Press; 1981.

10. Bouillaud JB. New Researches on Acute Articular Rheumatism in General; and Especially on the Law of Coincidence of Pericarditis and Endocarditis with This Disease, as Well as on the Efficacy of the Method of Treating it by Repeated Blood-Letting at Short Intervals, trans. James Kitchen. Philadelphia: Haswell, Barrington, and Haswell; 1837.

11. Herrick JB. Jean-Baptiste Bouillaud and his Contributions to Cardiology. Bull Soc Med Hist Chicago. 1940;5:230-46.

12. Ackerknecht, Medicine at the Paris Hospital; Toby Gelfand, Professionalizing Modern Medicine: Paris Surgeons and Medical Science and Institutions in the 18th Century. Westport, Conn.: Greenwood Press; 1980.

13. Pamela Bright, Dr Richard Bright (1789-1858) (London: Bodley Head, 1983); and Diana Freeman Berry and Campbell Mackenzie, Richard Bright (1789-1858): Physician in an Age of Revolution and Reform. London: Royal Society of Medicine; 1992.

14. Bright R. Cases of Spasmodic Disease Accompanying Affections of the Pericardium. Medico-Chirurg Transact. 1839;22:1-19.

15. Cunningham A. Thomas Sydenham: Epidemics, Experiment, and the 'Good Old Cause,' The Medical Revolution of the Seventeenth Century, ed. Roger French and Andrew Wear. Cambridge: Cambridge University Press; 1989. pp. 164-90.

16. Cullen W. First Lines of the Practice of Physic, for the Use of Students in the University of Edinburgh, 2nd edition. Philadelphia: Steiner and Cist; 1781. p. 156.

17. van Swieten B. Commentaries upon Boerhaave's Aphorisms Concerning the Knowledge and Cure of Diseases. Edinburgh: Charles Elliot; 1776;13(32):88.

18. Balfour W. Observations on the Pathology and Cure of Rheumatism. Edinburgh Med Surg J. 1815;11:168-87.

19. Seymour EJ. On the Most Effectual Treatment of Acute Rheumatism in Hospital Practice in the Last Eight Years. Medico-Chirurgical Rev J Pract Med. 1838;29:657-60.

20. Haygarth J. A Clinical History of Diseases. 1. A Clinical History of the Acute Rheumatism. 2. A Clinical History of the Nodosity of the Joints, 1805, reprinted with an introduction by Lawrence A. May. Oceanside, N.Y.: Dabor Science Publications; 1977.

21. Stillé A. Case of Rheumatism, Endo-pericarditis, Pleurisy, and Double Pneumonia, with Autopsy. Med Examin. 1840;3:21-5.

22. Jarcho S. Pericarditis Supervening on Rheumatism (Roots, 1836). Am J Cardiol. 1966;18:594-8.

23. Dr Yonge. Case of Cerebral Disturbance: Dependent upon Disease of the Pericardium. Guy's Hospital Reports. 1840;5:276-81.

24. Sydenham T. The Works of Thomas Sydenham, trans. from the Latin edition of Dr. Greenhill (Sydenham Society London). 1848;2:257-8.

25. Cheadle WB. Harveian Lectures on the Various Manifestations of the Rheumatic State: As Exemplified in Childhood and Early Life. Lancet. 1889;1:821-7, 871-7, 921-7.

26. Clay C. Sulphur in Rheumatic Affections. Lancet. 1839-40;2:783-4.

27. De Roches JJ. Two Cases of Acute Rheumatism, Treated with Opium: and Some Observations on the Comparative Merits of that Method, and of the Treatment Which is Founded on the Principle of Depletion. Edinburgh Med Surg J. 1805;1:154-9.

28. Fish S. Corroborative Testimony in Favor of Large Doses of Opium in Rheumatism. Boston Med Surg J. 1837;16:330-2.

29. Banks JT. Acute Rheumatism: Endocarditis Followed by Pericarditis and Pleuropneumonia. Dublin Hospital Gazette. 1854-55;1:53-5.

30. Corrigan DJ. Observations on the Treatment of Acute Rheumatism by Opium. Dublin J Med Sci. 1840;16:256-77.

31. Church WS. An Examination of Nearly Seven Hundred Cases of Acute Rheumatism: Chiefly with a View to Determining the Frequency of Cardiac Affections, and Especially Pericarditis, at the Present Time. St. Bartholomew's Hospital Reports. 1887;23:269-87.

32. Bury GW. A Statistical Account of Four Hundred Cases of Acute Rheumatism Admitted into the Wards of the Middlesex Hospital during the Years 1853-59. Br Foreign Medico-Chirurg Rev. 1861;28:194-8.

33. Pye-Smith PH. Analysis of the Cases of Rheumatism, and Other Diseases of Joints, Which have Occurred in the Hospital during

Three Consecutive Years: With Remarks on the Pathological Alliances of Rheumatic Fever. Guy's Hospital Reports. 1874;19: 311-56.

34. Maclagan T. The Treatment of Acute Rheumatism by Salicin. Lancet. 1876;1:342-3, 2:601-4.

35. Murphy GE. Salicylate and Rheumatic Activity: An Objective Clinical-Histologic Study of the Effect of Salicylate on Rheumatic Lesions, Those of Joints and Tendon Sheaths in Particular. Bull Johns Hopkins Hospital. 1945;77:1-42.

36. Taussig HB. Acute Rheumatic Fever: The Significance and Treatment of Various Manifestations. J Pediatrics. 1939;14:581-92.

37. Coburn AF. Salicylate Therapy in Rheumatic Fever: A Rational Technique. Bull Johns Hopkins Hospital. 1943;73:435-64.

38. Jager BV, Alway R. The Treatment of Acute Rheumatic Fever with Large Doses of Sodium Salicylate, with Special Reference to Dose Management and Toxic Manifestations. Am J Med Sci. 1946;211:273-85.

39. Smull K, Wégria R, Leland J. The Effect of Sodium Bicarbonate on the Serum Salicylate Level: During Salicylate Therapy of Patients with Acute Rheumatic Fever. J Am Med Assoc. 1944;125:1173-5.

40. Sable HZ. Toxic Reactions Following Salicylate Therapy: A Review of the Literature and Clinical Reports. Canadian Med Assoc J. 1945;52:153-9.

41. Keith JD, Ross A. Observations on the Salicylate Therapy in Rheumatic Fever. Canad Med Assoc J. 1945;52:554-9.

42. Warren HA, Higley CS, Coombs FS. The Effect of Salicylates on Acute Rheumatic Fever. Am Heart J. 1946;32:311-26.

43. Levy RL, Golden R. Roentgen Therapy of Active Rheumatic Heart Disease: A Summary of Eleven Years' Experience. Am J Med Sci. 1937;194:597-601.

44. Griffith GC, Halley EP. The Treatment of Rheumatic Fever by Roentgen-Ray Irradiation. Ann Intern Med. 1946;24:1039-42.

45. Schwartz SP, Weiss MM. Digitalis Studies on Children with Heart Disease: Effects of Digitalis on the Electrocardiograms of Children with Rheumatic Fever and Chronic Valvular Disease. Am J Dis Child. 1929;38:699-714.

46. Sutton LP, Wyckoff J. Digitalis: Its Value in the Treatment of Children with Rheumatic Heart Disease. Am J Dis Child. 1931;41:801-15.

47. Walsh BJ, Sprague HB. The Treatment of Congestive Failure in Children with Active Rheumatic Fever. J Am Med Assoc. 1941;116:560-2.

48. Taranta A, Markkowitz M. Rheumatic fever. London: MTP Press Boston; 1981.

49. Ward H, Lyons C. Studies on the hemolytic streptococcus of human origin. I. Observations on the virulent, attenuated, and avirulent variants. J Exp Med. 1935;61:515-29.

50. Lancefield RC. Current knowledge of the type specific M antigens of group A streptococci. J Immunol. 1962;89:307-13.

51. Todd E, Lancefield R. Variants of hemolytic streptococci; their relation to type-specific substance, virulence, and toxin. J Exp Med. 1928;48:751-67.

52. Lancefield R, Todd E. Antigenic differences between matt hemolytic colonies and their glossy variants. J Exp Med. 1928;48:769-90.

53. Kaplan MH, Meyeserian M. An Immunological Cross-reaction between Group-A Streptococcal Cells and Human Heart Tissue. Lancet. 1962;1:706-10.

54. Rodman Paul J. The Epidemiology of Rheumatic Fever: A Preliminary Report with special reference to Environmental Factors in Rheumatic Heart Disease and Recommendations for Future Investigation. New York: Metropolitan Life Insurance Co.; 1930. p. 30.

55. Hench PS. Recent Studies on Arthritis and Rheumatism in the United States. Ann Rheumatic Dis. 1941;2:172-92.

56. Coombs CF. The Diagnosis and Treatment of Rheumatic Heart Disease in its Early Stages. Br Med J. 1930;1:227-30.

57. Fred Hiss JG. A Plan for Rehabilitation for Rheumatic Subjects. J Pediatr. 1945;26:230-6.

58. Massell BF, Warren JE, Sturgis GP, Hall B, Craige E. The Clinical Response of Rheumatic Fever and Acute Carditis to ACTH. N Engl J Med. 1950;242:641-7, 692-8.

59. Hench PS, Kendall EC, Slocumb CH, Polley HF. Effects of Cortisone Acetate and Pituitary ACTH on Rheumatoid Arthritis, Rheumatic Fever, and Certain Other Conditions: A Study in Clinical Physiology. Arch Internal Med. 1950;85:545-66.

60. Barnes AR, Smith HL, Slocumb CH, Polley HF, Hench PS. Effect of Cortisone and Corticotropin (ACTH), on the Acute Phase of Rheumatic Fever: Further Observations. Am J Dis Child. 1951;82:397-425.

61. Barnes AR, Smith HL, Slocum C, Polley HF, Hench PS. Acute Rheumatic Fever Treated with Cortisone and Corticotropin. In: Thomas L (Ed). Rheumatic Fever: A Symposium. Minneapolis: University of Minnesota Press; 1952. pp. 274-90.

62. Bunim JJ, Kuttner AG, Baldwin JS, McEwen C. Cortisone and Corticotropin in Rheumatic Fever and Juvenile Rheumatoid Arthritis. J Am Med Assoc. 1952;150:1273-8.

63. Spain DM, Roth D. Effect of Cortisone and ACTH on the Histopathology of Rheumatic Carditis: Report of a Necropsied Case. Am J Med. 1951;11:128-31.

64. Parascandola. The Introduction of Antibiotics into Therapeutics. in: Kawakita Y, Sakai S, Otsuka Y (Eds). History of Therapy. Tokyo: Ishiyaku EuroAmerica; 1990. pp. 261-81.

65. Denny FW, Wannamaker LW, Brink WR, Rammelkamp Jr CH, Custer EA. Prevention of Rheumatic Fever: Treatment of the Preceding Streptococcic Infection. J Am Med Assoc. 1950;143:151-3.

66. American Heart Association. Prevention of Rheumatic Fever. Lancet. 1953;1:285-6.

67. Catanzaro FJ, Stetson CA, Morris AJ, Chamovitz R, Rammelkamp Jr CH, Stolzer BL, et al. The Role of the Strepococcus in the Pathogenesis of Rheumatic Fever. Am J Med. 1954;17:749-56.

68. Chamovitz R, Catanzaro FJ, Stetson CA, Rammelkamp Jr CH. Prevention of Rheumatic Fever by Treatment of Previous Streptococcal Infections: I. Evaluation of Benzathine Penicillin G. N Engl J Med. 1954;251:466-71.

69. Frank PF, Stollerman GH, Miller LF. Protection of a Military Population from Rheumatic Fever: Routine Administration of Benzathine Penicillin G to Healthy Individuals. J Am Med Assoc. 1965;193:775-83.

70. Morris AJ, Chamovitz R, Catanzaro FJ, Rammelkamp Jr CH. Prevention of Rheumatic Fever by the Treatment of Previous Streptococci Infections: Effect of Sulfadiazine. J Am Med Assoc. 1956;160:114-6.

71. Massell BF, Sturgis GP, Knobloch JD, Streeper RB, Hall TN, Norcross P. Prevention of Rheumatic Fever by Prompt Penicillin Therapy of Hemolytic Streptococci Respiratory Infections. J Am Med Assoc. 1951;146:1469-74.

72. Pitt Evans JA. Oral Penicillin in the Prophylaxis of Streptococcal Infection and Rheumatic Relapse. Proceed Royal Soc Med. 1950;43:206-8.

73. Gale AH, Gillespie WA, Perry CB. Oral Penicillin in the Prophylaxis of Streptococcal Infection in Rheumatic Children. Lancet. 1952;2:61-3.

74. Kohn KH, Milzer A, Maclean H. Prophylaxis of Recurrences of Rheumatic Fever with Penicillin Given Orally: Final Report of a Five Year Study. J Am Med Assoc. 1953;151:347-51.

75. Roberts E. Use of Sulfonamides and Penicillin to Prevent Recurrence of Rheumatic Fever: A Twelve Year Study. Am J Dis Child. 1953;85:643-7.
76. Stollerman GH, Rusoff JH. Prophylaxis against Group A Streptococcal Infections in Rheumatic Fever Patients: Use of New Repository Penicillin Preparation. J Am Med Assoc. 1952;150:1571-5.
77. Lim WN, Wilson MG. Comparison of the Recurrence Rate of Rheumatic Carditis among Children Receiving Penicillin by Mouth Prophylactically or on Indication: A Six-Year Study. N Engl J Med. 1960;262:321-5.
78. Stollerman GH. The Prevention of Rheumatic Fever by the Use of Antibiotics. Bull N Y Acad Med. 1955;31:165-80.
79. Kuttner AG, Mayer FE. Carditis during Second Attacks of Rheumatic Fever: Its Incidence in Patients without Clinical Evidence of Cardiac Involvement in Their Initial Rheumatic Episode. N Engl J Med. 1963;268:1259-61.
80. Johnson EE, Stollerman GH, Grossman BJ. Rheumatic Recurrences in Patients Not Receiving Continuous Prophylaxis. J Am Med Assoc. 1964;190:407-13.
81. American Heart Association. Prevention of Rheumatic Fever. Circulation. 1965;31:948-52.
82. Miller JM, Massell BF. Studies of Bacterial Throat Flora during Chemoprophylaxis of Rheumatic Fever. N Engl J Med. 1956;254:149-53.
83. Naimon RA, Barrow JG. Penicillin-Resistant Bacteria in the Mouths and Throats of Children Receiving Continuous Prophylaxis against Rheumatic Fever. Ann Intern Med. 1963;58:768-72.
84. Smith MA, Fried AR, Morris EM, Robbins LC, Zukel WJ. Rheumatic Fever Prophylaxis: A Community Program through the Private Physician. J Am Med Assoc. 1952;149:636-9.
85. Bunn WH, Bennett HN. Community Control of Rheumatic Fever. J Am Med Assoc. 1955;157:986-9.
86. McGuinness AC. The National Attack on Rheumatic Fever. Public Health Reports. 1959;74:870-2.
87. Zagala JG, Feinstein AR. The Preceding Illness of Acute Rheumatic Fever. J Am Med Assoc. 1962;179:863-6.
88. Mario Spagnuolo F, Wood HF, Taranta A, Tursky E, Kleinberg E. Rheumatic Fever in Children and Adolescents: A Long-term Epidemiologic Study of Subsequent Prophylaxis, Streptococcal Infections, and Clinical Sequelae: VI. Clinical Features of Streptococcal Infections and Rheumatic Occurrences. Ann Intern Med. 1964;60(suppl 5):68-86.
89. Czoniczer G, Lees M, Massell BF. Streptococcal Infection: The Need for Improved Recognition and Treatment for the Prevention of Rheumatic Fever. N Engl J Med. 1961;265:951-2.
90. Grossman BJ, Stamler J. Potential Preventability of First Attacks of Acute Rheumatic Fever in Children. J Am Med Assoc. 1963;183:985-8.
91. Marienfeld CJ, Robins M, Sandige RP, Findlan C. Rheumatic Fever and Rheumatic Heart Disease among US College Freshmen, 1956-60. Public Health Reports. 1964;79:789-811.
92. RuDusky BM. Heart Murmurs in Youths of Military Age: Evidence of Inadequate Rheumatic Fever Prophylaxis. J Am Med Assoc. 1963;185:1004-7.
93. Fischel EE, Frank CW, Ragan C. Observations on the Treatment of Rheumatic Fever with Salicylate, ACTH, and Cortisone: I. Appraisal of Signs of Systemic and Local Inflammatory Reaction during Treatment, the Rebound Period, and Chronic Activity. Medicine. 1952;31:331-55.
94. Rowe RD, McKelvey AD, Keith JD. The Use of ACTH, Cortisone, and Salicylates in the Treatment of Acute Rheumatic Fever. Canad Med Assoc J. 1953;68:15-20.
95. Illingworth H, John Rendle-Short L. Cortisone and Salicylates in Rheumatic Fever. Lancet. 1954;2:1144-8.
96. Massell BF. The Medicinal Treatment of Acute Rheumatic Fever. Med Clin North Am. 1953;37:1215-34.
97. Swift HF, Moen JK, Hirst GK. The Action of Sulfanilamide in Rheumatic Fever. J Am Med Assoc. 1938;110:426-34.
98. Coburn AF, Moore LV. The Prophylactic Use of Sulfanilamide in Streptococcal Respiratory Infections, with Especial Reference to Rheumatic Fever. J Clin Invest. 1939;18:147-55.
99. Thomas CB, France R. A Preliminary Report of the Prophylactic Use of Sulfanilamide in Patients Susceptible to Rheumatic Fever. Bull Johns Hopkins Hospital. 1939;64:67-77.
100. Coburn AF, Young DC. The Epidemiology of Hemolytic Streptococcus during World War II in the United States Navy. Baltimore: Williams and Wilkins; 1949.
101. Wilson AT. The relative importance of the capsule and the M antigen in determining colony form of group A streptococci. J Exp Med. 1959;109:257-70.
102. Lancefield R, Todd E. Antigenic differences between matt hemolytic colonies and their glossy variants. J Exp Med. 1928;48:769-90.
103. Foley MJ, Wood Jr WB. Studies on the pathogenicity of group A streptococci. II. The antiphagocytic effects of the M protein and the capsular gel. J Exp Med. 1959;110:617-28.
104. Gray GC, Escamilla J, Hyams KC, Struewing JP, Kaplan EL, Tupponce AK. Hyperendemic Streptococcus pyogenes infection despite prophylaxis with penicillin G benzathine. N Engl J Med. 1991;325:92-7.
105. Heggie AD, Jacobs MR, Linz PE, Han DP, Kaplan EL, Boxerbaum B. Prevalence and characteristics of pharyngeal group A beta-hemolytic streptococci in US Navy recruits receiving benzathine penicillin prophylaxis. J Infect Dis. 1992;166:1006-13.
106. Siegel AC, Johnson EE, Stollerman GH. Controlled studies of Streptococcal pharyngitis in a pediatric population. 2. Behavior of the type specific immune response. N Engl J Med. 1961; 265:566-71.
107. Stollerman GH, Ekstedt R. Long chain formation by strains of Group A streptococci in the presence of homologous antiserum: a type-specific reaction. J Exp Med. 1957;106:345-56.
108. Cohen IR, Stollerman GH. Non-type specific resistance to group A streptococci in germ free and conventional mice. Proc Soc Exp Biol Med. 1963;114:202-5.
109. Stollerman GH, Ekstedt RD, Cohen IR. Natural resistance of Germfree mice and colostrum-deprived piglets to group A streptococci. J Immunol. 1965;95:131-40.
110. Rothbard S, Watson R. Variation occurring in group A streptococci during human infections: Progressive loss of M substance correlated with increasing susceptibility to bacteriostasis. J Exp Med. 1948;87:521-33.
111. Rothbard S. Protective effect of hyaluronidase and type-specific anti-M serum on experimental group A infections in mice. J Exp Med. 1948;88:325-37.
112. Stollerman G. Factors determining the attack rate of rheumatic fever. JAMA. 1961;177:823-8.
113. Kaplan EL, Top FH Jr, Dudding BA, Wannamaker LW. Diagnosis of streptococcal pharyngitis: differentiation of active infection from the carrier state in the symptomatic child. J Infect Dis. 1971;123:490-501.

114. Stollerman GH, Siegel AC, Johnson EE. Variable epidemiology of Streptococcal disease and the changing pattern of rheumatic fever. Mod Concepts Cardiovasc Dis. 1965;34:45-8.

115. Stollerman GH. Rheumatic fever and streptococcal infection. New York: Stratton G; 1975.

116. Stollerman GH. Nephritogenic and rheumatogenic group A streptococci. J Infect Dis. 1969;120:258-63.

117. Stollerman G. The relative rheumatogenicity of strains of group A streptococci. Mod Concepts Cardiovasc Dis. 1975;44:35-40.

118. Bisno AL. The concept of rheumatogenic and non-rheumatogenic group A streptococci. In: Reed SE, Zabriskie JB (Eds). Streptococcal diseases and the immune response. New York: Academic Press; 1980. pp. 789-803.

119. Facklam RF, Martin DR, Lovgren M, Johnson DR, Efstratiou A, Thompson TA, et al. Extension of the Lancefield classification for group A streptococci by addition of 22 New M protein gene sequence types from clinical isolates: emm103 to emm124. Clin Infect Dis. 2002;34:28-38.

120. Veasy LG, Wiedmeier SE, Orsmond GS, Ruttenberg HD, Boucek MM, Roth SJ, et al. Resurgence of acute rheumatic fever in the intermountain region of the United States. N Engl J Med. 1987;316:421-7.

121. Centers for Disease Control. Acute rheumatic fever—Utah. MMWR Morb Mortal Wkly Rep. 1987;36:108-10.

122. Congeni B, Rizzo C, Congeni J, Sreenivasan VV. Outbreak of acute rheumatic fever in northeast Ohio. J Pediatr. 1987;111:176-9.

123. Wald ER, Dashefsky B, Feidt Chiponis D, Byers C. Acute Rheumatic fever in western Pennsylvania and the tristate area. Pediatrics. 1987;80:371-4.

124. Centers for Disease Control. Acute rheumatic fever at a Navy Training center—San Diego, California. MMWR Morb Mortal Wkly Rep. 1988;37:101-4.

125. Centers for Disease Control. Acute rheumatic fever among Army Trainees—Fort Leonard Wood, Missouri 1987-1988. MMWR Morb Mortal Wkly Rep. 1988;37:519-22.

126. Kaplan EL, Johnson DR, Cleary PP. Group A streptococcal Serotypes isolated from patients and sibling contacts during the resurgence of rheumatic fever in the United States in the mid-1980s. J Infect Dis. 1989;159:101-3.

127. Stollerman GH. Rheumatogenic group A streptococci and the return of rheumatic fever. Adv Intern Med. 1990;35:1-25.

128. Johnson DR, Stevens DL, Kaplan EL. Epidemiologic analysis of Group A streptococcal serotypes associated with severe systemic infections, rheumatic fever, or uncomplicated pharyngitis. J Infect Dis. 1992;166:374-82.

129. Veasy LG, Tani LY, Daly JA, Korgenski K, Miner L, Bale J, et al. Temporal association of the appearance of mucoid strains of Streptococcus pyogenes with a Continuing high incidence of rheumatic fever in Utah. Pediatrics. 2004;113:168-72.

130. Smoot JC, Korgenski EK, Daly JA, Veasy LG, Musser JM. Molecular analysis of group A streptococcus type emm18 isolates temporally associated with acute rheumatic fever outbreaks in Salt Lake City, Utah. J Clin Microbiol. 2002;40:1805-10.

131. Smoot JC, Barbian KD, Van Gompel JJ, Smoot LM, Chaussee MS, Sylva GL, et al. Genome sequence and comparative microarray analysis of serotype M18 group A Streptococcus strains associated with acute rheumatic fever outbreaks. Proc Natl Acad Sci U S A. 2002;99:4668-73.

132. Cockerill FR 3rd, MacDonald KL, Thompson RL, Roberson F, Kohner PC, Besser-Wiek J, et al. An outbreak of invasive group A streptococcal disease associated with high carriage rates of the invasive clone among school-aged children. JAMA. 1997;277:38-43.

133. Beachey EH, Ofek I. Epithelial cell binding of group A streptococci by lipoteichoic acid on fimbriae denuded of M protein. J Exp Med. 1976;143:759-71.

134. Ofek I, Beachey EH, Jefferson W, Campbell GL. Cell membrane-Binding properties of group A streptococcal lipoteichoic acid. J Exp Med. 1975;141:990-1003.

135. Hanski E, Caparon M, Protein F. a fibronectin binding protein, is an adhesin of the group A streptococcus. Proc Natl Acad Sci USA. 1992;89:6172-6.

136. Schrager HM, Albertí S, Cywes C, Dougherty GJ, Wessels MR. Hyaluronic acid capsule modulates M protein-mediated adherence and acts as a ligand for attachment of group A streptococcus to CD44 on human keratinocytes. J Clin Invest. 1998;101:1708-16.

137. Cywes C, Stamenkovic I, Wessels MR. CD44 as a receptor for Colonization of the pharynx by group A streptococcus. J Clin Invest. 2000;106:995-1002.

138. Cywes C, Wessels MR. Group A Streptococcus tissue invasion by CD44-mediated cell signalling. Nature. 2001;414:648-52.

139. Wessels MR, Bronze MS. Critical role of the group A streptococcal capsule in pharyngeal colonization and infection in mice. Proc Natl Acad Sci USA. 1994;91:12238-42.

140. Dinkla K, Rohde M, Jansen WT, Kaplan EL, Chhatwal GS, Talay SR. Rheumatic fever-associated Streptococcus pyogenes isolates Aggregate collagen. J Clin Invest. 2003;111:1905-12.

141. Varco RL, Baronofsky ID. The Surgical Problem in Rheumatic Valvular Heart Disease in Rheumatic Fever: A Symposium Minneapolis: Lewis Thomas University of Minnesota Press; 1952. pp. 249-64.

142. Gillum FR. Trends in Acute Rheumatic Fever and Chronic Rheumatic Heart Disease: A National Perspective. Am Heart J. 1986;111:430-2.

143. Bland EF. Rheumatic Fever: The Way it Was. Circulation. 1987;76:1190-5.

144. Rantz. "Rheumatic Fever," in Internal Medicine in World War II. In: Coates JB Jr (Ed). Infectious Diseases. Washington, D.C.: Office of the Surgeon General; 1963. pp. 225-38.

145. Denny FW. T Duckett Jones and Rheumatic Fever in 1986. Circulation. 1987;76:963-70.

146. Vijayalakshmi IB, Mithravinda Deva J, Prabhu AN. Role of Echocardiography in diagnosing Carditis in the setting of acute rheumatic fever. Cardiology in the Young. 2005;15:583-8.

147. Vijayalakshmi IB, Vishnuprabhu RO, Chitra N, Rajasri R, Anuradha TV. The efficacy of echocardiographic criterions for the diagnosis of carditis in acute rheumatic fever. Cardiol Young. 2008;18:586-92.

2

Rheumatic Fever and Rheumatic Heart Disease: A 4-century Review with Special Reference to India

*Late S Padmavati, IB Vijayalakshmi,
Monica Kher*

> *"To understand a science, it is necessary to know its history."*
>
> —**Auguste Comte** (1798–1857)
> (French Philosopher and Sociologist and
> Founder of Positivism)

INTRODUCTION

The word rheumatism, of course, derives from the Greek "pew" and refers to the flowing of humors into the joints of affected persons. Rheumatism is a disease well known to medical antiquity and one of the earliest historical accounts we have of the condition is attributed by Guillaume Baillou[1] in 1616 to Hippocrates whom he quotes as follows: "In those in whom pains and swellings come and go around the joints, and these not after the manner of gout in the foot, one will find large viscera and in the urine, a white sediment."

Some 30 million people are currently thought to be affected by rheumatic heart disease (RHD) globally,[2] and in 2015, RHD was estimated to have been responsible for 305,000 deaths and 11.5 million disability-adjusted life years lost. Of these deaths, 60% occurred prematurely (i.e., before the age of 70 years), although these figures are very uncertain owing to incomplete data in many countries. Despite the availability of effective measures for prevention and treatment, there has been little change in the contribution of RHD to overall global mortality between 2000 and 2015.[3] Other organizations, which have been active in control, are the World Heart Federation (WHF), which has a committee on rheumatic fever (RF)/RHD among its councils, the International Lancefield Society, the American Heart Association (AHA), and the Indian Council of Medical Research (ICMR).

This malady has ravaged the world for the past four centuries, although diagnosed and treated only since the 20th century. In spite of much research, the link between "the throat and the heart" remains elusive. Unless this is established, full control of the disease may not be possible. This review highlights the changes that have occurred in the area of RF/RHD in four centuries with emphasis on Indian situation.

HISTORICAL DATA

Industrialized Countries

History of Clinical Manifestations and Diagnosis of Rheumatic Fever

The major clinical manifestations of RF were not well recognized until Thomas Sydenham (1624–1689), an English physician distinguished an acute, febrile polyarthritis in 1685. He recognized that it was "chiefly attacking the young and vigorous" and different from gout. 1 year later, he described "St. Vitus' dance" the neurological disorder that is now called "Sydenham's chorea."[4]

Richard Bright (1789–1858), a British physician, who was the first to describe the clinical manifestations of the kidney disorder known as Bright's disease or nephritis, was also the first, who in 1839 connected the febrile polyarthritis with RF.[5]

In 1797, Matthew Baillie (1761–1783), a Scottish-born physician and pathologist and pupil of his uncle, the anatomist John Hunter, had noted in 1797 a thickening of some heart valves in autopsies of patients who had had acute rheumatism. 4 years later, William Charles Wells (1757–1817), a Scottish-American physician and printer, published a series of 16 cases of "rheumatism of the heart" (median age 15 years) and addled the description of subcutaneous nodules.[6]

Laennec had described murmurs caused by deformities of the mitral valves. A few years later in 1835, James Hope (1801–1841), an English physician known for discovering the early diastolic murmur of mitral stenosis in 1829, who has been called "the first cardiologist" according to Wikipedia,[7] described murmurs that originated from the other valves and concluded that RF is the most frequent cause.[8]

A French physician Jean-Baptiste Bouillaud (1796–1881) soon confirmed this opinion. Bouillaud, who performed studies of "heart sounds", is known for providing a correlation between rheumatism and heart disease, and a French medical dictionary still refers to acute rheumatic carditis as "Bouillaud's disease."

The "Aschoff nodule," the myocardial granuloma that came to be considered pathognomonic of rheumatic carditis, had been recognized as early as 1883 but was described definitively by a German physician and pathologist Ludwig Aschoff (1866–1942) in 1904.[6]

There is no single confirmatory clinical sign or laboratory test for the diagnosis of acute rheumatic fever. In 1944, T Duckett Jones, who was Director of research in RF and RHD at the House of Good Samaritan Hospital in Boston for 20 years, established the first clinical criteria for its diagnosis. These criteria known as the "Jones Criteria" remained the benchmark for acute rheumatic fever diagnosis for over 50 years.[9,10]

Thus, RF as we know it today is the result of the fitting together of entities, which appear unrelated. The relationship between GAS and RF was established only in 1931 by Collis (England) and Coburn (USA). The prevention of rheumatic recurrences by antistreptococcal medication was confirmed by Coburnand Moore in 1929 and the prevention of first attack of RF by the treatment of GAS Pharyngitis in 1949 by Massell and Wannamaker.[11] RF was a notifiable disease in Denmark since 1860 and has shown a steady decline since then, even before the antibiotic era. The same trend was seen in the USA.[11]

The decline in western countries has been attributed to improvement in standards of living with less overcrowding, early access to medical care, use of antibiotics, and most importantly to change in the virulence of the organism. The last aspect was strikingly brought out in the 1987 outbreak in parts of the USA, when white patients with easy access to medical care were affected. Today, the disease is practically absent in the western world. School surveys show a prevalence well below 0.5 per thousand.[11,12]

Developing Countries

Again, much of the data is between 1940 and 1970, when RHD accounted for the majority of cardiac cases and when the prevalence in schoolchildren was high. This was true of countries in north and south Africa, the middle East, the Maoris of New Zealand and Aborigines of Australia, the Philippines, Indonesia, Pakistan, India, Burma and Singapore. Even in these countries, there was an ethnic divide with underprivileged groups being more affected. Subsequently, the situation improved in some economies, which are now in the developed category (Singapore, Israel, and Japan).[12] The highest prevalence is in Sub-Saharan Africa and the Pacific islands (where incidentally the WHF has active control programs) followed by many parts of Asia, the Middle East, and least in industrialized countries, e.g., USA.

India

About 100 years back, RF/RHD was believed to be a disease of "temperate climate". In 1835, Malcomson observed that rheumatism was prevalent among sepoys[13] and in 1870, Moore[14] reported numerous cases of rheumatism in Rajasthan. Rogers[15] indicated absence of RF in India as except one possible case he did not find RHD in 4,800 postmortem records in 37 years in Calcutta (Kolkata) in spite of 25 cases of mitral stenosis which he labeled as nonrheumatic. Megaw[16] reported RHD from plains of India but felt that it was less common than seen in colder climates. Clark[17] reported absence of hemolytic streptococcal infections and low prevalence of RF/RHD in tropics. Keats[18] did not find a single case of RHD in 600 autopsies in Amritsar. Drury[19] found mitral valve disease in 62% and mitral stenosis in 10% in an analysis of 319 clinically diagnosed cases of heart disease admitted to the Medical College Hospital in Calcutta (Kolkata). Basu[20] found 8.3% cases of rheumatic carditis and pericarditis in 446 patients of acquired heart disease. Hughes and Yusuf[21] referred to mitral stenosis in an article on heart disease in Punjab.[21]

■ INDIAN PERSPECTIVE

Situation in India (Tables 1 and 2)

The first clinical evidence of RF came from Punjab by Wig in 1935[22] and on rheumatism in childhood and adolescence by Kutumbiah in 1940.[23] This was followed by a large number of hospital-based surveys for the relatively "new" disease accounting for 20–50% admissions in hospitals in various parts of the country. With the results, RF was labeled as severe or malignant in India with multivalve involvement and congestive cardiac failure even in the initial attack of

TABLE 1: Prevalence of RF/RHD in India (per thousand).

Years	*Sources*	*Prevalence*
Before WW I and II	*Autopsies*	*Probably low; Opinion divided*
1940–1983	All India Survey School Children	1.8–11 (Average 6)
1984–1995	School Surveys	1–3.9
2000	Isolated School Survey, Kanpur	4.54
2003	School Survey, Vellore	0.68
2006	School Suvey, Gorakhpur	0.50
2003–2006	School Survey, Bikaner	0.67

(RF: rheumatic fever; RHD: rheumatic heart disease; WW: World War)

TABLE 2: Collaborative research projects on RF/RHD in India.

Source	*Year*	*Title*
RF/RHD		
PL-480 01-800-2	1966–1974	Effects of drugs prophylaxis on the incidence of rheumatic fever in Delhi
ICMR	1972–1975	Collaborative study of epidemiology of rheumatic fever and rheumatic heart disease in India
WHO	1972–1977	WHO cooperative RF prophylaxis study and criteria study
ICMR	1975–1979	Secondary prophylaxis of rheumatic fever, rheumatic heart disease collaborative study
DST	1979–1984	RF/RHD and streptococcal infections—factor analysis of prevalence and evaluation of current methods of surveillance and research into alternate approaches for control
ICMR	1984–1990	Pilot study on the feasibility of utilizing the existing school health services in Delhi and PHCs for the control of RF/RHD
ICMR	2002–2006	Jai Vigyan Project (Vellore and Chandigarh)
NIAID	2006–2014	Registry-based (Chandigarh and Vellore)
NCT342199		
Additional measures		
Government of India	1966–1971	Inclusion in fourth 5-year plan
Streptococcal reference laboratory	1974	Delhi and Vellore
ICMR	1987, 1993	Transfer of technology to states

(DST: Department of Science and Technology; ICMR: Indian Council of Medical Research; NIAID: National Institute of Allergy and Infectious Diseases; RF: rheumatic fever; RHD: rheumatic heart disease)

RF.[24] Roy delineated the features of RF and compared with features seen in Boston (USA). The presence of RF/RHD was not only established but also considered to be the most common heart disease in the country by mid-1950s.

So, acute was the problem that several research programs funded by WHO and the ICMR were set-up to investigate it. The introduction of echocardiography as a tool in diagnosis changed the picture considerably. There have been reports of a decline in RF/RHD from isolated school surveys in recent years. The evidence for and against is given here.

Rheumatic heart disease was made into a program of the fourth 5-year plan, but not subsequently. A streptococcal reference lab was set up in 1974 in Delhi and Vellore, which used to hold annual conferences for grassroots workers. It held transfer of technology sessions in 1987 and 1993, but these proved ineffective as there was no timely support from the Central or State government. There is no doubt, however, that increased awareness has been created throughout India. Sore throats are referred to doctors and some states have started School Health Services (Tamil Nadu). The fear of penicillin injection has been diminished. Of the many reasons cited for decline in RF/RHD in other parts of the world, e.g., improved socioeconomic conditions seem least likely in India as the below poverty line (BPL) population in India has been estimated between 40 and 70%.

GLOBAL AND ASIAN BURDEN OF RHEUMATIC FEVER/RHEUMATIC HEART DISEASE

The burden of RF/RHD has been described in detail by Carapetis and colleagues.[25,26] Excluding developed economies, the global burden of RHD in the 5–14 year old children was estimated to be 0.8–5.7/1,000 with a median of 1.3/1,000. Subsequent data from studies in Asia suggested that the number of children with RHD in Asia could be between 1.96 and 2.21 million. The findings were extrapolated to include all ages and estimated that globally there were 15.6–19.6 million patients. In the study of Asian countries, the burden of RHD was estimated to be 10.8–15.9 million patients. The estimates of RHD in Asian countries indicate that the global burden is significantly higher than the earlier estimates for children as well as all age groups **(Table 3)**.

These estimates do not take into account subclinical carditis identified on the basis of echocardiography and Doppler studies in surveys of school children **(Table 4)**. Can we identify children with subclinical carditis and not put them on secondary prophylaxis?

Decline of RHD in India: Is it Real?

Systematic review of available data across the country by individual authors and ICMR lead multicentric survey studies and suggest declining trends especially after 2,000 onwards.

Trends of changes in prevalence of RF/RHD from early 1990s to late 2,000 using clinical screening confirmed with echocardiography **(Fig. 1)**.[31]

It is important to recognize that India is witnessing transitions in socioeconomic and healthcare sector and also there is a rapid urbanization. Unfortunately, no temporal data are available from states with poor health indicators to get insights about the disease trends.

However, the large number of young cases undergoing balloon mitral valvuloplasty (BMV) in government hospitals (to which the poor go) and with it being the most important noncoronary intervention in India and the number of very young patients undergoing valve replacement (MVR and DVR) do not suggest a decline.[32] The preoccupation with IHD, which is now a major killer, may be another reason for lack of interest in RHD as a cardiac problem.

TABLE 4: Prevalence of subclinical carditis in echo studies of school children.[27-30]

Place	n	Clinical	Echo	Subclinical
Nicaragua	3,150	13 (4)	150 (48)	137 (44)
Tonga	5,053	78 (15.4)	169 (33.4)	91 (18)
Cambodia	3,677	8 (2.2)	79 (21.5)	71 (19.3)
Mozambique	2,170	5 (2.3)	66 (3.4)	61 (28.1)
India	627	5 (0.8)	128 (20.4)	123 (19.6)
Tonga auscultation positive 46% silent 54% (figures calculated)				
Figures in parenthesis are per 1,000				

TABLE 3: Global and Asian magnitude of RF/RHD[25,26] (excluding developed economies).

RHD	Age (years)	Number of patients (million)
Global	5–14	2.4
Asia	5–14	01.96–19.6
Global	All ages	15.6–19.6
Asia	All ages	10.8–15.9
Acute RF		**n/year**
Global	5–14	336,000
	All ages	471,000
If 282 60% have RHD	282,000 new cases	
188.4 40% potential RHD	189,000	
Estimated deaths	**Rate/year (%)**	**n/year**
Global	1.5	233,000–294,000
Asia	3.3	356,000–524,000
(RF: rheumatic fever; RHD: rheumatic heart disease)		

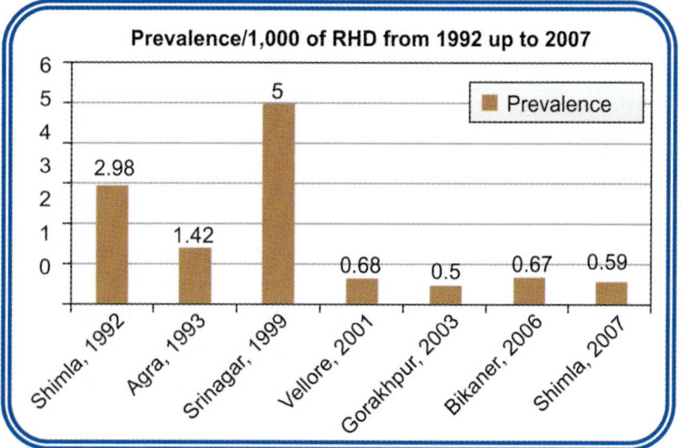

FIG. 1: Prevalence/1,000 of RHD from 1992 up to 2007.

(RHD: rheumatic heart disease)

Results of Research Programs

Clinical Profile

The criteria for the diagnosis enunciated by Dr T Duckett Jones' have been modified, revised, and updated by the AHA.[33] However, physicians have a right to make a diagnosis of RF on the basis of clinical judgment even if the updated criteria are not satisfied. This may be due to—(1) absence of history suggestive of RF in almost 50% patients of RHD and (2) identification of subclinical carditis by echocardiographic studies, indicating inadequacy of clinical diagnosis. Severe disease with accelerated progression, multivalvular involvement, and "Juvenile mitral stenosis" have all been described in earlier studies. Today, one still sees juvenile mitral stenosis in significant numbers needing BMV.[34-36]

Treatment

There has been little or no change in treatment since the 1950s, except for the addition of new antibiotics. Penicillin remains the drug of choice.[37]

Prevention

The prevention, control, and elimination or eradication of RHD are increasingly being recognized as an important developmental issue by Member States. WHO whose programs have been most widespread has suggested primary prevention whenever possible, secondary prevention in all programs and technical procedures (personal training, medical information, health education community participation and improving medical care of children, particularly RF/RHD patients). In addition, it has also suggested integration in the routine health care services of the country.[38]

This advice has been followed in several countries with good results (Thailand, Saudi Arabia, Israel, and Singapore) to mention a few. In India also, the programs in integration have been successful. Implementation over a wide area is lacking.[39-42] The methods of primary and secondary prevention have been comprehensively listed in the AHA Scientific Statement. Every doctor in practice should be aware of this.

Rheumatic Fever Vaccine

Development of a vaccine for RHD started in the early 1960s with crude cell wall to purified M proteins.[43] Nevertheless, there is no protective vaccine available yet to prevent GAS infection. Recently, the proteomic approach combined with two other technologies (protein array and FACS) helps to identify well-expressed, highly conserved cell surface/secreted proteins, which are considered to be important characteristics of protective antigens.[44] This combined prescreening strategy has the great advantage of reducing a large number of protein antigens undergoing animal testing in a genome-based vaccine identification method such as reverse vaccinology (RV). Various advances have been made to the classical RV approach, such as subtractive RV and pan-genome RV.[44]

Recent 30-valent vaccines based on M protein, which are shown to be protective against RHD in the US and European population,[45] are undergoing clinical trials. A global vaccine that covers other regions of the world, especially low-income countries, would be extremely helpful to eradicate RHD completely.

In the meantime, early diagnosis and time-tested methods of treatment and of primary and secondary prevention should continue at the practitioner level and whenever possible, integrate these into school health services and primary health centers.

GLOBAL AGENDA

During the 71st World Health Assembly in May 2018, Member States of the World Health Organization unanimously adopted a global resolution on RF and RHD.[46] Ensuring global leadership in RHD has been challenging. RHD has been neglected by policymakers and civil society because it does not sit in a single department (e.g., at WHO) nor is it amenable to single-intervention strategies. Additionally, people living with RHD are often socially vulnerable and have few opportunities to share their lived experiences. The Listen to My Heart program[47] is one promising model of patient engagement and empowerment.

The goal of universal health coverage, which all countries have endorsed as part of United Nations Sustainable Development Goal 3,[48] holds promise for improving access to and the affordability of RHD-related care. As we can narrow down and fill the gaps of understanding of disease with new research and carry out better implementation in healthcare delivery, we are heading in the right direction to control or even think of eradication the disease.

REFERENCES

1. Baillou G. de. Liber de Rheumatismo. Opera Medica Omnia. Geneva: De Tournes; 1762. p. 314.

2. Global Burden of Disease Collaborative Network. Global Burden of Disease Study 2016 (GBD 2016) Results. Seattle, United States: Institute for Health Metrics and Evaluation (IHME); 2017. [online] Available from http://ghdx.healthdata.org/gbdresults-tool. [Last accessed August, 2022].

3. World Health Organization. (2016). Global Health Estimates, 2015. [online] Available from http://www.who.int/healthinfo/global_burden_disease/estimates/en/index1.html. [Last accessed August, 2022].

4. Murphy GE. The evolution of our knowledge of rheumatic fever. An historical survey with particular emphasis on rheumatic heart disease. Bull Hist Med. 1943;14:123-47.

5. Schechter DC. St. Vitus' dance and rheumatic disease. N Y State J Med. 1975;75:1091-102.

6. Benedek TG. Subcutaneous nodules and the differentiation of rheumatoid arthritis from rheumatic fever. Semin Arthritis Rheum. 1984;13:305-21.

7. Hajar R. Heart Views. 2016 Jul-Sep;17(3):120-126. doi: 10.4103/1995-705X.192572. PMID: 27867464

8. Hope J. A Treatise on the Diseases of the Heart and Great Vessels, and on the Affections which may be Mistaken for Them, 3rd London edition. USA, Philadelphia: 1846.

9. Seckeler MD, Hoke TR. The worldwide epidemiology of acute rheumatic fever and rheumatic heart disease. Clin Epidemiol. 2011;3:67-84.

10. Jones TD. The diagnosis of rheumatic fever. JAMA. 1944;126:481-4.

11. Taranta A, Markowitz M. Rheumatic fever. MTP Press Boston; London: 1981.

12. Agarwal BL. Rheumatic fever and rheumatic heart disease in developing countries. London: Arnold Publishers; 1988.

13. Kutumbiah P. Rheumatic fever and rheumatic heart disease in India; review of 25 years of study and progress. Indian J Pediatr. 1958;25:240-5.

14. Moore WJ. A month's practice in a small Indian dispensary. Indian Med Gaz. 1870;5:207-11.

15. Rogers L. Gleanings from the Calcutta post mortem records III-Diseases of the circulatory system. Indian Med Gaz. 1910;45:84-90.

16. Megaw JWD. Note on the causation of diseases of the heart and aorta in Europeans in India. Indian Med Gaz. 1910;45:81-4.

17. Clark JT. The geographical distribution of rheumatic fever. J Trop Med Hyg. 1930;33:249-58.

18. Keates HC. Rheumatic fever and the tropics. Br Med J. 1932;ii:900.

19. Drury FJ. Circulatory disease in India. Indian Med Gaz. 1910;45:41-5.

20. Basu UP. Preliminary observations on acquired diseases of the heart and aorta as met with in Bengal. Indian Med Gaz. 1925;60:307-10.

21. Hughes TA, Yusuf M. Heart disease in the Punjab with special reference to mitral stenosis. Indian Med Gaz. 1930;65:483.

22. Wig KL. Clinical evidence of rheumatic fever in the Punjab. Indian Med Gaz. 1935;70:260-3.

23. Kutumbiah P. A study of the lesions in rheumatic heart disease in South India. Indian J Med Res. 1940;27:631-41.

24. Padmavati S. Epidemiology of cardiovascular disease in India. I. Rheumatic heart disease. Circulation. 1962;25:703-10.

25. Carapetis JR, Steer AC, Mulholland EK, Weber M. The global burden of group: A streptococcal disease. Lancet Infect Dis. 2005;5:685-94.

26. Carapetis JR. Rheumatic heart disease in Asia. Circulation. 2008;118:2748-53.

27. Paar JA, Berrios NM, Rose JD, Cáceres M, Peña R, Pérez W, et al. Prevalence of rheumatic heart disease in children and young adults in Nicaragua. Am J Cardiol. 2010;105:1809-14.

28. Carapetis JR, Hardy M, Fakakovikaetau T, Taib R, Wilkinson L, Penny DJ, et al. Evaluation of a screening protocol using auscultation and portable echocardiography to detect asymptomatic rheumatic heart disease in Tongan school children. Nat Clin Pract Cardiovascu Med. 2008;5:411-7.

29. Marijon E, Ou P, Celermajer DS, Ferreira B, Mocumbi AO, Jani D, et al. Prevalence of rheumatic heart disease detected by echocardiographic screening. N Eng J Med. 2007;357:470-6.

30. Saxena A, Ramakrishnan S, Roy A, Sethi S, Krishnan A, Misra P, et al. Prevalence and outcome of subclinical rheumatic heart disease in India. The RHEUMATIC (Rheumatic Heart Echo Utilisation and Monitoring Actuarial Tends in Indian Children) Study. Heart. 2011;97:2018-22.

31. Negi PC, Sondhi S, Asotra S, Mahajan K, Mehta A. Current status of rheumatic heart disease in India. Indian Heart J. 2019;71(1):85-90.

32. Padmavati S. International cardiology worldwide: An Indian perspective. J Int Cardiol. 1995;8:39-42.

33. American Heart Association. Guidelines for the diagnosis of rheumatic fever. Jone criteria. 1992 update. Special Writing Group of the Committee on Rheumatic fever, Endocarditis and Kawasaki disease of the Council on Cardiovascular Disease in the young of the American Heart Association. JAMA. 1992;268:2069-73.

34. Padmavati S. Rheumatic fever and rheumatic heart disease in India. Progress Cardiol. 1987:169-83.

35. Padmavati S. Rheumatic fever and rheumatic heart disease in India at the turn of the Century. IHJ. 2001:53:35-7.

36. Padmavati S. Rheumatic heart disease in the SAARC countries: past, present and future Directions Quarterly. J Cardiol. 2002:1;A-3A.

37. Prevention of rheumatic fever and Diagnosis and treatment of acute streptococcal pharyngitis. AHA Scientific Statement. Circulation. 2009;119:1541-51.

38. Porfirio N. RF/RHD Prevention: Lessons Learned. [online] Available from http://www.fac.org.ar/scvc/llave/epi/nordet/nordeti.htm. [Last accessed August, 2022].

39. Padmavati S, Bhatia D. Control of Rheumatic Fever and Rheumatic Heart Disease in India through School Health Services. ICMR Pilot Project. 1984–1990. [online] Available from www.icmr.nic.in [Last accessed August, 2022].

40. Sharma KB, Kunti P. Community control of Rheumatic Fever and Rheumatic Heart Disease. 1982/1990. ICMR; India: 1994.

41. Padmavati S. Rheumatic heart disease: prevalence and preventive measures in the Indian subcontinent. Heart. 2001;86(2):127.

42. Indian Council of Medical Research. Community Control of RF/RHD. ICMR Report; New Delhi; 1994.

43. Cunningham MW. Pathogenesis of group A streptococcal infections. Clin Microbiol Rev. 2000;13(3):470-511.

44. Bensi G, Mora M, Tuscano G, Biagini M, Chiarot E, Bombaci M, et al. Multi high-throughput approach for highly selective identification of vaccine candidates: The Group A *Streptococcus* case. Mol Cell Proteomics. 2012;11(6):M111015693.

45. Dale JB, Penfound TA, Chiang EY, Walton WJ. New 30-valent M protein-based vaccine evokes cross-opsonic antibodies against non-vaccine serotypes of group A streptococci. Vaccine. 2011; 29(46):8175-8.

46. WHO. Executive Board, 141st Session: Resolutions and Decisions, Annexes, Summary Records. Geneva: World Health Organization; 2017.

47. Zuhlke L, Perkins S, Cembi S. Rheumatic heart disease patient event: Cape Town hosts 4th Annual Listen to My Heart Rheumatic Heart Disease for patients at the South African Heart Association meeting in 2017. Eur Heart J. 2018;39:1669-71.

48. United Nations. Sustainable Development Goals: 17 Goals to Transform Our World. Goal 3: Ensure Healthy Lives and Promote Well-Being for All at All Ages. New York: United Nations; 2016.

3

Epidemiology of Group A Streptococcal Infections, Rheumatic Fever, and Rheumatic Heart Disease

S Pruthvish

> *"Medical science must cease to regard its function as primarily curative and preventive. It must rid itself of its obsession that its chief responsibility is to the individual rather than society."*
>
> —**Earnest Albert Hooton** (1887–1954)
> (US Anthropologist)

INTRODUCTION

Group A *Streptococcus* (GAS) causes a broad spectrum of disease, from mild superficial infections of the throat or skin to infections such as cellulitis and erysipelas, severe invasive infections including bacteremia and necrotizing fasciitis (often complicated by the streptococcal toxic shock syndrome), and the poststreptococcal complications of acute rheumatic fever (ARF) and acute poststreptococcal glomerulonephritis (APSGN). All group A streptococcal diseases are most common in settings of poverty, where living conditions promote transmission of the organism and prevention, and treatment programs are less likely to be present or effective. These settings also rarely have efficient systems for collecting disease burden data.

EPIDEMIOLOGY OF GROUP A STREPTOCOCCAL INFECTIONS

Rheumatic fever (RF) and rheumatic heart disease (RHD) are nonsuppurative complications of Group A streptococcal pharyngitis due to a delayed immune response. Although RF and RHD are rare in developed countries, they are still major public health problems among children and young adults in developing countries.[1-6] The economic effects of the disability and premature death caused by these diseases are felt at both the individual and national levels through higher direct and indirect healthcare costs.

Beta hemolytic streptococci can be divided into a number of serological groups on the basis of their cell wall polysaccharide antigen. Those in serological group A (*Streptococcus pyogenes*) can be further subdivided into more than 130 distinct M types and are responsible for the vast majority of infections in humans.[7-9] Furthermore, only pharyngitis caused by group A streptococci has been linked with the etiopathogenesis of RF and RHD. Other streptococcal groups (e.g., B, C, G, and F) have been isolated from human subjects and are sometimes associated with infection and streptococci in groups C and G can produce extracellular antigens (including streptolysin-O) with similar characteristics to that produced by group A streptococci.[7-9] Nevertheless, the available evidence does not link streptococci in non-group A types with the pathogenesis of RF and RHD, although further studies are warranted into the role of groups C and G in the pathogenesis of RF.[1,2,7-9] In both developing and developed countries, pharyngitis and skin infection (impetigo) are the most common infections caused by group A streptococci. Group A streptococci are the most common bacterial cause of pharyngitis, with a peak incidence in children 5–15 years of age **(Table 1)**.[3,5,7,9] Streptococcal pharyngitis is less frequent among children in the first 3 years of life and among adults. It has been estimated that most children develop at least one episode

TABLE 1: Make-up of regions as defined for this study.

Regions as defined for this study	Regions for UN population division included*	Corresponding WHO region
Sub-Saharan Africa	Eastern Africa, Middle Africa, Central Africa, Southern Africa	AFRO, EMRO
South-Central Asia	South-Central Asia	SEARO, EMRO
Asia other	Eastern Asia, South-Eastern Asia, excluding China and Japan	SEARO, WPRO
Latin America	Caribbean, Central America, South America	PAHO
ME and North Africa	Northern Africa, Western Asia	EMRO
Eastern Europe	Eastern Europe	EURO
Pacific and indigenous Australia/NZ	Melanesia, Micronesia, Polynesia plus indigenous Australians and Maori/Pacific Islanders in New Zealand	WPRO
Established market economies	Japan, non-indigenous Australia and New Zealand, Northern Europe, Southern Europe, Western Europe, Northern America	PAHO, EURO, WPRO
China	China	WPRO

*The countries making up each region are detailed on the UN Population Division website (http://esa.un.org/unpp/definition.html)

of pharyngitis per year, 15–20% of which are caused by group A streptococci and nearly 80% by viral pathogens.[1,2,7,9] The incidence of pharyngeal beta hemolytic streptococcal infections can vary between countries and within the same country, depending upon season, age group, socioeconomic conditions, environmental factors, and the quality of health care.[1-3,5,10,11] Surveys of healthy schoolchildren 6–10 years of age, for example, found antistreptolysin-O titers >200 Todd units in 15–70% of the children,[2] while other studies reported beta hemolytic streptococci carrier rates of 10–50% for asymptomatic schoolchildren.[1,2] In temperate countries, 50–60% of streptococci isolated from asymptomatic children belong to serological group A, while streptococci in serological groups C and G together occur in <30% of the children. Conversely, in many tropical countries, groups C and G streptococci occur with rates as high as 60–70% in asymptomatic carriers.[1-3,5,11] The presence of group A streptococci in the upper respiratory tract (URT) may reflect either true infection or a carrier state. In either state, the patient harbors the organism, but only in the case of a true infection does the patient show a rising antibody response. In the carrier state, there is no rising antibody response. It is thought that a patient with a true infection is at risk of developing RF and of spreading the organism to close contacts, while this is not thought to be the case with carriers.[1,5,10,12-18] Therefore, many professionals feel that only patients with true infections need to be given antibiotics. Group A streptococci are highly transmissible and spread rapidly in families and communities, with the predominant M types constantly changing. However, in publications about RF outbreaks, including recent ones in the United States of America (USA), it was reported that only a limited number of streptococcal stereotypes (i.e., M serotypes 1, 3, 5, 6, 18, 19, and 24) were obtained from the throat cultures of children in the affected communities.[2,3,5,7,19-23] Although no longitudinal studies have examined trends in group A streptococcal pharyngitis, nor in the asymptomatic carrier rates, available data suggest that pharyngitis and asymptomatic carrier rates have remained more or less stable in most countries.[3,5] However, in the last 20 years, some countries have reported changes in the M types, severity, and other characteristics of group A streptococci. More virulent strains have re-emerged and non-M type streptococci have been detected.[1-3,5,7,11,22] In the USA, despite a remarkable reduction in the incidence of RF since the 1950s, the incidence of infections caused by group A streptococci has not declined.[1-3,5,20,23] In the mid-1980s, the virulence, severity, and sequelae of these infections also appear to have changed remarkably. Outbreaks of ARF have been described from widely separated areas of the country and complications of streptococcal infections have been reported, including necrotizing fasciitis, streptococcal myositis, streptococcal bacteremia, and streptococcal toxic shock syndrome.[3,20,22,23] These outbreaks have not been confined to socially and economically disadvantaged populations.

Report of WHO concludes that approximately 18.1 million people currently suffer from a serious GAS disease, another 1.78 million new cases occur each year and these diseases are responsible for over 500,000 deaths each year. Added to this are over 111 million prevalent cases of streptococcal pyoderma and 616 million new cases of GAS pharyngitis each year.[15] The vast majority of all these cases came from less developed countries (79% of RHD cases, 95% of ARF cases, 97% of APSGN cases, 97% of invasive GAS cases) **(Tables 1 to 5)**. We have used relatively conservative assumptions at each step, so these are minimum summary estimates of the burden of GAS diseases.

■ RHEUMATIC FEVER/RHEUMATIC HEART DISEASE: MORBIDITY AND MORTALITY

In 1994, it was estimated that 12 million individuals suffered from RF and RHD worldwide[6] and at least 3 million had congestive heart failure (CHF) that required repeated hospitalization.[24] A large proportion of the individuals with CHF required cardiac valve surgery within 5–10 years.[4,6,24] The mortality rate for RHD varied from 0.5 per 100,000

TABLE 2: Estimated number of rheumatic heart disease cases in children aged 5–14 years.

Region	Number of studies (number using echo)	Median (IQR) RHD prevalence (per thousand)	Types of studies used for calculations*	Number of denominator (screened)	Number of RHD cases found	Calculated regional RHD prevalence (per thousand)	Population 5–14 years (thousands)	Estimated RHD cases aged 5–14 years
Sub-Saharan Africa	14 (10)	3.0 (2.7–6.4)	E	92,823	528	5.7	177,244,000	1,008,207
South-Central Asia	14 (12)	1.6 (1.3–2.4)	E	12,9300	279	2.2	340,530,000	734,786
Asia other	6 (0)	1.1 (0.8–1.3)	A	243,668	199	0.8	124,677,000	101,822
Latin America	7 (4)	3.0 (2.0–4.1)	E	45,850	58	1.3	108,278,000	136,971
ME and North Africa	7 (4)	1.9 (0.8–2.4)	E	28,404	52	1.8	83,956,000	153,679
Eastern Europe**	1 (0)	1.0	A	228,958	225	1.0	41,076,000	40,366
Pacific and India	7 (6)	7.6 (2.7–13.5)	E	32,742	116	3.5	2,185,798	7,744
Australia/NZ								
Established market economics	1 (1)	0.3	E	385,000	116	0.3	110,621,202	33,330
China	1 (0)	0.8	A	31,180	25	0.8	220,226,000	176,576
Total				1,217,929	1,598	1.3	1,208,794,000	2,393,482

(IQR: interquartile range; RHD: rheumatic heart disease)

*E, only included studies using echocardiographic confirmation RHD lesions; A, all studies included.

**For Eastern Europe, 1998 data from Romania were used, based on prevalence cited in regions where RHD registers not operating. Numerators and denominators are not available. 1994 government statistics from Russia cite a prevalence of 5 per 1,000 in schoolchildren, but the more conservative Romanian estimate was used. See text for details and references.

TABLE 3: Estimated number of cases of acute poststreptococcal glomerulonephritis.

Region	APSGN incidence in children"	Population aged <15 years (thousands)	Annual number of APSGN cases in children	APSGN incidence adults*	Population aged >5 years (thousands)	Annual number APSGN cases in adults	Total APSGN cases all ages
Less developed countries	24.3	1,609,317	391,064	2	3,267,392	65,348	456,412
More developed countries	6	218,859	13,132	0.3	975,013	2,925	16,057
Total		1,828,176	404,196		4,242,405		472,468

(APSGN: acute poststreptococcal glomerulonephritis)

*See text for details of how incidences calculated.

population in Denmark, to 8.2 per 100,000 population in China[25] and the estimated annual number of deaths from RHD for 2,000 was 332,000 worldwide.[26] The mortality rate per 100,000 population varied from 1.8 in the WHO Region of the Americas to 7.6 in WHO South East Asia Region. The disability-adjusted life years (DALYs) lost to RHD ranged from 27[4] DALYs per 100,000 population in the WHO Region of the Americas to 173.4 per 100,000 population in the WHO Southeast Asia Region. An estimated 6.6 million DALYs are lost per year worldwide. Data from developing

TABLE 4: Recent population-based studies of the incidence of symptomatic group A streptococcal pharyngitis.

Year	Place	Age	Number of subjects	GAS pharyngitis incidence (per person-year)	Serological confirmation
1988	Kuwait	5–14	28,920	0.03	No
1995–1996	India	5–15	536	0.95	No
1998	New Zealand	School-age	~24,000	0.50	No
2001-2002	Australia	All	852	0.14 < 18 years	Yes
				0.14 > 18 years	

TABLE 5: Recent studies documenting the incidence of acute rheumatic fever in children and adolescents.

Year of study	Place	Age	ARF incidence (per 100,000 per year)
Asia other:			
1981–1990	Malaysia, Kuala Lumpur	Children	21.2
Eastern Europe:			
1982–1987	Yugoslavia, Belgrade	0–19	9.2 (1982), 3.3 (1987)
1990–1991	Slovenia	0–14	0.7
1982	Serbia	5–14	11.1
1999	Romania	5–15	16.5
1994	Russia	Children	18
Established market economies:			
1984–1988	USA, Hawaii	4–18	9.5 (All)
1982–1997	New Zealand, Auckland	5–15	<10 (European descent)
1988–1997	New Zealand	5–14	16.7 (All)
Indian subcontinent:			
1984–1995	India	5–14	54
Latin America and Caribbean:			
1982–1992	Martinique and Guadeloupe	<20	17.4–19.6 (1982)
1996	Cuba, Pinar del Rio	5–14	2.7
1986–1990	Barbados	0–19	8
1982	Cuba, Havana	5–14	10.5
1986	Cuba, Santiago, and Pinar del Rio	5–14	21.0 (Santiago)
			28.4 (Pinar)
1987–1991	Martinique	5–14	53
1994–1999	Mexico	5–20	70
1992	Brazil, Belo Horizonte	10–20	360
Middle East and North Africa:			
1997–2000	Algeria	4–19	11.1 (1997), 6.2 (2000)
166–84	Israel	5–15	4.4
1988–1997	Israel	5–35	5
1984–1994	Qatar	4–14	11.2
1980–1990	Israel, Tel Aviv	5–15	15.5
1980–1983	Kuwait	Children	19.6

Continued

Continued

Year of study	Place	Age	ARF incidence (per 100,000 per year)
1984–1988	Kuwait	5–14	29
1990	Tunisia	School age	30
1997	Oman	6–18	40
Pacific and Indigenous Australia/New Zealand:			
1982–1997	New Zealand, Auckland	5–15	80–100 (Pacific Islanders)
			40-80 (Maori)
1984–1988	USA, Hawaii	4–18	195 (Hawaiian Samoans)
2002	Australia, Aboriginal	5–14	374
1988–1992	Australia, Aboriginal	5–14	375
1987–1996	Australia, Aboriginal	5–14	508
1978–1987	Australia, Aboriginal	5–14	815
(ARF: acute rheumatic fever)			

TABLE 6: Estimated global number of rheumatic heart disease cases and inferred RHD prevalence in all age groups.

Age group and assumption	Estimated global number of RHD cases	Inferred all age prevalence of RHD in less developed countries* (per thousand)
5–14 years (from **Table 2**)	2,393,482	
All ages, assuming 5.5 times the number of 5–14 years cases in older age groups	15,557,632	2.5
All ages, assuming 7.2 times the number of 5–14 years cases in older age groups	19,626,551	3.2

(RHD: rheumatic heart disease)

*Assumes 79% of all RHD cases in less developed countries (see text for details and population in less developed countries is 4,876 million) (from UN Population Division website)

TABLE 7: Estimated global deaths due to rheumatic heart disease each year, based on estimated of mortality rates of existing RHD patients.

Estimated of RHD cases (from Table 6)	Estimated global number of RHD cases	Number of RHD deaths each year (assuming 1.5% per year)
Low range estimated	15,557,632	233,364
High range estimated	19,626,551	294,398

countries (e.g., Brazil and India), as well as some indigenous populations in wealthy countries (Australia and New Zealand). Moreover, migration from low-income to high-income settings might be responsible for a new burden of RHD in high-income countries where the disease has been largely eliminated (World Heart Federation, 2013).

- Rheumatic heart disease claims over 291,000 lives each year—the large majority in low- or middle-income countries (WHO, 2020).

countries suggest that mortality due to ARF and 1 DALYs lost is the sum of years of life lost owing to premature death, plus the years lived with disability adjusted for the severity of the disability.[24] RHD remains a problem and children and young adults still die from ARF **(Tables 6 and 7)**.[4-6,14,24-26]

- RHD remains the most common cardiovascular disease in young people aged <25 years. RF and RHD have been almost eradicated in areas with establish economies. But, RF and RHD are endemic in developing countries and are also common in poorer populations in middle-income

■ INCIDENCE AND PREVALENCE OF ACUTE RHEUMATIC FEVER/ RHEUMATIC HEART DISEASE

Reliable data on the incidence of ARF are scarce. In some countries, however, local data obtained from ARF registers of schoolchildren provide useful information on trends **(Tables 1, 2 and 5)**. The annual incidence of RF in developed countries began to decrease in the 20th century, with a marked decrease after the 1950s; it is now below 1.0 per 100,000.[6] A few studies conducted in developing countries report incidence rates ranging from 1.0 per 100,000 school-age children in Costa Rica,[27] 72.2 per 100,000 in French Polynesia, 100 per 100,000 in Sudan, to 150 per 100,000 in China.[6] Crowding and socioeconomic conditions adversely affect RF incidence **(Table 8)**.[1-7,14,22,23]

The prevalence of RHD has also been estimated in surveys, mainly of school-age children. The surveys results showed there was wide variation between countries, ranging from 0.2 per 1000 school children in Havana, Cuba to 77.8 per 1,000 in Samoa.[1,28-45] The prevalence of RF and RHD and the mortality rates varied widely between countries and between population groups in the same country, such as between Maoris and non-Maoris in New Zealand, Samoans, and Chinese in Hawaii and Aboriginals and non-Aboriginals in Northern Australia.[1,2,5,6,12,17] Although it is known that hospital morbidity data often give biased information about the magnitude of diseases, they are the only data available in many developing countries. Based on such data, RHD accounts for 12–65% of hospital admissions related to cardiovascular disease and for 2.0–9.9% of all hospital discharges in some developing countries.[5,6,46] There has been a marked decrease in the mortality, incidence, prevalence, hospital morbidity, and severity of RF and RHD in some places that have implemented prevention programs, such as Havana, Cuba, Costa Rica, Cairo, Egypt, Martinique, and Guadeloupe.[1,2,5,6,27,44,47-53]

According to Dr Padmavati,[39] the burden of RF and RHD that occur globally is large, particularly in developing countries. In India, about 6 million children are suffering from RHD—a number nearly equivalent to twice the total population of New Zealand. RHD is estimated to cause around 0.5 million deaths per year globally **(Tables 2, 6, and 7)**.

REDUCING THE BURDEN OF THE DISEASE

For at least five decades, this unique nonsuppurative sequela to group A streptococcal infections has been a concern of the WHO and its member countries. Sentinel studies conducted under the auspices of the WHO during the last four decades clearly documented that the control of the preceding infections and their sequelae is both cost-effective and inexpensive. Without doubt, appropriate public health control programs and optimal medical care reduce the burden of disease. Although, the responsible pathogenic mechanism(s) still remain(s) incompletely defined, methods for optimal prevention and management have changed during the past 15 years.

A report of WHO, Western pacific region says RF and RHDs are still major health issues in some parts of China, the Lao People's Democratic Republic, Mongolia, the Philippines, Tonga, and Vietnam.[52]

A review of the available statistics reveals that from 1960 to 1970 in the (former) United Socialist Soviet Republic

TABLE 8: Studies comparing risk of rheumatic heart disease in rural compared to urban residents, or in different socioeconomic strata.

Year and reference	Country	Age group	Risk ratio for RHD rural compared to urban	Other findings related to socioeconomic status
Early 1990[6]	Myanmar	>15	3.25 rural vs. urban	
1997[12]	Australia	All	2.1 rural vs. urban	
1997[13]	Samoa	5–17	1.9 rural vs. urban	
Late 1980s[14]	Saudi Arabia	6–15	1.5 rural vs. urban	
Mid 1990s[15,16]	India	5–16	1.8 rural vs. urban	RR 1.6 urban government
			Government schools	Schools vs. private schools
Early 1990s[17]	Bangladesh	5–15	0.3 rural vs. urban	
1989–1990[18]	Algeria	6–19	0.3 rural vs. urban	
1989–1990[19]	India	5–15		6.8 slums vs. other urban
1996[20]	Zaire	5–16		RR 0.2 rural vs. slums RR 3.6
				Low SES vs. upper SES
Early 1990s[21]	India	6–16		Prevalence RHD
				Poor SES: 3.6
				Average SES: 2.4
				Good SES: 0.4
				V good SES: 0.0
(RHD: rheumatic heart disease; SES: socioeconomic status)				

(USSR), the rate of RF incidence was 20–30 cases per 1,000 population.[53] With the improvement in quality of life and increased awareness of importance of health among the general population, the incidence of ARF has decreased. In USSR, at the beginning of the 1990s, the frequency of RF in Kyrgyzstan began to rise. Annual reports on children and adults, produced by rheumatologists between 1998 and 2006 for the public health sector, demonstrated a high incidence of cardiac involvement and high recurrence rates of RF. Among the general population, the incidence of RF/RHD increased by 5.6–6.4 per 1,000 population during this period. ARF is a leading cause of cardiovascular disease among children in the RF-/RHD-positive population of Kyrgyzstan. In 2005 alone, there was a distinct increase in cases of RF, from 0.8 to 2.3 per 1,000 children (+151.4%). Notably, a large number of these patients were from rural areas, which have a primarily ethnic Kyrgyz population. Since ARF is one of the complications of tonsillopharyngitis, caused by group A β-hemolytic *Streptococcus* (GABHS), investigating the prevalence of GABHS pharyngitis in Kyrgyzstan is necessary. About 3% of patients with untreated streptococcal tonsillopharyngitis experience complications from RF **(Table 8)**, while RHDs that develop as complications of RF comprise 35–40% of all hospitalizations of cardiovascular disease.

◼ RESEARCH IN THE AREA OF GABHS/ RF/RHD

Landmark research has been undertaken during the first half of the 20th century. This research provided the foundations for understanding the pathogenesis and epidemiology of streptococcal diseases. Lancefield identified structural differences in organisms that allowed her to classify streptococci into serogroups and serotypes and led her to define the biologic significance of M protein on group A streptococci. WHO by careful epidemiologic study demonstrated that treatment of a streptococcal sore throat with penicillin could prevent RF. The second half of the 20th century saw the increasing development of techniques for dissecting the structure and function of streptococci, explaining the pathogenesis of streptococcal disease, and describing the epidemiology of disease manifestations. In 1999, the Group A *Streptococcus* had just been sequenced. By 2002, Professor Jo Ferretti and others had done sequencing of eight different strains representing a number of streptococcal species. This work opens the door to comparative genomics and to understand the relationships and distinctions between and within species. It should now be possible to better understand cell physiology and metabolism, identify bacterial virulence factors, determine antimicrobial resistance mechanisms, explore the impact of gene acquisitions and deletions, identify phage-determined activities, detect alternative vaccine candidates, and help to explain bacterial evolution.

The production and utilization of vaccines first require well-developed surveillance systems. Such systems inform on the frequency and distribution of strains causing disease, inform public health intervention strategies, and provide the information against which vaccines can be developed and their effectiveness measured. Predominant group A strain types vary according to geography. Types occurring in the industrialized nations of the Northern Hemisphere are distinct from those causing the same disease in developing countries of the world. Within Australia, a similar dichotomy occurs with differences in disease presentations between the tropical north and the more populated region of southern Australia.

The need to understand what strain types are causing disease and where is of paramount importance for both serogroup A and serogroup B streptococci, since vaccines based on type specific polysaccharides or proteins would need to be tailor made to fit the circumstance.

Lessons from Africa

A study indicates that preventive program that relies almost exclusively on secondary prevention, such as the one advocated by the WHO could not reduce the burden of RF and RHD in Africa. A strategy consisting of educating health personnel to recognize bacterial sore throat using simple clinical algorithms (instead of relying on a bacteriologic diagnosis), followed by a single injection of benzathine penicillin for the treatment of suspected cases, has been shown to be effective.[54,55] The implementation of such a strategy through the existing health care infrastructure may be efficient and cost-effective and has the potential to reduce the burden of RF/RHD. The recently devised Awareness Surveillance Advocacy Prevention (ASAP) program is the first step toward implementing such a comprehensive preventive strategy in Africa. The initial effort and expense in integrating primary prevention into national RHD programs can be expected to be more than offset by the reduction in the number of patients with severe valvular disease who will subsequently require expensive tertiary care. Finally, it cannot be overemphasized that RF/RHD is a disease of poverty. Therefore, over and above the preventive strategies, living conditions and access to healthcare must improve substantially in order to reduce disease burden in sub-Saharan Africa.[29,30,46]

Lessons from India

The population of India is over 1 billion people, representing nearly 25% of the world's population. Information on GAS epidemiology from India is scant to say the least and it is sorely needed. We now know that streptococcal toxic shock syndrome and fasciitis that have occurred in the US, Europe, Australia, and Japan, with greater frequency in recent years, are caused by several genetically similar emm types of GABHS.[56] The implication of such genetic and epidemiologic data is that these genetically related strains have spread worldwide. Current information from India is far too limited to know if these virulent strains of GAS occur in India and if they do, to what extent might they be the cause of frequent invasive disease in hospitalized patients.

A community-based RF/RHD cohort study indicates that RF/RHD control program can be sustained within the primary healthcare system and the case registry can be utilized not only for monitoring the program but also to gain insight into the epidemiology of the disease.[57] A cross-sectional and follow-up study of epidemiology of group A streptococcal pharyngitis and impetigo in a rural community of northern India indicated that in north India, pharyngitis was more common than impetigo. Most prevalent emm types of GAS in this region differ from those included in M protein-based vaccines.

The new program by Government of India since September 2018 "*Ayushman Bharat*" will be a boon to people of India specially to cover tertiary care for people living in lower socioeconomic status.

Lessons from Africa

Rheumatic heart disease remains a public health priority in Africa, despite being nearly eliminated in high-income countries. Basic science research remains critical in understanding the unexplained susceptibility seen in some individuals who proceed to develop RHD. Adherence to penicillin prophylaxis remains a major concern in Africa. Multidisciplinary cooperation, preconception, and antenatal care have been proposed as the key measures to improve the pregnancy outcomes of RHD patients.[58]

Lessons from Australia

Rheumatic heart disease incidence increased in the region from 4.7/100,000/year in 1997 to 49.4/100,000/year in 2017 ($p < 0.001$). In 2017, the prevalence of RHD was 12/1,000 in the Indigenous population and 2/1,000 in the non-Indigenous population ($p < 0.001$). The incidence of RHD, RHD-related hospitalizations, and RHD-related surgery continues to rise in FNQ. While this is partly explained by increased disease recognition and improved delivery of care, the burden of RHD remains unacceptably high and is disproportionately borne by the socioeconomically disadvantaged Indigenous population.[59]

■ WORK OF WHO

In the early years of WHO, activities in the area of cardiovascular disease also concentrated on research on etiology, standardization of clinical and pathological criteria, and prevention of RF/RHD. Special attention was given to efficient prophylaxis for RF/RHDs. Penicillin is effective for treatment of acute hemolytic streptococcal infection, which may cause RF/RHD.[60] Adequate treatment of acute hemolytic streptococcal infection by penicillin was widely recommended for prevention of RF/RHD. In 1966, the WHO expert committee recommended the establishment of pilot centers to carry out preventive programs against RF and a network of WHO reference laboratories for bacteriological and serological diagnosis of group A streptococcal infections.

World Health Organization has made the following recommendations[61,62] for improved prevention of RF/RHD:

- Coordination between different organizations and with WHO for better control of RHD
- Quality control of benzathine penicillin, universal availability, and affordable pricing
- Health education of population and training of personnel
- Establishing algorithms for diagnosing streptococcal sore throat and treating it
- Use of Doppler ECHO for diagnosing carditis
- Urging the scientific committee to intensify research efforts towards vaccine
- Improving RHD surveillance and statistics collection
- Involving schools in control program—educating children, screening for RF/RHD and also streptococcal infection and improve adherence to secondary prophylaxis.

World Health Organization has decided to play particular attention to those countries which are currently experiencing a "double burden" of disease, i.e., levels of noncommunicable diseases are rising, while communicable diseases remain at high levels. Development of national policies and a program on prevention and control of cardiovascular diseases and other noncommunicable diseases will be further supported in countries where such policies and programs have not yet been formulated. Primary prevention will be stressed. WHO will redefine the roles of primary healthcare workers to include prevention and control of noncommunicable diseases and prepare guidelines on the prevention and control of noncommunicable diseases for such workers. Secondary prevention of noncommunicable diseases in the community especially RF/RHDs in schools will be further developed.

Latest from WHO[63]

Despite it being eradicated in many parts of the world, the disease remains prevalent in sub-Saharan Africa, the Middle East, Central and South Asia, the South Pacific, and among immigrants and older adults in high-income countries, especially in indigenous peoples.

In 2018, the World Health Assembly adopted resolution WHA71.14 calling for WHO to launch a coordinated global response to RHD and RF. The organization is working to develop clinical guidelines for RHD and with the help of WHO regional offices, a workplan is being developed to put interventions in place to prevent RHD and care for people already living with it.

Ensuring a steady, quality supply of benzathine penicillin is also a key priority in the 13th WHO General Program of Work, specifically the strategic priority on universal health coverage, access to medicines, vaccines, and health products. Additionally, the WHO Roadmap for access to medicines, vaccines, and other health products 2019–2023 and the WHO

Benzathine Penicillin Technical Working Group are working to address global supply and demand issues for benzathine penicillin and ensure a quality-assured, safe, and effective product is available on the shelves when needed.

Recommendations in the resolution on rheumatic fever and rheumatic heart disease (2018):

The resolution calls on member states to take action in five areas:

1. Improve access to primary healthcare
2. Strengthen data collection and knowledge of RHD prevalence in endemic countries
3. Ensure affordable and reliable access to technologies and medicine
4. Strengthen national and international cooperation
5. Tackle the root determinants of RF and RHD

the epidemiological shift in the past 50 years, improved data is needed from developing countries. RF and RHD do not receive due attention. There is an urgent need for the global effort to prevent RF and RHD. Immediate priority is to be given to establish comprehensive and sustainable surveillance systems for the disease. Group A streptococcal vaccines are still years away from being available and even if the obstacles of serotype coverage and safety can be overcome, their cost could make them inaccessible to the populations that need them the most. Due to the limitations of primary prophylaxis as a population-based strategy, new approaches to primary prevention are needed. The most effective approach for control of RF and RHD is secondary prophylaxis as part of a National Control program.

■ CONCLUSION

The RF and RHD still remain a major public health problem. Though there is a significant decline of RF/RHD cases in the developed world, RF remains highly prevalent in the developing nations, where overcrowding, poor hygiene, and limited access to healthcare persist. Due to

■ ACKNOWLEDGMENT

WHO Sources: Experiences during Lancefield workshop Goa 2002; Experiences interacting with Community Medicine Department, PGI, Chandigarh, India ; Experiences interacting with Community Medicine Dept , MS Ramaiah Medical College, Bengaluru, India

■ REFERENCES

1. World Health Organization. Rheumatic fever and rheumatic heart disease. Report of a WHO Study Group. Geneva; World Health Organization: 1988 (Technical Report Series, No. 764).
2. Taranta A, Markowitz M. Rheumatic fever. Boston: Kluwer Academic Publishers; 1989. pp. 1-18.
3. Kaplan E. Recent epidemiology of Group A streptococcal infections in North America and abroad: an overview. Pediatrics. 1996;97(6):S945-S948.
4. World Health Report. Conquering suffering. Enriching humanity. Geneva: World Health Organization; 1997. pp. 43-4.
5. Krishna Kumar R, et al. Epidemiology of streptococcal pharyngitis, rheumatic fever and rheumatic heart disease. In: Narula J, et al (Eds). Rheumatic Fever. Washington, DC: American Registry of Pathology Publisher; 1999. pp. 41-78.
6. World Health Organization. Joint WHO/ISFC meeting on RF/RHD control with emphasis on primary prevention, Geneva, 7–9 September 1994. Geneva: World Health Organization; 1994 (WHO Document WHO/CVD 94.1).
7. Bisno AL. Acute pharyngitis: etiology and diagnosis. Pediatrics. 1996;97(6):S949-S954.
8. Carapetis JR, Currie BJ, Kaplan EL. Epidemiology and prevention of group A streptococcal infection: acute respiratory tract infections, skin infections, and their sequelae at the close of the twentieth century. Clin Infect Dis. 1999;28:205-10.
9. Shulman ST, et al. Streptococcal infections. In: Stevens D, Kaplan E (Eds). Clinical Aspects, Microbiology, and Molecular Pathogenesis. New York: Oxford University Press; 2000. pp. 76-101.
10. Kaplan EL. The group A streptococcal upper respiratory tract carrier state: an enigma. J Pediatr. 1980;97(3):337-45.
11. Pruksakorn S, Sittisombut N, Phornphutkul C, Pruksachatkunakorn C, Good MF, Brandt E. Epidemiological analysis of non-M-typeable group A *Streptococcus* isolates from a Thai population in Northern Thailand. J Clin Microbiol. 2000;38(3):1250-4.
12. Nandi S, Kumar R, Ray P, Vohra H, Ganguly NK. Group A streptococcal sore throat in a periurban population of Northern India: a one-year prospective study. Bull World Health Organ. 2001;79:528-33.
13. Begovac J, Bobinac E, Benic B, Desnica B, Maretic T, Basnec A, et al. Asymptomatic pharyngeal carriage of beta-haemolytic streptococci and streptococcal pharyngitis among patients at an urban hospital in Croatia. Eur J Epidemiol. 1993;9(4):405-10.
14. Fraser GE. A review of the epidemiology and prevention of rheumatic heart disease: Part II. Features and epidemiology of streptococci. Cardiovasc Rev Rep. 1996;17(4):7-23.
15. Nordet P, et al. Amigdalofaringitis aguda. Estudio clinico-bacteriologico y terapeutico. [Acute tonsillopharyngitis. Clinical, bacteriological and therapeutic study.] Revista Cubana Pediatria. Cuban J Pediatr. 1989;61(6):821-33.
16. Steihoff MC, Abd el Khalek MK, Khallaf N, Hamza HS, el Ayadi A, Orabi A, et al. Effectiveness of clinical guidelines for the presumptive treatment of streptococcal pharyngitis in Egyptian children. The Lancet. 1997;350:918-21.
17. Dagnelie CF, Touw-Otten FW, Kuyvenhoven MM, Rozenberg-Arska M, de Melker RA. Bacterial flora in patients presenting with sore throat in Dutch general practice. Fam Pract. 1993;10(4):371-7.
18. Dagnelie CF, Bartelink ML, van der Graaf Y, Goessens W, de Melker RA. Towards a better diagnosis of throat infections (with group A beta-haemolytic *Streptococcus*) in general practice. Br J Gen Pract. 1998;427:959-62.
19. Anthony BF, Kaplan EL, Wannamaker LW, Chapman SS. The dynamics of streptococcal infections in a defined population

of children: serotypes associated with skin and respiratory infections. Am J Epidemiol. 1976;104:652-66.

20. Kaplan EL, Johnson DR, Cleary PP. Group A streptococcal serotypes isolated from patients and siblings contact during the resurgence of rheumatic fever in the United States in the mid-80s. J Infect Dis. 1989;159:101-3.

21. Veasy LG, Tani LY, Hill HR. Persistence of acute rheumatic fever in the intermountain area of the United States. J Pediatr. 1994;124:9-16.

22. Bronze MS, Dale JB. The re-emergence of serious group A streptococcal infections and acute rheumatic fever. Am J Med Sci. 1996;311(1):41-54.

23. World Health Organization. The WHO Programme on Streptococcal Disease Complex. Report of a Consultation. Geneva: WHO: 16–19 February 1998. Geneva: World Health Organization; 1998 (WHO document EMC/BAC/98.7).

24. Murray CJ, Lopez AD. Global health statistics. Cambridge: Harvard University Press; 1996. pp. 64-67. (See also: Murray CJ, Lopez AD. Global burden of disease and injury series. Cambridge: Harvard University Press; 1996:643-45).

25. World Health Organization. World Health Statistical Annual 1990–2000. Geneva: World Health Organization; 2000.

26. World Health Organization. Health system: improving performance. The World Health Report, 2001. Geneva: World Health Organization; 2001. pp. 144-55.

27. Arguedas A, Mohs E. Prevention of rheumatic fever in Costa Rica. J Pediatr. 1992;121(4):569-72.

28. Anabwani GM, Bonhoeffer P. Prevalence of heart disease in school children in rural Kenya using colour-flow echocardiograph. East Afr Med J. 1996;73(4):215-17.

29. Mukelabai K, Pobee JOM, Shilalukey-Ngoma M, Malek ANA, Pankajam MI, Mupela M. Rheumatic heart disease in a sub-Saharan African city: epidemiology, prophylaxis and health education. Cardiologie Tropicale. Tropical Cardiol. 2000;26(102): 25-8.

30. Oli K, Porteous J. Prevalence of rheumatic heart disease among school children in Addis Ababa. East Afr Med J. 1999;76(11):601-5.

31. Toure S, Balde MD, Balde OD, Sow T, Toure A, Conde A, et al. Enquête sur les cardiopaties en mielieu scolaire et universitaire ã Conakry, R. de Guinée. [Prevalence of cardiopathies in primary school, secondary school and university in Conakri, R. Guinéa.] Cardiol Trop [Trop Cardiol]. 1992;18(72):205-10.

32. Longo-Mbenza B, Bayekula M, Ngiyulu R, Kintoki VE, Bikangi NF, Seghers KV, et al. Survey of rheumatic heart disease in schoolchildren of Kinshasa town. Int J Cardiol. 1998;63(3):287-94.

33. Nordet P, Lopez R, Sarmiento L, Dueñas A. Fiebre reumática en Cuba: incidencia, prevalencia, mortalidady caracteristicas clinicas. Rheumatic fever and rheumatic hear disease in Cuba: incidence, prevalence mortality and clinical characteristics. Revista Cubana de Cardiologia y Cirugia Cardiovascular. Cuban J Cardiol Cardiovasc Surg. 1991;5(1):25-33.

34. WHO/CVD Unit. WHO programme for the prevention of rheumatic fever/rheumatic heart disease in 16 developing countries (AGFUND). Report from Phase I (1986–1990). Bull World Health Organ. 1982;70(2):213-8.

35. Le rhumatisme articulaire aigu: réalités et perspectives au Maroc. L' Objectif médical, Edition Maroc. Numéro spécial et hors série, 1990.

36. Al-Sekait MA, et al. Rheumatic fever and chronic rheumatic heart disease in schoolchildren in Saudi Arabia. Saudi Med J. 1991;12:407-10.

37. Kechrid A, Kharrat H, Bousnina S, Kriz P, Kaplan EL. Acute rheumatic fever in Tunisia. In: Horoued, Bouvet A, Leclercq R, Montclos H, Sicard M (Eds). Streptococci and the host. New York: Plenum Press Publishers; 1997. pp. 121-3.

38. Thakur JS, Negi PC, Ahluwalia SK, Vaidya NK. Epidemiological survey of rheumatic heart disease among school children in the Shimla Hills of northern India: prevalence and risk factors. J Epidemiol Community Health. 1996;50(1):62-7.

39. Padmavati S. Rheumatic heart disease: Prevalence and preventive measures in the Indian subcontinent. Heart. 2001;86:127.

40. Prakash RR, Pandey MR. Prevalence of rheumatic fever and rheumatic heart disease in school children of Kathmandu city. Indian Heart J. 1997;49:518-20.

41. Mendis S, Nasser M, Perera K. A study of rheumatic heart disease and rheumatic fever in a defined population in Sri Lanka. Ceylon J Med Sci. 1998;40(2):31-7.

42. Talbot RG. Rheumatic fever and rheumatic heart disease in the Hamilton health district: an epidemiological survey. NZ Med J. 1984;97:630-4.

43. Carapetis JR, Wolff DR, Currie BJ. Acute rheumatic fever and rheumatic heart disease in the top end of Australia's Northern Territory. Med J Aust. 1996;164(3):146-9.

44. Nordet P, Gilberto LL, Hugo L, Plácido A, Rodríguez L, Lidia RN. Fiebre reumatica in Ciudad de la Habana. Prevalencia y caracteristicas, 1972–1987. Rheumatic fever in Havana. Prevalence and characteristics, 1972–1987. Revista Cubana Pediatria. Cuban J Pediatr. 1989;61(2):228-37.

45. Steer A. Rheumatic heart disease in schoolchildren in Samoa. Arch Dis Child. 1999;81(4):373-4.

46. Bertrand E. Morbidité Cardiovasculaire en Afrique Subsaharienne en 1990–2000. Cardiovascular morbidity in sub-Saharan Africa between 1990–2000. Cardiol Trop [Trop Cardiol]. 2000;26(104): 88-9.

47. Gordis L. The virtual disappearance of rheumatic fever in the United States: lessons in the rise and fall of disease. Circulation. 1985;72(6):1155-62.

48. Strasser T, et al. The community control of rheumatic fever and rheumatic heart disease: report of a WHO international cooperative project. Bull World Health Organ. 1981;59(2): 285-94.

49. Flight RJ. The Northland rheumatic fever register. NZ Med J 1984;97:671-3.

50. Bach JF, Chalons S, Forier E, Elana G, Jouanelle J, Kayemba S, et al. Ten-year educational programme aimed at rheumatic fever in two French Caribbean islands. Lancet. 1996;347:644-8.

51. Bitar FF, Hayek P, Obeid M, Gharzeddine W, Mikati M, Dbaibo GS. Rheumatic fever in children: a 15-year experience in a developing country. Pediatr Cardiol. 2000;21(2):119-22.

52. National Institute of Allergy and Infectious Diseases (NIAID). World Health Organization, WPRO "Fifty years of WHO in the Western Pacific Region". Indian J Med Res. 2004;119:ix-xi.

53. Nakajima T, Yamano Y, Sato T, Izumi T, Azakami K, Hasegawa D, Fujii R, et al. Increased prevalence of group A β-hemolytic *Streptococcus* among an ethnic population in Kyrgyzstan detected by the rapid antigen detection test. Institute of Medical, Science, St. Marianna University, School of Medicine, 2-16-1 Sugao, Miyamae-ku, Kawasaki, Kanagawa 216-8512, Japan. Mol Med Rep. 2008;1(6):869-74.

54. Karthikeyan G, Mayosi BM. Is Primary Prevention of Rheumatic Fever the Missing Link in the Control of Rheumatic Heart Disease in Africa. Circulation. 2009;120(8):709-13.

55. WHO. "A Review of the Technical Basis for the Control of Conditions Associated with Group A Streptococcal Infections" Discussion papers on Child Health WHO/FCH/CAH/05.08. Geneva: World Health Organization; 2005.

56. Taranta A, Markowitz M. Rheumatic fever. Boston, Kluwer Academic Publishers, 1989:1-18. Kaplan E. Recent epidemiology of Group A streptococcal infections in North America and abroad: an overview. Pediatrics. 1996;97(6):S945-48.

57. Kumar R, Raizada A, Aggarwal AK, Ganguly NK. A community-based rheumatic fever/rheumatic heart disease cohort: twelve-year experience. Department of Community Medicine, Postgraduate Institute of Medical Education and Research, Chandigarh. Indian Heart J. 2002;54(1):54-8.

58. Muhamed B, Mutithu D, Aremu O, Zühlke L, Sliwa K. Rheumatic fever and rheumatic heart disease: Facts and research progress in Africa. Int J Cardiol. 2019;295:48-55.

59. Kang K, Chau KWT, Howell E, Anderson M, Smith S, Davis TJ, et al. The temporospatial epidemiology of rheumatic heart disease in Far North Queensland, tropical Australia 1997–2017; impact of socioeconomic status on disease burden, severity and access to care. PLoS Negl Trop Dis. 2021;15(1):e0008990. World Health Organization.

60. Kumar R, Vohra H, Chakraborty A, Sharma YP, Bandhopadhya S, Dhanda V, et al. A cross-sectional and follow up study Epidemiology of group a streptococcal pharyngitis and impetigo in a rural community of northern India. School of Public Health, Departments of Experimental Medicine & Biotechnology & Cardiology Postgraduate Institute of Medical Education & Research, Chandigarh, & Indian Council of Medical Research, New Delhi, India. Indian J Med Res. 2009;130(6):765.

61. The WHO global programme for the prevention of RF/RHD. Report of a consultation to review progress and develop future activities. Geneva: World Health Organization; 2000 (WHO/CVD/00.1).

62. WHO. "The Current Evidence for the Burden of Group A Streptococcal Diseases" Discussion papers on Child Health "WHO/FCH/CAH/05.07.17. Rheumatic fever and rheumatic heart disease. Report of WHO study group. Geneva: World Health Organization; 2004. (TRS Series No. 923).

63. WWW.who.int as accessed on 21 January 2021.

4

Can We Change the Epidemiological Trend of Rheumatic Heart Disease in India?

Smita Mishra

■ INTRODUCTION

Rheumatic fever (RF) is an immunologically mediated sequelae of relatively innocuous Group A β-hemolytic *Streptococci* (GABHS or GAS) throat infection. It is characterized by an inflammatory process involving collagen fibrils, which often results in pericardial inflammation and a lasting damage to heart valves.[1,2] The irreversible valvular damage, also known as rheumatic heart disease (RHD), is an important cause of cardiac failure and related premature mortality. Notably, streptococcal pharyngitis, a prerequisite to acute rheumatic fever (ARF), is the only common childhood bacterial disease without an effective vaccine. In this article, we will discuss the identifiable epidemiological determinants of ARF/RHD and analyze their potential to become the instrumental to induce a downward trend in the prevalence of the disease in India. Enlisted candidates for the task include factors responsible for virulence of the streptococci, environmental factors, and vulnerabilities of the human host. In last decade, many outstanding initiatives were taken to change the perspective largely. In this chapter, we will discuss how the collective efforts have made a difference in epidemiological trend of RF-RHD.

■ EPIDEMIOLOGICAL ASPECTS OF ACUTE RHEUMATIC FEVER AND RHEUMATIC HEART DISEASE: RECENT TRENDS

Because of the inhomogeneous healthcare delivery systems across the country, the magnitude of the problem remains obscured. According to a recently published report, RHD affects over 33 million individuals worldwide and has resulted in approximately 350,000 premature deaths/year.[3] In last two to three decades, a significant decline in clinical RF-RHD has been seen **(Table 1)**.[3-12] The Global Burden of Disease Study (GBDS) 1990–2016 showed a remarkable increase in prevalence of ischemic cardiovascular diseases and stroke in India between the aforementioned period; whereas there was decrease in the age-standardized disability-adjusted life-years (DALYs) rate of RHD, in all epidemiological transition level (ETL) state groups[4] **(Fig. 1A)**. Yet, when compared to the global average, RHD DAILY rate was 2.4 times of global average.[4] Lately, in studies using echo screening, a statistically significant higher prevalence of subclinical carditis (SCC) has been demonstrated, contesting the claim made by clinical studies

TABLE 1: Epidemiological study and RHD prevalence in India.

Author	Place	Year	Age (years)	Population studied	Prevalence (per 1,000)
ICMR[5]	Ballabhgarh (rural)	1982–1990	5–15	13,509	2.9
Padmavati[6]	Delhi (urban)	1984–1994	5–10	40,000	3.9
Agarwal et al.[7]	Aligarh	1995	All	3,760	6.4
Grover et al.[8]	Ambala (rural)	1988–1991	5–15	31,200	2.1
Lalchandani et al.[9]	Kanpur (combined)	2,000	7–15	3,953	4.5 (rural: 7.4) (urban: 1.2)
Jose and Gomathi et al.[10]	Vellore (rural)	2001–2002	5–18	229,829	0.68
Mishra et al.[11]	Gorakhpur (urban)	2003–2006	4–18	118,212	0.5
A Bharani et al.[12]	Indore (urban)	2004–2007	5–15	25,676	0.46

(ICMR: Indian Council of Medical Research; RHD: rheumatic heart disease)

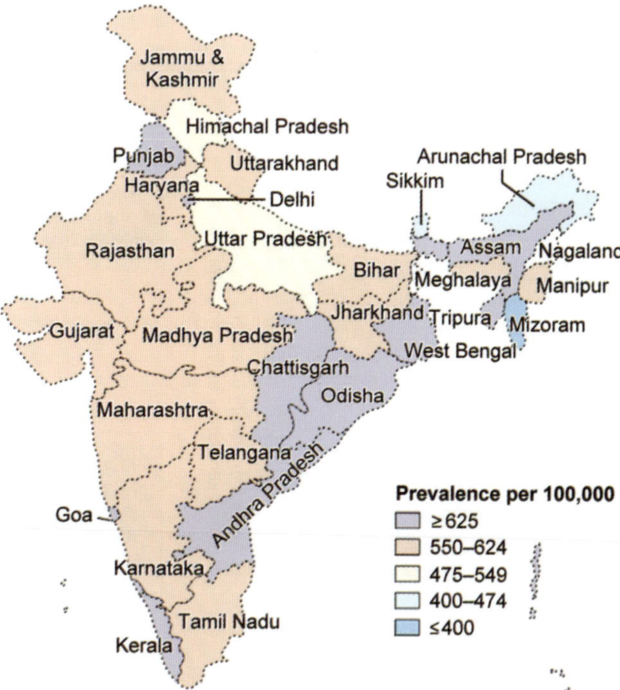

FIG. 1A: Rheumatic Heart Disease in India: Global Disease Burden studies 2016[4].
Source: India State-Level Disease Burden Initiative CVD Collaborators. The changing patterns of cardiovascular diseases and their risk factors in the states of India: the Global Burden of Disease Study 1990-2016. Lancet Glob Health. 2018;6(12):e1339-51

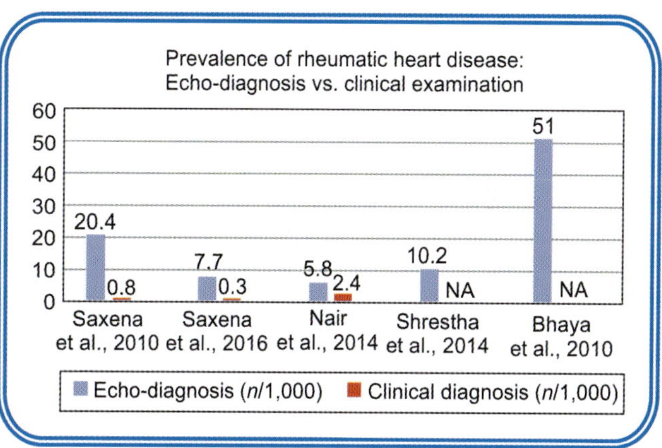

FIG. 1B: Comparative Data of Prevalence of carditis: Echo-diagnosis and clinical diagnosis.[13-17]

the improvement in the socioeconomic state, access, and affordability of healthcare services, change in health-seeking behavior of the community leading to timely treatment of acute pharyngitis. It has been observed that concerted ICMR (Indian Council of Medical Research) studies led to change in health-seeking behavior of the concerned population. Arguably, indices of human development are the major determinants of the RF prevalence and they grossly vary across the country. Therefore, available Indian data from the selective studies may not be considered as reasonable representation of the country as a whole.[4,16-18]

Rationally, Australian New Zealand guidelines of ARF/RHD altered the Jones clinical criteria to improve the sensitivity, in the area with high prevalence.[19,20] No such consideration has been shown in Indian studies done before the creation of World Heart Foundation.

PATHOGENESIS (FIGS. 2 AND 3)

Primarily, RF is related to the GABHS throat infection but some case series have found a relationship with streptococci causing pyoderma and reactive arthritis, particularly

that prevalence of RF-RHD has substantially gone <1/1,000 population.[13-17] But, a downward trend has been observed in prevalence of SCC [20.3/1,000 (2010) vs. 7.7/1,000 (2016)] when study was resumed in same area after 5–6 years **(Fig. 1B)**.[14,17] Correspondingly, Negi et al. reported a two-point survey study, carried out among the school children (urban and rural area) of Shimla, over a gap of about 15 years and confirmed five-fold decline in the prevalence of RF-RHD.[18] Authors attributed the declining trend to

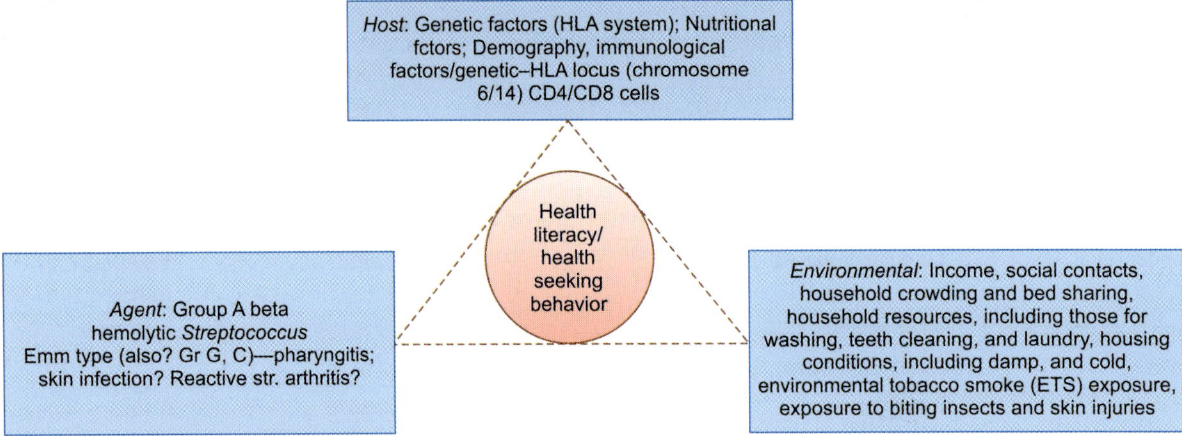

FIG. 2: Rheumatic fever—epidemiological triangle and determinants of disease.[19-21]

(HLA: human leukocyte antigen)

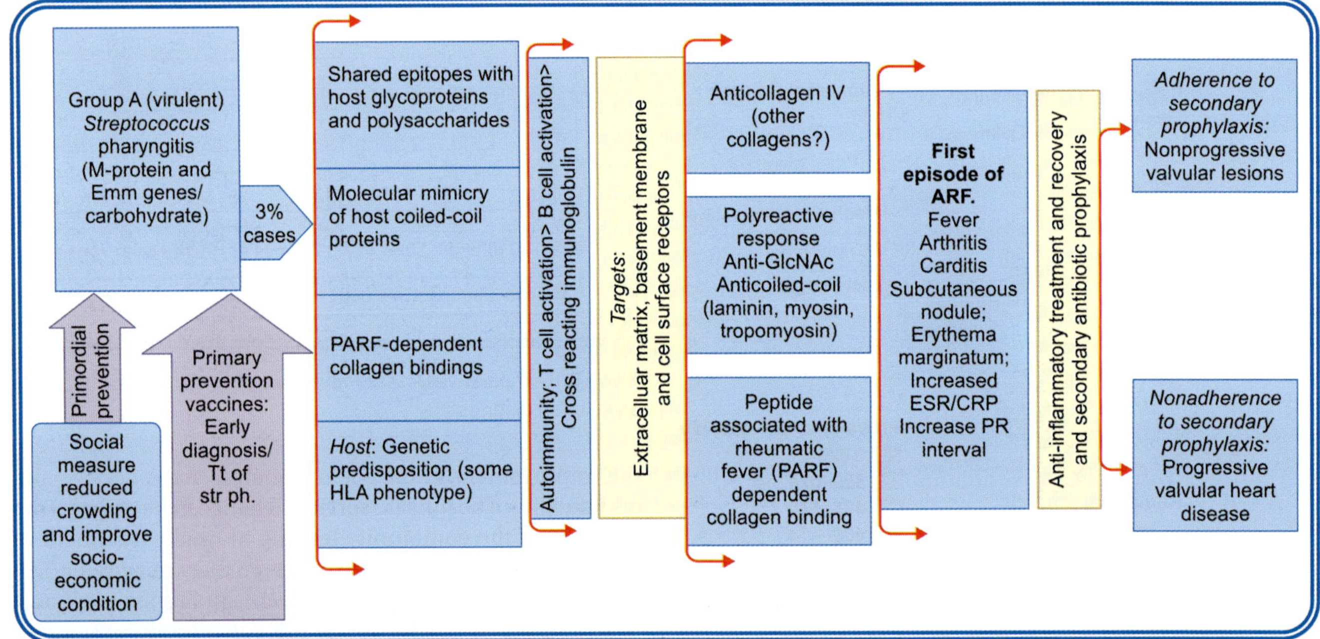

FIG. 3: Pathogenesis of rheumatic fever and level of prevention.[19-21]

(ARF: acute rheumatic fever; CRP: C-reactive protein; ESR: erythrocyte sedimentation rate)

in aborigine population of Australia and New Zealand **(Fig. 2)**. Pathogenesis of ARF/RHD is discussed elsewhere in book, but it is well established now that the RF results from amplified immunological response against the many candidate proteins of host, having molecular mimicry with GABHS bacterial protein **(Figs. 2 and 3)**.[19-24] Classical epidemiological triad (agent, host, and environment) is difficult to discern in ARF as agent leaves immunological trail and remains invisible at the time of clinical appearance of the ailment. Moreover, understanding of epidemiological model is important to strategize an effective control program. Additionally, ARF has a variance in the outcome of different organs passing through the analogous inflammatory process. Presence of the autoantibodies against the collagen I of the cardiac valves indicated possibility of alternative pathways responsible for valvular damage in ARF-RHD.

Host Factor and Role of Genetics

Several inheritable factors augmenting or altering the immunological response have been identified, explaining the prevalence of RF in only 3% population exposed to GABHS pharyngitis.[19-24] Auckland et al. reported a major susceptibility locus for RHD in human leukocyte antigen

(HLA) region (human HLA locus, on chromosome-6) of Indian and Fijian population.[24]

VANISHING ACT OF RHEUMATIC FEVER IN DEVELOPED WORLD: LESSON LEARNED

World Health Organization describes ARF–RHD as a disease grounded in the poverty.[25,26] The virtual disappearance of ARF/RHD in western world has been a landmark, which could not be replicated in a few of developed countries and in most of the developing countries. Industrialized nations now have an average annual RF incidence of <0.5/100,000 and RHD prevalence of <0.05/1,000.[19-26] Knowing the complex nature of RF–RHD and its unabated presence in other part of world needed a thorough analysis particularly in view of the fact that RHD-related mortality dipped-down by 50% before the advent of effective antibiotics such as sulfonamide and penicillin **(Fig. 4)**.[27] Following theories were put forward by Dr L Gordis:[27] (1) Decreased prevalence of streptococci, in general in USA; (2) decreased prevalence of rheumatogenic variants; (3) decreased virulence of bacteria as was evident by decreased severity of then prevailed scarlet fever; (4) disappearance of cofactors needed to produce RF; (5) emergence of effective antibiotic therapy; (6) better medical care; and (7) host factors including nutrition, genetic predisposition, etc. There was an upswing in incidence after 1985, drawing attention to the temporal shift of virulent strains and also identification of type of M proteins associated with carditis.[28]

CONTROL OF RHEUMATIC FEVER IN DEVELOPING WORLD

For a country such as India, primordial prevention, i.e., controlling environmental, economic determinants or sledge–hammer use of antibiotics for pharyngitis without getting into discretion of exact diagnosis, has feasibility issues. Hence, ARF–RHD control program has targeted so for, the re-infection with agent or GABHS. **Table 2** is the comprehensive review of these factors.[17-24]

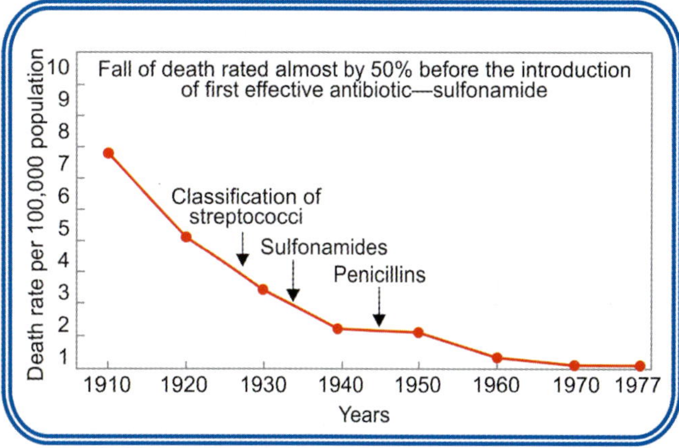

FIG. 4: Crude death rates from the ARF/RHD (USA) 1910–1977.

Source: Gordis L. The virtual disappearance of rheumatic fever in the United States: Lessons in the rise and fall of disease: T. Duckett Jones Memorial Lecture. Circulation. 1985;72:1155-62.

TABLE 2: Agent, host, environment, and health system: the determinants of diseases.

Direct and indirect results of interaction of the environmental/agent/host health system determinants on rheumatic fever and rheumatic heart disease[4]

Determinants	Effects	Impact on RF and RHD burden
Socioeconomic and environmental factors (poverty, undernutrition, overcrowding, and poor housing)	• Rapid spread of group A streptococcal strains • Difficulties in accessing healthcare	• Higher incidence of acute streptococcal pharyngitis and suppurative complications • Higher incidence of acute RF Higher rates of recurrent attacks
Health system-related factors: • Shortage of resources for health care • Inadequate expertise of healthcare providers • Low level awareness of the disease in the community	• Inadequate diagnosis and treatment of streptococcal pharyngitis • Misdiagnosis or late diagnosis of acute RF • Inadequate secondary prophylaxis and/or noncompliance with secondary prophylaxis	• Higher incidence of acute RF and its recurrence • Patients unaware of the first RF episodes • More severe evolution of disease • Untimely initiation or lack of secondary prophylaxis • Higher rates of recurrent attacks with more frequent and severe heart valve involvement and higher rates of repeated hospital admissions and expensive surgical interventions
Virulence of bacteria (M protein 1, 3, 5, 6, 14, 18, 19, 24, Emm variety, etc.)	Predisposes for immunological response	Increased chances of ARF
Vulnerable host (genetic predisposition, malnutrition, etc.)	Valvular disease	Higher rates of recurrent attacks with more frequent and severe heart valve involvement
(ARF: acute rheumatic fever; RF: rheumatic fever; RHD: rheumatic heart disease)		

In order to define relationship between GABHS infection, ARF–RHD and socioeconomical determinants, Coffey et al. made an extensive and systematic literature review of 1,164 relevant observational and experimental studies.[29] Significant associations between socioeconomic factors and risk of Group A streptococci and ARF/RHD were found in 57.1%, and 50% studies, respectively. The majority of studies included in this meta-analysis found reasonable causal association with nutritional status, crowding, dwelling characteristics, education, and employment status of parents or patients, despite of heterogeneity in quality of evidence.

A DECADE OF EMERGING GLOBAL LEADERSHIP TO CONTROL RHEUMATIC FEVER: POLICY, GUIDELINES, AND DATA COLLECTION (2011–2020)

In 2010–2011, while writing this chapter, we discussed multiple barriers posing as the gaps in the policies, guidelines, and health delivery system. However, in last 10 years, developing world has seen the joint-leadership coming from Australia, New Zealand, India, South Africa and many other countries leading to coordinated efforts and tandem walking with the various global agencies. This new uprising in the public health perspectives brought in a new zeal and energy while pursuing the goals, which were once thought to be unachievable. This enterprising global leadership perhaps may be tributed for the negative epidemiological trends in India and other places. Many important events, which have empowered the efforts to control RF-RHD, are as follows:

- Publication of new guidelines from Australia and New Zealand dissociating itself from the traditional approach of American Heart Association (AHA)/WHO/Indian guidelines.[19,20]
- Onset of Global Burden of Diseases, studies and massive collection of epidemiological data allowing comprehensive analysis of the etiological and pathological factors.[4]
- Carapetis et al., while collecting, comprehending, and coordinating related data from all parts of globe, steered a constructive drive among the developing countries, which has dodged the "savior" role of developed countries.[19,20-23]
- World Heart Federation emerged as the biggest challenger for the traditional dominance of west as the policymakers. WHF has the moto to reduce death by 25% in under 25 years age group from RHD up to 2025.[30,31]
- Echocardiography, which was unjustly denied its promising role in the RF control/prevention program, could be recruited in the toolbox of clinical Jones criteria.[13-20,30,32]
- *Portable echocardiographic machines*: India suffered a setback due to rising female feticide prevalence, which culminated into preconception—Prenatal Sex Determination (PNDT) Test Act, prohibiting generous use and portability of ultrasound (US) machines. However, countries with poor health infrastructure were benefitted by introduction of handy, portable US machine.
- *Publication of revised Jones criteria 2015 by AHA*: These criteria are inspired by global trends as discussed above and are evidence of path-breaking transformation in policymaking and advocacy.[32]
- *Role of institutions in India*: Formation of rheumatic consortium (2014), an initiative by All India Institute of Medical sciences under the banner of Pediatric Cardiology Society of India and Cardiology Society of India, is another milestone to create an advocacy for the RF/RHD in India and neighboring countries.[33]
- CSI (Cardiology Society of India) position paper on heart failure guidelines was a unified Indian effort to gather data on specific conditions relevant to the Indian context, which included RF and heart disease.[34]
- *United Nation's Sustainable Development Goals*:[35,36] We will discuss subsequently that how Sustainable Developmental Goal-2030 (SDG-2030) and SDG score are the wholesome package to control RF–RHD without even mentioning it.

DESIGN OF A COMMUNITY OUTREACH MODULE[19-26]

Management of GABHS Pharyngitis[19,20-23,37]

Early recognition and treatment with appropriate antibiotics for desired duration is utmost important both for the general population and part of prevention strategy for recurrence of RF. Yet, a sledgehammer approach to treat all cases of sore throat as GABHS pharyngitis cannot be advocated.[21]

Epidemiological Module[19-23,37]

Tables 2, to 4 provide comprehensive compilation of various epidemiological determinants of RF-RHD and preventive/management strategies.

A successful model is desired for dispensing the epidemiological information and solutions for RF–RHD. Restricted access of the healthcare delivery systems in certain territories may be responsible for both—presence of statistical blind spots for epidemiological data and undulating prevalence status of RF–RHD. Specially designed, unit-specific, module-based investigational and interventional programs are needed to meet the need of tribal colonies, urban slums, and remote rural India. These regions with the poorest healthcare infrastructure need to be prioritized. An ideal Community Outreach Module has to have following components:[36]

- The proactive, sensitized state, and central government
- Medical colleges/civil hospitals and associated ancillary services recruitment in the program

- Involvement of professional academic association such as Indian Academy of Paediatrics, Cardiological Society of India, Pediatric Cardiological Society of India, and Indian Medical Association

- Paramedic training for benzathine penicillin G (BPG) injection and anaphylaxis management
- Role of research organizations such as Indian Council of Medical Research in collecting epidemiological data and improving the health-seeking behavior of society
- Tertiary prevention of progressive VHD with timely intervention is also important. It also gives opportunity to secure native valve for longer duration avoiding the financial burden and need of long-term anticoagulation
- To provide patient education for strict INR monitoring to avoid restenosis of prosthesis as well as overt episodes of accidental bleeding.

TABLE 3: Prevention of ARF-RHD.[3,15,17,19-27]	
Collection of epidemiological data	In view of AHA 2015 revised clinical criteria, risk stratification of a population in a geographical area is required and therefore epidemiological accurate data collection is utmost important to design and execute a control program of ARF and RHD
Prevention of ARF and RHD	I. *Primordial prevention*: By modulating socioeconomic factors—alleviation of poverty, better housing, avoid crowding as spelled out in sustainable development goals adopted by UN
	II. *Primary prevention*: This can be done by developing and researching for a cost-effective vaccine, early diagnosis and adequate treatment of sore throat by GABHS infection
	III. *Secondary prevention*: Early diagnosis of RF and secondary prophylaxis preferably with benzathine penicillin G and to ensure the adherence
	IV. *Tertiary prevention*: The goal of early, effective and adequate anti-inflammatory treatment and management of valvular heart disease

(ARF: Acute rheumatic fever; GABHS: group A β-hemolytic *Streptococcus*; UN: United Nations; RHD: rheumatic heart disease)

Feasibility and Scope of RF/RHD Control Program in the Time of Pandemic COVID-19

Pandemic 2019 has brought socioeconomic crisis in addition to the health calamities. It has decreased gross domestic product (GDP) by −23% in India and increased the number of people below poverty line and hampered the screening programs.[38]

On the other hand, it improved the hygiene, blocking the transmission of droplet infection, due to increased use of masks and hand-hygiene. During the pandemic, resilience of health infrastructure in India was also proved to be fairly good. Therefore, scope of primordial prevention has risen recently like never before.

■ ROLE OF WORLD HEALTH ORGANIZATION[24,25]

In 2018, World Health Assembly launched a coordinated program to respond the zealous global drive, and to upgrade

TABLE 4: ARF/RHD prevention and control program: Role allocation.			
Role of government	**Role of medical colleges/civil hospitals and associated ancillary services**	**Role of IAP and pediatricians**	**Role of paramedics**
- RF-RHD prevention program needs to be accepted as government program - Set-up goals and budget allocation - Sensitize healthcare system - Procure BPG and ensure turnover - Cardiac patients must be considered as physically handicapped and given facilities for treatment - Introduce insurance policies	- To run RHD prevention program - To run regular rheumatic clinic from pediatric department - Training program for medical and paramedical staff - To sensitize them for secondary prophylaxis - Research/thesis at 5–7 years interval or creation of registries	*Role of IAP*: - To ensure the participation at all levels - To improve awareness by publications - IAP branches can bring out their program for helping the patients *Role of pediatricians*: Only pediatricians can successful run supervised RHD prevention program	*Must know*: - Doses and how to dilute the benzathine penicillin - Be trained for IM injection and learn precautions - How to do sensitivity test - Be trained in recognizing and managing anaphylaxis - Be trained to handle life support - Record keeping - *RHD card*: Entry for every injection like in vaccination/INR monitoring card

(ARF: acute rheumatic fever; BPG: benzathine penicillin G; IAP: Indian Academy of Pediatrics; RHD: rheumatic heart disease)

and accelerate the preventive program. WHO has taken following initiatives:

- To establish RF/RHD prevention and health promotion in schoolchildren in as many countries as possible, wherever RF/RHD remains a major public health problem
- To urge Ministries of Health in all of these countries, as well as nongovernmental organizations and donor agencies, to intensify their efforts to promote and support the establishment of at least a local/provincial program on RF/RHD prevention and control
- It is working on developing and upgrading guidelines in view of recent publications
- WHO has owned the responsibility to ensure a steady, quality supply of BPG.

INITIATIVE TAKEN BY INDIAN ACADEMIC OF PEDIATRICS[37]

Indian Academy of Pediatrics (IAP) took the initiative by organizing a consensus meeting on pediatric RF–RHD (2007) and published its guidelines (2008) based on the survey among the pediatricians about the knowledge attitude and practice. Pediatricians are major stakeholders for the efficient implementation of RF control program as this disease mostly affects pediatric (<20 years) population. Following recommendations were made:

- Recognition and prompt treatment of GABHS pharyngitis
- Early recognition of ARF–RHD
- Secondary prophylaxis (SP) preferably with long-acting BPG. Alternative treatment with oral penicillin and erythromycin was recommended in penicillin-sensitive patients.
- It also provided guidelines on diagnosis and management of valvular lesions, infective endocarditis, rhythm issues, etc.
- Consensus guidelines were published in "Indian Paediatrics" a journal religiously followed by all pediatricians of country.
- IAP also approached to various pharmaceutical companies, ICMR, and government to improve the supply of BPG in the country.
- On behest of IAP, BPG was included in the list of essential drugs in 2011.[39]

ROLE OF INDIAN COUNCIL OF MEDICAL RESEARCH AND JAI VIGYAN MISSION MODE PROJECT AND NATIONAL HEALTH MISSION[4,18,21,40,41]

The Indian Council of Medical Research initiated community control and prevention of RF/RHD through hospital-based passive surveillance and implementation of SP under Jai Vigyan Mission Mode Project from 2000 to 2010. Changing socioeconomic state, improved living conditions, and improving connectivity and access to healthcare centers after liberal economic policies and introduction of National Rural Health Mission (Now—National Health Mission) helped in better delivery of healthcare system. Jai Vigyan Mission Mode Project on community control of RF/RHD had four arms—(a) epidemiology; (b) molecular typing of rheumatogenic strains; (c) RF/RHD registries; and (d) development of a vaccine against streptococci.

Nevertheless, none of the ICMR research projects were based on troubled and under developed states such as Bihar, UP, MP, North Eastern regions and Jammu and Kashmir state or the tribal belts. The results of the molecular and vaccine-related research remained unknown.

SUSTAINABLE DEVELOPMENTAL GOAL 2030, SDG SCORE, AND RF CONTROL PROGRAM[35,36]

The RF/RHD is both a biological and a social problem. Its public health importance is not only a direct result of its high occurrence rates (mortality, prevalence, and incidence), but also the population affected (children and young adults). Its economic consequences, both in healthcare related costs and in indirect costs to society (often resulting in premature death or disability), are very significant.[41]

The United Nations (UN-1945) is an international organization currently made up of 193 countries, which takes an active role in designing and developing the global policy issues. Sustainable Developmental agenda 2030 (2015) is an ambitious 17th point plan to promote sustainable development in all countries of the world. It has been broadly accepted that to have a sustained development, world has to have a multilayered proposal to sort-out the intertwined issues related to the health, education, climate change, poverty, and economic growth **(Box 1)**.

Mitigation of the poverty, the food security (Goals 1 and 2), reducing maternal mortality rate (target 3.1), universal health coverage (target 3.8), improving housing, and hygiene (Goal 11) are grossly desired goals to reduce the transmission of streptococci and prevalence of ARF/RHD. Eventually, control of any endemic issue depends on engagement of committed people, well-researched, and precise policies, which must convert into carefully defined programs. It has been appreciated globally that the good policies have a lot of impact globally, regionally, and nationally when they dribble down into good action and execution, locally.

It is important to acknowledge that India is in endemic RF zone, carrying the moderate-to-high risk for RF. India secured 117th position in global SDG scale much lower in comparison with most of its neighboring countries: Shri Lanka—94th; Nepal—96th; Myanmar—104th; and Bangladesh—109th.[36] All developed countries and China stand within the SDG score of 50, which also implicates better human development indices in these countries.

BOX 1	**Proposed health-related targets:**[35,36] **Sustainable Development Goal, 2030.**

- *Goal 1*: End poverty in all its forms everywhere
- *Goal 2*: End hunger, achieve food security and improved nutrition and promote sustainable agriculture

Sustainable Development Goal 3: Ensure healthy lives and promote well-being for all ages:

- *3.1* by 2030 reduce the global maternal mortality ratio to less than 70 per 100,000 live births
- *3.3* by 2030 end the epidemics of AIDS, tuberculosis, malaria, and neglected tropical diseases and combat hepatitis, water-borne diseases, and other communicable diseases
- *3.4* by 2030 reduce by one-third premature mortality from noncommunicable diseases (NCDs) through prevention and treatment, and promote mental health and wellbeing
- *3.b* support research and development of vaccines and medicines for the communicable and noncommunicable diseases that primarily affect developing countries, provide access to affordable essential medicines and vaccines, in accordance with the Doha declaration which affirms the right of developing countries to use to the full the provisions in the TRIPS agreement regarding flexibilities to protect public health and, in particular, provide access to medicines for all
- *3.c* increase substantially health financing and the recruitment, development and training and retention of the health workforce in developing countries, especially in LDCs and SIDS
- *3.d* strengthen the capacity of all countries, particularly developing countries, for early warning, risk reduction, and management of national and global health risks
- *11. Make cities and human settlements inclusive, safe, resilient, and sustainable*

Source: https://rhdaction.org/prevention/primordial-prevention

■ ROLE OF ADVOCACY AND NEW GUIDELINES

Jones Clinical Criteria: The Holy Grail for Rheumatic Fever

"Rheumatic heart disease is a global health issue which should not even exist in the 21st century, yet it continues to limit the lives and opportunities of individuals across the world. We must seize every opportunity we can to eliminate this preventable disease."

—Dr Salim Yusuf, President World Heart Federation[30,31]

Clinical Jones criteria, revised or modified several times in last many decades, are the pivotal for clinical diagnosis.[32,42] In a nutshell, review of various publications suggests following limitations of the jones criteria.[4,17-33]

- These major and minor criteria were not universally present. Even if they were present but were not conspicuous enough to be identified easily.[19,20,32]

- *Diagnosis of pancarditis*: It is known since beginning that ARF affects all three layers of heart but essentially valvulitis is the hallmark of rheumatic carditis. The pericarditis and myocarditis in isolation are not specific for RF. The clinical Jones criteria for carditis had described murmur of ARF as follows: (i) an apical systolic murmur, which does not change with posture or respiration; (ii) parasternal high-pitch diastolic murmur (aortic regurgitation); (iii) a third murmur—mid-diastolic apical [carry Coomb's or murmur of mitral stenosis (MS)]. The issues with diagnosis of carditis were multiple: (a) early carditis usually does not produce classical murmur; (b) there is gradual decline in auscultatory skills of physicians; (c) the murmurs may not be of rheumatic origin in about 60% pediatric population even in endemic zones due to high prevalence of benign (Still's murmur) and small ventricular septal defects; (d) unjust prescription of secondary BPG prophylaxis by zealous physicians while other physicians may ignore presence of several fold higher incidences of SCC (by echo imaging) in comparison to the clinical carditis; (e) RF may present only with fever and subclinical valvulitis and may be missed initially. It may present subsequently with MS, a late sequelae, which occur very quickly following RF in 40–50% cases. The patients with MS may not have other components of clinical criteria.
- Polyarthralgia is common than the polyarthritis in the high-prevalent area.
- Chorea is usually associated with carditis but it has a late and insidious onset and does not give opportunity to diagnose carditis early.
- Erythema marginatum and subcutaneous nodule are specific but are relatively infrequent. They are likely to be missed in routine clinical examination.

Judicious Application of Echo Imaging: Role of World Heart Federation (Table 5)

The American Heart Association and WHO guidelines declined the idea to include echo imaging for the diagnosis of carditis for following reasons: (1) overestimation of regurgitant lesions due to the absence of guidelines to differentiate the physiological and pathological valvular lesions; (2) cost escalation of mass screening due to echocardiography.

These contradictions and controversies compelled researchers, cardiologists, pediatric cardiologists, and epidemiologists to come under one umbrella and develop the recommendations applicable in the diverse group of patient population.[32,33] Carapetis J and group became key to create a combined group of researchers, pediatric/adult cardiologists, epidemiologists, and specialists from all relevant specialties. Over the period of time, multiple epidemiological studies from the affected countries emphatically demonstrated:[13-23,30,31] (1) prevalence of SCC is several folds higher than the clinical carditis; (2) the SCC has a potential to progress into moderate-to-severe carditis

TABLE 5: World Heart Federation criteria for echocardiographic diagnosis of RHD (2012).[31]

Echocardiographic criteria for individuals aged ≤20 years:

Definite RHD (either A, B, C, or D)	A. Pathological MR and at least two morphological features of RHD of the MV B. MS mean gradient ≥4 mm Hg* C. Pathological AR and at least two morphological features of RHD of the AV D. Borderline disease of both the AV and MV
Borderline RHD (either A, B, or C)	A. At least two morphological features of RHD of the MV without pathological MR or MS B. Pathological MR C. Pathological AR
Normal echocardiographic findings (all of A, B, C, and D)	A. MR that does not meet all four Doppler echocardiographic criteria (physiological MR) B. AR that does not meet all four Doppler echocardiographic criteria (physiological AR) C. An isolated morphological feature of RHD of the MV (for example, valvular thickening) without any associated pathological stenosis or regurgitation D. Morphological feature of RHD of the AV (for example, valvular thickening) without any associated pathological stenosis or regurgitation echocardiographic criteria for individuals aged >20 years

Echocardiographic criteria for individuals aged >20 years:

Definite RHD (either A, B, C, or D)	A. Pathological MR and at least two morphological features of RHD of the MV B. MS mean gradient ≥4 mm Hg* C. Pathological AR and at least two morphological features of RHD of the AV, only in individuals aged <35 years‡ D. Pathological AR and at least two morphological features of RHD of the MV

(MR: mitral regurgitation; MS: mitral stenosis; RHD: rheumatic heart disease)

*Congenital MS must be ruled out.

‡ Rule out bicuspid AV.

The World Heart Federation collected epidemiological data from the concerned countries and published the precise echocardiographic criteria.[30,31] The revised Jones criterion was subsequently published in 2015 by AHA accommodating the echo imaging.[32] AHA also yielded to relax the criteria in endemic areas in line with the previously published Australian guidelines.

Highlights of WHF echo criteria are as follows:

- *Less than 20 years of age:* Prevalence of ambiguity of RF–RHD diagnosis is more in comparison to the patient population >20 years of age.
- WHF echo criteria are divided in twogroups based on age groups.
- These groups are further divided in subgroups **Table 5**.
- WHF preconditioned the image optimization. Accordingly, color Doppler assessment must be done with maximized scale and harmonics must not be used during the evaluation of chordal and valvular thickness. Following pathomorphological features need to present for a diagnosis of RF–RHD:
  ○ Definition of rheumatic disease of mitral valve: (i) Increased mitral valve thickening ≥3 mm (age-specific); (ii) chordal thickening; (iii) restricted leaflet motion; and (iv) excessive leaflet tip motion during systole.
  ○ Definition of rheumatic disease of aortic valve—may have following features: (i) irregular or focal thickening; (ii) coaptation defect; (iii) restricted leaflet motion, prolapse.

Revised Jones Criteria 2015:[32] A Course Correction to Drop Down Restriction (Table 6)

Many shortcomings narrated before are now addressed well in AHA revised Jones criteria 2015. Moreover, AHA conceded to the fact that the RF has the global heterogeneity and conventional stringent universal Jones criteria had the potential to miss a diagnosis in the most vulnerable population. Therefore, a definition of low- and high-risk population was accepted as follows:

High- and low-risk population based on prevalence of RF–RHD:

- A population with ARF incidence <2 per 100,000 school-aged children (5–14 years old) per year, or an all-age prevalence of RHD of ≤1 per 1,000 population per year is defined as low risk (Class IIa, Level of Evidence C).
- Depending on their reference population, children not from low-risk population have moderate to high risk (Class I, Level of Evidence C).

Revised criteria conceded that carditis and arthritis are most prevalent major manifestations while chorea, subcutaneous nodule, and erythema marginatum are specific but are less likely to be seen.

Diagnosis of carditis: Revised criteria (2015) have accepted echo imaging as the class I indication for the following:

- For all cases of confirmed and suspected ARF (Level of Evidence B)

in 4–12% of cases; (3) early diagnosis is a tactical tool for control of RF-RHD as we have a method to control the valvular lesions because SP with BPG has shown emphatic role in prevention of the progression of RHD; (4) frequent echo monitoring may obviate the need of secondary BPG prophylaxis in mild/borderline or suspected but unproven cases; and (5) echo is the best modality to monitor the existing valvular lesions.

TABLE 6: AHA's (American Heart Association) revised Jones Criteria, 2015.[32]

Evidence of preceding GAS infection (at least one of the following):

1. Increased or rising anti-streptolysin O titer or other streptococcal antibodies (*anti-DNase B*). A rise in titer is better evidence than a single titer result
2. A positive throat culture for group A β-hemolytic streptococci
3. A positive rapid group A streptococcal carbohydrate antigen test in a child whose clinical presentation suggests a high pre-test probability of streptococcal pharyngitis

Major criteria:

Low-risk population (ARF incidence ≤ 2 per 100,000 school-aged children or all-age RHD prevalence of ≤ 1 per 1,000 population year population)	Moderate-/high-risk population (children not clearly from a low-risk population)
Clinical and/or subclinical carditis	Clinical and/or subclinical carditis
Polyarthritis	Monoarthritis, polyarthritis, and/or polyarthralgia
Chorea	Chorea
Erythema marginatum	Erythema marginatum
Subcutaneous nodules	Subcutaneous nodules

Minor criteria:

Prolonged PR interval	Prolonged PR interval
Polyarthralgia	Monoarthralgia
≥38.5°C	≥38°C
Peak ESR ≥ 60 mm in 1 hour and/or CRP ≥ 3.0 mg/dL	Peak ESR ≥ 30 mm in 1 hour and/or CRP ≥ 3.0 mg/dL

(ARF: acute rheumatic fever; CRP: C-reactive protein; ESR: erythrocyte sedimentation rate; RHD: rheumatic heart disease)

- Serial echo screening would be justified in suspected or diagnosed patients of RF with no evidence of carditis to begin with (Level of Evidence C).
- Echocardiography/Doppler testing should be performed to assess whether carditis is present even in the absence of auscultatory findings, particularly in moderate- to high-risk populations and when ARF is considered likely (Level of Evidence B).
- Specific criteria for valvulitis incriminated are as follows:
  ○ *Mitral regurgitation (MR)*—seen in ≥2 views, jet length ≥2 cm, peak velocity >3 m/s, pansystolic
  ○ *Aortic regurgitation (all four)*—seen in ≥2 views, jet length ≥1 cm, peak velocity >3 m/s, pandiastolic

Diagnosis of joint involvement: In high-risk population, any of following—monopoly arthritis or polyarthritis, or polyarthralgia, is accepted as the major and monoarthralgia as the minor criteria. For low-risk population, only polyarthritis has to be considered as the major and polyarthralgia as the minor criteria.

Other minor criteria: Besides the joint involvement, following criteria were included as minor criteria—fever (≥38.5°F), sedimentation rate ≥30 mm and/or C-reactive protein (CRP) ≥3.0 mg/dL, and prolonged PR interval (unless carditis is a major criterion).

Revised criteria 2015 now take a cut-off erythrocyte sedimentation rate (ESR) as 60 mm/1st hour for low risk and 30 mm/1st hour in high-risk population.

Evidence of preceding Streptococcal infection:

Any one of the following can serve as Class I level indication of preceding infection:

- *Raised anti-streptolysin O titer or anti-DNase B*: A rising titer is better indicator (Level of Evidence B)
- Throat swab culture positive for group A β-hemolytic *Streptococci* (Level of Evidence B)
- Rapid group A *Streptococcal* carbohydrate antigen test positive in a child who have high probability of *Streptococcal* sore throat (Level of Evidence B).

ARF diagnosis in high-risk population: First episode of RF is diagnosed by presence of two major or one major + two minor criteria; Now, polyarthralgia and monoarthritis are included as major criteria for high-risk population..

Subsequent episode: Patients with a history of ARF or RHD are at high risk for recurrent attacks if re-infected with group A *Streptococci*. In cases with past history of RF or established RHD, if GABHS infection has been documented, two major, one major and two minor, or three minor manifestations may be sufficient for a presumptive diagnosis. In the cases where none of the major criteria is present, a meticulous effort to be made to rule out the other possible diagnosis.

Rheumatic chorea and insidious onset rheumatic carditis: No requirement of other major manifestations or supportive evidence of streptococcal sore throat infection.

Chronic valve lesions of RHD (patient presenting with pure MS or MS/MR with or without aortic valve disease): Do not require any other criteria to diagnose as RHD.

With publication of AHA guidelines and new Australian guidelines, a tremendous hope has been generated and now India and other countries are in better position to have an early diagnosis, better monitoring, and discretion to implement an effective epidemiological control program of RF-RHD.

▪ FUTURE OF CONTROL PROGRAM: ROLE OF PRIMORDIAL, PRIMARY, AND SECONDARY PREVENTION

Vaccines[19,20-23,42-45] (Table 7)

"A safe, globally effective and affordable GAS vaccine is needed to prevent and potentially eliminate acute GAS infections (pharyngitis, skin infections, cellulitis, and invasive disease) and associated antibiotic use, immune-mediated sequelae (kidney disease, RF and RHD) and associated mortality."

—**WHO, Vision statement 2018[43]**

TABLE 7: Vaccines against the Group A β-hemolyticus Streptococci.*

Antigen	Comments
Non-M protein vaccine:	
Group A carbohydrate GAC	*Preclinical stage*: Ag conserved in species of *Streptococcus* pyogenes
C5a peptidase	*Preclinical stage*: Potentially, high emm type coverage and cross-protection against other streptococcal pathogens
Type-specific M protein vaccines: N-terminus based:	
Hexavalent tandem Antigen	Clinical trial phase II, protective in humans but low emm coverage
26-valent combination of tandem antigens (StreptAvax™)	Clinical trial stage II completed. Protective but low emm coverage
30-valent combination of tandem antigens	Preclinical. Increased emm coverage
M protein vaccines—conserved C-repeat based:	
C-terminal protective epitope StreptInCor	Preclinical, capable of inducing cellular and humoral responses, mucosal IgA and systemic IgG production in mice
P145 and derivatives J8 and J14	Preclinical stage; human antibodies against P145 cross-react with different emm types
Multivalent J14	Preclinical; broader emm coverage
*Adapted from reference 44	

Primordial and primary prevention of RF is highly desirable but hardly feasible as if now. An effective vaccine is expected to be an asset to the world and India as it would reduce the cost for diagnostic procedures, antibiotics, and eventually interventional management for valvular heart diseases. We must appreciate that polyarthritis and chorea are benign and inconsequential in long term, but they cause significant transient disability to the affected person.

Recently, we have seen quick evolution of multiple vaccines in short duration, against the COVID-19 [Severe Acute Respiratory Syndrome Corona Virus (SARS-COV-2)].

Whereas, development of the streptococcal vaccine remained an elusive project despite of catching attention of many laboratories worldwide, but no interest has been shown by the corporates. The reason for this probably lies in the inability to find out a promising project for the profit-seeking industry, with the conclusively proven streptococcal molecules responsible for the cardiac cross-reactive antibodies found in the patients with RF. Besides, there is no ideal cost-effective animal model other than nonhuman primates. Research laboratories have very limited access to the monkey model for various reasons, which includes tremendous cost escalation. Finally, selection of a safe and effective delivery system/adjuvant is also a challenging task. Besides these technical issues, it can also be argued that

lack of initiatives from developed nations is a root cause for lack of enthusiasm and prevailing ignorance towards the potential of an effective vaccine against the GABHS.

Nonetheless, there are multiple antigenic components of streptococci speculated to be good candidate for vaccine. Moreover, use of technical "reverse vaccinology" (use of genome, transcriptome, and proteome data) for identification of vaccine antigens may shorten the time in picking up candidate antigen.[45]

Presently, expectation of addition of vaccines in the armor of RF–RHD program is a far-fetched dream though any such efforts may be a big gift to the vulnerable population.

Secondary Prophylaxis with Antibiotics: Glittering Gold or Else?

Long-acting BPG is the backbone of RF prevention program. Addition of benzathine counterion to the penicillin sodium creates a compound, which has low solubility in water. Intramuscular administration of BPG has tendency to be released slowly over the time of 3–4 weeks and, therefore, maintaining the blood levels sufficient to kill GABHS acquired during this period.[46] Long-acting BPG provides opportunity to supervised injection at 3–4 weeks interval and with good adherence (>80%) recurrence of RF can be prevented and RHD related morbidity and morbidity can be reduced drastically. BPG prophylaxis is the Grade 1A indication (AHA guidelines 2010).[19,20,32,37,46]

However, in a recent publication, none of children had benzylpenicillin concentrations >0.02 mg/L for the full time between doses.[47] This observation has shown a major knowledge gap relating to pharmacokinetic/pharmacodynamic relationships between BPG and clinical outcomes. BPG was included in WHO list of essential drugs in 2011.[39] Oral penicillin is not equally effective.[46] Oral erythromycin is prescribed to the patients allergic to the penicillin. There are studies to suggest that erythromycin- and tetracycline-resistant strains are emerging.[48] However, following issues related to the BPG must be debated and resolved:

- *Role of liquid penicillin*: BPG salt had poor water solubility. It may block the needle during the intramuscular injection. To overcome that liquid (prediluted), penicillin was introduced. This development led to shortage of regular BPG in India and many other countries. Furthermore, it was costlier and required cold chain. IAP took up this matter to the central ministry and subsequently BPG (0.6 million IU and 1.2 million IU doses) was included in the list of essential drugs (2011 edition) in India. Year 2000 onwards, penicillin supply was erratic. Recently, WHO has taken responsibility to maintain supply of BPG consistent.
- *BPG sensitivity test* has also problem. It is not advised in many countries but India sensitivity testing is recommended. Being a lipid-soluble agent and poor water solubility, it cannot be diluted to the lowest strength

required for skin sensitivity test and being a long-acting agent, it may not reflect response in stipulated time.[37]

- *Safety of BPG injections* need to be established. Respective reported incidence of allergic reaction and anaphylactic reaction is 3.2% and 0.2%. It is advisable that first injection must be administered in a hospital set-up. However, emerging data suggests that anaphylaxis may not be as common as it was thought to be and many other factors may be responsible for the life-threatening events.[48] Fear for anaphylaxis has led to ban on BPG in few of the Indian states (Kerala and Tamil Nadu).[49]
- *Mitigation of pain during the intramuscular injection:* BPG injection is painful and may cause decompensation of cardiac status in few patients causing life-threatening events.[46] The possibility exists that inadequate dose gets administered.
- *Reformulation of drug:* To improve the solubility, emulsifying agents are often added to the BPG, which may include substance such as soy lecithin, responsible for allergic reaction.

  Few studies came out with innovative suggestions for reformulation of the BPG, which include microemulsions, nanoparticles, and implantable drug monoliths.[50] Finally, global efforts are on, to develop a safe, quality assured BPG, which is critical to establish an RF control program.
- *Duration of SP:* Recent publications advocate duration of SP up to 21 years or 10 years from the day of first diagnosis, whichever is longer, if there are no established valvular lesions. There is no unanimity about duration of SP (35 or 40 years or lifelong) for patients with established valvular lesions.[13-23,37]
- *Dose of BPG and body weight criteria:*[13-23,37] Though there is uniformity about the doses of BPG (1.2 million IU or 900 mg for adults and 0.6 million IU or 450 mg for children) but cut-off value of body weight has variation as follows: Australian–New Zealand guidelines—20 kg, Indian, AHA guidelines—27 kg, and WHO guidelines—30 kg. Indian guidelines proposed 2 weeks interval between two injections for children who are receiving low (0.6 million IU) doses. The BPG levels may be suboptimal in many patients predisposing them to the recurrent GABHS infection. A serious discussion is warranted to establish the right cut-off values for body weight and duration of SP.[47]
- *Compulsory training of paramedic for administration of BPG:* It is important, therefore, a training program and guidelines for the paramedics that how to administer BPG and how to take care of anaphylactic reaction. It is important to give first injection in hospital setting where prefilled syringes with adrenaline and steroids are available.

■ CONCLUSION

With the available statistical data, we can say that there has been a conscientious effort to fill-up the gaps and overcome barriers in the healthcare delivery system, which has allowed us to create a better preventive strategy in India. However, more aggressive approach is needed to access remote area and to get a more realistic epidemiological picture of the problem. Although introduction of a suitable cost-effective vaccine is the best preventive armor, it is not expected in recent future due to varied reasons. It is difficult to envisage that agent (GABHS) can be eradicated or environment can be modulated drastically in India. Yet, with the help of community outreach and adherence to SP program, India can achieve the major epidemiological breakthrough to decrease mortality and morbidity associated with RHD. Securing and providing the good-quality BPG is a task, which must be prioritized on all the fronts. Utility, efficacy, and cost of liquid BPG need to be titrated in a balance of cost and benefits. Finally, sensitivity testing of BPG, dosing schedule, and dose interval need a consensus across the board to keep BPG SP effective and fruitful.

■ REFERENCES

1. English PC. Rheumatic fever in America and Britain. A biological, epidemiological and medical history. New Jersey: Rutgers University Press; 1999. pp. 17-52.
2. Stollerman GH, Lewis AJ, Schultz I, Taranta A. Relationship of immune response to group A streptococci to the course of acute, chronic and recurrent rheumatic fever. Am J Med. 1956;20:163-9.
3. Watkins DA, Johnson CO, Colquhoun SM, Karthikeyan G, Beaton A, Bukhman G, et al. Global, regional, and national burden of rheumatic heart disease, 1990–2015. N Engl J Med. 2017;377:713-22.
4. India State-Level Disease Burden Initiative CVD Collaborators. The changing patterns of cardiovascular diseases and their risk factors in the states of India: the Global Burden of Disease Study 1990-2016. Lancet Glob Health. 2018;6(12):e1339-51.
5. ICMR. Community control of rheumatic fever and rheumatic heart disease. New Delhi: Report of ICMR Task Force study, ICMR; 1994.
6. Padmavati S. Rheumatic fever and rheumatic heart disease in India at the turn of the century. Indian Heart J. 2001;53:35-7.
7. Agarwal AK, Yunus M, Ahmad J, Khan A. Rheumatic heart disease in India. JR Soc Health. 1995;115:303-9.
8. Grover A, Dhawan A, Iyengar SD, Anand IS, Wahi PL, Ganguly NK. Epidemilogy of rheumatic fever and rheumatic heart disease in a rural community in northern India. Bull WHO. 1993;71:59-66.
9. Jacob Jose V, Gomathi M. Declining prevalence of rheumatic heart disease in rural schoolchildren in India: 2001-2002. Indian Heart J. 2003;55:158-60.
10. Lalchandani A, Kumar HRP, Alam SM. Prevalence of rheumatic fever and rheumatic heart disease in rural and urban schoolchildren of district Kanpur. Indian Heart J. 2000;50:672.

11. Misra M, Mittal M, Singh RK, Verma AM, Rai R, Chandra G, et al. Prevalence of rheumatic heart disease in school-going children of Eastern Uttar Pradesh. Indian Heart J. 2007;59:42-3.

12. Bharani A. Prevalence of rheumatic fever/rheumatic heart disease in India: lessons from active surveillance and a passive registry JACC. 2010;55(10A):E1415.

13. Bhaya M, Panwar S, Beniwal R, Panwar RB. High prevalence of rheumatic heart disease detected by echocardiography in school children. Echocardiography. 2010;27:448-53.

14. Saxena A, Ramakrishnan S, Roy A. Prevalence and outcome of subclinical rheumatic heart disease in India: the rheumatic study. Heart. 2011;97:2018-22.

15. Nair B, Vishwanthan S, Krisy G, Gupta PN, Nair N, Thakkar A. Rheumatic heart disease in Kerala: a vanishing entity. An echo Doppler study in 5-15years schoolchildren. Int J Cardiol. 2015;2015:930790.

16. Shrestha NR, Karki P, Mahto R. Prevalence of subclinical rheumatic heart disease in eastern Nepal: a school-based cross-sectional study. JAMA Cardiol. 2016;1:89-96.

17. Saxena A, Desai A, Narvencar K. Echocardiographic prevalence of rheumatic heart disease in Indian school children using World Heart Federation criteria: a multi site extension of rheumatic study (the e-rheumatic study). Int J Cardiol. 2017;249:438-42.

18. Negi PC, Kanwar A, Chauhan R, Asotra S, Thakur JS, Bhardwaj AK. Epidemiological trends in RF/RHD in school children of Shimla in north India. Indian J Med Res. 2013;137:1121-7.

19. RHD Australia (ARF/RHD Writing Group), National Heart Foundation of Australia, the Cardiac Society of Australia and New Zealand. (2012). Australian guideline for prevention, diagnosis and management of acute rheumatic fever and rheumatic heart disease, 2nd edition. [online] Available from http://www.apsu.org.au/assets/past-studies/www.rhdaustralia.org.au-sites-default-files-guideline-0.pdf. [Last accessed August, 2022].

20. Baker MG, Gurney J, Oliver J, Moreland NJ, Williamson DA, Pierse N, et al. Risk Factors for Acute Rheumatic Fever: Literature Review and Protocol for a Case-Control Study in New Zealand. Int J Environment Res Public Health. 2019;16:4515.

21. Kumar RK, Tandon R. Rheumatic fever & rheumatic heart disease: The last 50 years. Indian J Med Res. 2013;137:643-58.

22. Cunningham MW. Rheumatic fever, autoimmunity, and molecular mimicry: the streptococcal connection. Int Rev Immunol. 2014;33(4):314-29.

23. Herath VCK, Carapetis J. Rheumatic fever: What is new? Curr Ped Rep. 2015;3:211-8.

24. Auckland K, Mittal B, Cairn BJ, Naveen G, Kumar S, Mentzer AJ, et al. The Human Leukocyte locus and rheumatic heart disease susceptibility in south Asians and Europeans. Sci Rep. 2020;10(1):9004.

25. World Health Organization. Rheumatic fever and rheumatic heart disease. Report of a WHO Expert Consultation. Geneva: World Health Organization; 2004 (Technical Report Series No. 923).

26. WHO. (2020). Rheumatic Heart Disease. [online] Available from https://www.who.int/news-room/fact-sheets/detail/rheumatic-heart-disease. [Last accessed August, 2022].

27. Gordis L. The virtual disappearance of rheumatic fever in the United States: Lessons in the rise and fall of disease: T. Duckett Jones Memorial Lecture. Circulation. 1985;72:1155-62.

28. Shulman ST, Stollerman G, Beall B, Dale JB, Tanz RR. Temporal changes in Streptococcal M protein types and the near-disappearance of acute rheumatic fever in the United States. Clin Infect Dis. 2006;42(4):441-7.

29. Coffey PM, Ralph AP, Krause VL. The role of social determinants of health in the risk and prevention of group A streptococcal infection, acute rheumatic fever and rheumatic heart disease: A systematic review. PLoS Negl Trop Dis. 2018;12(6):e0006577.

30. Remenye B, Carapetis J, Wyber R, Taubert K, Mayosi BM. Position statement of word heart federation on the prevention and control of rheumatic heart disease. Nat Rev Cardiol. 2013;10:284-92.

31. Reményi B, Wilson N, Steer A, Ferreira B, Kado J, Kumar K, et al. World Heart Federation criteria for echocardiographic diagnosis of rheumatic heart disease: an evidence-based guideline. Nat Rev Cardiol. 2012;9(5):297-309.

32. Gewitz MH, Baltimore RS, Tani LY, Sable CA, Shulman ST, Carapetis J, et al. American Heart Association Committee on rheumatic fever, endocarditis, and Kawasaki disease of the council on cardiovascular disease in the young. Revision of the Jones Criteria for the diagnosis of acute rheumatic fever in the era of Doppler echocardiography: a scientific statement from the American Heart Association. Circulation. 2015;131:1806-18.

33. Saxena A, Kumar RK. The National Rheumatic Heart Consortium: A nationwide initiative for the control of rheumatic heart disease in India. Natl Med J India. 2015;28(3):144-6.

34. Guha S, Harikrishnan S, Ray S, Sethi R, Ramakrishnan S, Banerjee S, et al. CSI position statement on management of heart failure in India. Indian Heart J. 2018;70(Suppl 1):S1-S72.

35. United Nations Development Programme. Sustainable Developmental Goals 2030 (UNDP). [online] available from https://www.undp.org/content/undp/en/home/sustainable-development-goals.html. [Last accessed August, 2022].

36. Sustainable Development Report. SDG Index score, 2020. [online] Available from https://dashboards.sdgindex.org/rankings. [Last accessed August, 2022].

37. Mishra S, Saxena A, Kumar RK, Mishra Y, Ahmed Z, Gera R, et al. Consensus Guidelines on Pediatric Acute Rheumatic Fever and Rheumatic Heart Disease IAP Working Group on Pediatric Acute Rheumatic Fever. Indian Pediatr. 2008;45(7):565-73.

38. India Today. GDP at historic low: Looking beyond the coronavirus shock (India today). [online] available from https://www.indiatoday.in/business/story/gdp-at-historic-low-looking-beyond-the-coronavirus-shock-1717439-2020-09-01. [Last accessed August, 2022].

39. India Go. (2011). National List of Essential Medicines of India. [online] Available from https://pharmaceuticals.gov.in/sites/default/files/NLEM.pdf. [Last accessed August, 2022].

40. ICMR. Highlights of ICMR Activities and Achievements. [online] Available from http://icmr.nic.in/highlights.htm#Non-communicable%20Diseases. [Last accessed August, 2022].

41. Nordet P. Rheumatic Fever. Clinical and epidemiological aspects. Havana, Cuba. 1972–1987. Thesis for Scientific Degree. Havana, Cuba: Cuban Ministry of Health; 1988.

42. Jones TD. Diagnosis of rheumatic fever. JAMA. 1944;126:481-4.

43. WHO. (2018). Road map-group A vaccine development (WHO vision statement 2018). [online] available from https://savac.ivi.int/documents/WHO-IVB-18.08-GAS%20Vaccine%20Develoment%20Technology%20Roadmap%202018.pdf. [Last accessed August, 2022]

44. Pritchard C, White M, Brown S. Life Sciences New Talent collection. R Soc Open Sci. 2022;9(1).

45. Sharma A, Nitsche-Schmitz DP. Challenges to developing effective streptococcal vaccines to prevent rheumatic fever and rheumatic heart disease. Devel Ther. 2014;4;39-54.

46. Marantelli S, Hand R, Carapetis J, Beaton A, Wyber R. Severe adverse events following benzathine penicillin G injection for rheumatic heart disease prophylaxis: cardiac compromise more likely than anaphylaxis. Heart Asia. 2019;11:e011191.

47. Hand RM, Salman S, Newall N, Vine J, Page-Sharp M, Bowen AC, et al. A population pharmacokinetic study of benzathine benzylpenicillin G administration in children and adolescents with rheumatic heart disease: new insights for improved secondary prophylaxis strategies. J Antimicrob Chemother. 2019;74(7):1984-91.

48. Bhardwaj N, Mathur P, Behera B, Mathur K, Kapil A, Misra MC. Antimicrobial resistance in beta-haemolytic streptococci in India: A four-year study. Indian J Med Res. 2018;147(1):81-7.

49. International Rheumatic Fever Study Group. Allergic reactions to long-term BPG prophylaxis for rheumatic fever. Lancet. 1991;337:1308-10.

50. RHD Action. RHD global status of BPG. [online] Available from https://rhdaction.org/sites/default/files/RHD%20Action_Global%20Status%20of%20BPG%20Report_Online%20Version.pdf. [Last accessed August, 2022].

5

Etiopathogenesis and Management of Streptococcal Infection

Usha Anand, IB Vijayalakshmi

INTRODUCTION

Group A streptococcal (GAS) infections of the pharynx are the precipitating cause of rheumatic fever. During epidemics over a half century ago, as many as 3% of untreated acute streptococcal sore throats were followed by rheumatic fever, and in endemic infections, the incidence of rheumatic fever is substantially less.[1] Appropriate antibiotic treatment of streptococcal pharyngitis prevents acute rheumatic fever (ARF) in most cases.[2] Unfortunately, at least one-third of episodes of ARF result from inapparent streptococcal infections.[3] In addition, some symptomatic patients do not seek medical care. In these instances, ARF is not preventable. Hence, proper understanding of etiopathogenesis, timely diagnosis, and treatment of GAS infection is very important.

BACKGROUND

Prevention of initial episodes of ARF requires accurate recognition and proper antibiotic treatment of GAS pharyngitis. Streptococcal skin infections (impetigo or pyoderma) have not been proven to lead to ARF. Acute pharyngitis is caused considerably more often by viruses than by bacteria. Viruses that commonly cause pharyngitis include influenza virus, parainfluenza virus, rhinovirus, coronavirus, adenovirus, respiratory syncytial virus, Epstein–Barr virus, enteroviruses, and herpes viruses. Other causes of acute pharyngitis include groups C and G streptococci, *Neisseria gonorrhoeae, Mycoplasma pneumoniae, Chlamydia pneumoniae, Arcanobacterium haemolyticum,* and human immunodeficiency virus (HIV).

Group A streptococcal pharyngitis is primarily a disease of children 5–15 years of age and in temperate climates, it usually occurs in the winter and early spring. GAS is an uncommon cause of pharyngitis in preschool children, but outbreaks in childcare settings have been reported.[4,5] However, rheumatic fever is rare in children <3 years of age. Initial attacks of rheumatic fever are also rare in adults, but recurrences are well documented.

EVOLUTION OF THE CONCEPT OF RHEUMATOGENIC STRAINS

The World War-II epidemics of ARF that occurred among military recruits, assembled from many different areas of the US, were shown to be caused by GAS strains belonging to but a few prominent M serotypes.[6-8] These epidemic strains were heavily encapsulated, M protein-rich variants. When introduced into the ranks of close living recruits, they spread rapidly, not by fomites but by droplet infection through close person-to-person contact. Infections by strains representing several M serotypes were associated with a strikingly similar postinfection ARF attack rate of approximately 3% in untreated individuals.[9] This attack rate varied with the intensity of the immune response.[10]

Nonrheumatogenic GAS

As early as the late 1930s, Alvin Coburn noted that ARF was not reactivated by throat infections due to strains representing certain M protein serotypes.[11] By the 1950s, it was further reported that strains within certain M types caused acute glomerulonephritis (AGN)[12] rather than ARF, the two complications very rarely occurring from the same antecedent infection. By the 1960s, GAS strains causing streptococcal pyoderma (impetigo), a primary skin infection, were shown to be different from those primarily infecting the throat. Some pyoderma strains caused AGN, but none caused ARF.[13-15] Therefore, the so-called "skin strains" must be regarded as nonrheumatogenic.

Properties of Known Rheumatogenic Strains

Some characteristics of the GAS strains clearly responsible for the great ARF epidemics of World War-II have been defined.[16] Briefly, they are very rich in M protein (i.e., have very large M molecules), are heavily encapsulated, and are highly mouse virulent. They produce striking "mucoid" colonies on blood agar plates. They are tropic primarily for the throat rather than the skin, infecting the latter only secondarily through wounds or skin lesions. They evoke strong type specific immune responses in humans and in mice, much more so than M type-specific responses from pyoderma strains. They do not contain the lipoproteinase commonly seen in skin strains (serum opacity factor). They have been found so far to be distributed among a limited number of serotypes, such as M 1, 3, 5, 6, 18, 19, and 24 and some others.[8]

It should be emphasized, however, that the M serotype alone does not equate with rheumatogenicity because strain variation is common within a given serotype. This fact has caused confusion and controversy about the concept of rheumatogenic M serotypes. On the other hand, very few studies have routinely assessed encapsulation and many strains identified as M positive may have relatively small or no capsules.

Why are rheumatogenic strains difficult to identify?

In a severe epidemic of GAS pharyngitis, one strain of a given M serotype often becomes prevalent. In such cases, the attack rate of ARF following such specific infections can be accurately calculated. In clinical practice, however, by the time ARF is diagnosed the infecting strain is usually not recoverable or the clones persisting in the patient's throat may have attenuated so that their M type may no longer be recognizable. Moreover, new GAS strains may have been acquired during the latent period between the antecedent infection and the onset of ARF.[17]

Acute rheumatic fever patients are often referred to centers (especially pediatric cardiology clinics) where in-depth studies of streptococcal strains are not usually performed. Reference laboratories often receive strains that dissociate during transfer and no longer express all the virulence factors. When clinical laboratories do the throat cultures, colony morphology is rarely observed or reported. Yet, the appearance of mucoid colonies in a cohort may signal danger. For example, in the late 1950s, in a prospective surveillance of throat cultures from naval recruits of the Great Lakes Naval Training Center, Great Lakes, Illinois, the sudden appearance of a predominant highly "mucoid" M type accurately predicted the onset of a severe epidemic of ARF.[18]

The Molecular Biology and Genetics of Well-known Rheumatogenic GAS

By the 1980s, the primary molecular structure of M protein was determined[19] and its type-specific antigen was shown to reside in its small terminal N-acetyl peptide.[20] Two highly conserved epitopes within M protein divide GAS immunologically into Class I (throat) and Class II (skin) strains.[21] All ARF strains fall clearly into Class I throat strains and individuals who had contracted ARF were shown to have higher than normal titers against the Class I epitope, whereas they lacked antibodies to the Class II epitope.[22] Moreover, in the large M protein molecules of Class I rheumatogenic strains, distinct epitopes were identified that cross-react with cardiac, synovial, and brain tissues and these were separable from the terminal type-specific antigen.

The genes of M protein (emm) have now been shown to be divided into four subfamilies of nucleotide sequences, arranged in five distinctive chromosomal patterns, identified as A-E.[23] By these genetic patterns, rheumatogenic pharyngitis strains are clearly differentiated from impetigo strains, but not yet clearly from all other throat strains. Whether epitopes that cross-react with host tissues are present exclusively in rheumatic fever strains is not clear. An attractive hypothesis is that the deposition of a heavy antigenic load of these cross-reactive epitopes in pharyngeal lymphoid tissues, already hypersensitized during early childhood by repeated streptococcal infections, causes a break in the immune tolerance of susceptible hosts that lead to the various stigmata of ARF.

Swallowing large amounts of such antigens seems to have a powerful immunizing effect. It is an old observation that streptococcal pharyngitis produces a more striking immune response to all streptococcal antigens in those who develop ARF compared to those who do not, whereas ARF patients respond normally to other common test antigens. After nasal administration of synthetic M vaccines, mice produce type-specific IgA antibodies and are protected from experimental systemic challenge with homologous M-type strains.[24] In addition, the adjuvant effect of the superantigenic properties of the proximal conserved part of the M protein may also promote exaggerated immune responses and autoimmunity.

Recently, the M protein genes and those of hyaluronic acid, streptolysin S, erythrogenic toxins, and others have been identified[25] and now provide a genomic approach to characterizing GAS strains. Other than quantitative features of virulence as measured by M protein and hyaluronate content,[26] molecular differences between rheumatogenic and nonrheumatogenic throat strains are not yet clear.

Group A *Streptococcus* Virulence

Group A *Streptococcus* is a natural pathogen only for human beings. Whereas all members of the species are identified by their group-specific carbohydrate cell wall, its outer surface is composed of tiny hair-like coiled projections by which the organism adheres to tissues.[27] In virulent strains, these structures contain an extractable and remarkably heterotypic antigen, the M protein.[28] More than 100 immunologically specific M serotypes have so far been identified. Immunity to virulent GAS infection is only M type specific, accounting for the frequency of GAS infections. When fully virulent, each chain of cocci is surrounded by a capsule of hyaluronic acid that is responsible for the "mucoid" appearance of GAS colonies on blood agar.[29] The larger the capsule, the smaller the chains.[30] The capsule is produced only during active growth of the organism. *Streptococcal hyaluronate* is chemically identical to that occurring ubiquitously in human connective tissues so that antibodies to it are not readily raised. Thus, anticapsular immunity does not occur and the host defense to virulent strains depends on anti-M antibodies.

Both components, M protein and capsule, are primarily responsible for the striking resistance of virulent strains of GAS to phagocytosis.[31] But, M protein and capsule are rapidly lost during convalescence from acute pharyngitis[32] or shortly after leaving the host, when landing on fomites or when grown in artificial media. After fresh isolation, strain virulence may be maintained, however, by frequent transfer through fresh human blood or by intraperitoneal mouse passage.

Once host defenses are penetrated, strains of GAS excrete many extracellular toxic substances that enhance tissue destruction and promote invasion (streptolysin S and O, streptokinase, DNA nucleases, hyaluronidase, erythrogenic toxins, anticomplementary proteins, etc.).

On blood agar cultures, clones of encapsulated variants form large "mucoid" colonies resembles a drop of oil, whereas loss of encapsulation results in colonies that are opaque and "pearly" in appearance.[29] In the past, their appearance in throat cultures from military cohorts who were under prospective surveillance regularly predicted severe epidemics of streptococcal pharyngitis and ARF.[18]

Throat carriage, however, may sometimes stubbornly persist during convalescence when strains have lost these virulence factors. Such persisters may retain mucosal adherence ligands such as surface lipoteichoic acid[27] and F proteins[33] that stimulate internalization of the organisms by epithelial cells.[34] Such internalization is actually inhibited by the hyaluronate capsule[35,36] whose genetic expression is associated with that of other virulence factors (e.g., M protein, streptolysins, and erythrogenic toxins), causing cellular injury and promoting the invasion of deeper tissues.[25,37,38] Thus, the human throat is readily colonized by a variety of GAS strains of varying virulence, accounting for a spectrum of infection ranging from an asymptomatic colonization to local inflammation and extension to deeper tissues. Confirmation of the diagnosis of actual streptococcal pharyngitis, therefore, requires more than positive cultures, a significant increase in the titer of streptococcal antibodies [e.g., antistreptolysin O (ASLO/ASO), anti-DNase B, etc.].

STREPTOCOCCAL PHARYNGITIS

Transmission is by droplet infection or through fomites. Incubation period is 2–5 days. Crowding such as in schools,

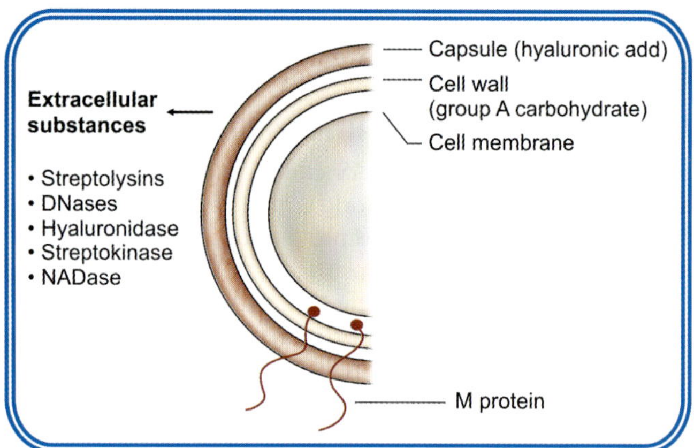

FIG. 1: Cellular and extracellular antigens of group A streptococci.

daycare centers, and military facilities increases the risk of transmission. Streptococcal pharyngitis may be strongly immunogenic when caused by strains of high virulence without producing severe symptoms. Streptococcal pharyngitis is self-limiting with duration of illness lasting for 5–7 days, even in the absence of specific treatment. A sore throat and a slight fever are soon forgotten. Direct throat swab culture and isolation of organism present a definitive evidence of GAS infection. The GAS produces various cellular and extracellular antigens as depicted in **Figure 1**. Direct antigen measurement or assays of specific antibodies in the infected patient are other methods of finding evidence of current and previous streptococcal infection, respectively.

Clinical features suggestive of streptococcal pharyngitis are sudden onset of sore throat, pain on swallowing, and fever. Other systemic symptoms such as headache, abdominal pain, nausea, and vomiting can occur in children. Signs include congestion of tonsils and the pharynx with or without exudates, anterior cervical lymphadenitis, petechiae on the soft palate (doughnut lesions) and sometimes a scarlatiniform rash **(Table 1 and Fig. 2)**. These features are not specific for streptococcal pharyngitis and can occur with other upper respiratory tract infections. These features are seen in patients >3 years of age. Children <3 years of age present with mucopurulent rhinitis, mild fever, and irritability. Presence of cough, coryza, diarrhea, hoarseness of voice, and conjunctivitis is all in favor of viral pharyngitis.[39] Scoring systems are proposed for clinical diagnosis. Higher the score, more likely the chance of having streptococcal pharyngitis.

Clinically, it is not possible to accurately differentiate streptococcal pharyngitis from viral pharyngitis.

Therefore, confirmation is required with a throat culture, antigen testing for present infection, and antibody testing for past evidence of infection.[40] Testing is not routinely required in children below 3 years of age and in adults. ARF is rare in these age groups. Laboratory test should be performed if clinical features are suggestive of streptococcal pharyngitis.

TABLE 1: Clinical presentation of streptococcal tonsillopharyngitis.

Common findings	Findings not suggesting GAS infection
Symptoms and signs:	
• Sudden onset of sore throat pain on swallowing • Fever headache • Abdominal pain, nausea, and vomiting • Tonsillopharyngeal erythema • Tonsillopharyngeal exudate • Soft palate petechiae ("doughnut" lesions) • Discrete ulcerative lesions • Beefy red, swollen uvula • Anterior cervical adenitis • Scarlatiniform rash	• Coryza • Hoarseness • Cough • Diarrhea • Conjunctivitis • Anterior stomatitis
Scoring systems:	
Centor criteria:	*Mcisaac criteria:*

• Tonsillar exudates—1
• Swollen tender cervical lymph nodes—1
• Fever—1
• No cough—1:
  ○ *0–1*: No testing or antibiotics
  ○ *2–3*: Rapid antigen test
  ○ *4*: No testing, empiric antibiotics
	• Tonsillar swelling or exudates—1
	• Swollen tender cervical lymph nodes—1
	• Temperature >38—1
	• No cough—1
	• Age 3–14 years—1
	• Age 14–44 years—0
	• Age > 44 years—1

(GAS: group A *Streptococcus*)	

If the clinical features are suggestive of viral origin, the pretest probability of isolating *Streptococcus* is low and testing need not to be performed.

Complications

- *Suppurative*: Peritonsillar abscess, retropharyngeal abscess, and mastoiditis
- *Nonsuppurative*: Acute glomerulonephritis, ARF, poststreptococcal reactive arthritis (PSRA), and pediatric autoimmune neuropsychiatric disorders associated with streptococcal infections (PANDAS)

Throat Culture

Throat culture is a standard method for establishing the diagnosis of streptococcal pharyngitis. It should be obtained properly by vigorous swabbing of pharyngeal wall and tonsils. Culture cannot differentiate between carrier state and true invasive infection.[41] Such carriers will asymptomatically harbor the organism in their upper respiratory tract and do not develop complication.[42,43]

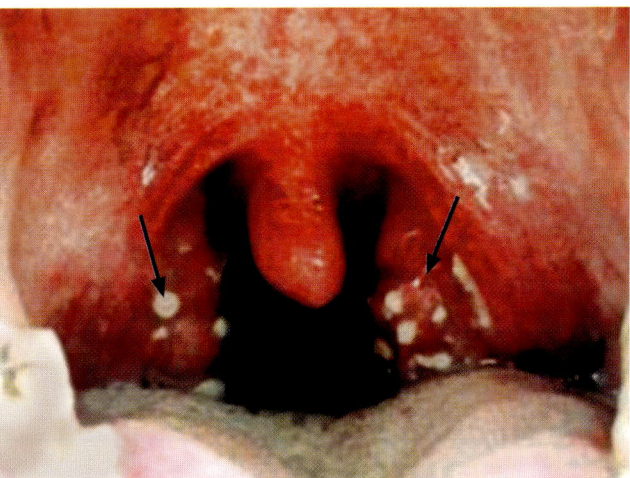

FIG. 2: Strep sore throat showing beefy red uvula with exudates on tonsils.

Quantification of growth from the throat swab culture does not differentiate carriage from infection, because sparse growth can also be associated with true infection. Throat swab cultures should be obtained from all household contacts of a child who has ARF and if the test results are positive, that contact should be treated.

Rapid Streptococcal Antigen Tests

Many rapid streptococcal antigen throat swab tests are available based on the carbohydrate antigen of the *Streptococcus*. These tests have a high degree of specificity, but their sensitivity is variable. Therefore, treatment is indicated for the patient with acute pharyngitis who has a positive test. There have been new tests with improved sensitivity but so far, there have been no studies in children to recommend that negative test need not require confirmation with throat culture.[44-46] Studies in adult have shown that the negative predictive value of the tests approaches 98% and hence negative test does not require confirmation with throat culture in adults.[47] Antigen tests can be positive in children who are carriers without invasive streptococcal infection.

Streptococcal Antibody Tests (Table 2)

During the case of an acute infection, diagnosis is made by clinical observation and then confirmed by rapid antigen tests or by isolation of group A streptococci from the site of infection. But when children present with nonsuppurative sequelae such as ARF and glomerulonephritis, it is not possible to recover the organism. The presence of a host immune response is the only evidence of the recent infection that remains. Measurement of antibodies to specific streptococcal antigens is, therefore, necessary to confirm the diagnosis of the preceding GAS infection.[48]

Various factors influence the antibody formation after GAS infection. The age of the patient, the endemicity of infection, site of infection, and promptness of antibiotic

TABLE 2: List of the group of commonly used streptococcal antibody tests.[48]

Antigen	Test
Extracellular	
Streptolysin O	Antistreptolysin O
Deoxyribonuclease B (DNase B)	Anti-DNase B
	Antistreptokinase
Streptokinase	Antistreptococcal
Hyaluronidase	Hyaluronidase*
Nicotinamide adenine dinucleotidase (NADase)	Anti-NADase*
Somatic/cellular	
Type-specific M-protein	Type-specific M antibody*
Group A carbohydrate	Anti-A carbohydrate*

*Not commercially available, but currently used in research and reference laboratories reference[48]

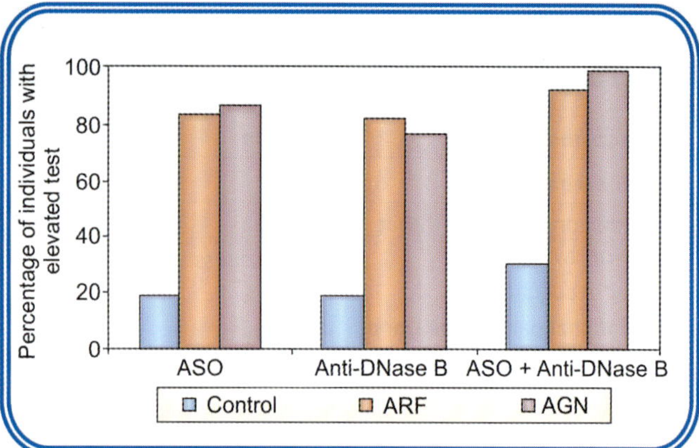

FIG. 3: Comparison of the percentage of individuals with acute rheumatic fever (ARF), acute glomerulonephritis (AGN), and healthy controls who have elevated streptococcal antibody titers. Note that when both ASO and anti-DNase B tests are done, the percentage of patients with ARF and AGN approach 92 and 98%, respectively. (ASO: antistreptolysin O)

TABLE 3: Age-stratified values of ASO and anti-DNase B in children between ages 2 years and 12 years.*

Age (years)	Geometric mean titer ASO	ULN ASO	Geometric mean anti-DNase B	ULN anti-DNase B
2	52	160	46	240
3	52	120	30	60
4	52	120	49	240
5	56	160	58	320
6	72	240	76	480
7	87	240	126	640
8	110	240	166	640
9	117	240	186	640
10	126	320	166	640
11	129	320	204	800
12	141	320	219	480

*Data from children residing in United States.

(ASO: antistreptolysin O; ULN: upper limit of normal)

therapy, all affect the level of titers. Episodes of infection are highest between 6 and 15 years who demonstrate higher level of antibodies than other age groups. Geographical areas with high endemicity have higher baseline antibody titers. The site of infection also alters the type and the briskness of the antibody response. The antibody response after streptococcal skin infection is not as strong when compared to that of upper respiratory infection. This is because the free cholesterol present in the skin binds to the streptolysin O molecule and decreases its antigenicity.[49]

Prompt initiation of antibiotic therapy will blunt the antibody response resulting in lower titers.[50] Demonstrating a rising titer from acute to convalescent sera will be a more accurate reflection of streptococcal infection.[51] Carriers do not experience a rise in streptococcal antibody titer when acute and convalescent sera are compared.[42]

Response to single antigen is seen in 80–85% of patients with rheumatic fever but 92–98% will show positive response when two antibodies are combined together.[52] Performing two tests will have higher predictive value for streptococcal infection than single test alone **(Fig. 3)**.

Practically, it may not be possible to show rising titers in all patients. Also, the patients might be in the convalescent phase at the time of first consultation. Hence, an "upper limit of normal (ULN)" value of antibody titers should be available for every population according to different age groups. It is defined as that titer exceeded by 20% of a normal population **(Table 3)**.[53]

The Antistreptolysin O Tests

The antibody produced against hemolytic toxin streptolysin O is the most widely available test. This antibody does not have a protective role in humans. The ASLO response starts after 1 week with maximal response being reached by 3–6 weeks after the infection.[54,55] The titer starts declining by 6–8 weeks after infection. Rarely, it can remain elevated indefinitely in the absence of recurrent streptococcal infection, the explanation for which is not clearly understood.

A single ASLO titer is generally considered to be modestly elevated if it is at least 240 Todd units in adults and 320 Todd units in children.[56]

The classic ASLO test is a neutralization assay where the antibodies in the serum neutralize the hemolytic activity of the streptolysin O toxin on RBCs. The highest dilution of the patient's serum showing no hemolysis is the endpoint. The reciprocal of this dilution is the titer given in Todd units or international units. The units depend on the reagent used whether Todd standard or the WHO international standard. Latex agglutination and nephelometric techniques are the recently available techniques, which are yet to be well standardized. Falsely high titers can be seen in chronic liver disease and hypercholesterolemia.

The Anti-DNase B Test

DNAases are extracellular antigens produced by Group A *Streptococcus* and are of mainly four types A, B, C, and D.[57] After infection titers begin to rise in 2 weeks and peak by 6–8 weeks. They remain elevated for a longer period than ASLO titers.[58]

Anti-DNase titers of 240 Todd units or greater in a school-aged patient and 120 Todd units or greater in an adult patient are viewed as elevated.[56] The same factors as age, geographical area, and endemicity that affect ASLO also affect anti-DNAase B. The difference is a stronger response after skin infection in case of anti-DNAase B. Their titers are not influenced liver disease, myeloma, or conditions resulting in hypercholesterolemic or hypergammaglobulinemic sera.

A false negative titer can be seen in acute hemorrhagic pancreatitis.[59]

The classic test is a neutralization assay where the antibodies to DNase B neutralize the enzymatic activity of DNase B. This prevents it from depolymerizing DNA that is bound to an indicator dye. Presently, there is no standardized universal reference serum available as there is for the ASLO test. Other less rigorously evaluated and standardized assay techniques have become available. The anti-DNase B test is more useful in glomerulonephritis that follows skin infection.

It can be used as an additional test in rheumatic fever when ASLO has not shown an adequate response. As described above, the addition of another test will increase the probability of finding past evidence of streptococcal infection **(Table 4)**.

Other Group A Streptococcal Extracellular Antibody Tests

Hyaluronidase is a substance secreted by the capsule of *Streptococcus* that elicits antibody response in the infected host. Streptokinase is another enzyme, which secretes and catalyzes the conversion of plasminogen to plasmin and

TABLE 4: Comparison of antistreptolysin (ASLO) O and anti-DNase B tests.[48]

	Antistreptolysin O	Anti-DNase B
Begins to rise:		
Peak	3–5 weeks	6–8 weeks
Decline	6–8 weeks	3 months
Response after infection:		
Upper respiratory infection	Good response	Good response
Skin infection	Feeble response	Good response
Influencing factors	False elevation	
Chronic liver disease	False elevation	
Hypergammaglobulinemia	False elevation	
Myeloma protein	False elevation	
High serum rheumatoid factor	False elevation	False low titer
Hypercholesterolemia Human serum DNases (as seen in pancreatitis) Clinical use	Evidence of preceding group A streptococcal infection in making a diagnosis of acute rheumatic fever or acute glomerulonephritis	Specifically useful in poststreptococcal glomerulonephritis following impetigo. Combined with ASLO gives a higher evidence of infection

thus has fibrinolytic properties.[60] The enzyme nicotinamide adenine dinucleotidase (NADase) has leukocytotoxic effects. However, antibody assay for above antigens is not commonly used for determination of GAS infection, because they are technically difficult to perform and are not commercially available. These tests are often available only in reference or research laboratories.[53,58,61]

Antibodies to Group A Streptococcal Somatic Antigens

The streptococcal cell wall has group A carbohydrate which forms the basis for Lancefield's classification. Studies have shown that following infection, titers of anti-A carbohydrate peak at 1–3 weeks and decline to normal levels 6–12 months later in most patients. However, in those patients with rheumatic valvular disease, elevated values persisted for 8 years or more.[62] This probably is due to antigen mimicry between these antigens and cardiac valvular tissue. This is also supported by the fact that the response is more brisk in rheumatic heart disease with valve involvement than in those without valvular involvement. As the reagent is not easily available, this test has limited use in clinical practice.

Streptococcal cell membrane contains the antigen M protein, which is responsible for different serotypes.

Presently, there are more than 100 known types. Hence, to use this test in clinical practice is not possible. The antibodies to M protein appear slowly over a period of several months. They have protective role in human host. Hence, they have been used in studies of M protein vaccines.[63]

Streptococcal antibody tests provide evidence only for an antecedent streptococcal infection. They are supportive and not diagnostic of ARF or poststreptococcal glomerulonephritis. Showing rising antibody titers in paired sera is definitive proof of a preceding streptococcal infection and when not feasible, occurrence of a single isolated titer that is high is also evidence of a previous streptococcal infection.

Use of these tests is not indicated in the management of routine uncomplicated streptococcal infections.

■ TREATMENT

Appropriate and timely therapy of streptococcal pharyngitis prevents an attack of rheumatic fever **(Table 5)**. Treatment makes the person noninfectious within 12 hours. Before selecting a treatment regimen, the clinical efficacy, compliance, cost, spectrum of activity, and side effects should be kept in mind. No regimen eradicates *Streptococcus*

TABLE 5: Primary prevention of rheumatic fever (treatment of streptococcal tonsillopharyngitis).[39]

Agent	Dose	Mode	Duration
Penicillins			
Penicillin V (phenoxymethyl penicillin)	Children: 250 mg 2–3 times daily for < 27 kg (60 lb); Children > 27 kg (60 lb), adolescents, and adults: 500 mg 2–3 times daily	Oral	10 days
	Or		
Amoxicillin	50 mg/kg once daily (maximum 1 g)	Oral	10 days
	Or		
Benzathine penicillin G	600,000 U for patients < 27 kg (60 lb); 1,200,000 U for patients > 27 kg (60 lb)	Intramuscular	Once
For individuals allergic to penicillin			
Narrow-spectrum cephalosporin[†] (cephalexin, cefadroxil)	Variable	Oral	10 days
	Or		
Clindamycin	20 mg/kg/day divided in 3 doses (maximum 1.8 g/day)	Oral	10 days
	Or		
Azithromycin	12 mg/kg once daily (maximum 500 mg)	Oral	5 days
	Or		
Clarithromycin	15 mg/kg/day divided into BID (maximum 250 mg BID)	Oral	10 days

The following are not acceptable: Sulfonamides, trimethoprim, tetracyclines, and fluoroquinolones.
[†]To be avoided in those with immediate (type I) hypersensitivity to a penicillin.

from the pharynx in 100% of treated patients, though in vitro susceptibility is 100% to β-lactam antibiotics.

Penicillins

Penicillins are the drugs of choice in treatment of streptococcal pharyngitis. The spectrum of activity of penicillin is narrow, resistance has never been demonstrated and it is inexpensive. They have been shown to be effective even when started after 9 days after the onset of acute illness. Hence, a delay of 24–48 hours, while awaiting culture results before initiating antibiotic therapy is started, does not increase the risk of rheumatic fever. Early diagnosis (e.g., by rapid antigen test) and therapy may reduce the period of infectivity and morbidity, which would allow the patient to return to normal activity sooner. Patients are noninfectious after 12–24 hours of antibiotic therapy. Intramuscular benzathine penicillin is the only drug that has been demonstrated in controlled studies to prevent initial attack of rheumatic fever.[64] Oral penicillins are equally effective though the level of evidence is lower.

Oral Penicillins

Oral penicillin V and amoxicillin are the oral antibiotics of choice, in those not allergic to penicillin. The dosage is 40 mg/kg/day (not to exceed 750 mg for those weighing < 27 kg) to be given in 2–3 divided doses. Usual recommendation is 250 mg twice daily for most children and for adolescents and adults, it is 500 mg two to three times daily. The duration is for total of 10 days, which should be strictly adhered to. Clinical trials have shown that once daily amoxicillin at the dose of 50 mg/kg (maximum 1,000 mg) for 10 days is effective for streptococcal pharyngitis.[65-68] This is relatively inexpensive and once daily dose will enhance the compliance.

Benzathine Penicillin G

Intramuscular benzathine penicillin G should be considered for those patients where adherence to 10 days of therapy is difficult and those with family history of rheumatic heart disease. Children who are at higher risk because of overcrowding and low socioeconomic condition should also be given the parenteral preparation. It should be administered as a single dose, 6 million units for those <27 kg and 12 million units for those >27 kg. It should be injected into large muscle mass. The injection is very painful. Warming the medication to room temperature before administration reduces the discomfort. Combinations with procaine penicillin are less painful. The combination of 900,000 U of benzathine penicillin G and 300,000 U of procaine penicillin G is the dose for smaller children.[69] The efficacy of this combination for teenagers and adults requires further investigation. Allergic reactions to parenteral penicillins are known to occur. It can be acute in the form of urticaria and angioedema or delayed serum sickness-like reaction. Reactions are more common in adults than in children.

Oral Cephalosporins

Cephalosporins are as effective as penicillins in eradication of streptococci from pharynx. They should not be used in patients who have shown immediate hypersensitivity reaction to penicillin. Cross-reaction occurs in 10% of patients allergic to penicillin. Narrow-spectrum cephalosporins such as cefadroxil and cephalexin are preferred as broad-spectrum cephalosporins such as cefuroxime, cefixime, cefdinir, and cefpodoxime induce antibiotic resistance. 10 days course of a narrow-spectrum oral cephalosporin is recommended for most penicillin allergic individuals. Some studies have shown that 5 days course of broad-spectrum cephalosporin is as equally effective as 10 days of oral penicillin.[70-73] These regimens have not been approved by the Food and Drug Administration (FDA).

Oral Clindamycin

Reported rate of clindamycin resistance among group A streptococci is <1% isolates in the United States and is a reasonable alternative for treating penicillin allergic patients.

Macrolides

For patients allergic to penicillin, macrolides are safe alternatives. Duration of treatment is 10 days for erythromycin and clindamycin and 5 days for azithromycin. Macrolides (erythromycin and clarithromycin) and, to a lesser extent, Azalides (azithromycin) may cause prolongation of the QT interval. The effect is dose dependent. Macrolides use cytochrome P-450 3A for metabolism. Those drugs that inhibit cytochrome P-450 3A such as azole antifungal agents, HIV protease inhibitors, and some selective serotonin reuptake inhibitor antidepressants should not be taken concurrently with macrolides.[74,75] Streptococci are developing resistance to macrolides and up to 5–8% isolates have demonstrated resistance resulting in treatment failure.[76]

Antibiotics Not Recommended

Tetracyclines should not be used because of the high prevalence of resistance. Sulfonamides and cotrimoxazole do not eradicate streptococci in patients with pharyngitis and should not be used to treat active infections.[77] Older fluoroquinolones such as ciprofloxacin have limited activity while newer fluoroquinolones are expensive and have an unnecessarily broad spectrum of activity and, therefore, they are not recommended for routine treatment.[78]

Repeat throat swab cultures are recommended in only those who remain symptomatic or those who have had rheumatic fever because of high risk of recurrence. It should be done 2–7 days post-treatment. Treatment failure can occur with oral penicillin than with benzathine penicillin. Carriers account for part of the treatment failure patients.[79] Asymptomatic patients with treatment failure should be given a second course only if they have had rheumatic fever in themselves or in the family. Symptomatic individuals who have persistent streptococci can be given an alternative oral agent or an intramuscular benzathine penicillin. Narrow-spectrum cephalosporins, clindamycin or amoxicillin–clavulanic acid, or the combination of penicillin with rifampin is reasonable alternative agents.

Following hand hygiene, respiratory etiquette reduces the spread of infection.

Carriers

Streptococcal carriers have no risk for development of rheumatic fever or suppurative complications. They do not have positive serological tests. They do not play a role in the spread of streptococci to people around them.[42] When they have superimposed viral pharyngitis, it is impossible to distinguish carriers from infected individuals. A single course of appropriate antibiotic therapy should be administered to any patient with acute pharyngitis and evidence of GAS by a throat swab culture or an antigen detection test. Asymptomatic chronic streptococcal carriers usually do not need to be identified or treated with antibiotics.

■ SECONDARY PREVENTION: PREVENTION OF RECURRENT ATTACKS OF RHEUMATIC FEVER

General Considerations

An individual with a past history of even a single episode of rheumatic fever, when he develops an episode of streptococcal pharyngitis, is at high risk for a recurrent attack of rheumatic fever. The recurrent attack can worsen the damage to cardiac tissue that occurred after the first attack or may cause new onset of rheumatic heart disease in those who did not develop cardiac involvement in first attack. The most effective way to prevent the development of severe rheumatic heart disease is by preventing repeat episodes of streptococcal pharyngitis. The repeat episode may be asymptomatic and even when symptomatic optimal treatment may not prevent the second attack of rheumatic fever. This is because the individual would have already developed some immune response to the first attack, which gets boosted with repeat infection. Prevention, therefore, requires continuous prophylaxis rather than prompt recognition and treatment of acute episodes. Therefore, children with past histories of rheumatic fever (including those with only Sydenham chorea) and those with rheumatic heart disease require continuous prophylaxis. A full course of penicillin (as outlined in **Table 5**) should be given to patients with ARF to eradicate residual organism, even if a throat culture is negative. All streptococcal infections that occur in family members of patients with rheumatic fever should be treated promptly.

Duration of Prophylaxis

Risk of recurrence of rheumatic fever depends on several factors. Risk of streptococcal pharyngitis is high in children, teachers, healthcare personnel, military recruits, and people living in crowded conditions and low socioeconomic status. Multiple previous attacks also increase the risk. The risk increases if the individual has had carditis in previous attack and more so if there was valvular involvement. When deciding the duration of prophylaxis, all the above factors must be taken into consideration **(Table 6)**. With each attack, the severity of cardiac involvement worsens.[80-82] Therefore, people with earlier episodes of carditis ideally require lifelong prophylaxis or at least till the age of 40 years. Those with carditis and no residual disease need prophylaxis for 10 years or till age of 21 years whichever is longer. People with rheumatic fever with no carditis should be given prophylaxis for 5 years or till 21 years of age whichever is longer.

Regimen for Prevention of Recurrent Rheumatic Fever (Table 7)

Intramuscular Benzathine Penicillin G

An injection of 12 million units or 6 million units based on weight every 3 weeks is the recommended regimen for secondary prevention.[83,84]

TABLE 6: Duration of secondary rheumatic fever prophylaxis.[39]

Category	Duration after last attack
Rheumatic fever with carditis and residual heart disease (persistent valvular disease*)	10 years or until 40 years of age (whichever is longer), sometimes lifelong prophylaxis if valve surgery or replacement
Rheumatic fever with mild carditis	10 years or until 25 years of age (whichever is longer)
Rheumatic fever without carditis	5 years or until 18 years of age (whichever is longer)

*Clinical or echocardiographic evidence.

TABLE 7: Secondary prevention of rheumatic fever (prevention of recurrent attacks).[39]

Agent	Dose	Mode
Benzathine penicillin G	600,000 U for children < 27 kg (60 lb), 1,200,000 U for those > 27 kg (60 lb) every 3 weeks	Intramuscular
Penicillin V	250 mg twice daily	Oral
Erythromycin	20 mg/kg/dose Maximum 500 mg—twice a day	Oral

Oral Antibiotics

Compliance is a major concern with oral agents as all of them need to be taken every day. Results of poor compliance can be tragic. Patients need careful and repeated instructions about the importance of continuing prophylaxis. Most failures of prophylaxis occur in nonadherent patients. Even with good compliance, the risk of recurrence is higher in individuals receiving oral prophylaxis.[79] Oral agents are more appropriate for patients at lower risk for rheumatic fever recurrence. It may be considered in patients when they have reached late adolescence or young adulthood and are free of rheumatic attacks for at least 5 years.

Penicillin V

The recommended oral agent is penicillin V at the dose of 250 mg twice daily to all age groups. There are no published data about the use of other penicillins, macrolides, azalides, or cephalosporins for the secondary prevention of rheumatic fever.

Macrolides

For the patients who are allergic to penicillin, an oral macrolide can be substituted. They have the problem of causing QT prolongation as mentioned earlier. Drug interaction should be kept in mind when combining with agents causing inhibition of cytochrome P-450 3A.[74,75]

Poststreptococcal Reactive Arthritis

Poststreptococcal reactive arthritis is defined as inflammatory arthritis of ≥1 joint associated with a recent GAS infection in a patient who does not fulfill the Jones criteria for the diagnosis of ARF.[85] The arthritis in rheumatic fever occurs in 14–21 days after an episode of pharyngitis and responds dramatically to aspirin. PSRA occurs 10 days after the streptococcal pharyngitis and does not respond readily to aspirin. Joint involvement is asymmetrical, more common in upper extremity, nonmigratory, and can involve small joints. Involvement of axial skeleton and sacroiliac joint is uncommon. It can be mono-, oligo-, or polyarthritis. The typical arthritis in ARF is migratory polyarthritis of large joints sparing the axial skeleton. Arthritis in PSRA is cumulative and persistent whereas that in rheumatic fever is transient. The age distribution of PSRA is bimodal with peak at ages of 8–14 years and another at age 21–37 years. The typical age for rheumatic fever is 5–15 years. Extra-articular manifestations of erythema nodosum, uveitis, and glomerulonephritis can occur. In some of the studies, 83% of isolates were group A *Streptococcus*. Significant numbers belonged to group B, group C, or G. There is a high prevalence of upper limb joint involvement in PSRA, which is uncommon in gonococcal arthritis or enteric related reactive arthritis.

Glomerulonephritis has been recorded in some cases of PSRA. This feature is not seen in rheumatic fever. But, it is important to observe all patients with PSRA for associated underlying carditis for several months, as some patients have been known to develop valvular disease.[86,87] Some authorities recommend prophylaxis for 1 year but the effectiveness is not well established. Prophylaxis can be discontinued at the end of 1 year if there is no evidence of valvular disease.

There is a lot of unanswered questions about PSRA. PSRA is a heterogeneous entity. It is a distinct syndrome or the manifestation of ARF is not clear.[87] It is the episode of pharyngitis or is it due to streptococcal infection has not yet been established.

◼ PEDIATRIC AUTOIMMUNE NEUROPSYCHIATRIC DISORDERS ASSOCIATED WITH STREPTOCOCCAL INFECTIONS

It has been found that some patients with obsessive compulsive and tic disorders have an autoimmune response to streptococcal infection.[88] Streptococcal antigens crossreacts with brain tissue in basal ganglia similar to occurrence of Sydenham's chorea. Working criteria for diagnosis of PANDAS have been proposed.

- Presence of diagnostic criteria for obsessive–compulsive disorder (OCD) and/or tic disorder
- Pediatric onset, between 3 years and the beginning of puberty
- Episodic course of symptom severity, characterized by acute, severe onset, and dramatic symptom exacerbations
- Temporal relationship between symptom onset and/or exacerbation and group A β-hemolytic streptococcal infections (GABHS)
- Association with neurologic abnormalities, such as motor hyperactivity, tics, or choreiform movements

Hence, if secondary prophylaxis can prevent recurrent episodes of chorea then we can postulate that recurrences of these disorders could also be prevented. Because of the autoimmune nature of the condition, there have been trials of immunotherapy in form of plasma exchange and immunoglobulin infusion. Till date, it is an unproven hypothesis. The causal relation between streptococcal infection and PANDAS is not established. There is no recommendation for routine testing for streptococcal infection, antimicrobial prophylaxis, or immunosuppressive therapy.[89,90]

◼ SUMMARY

Group A β-hemolytic streptococcal sore throat is the first event in the natural history of ARF. It should be diagnosed, differentiated from nonstreptococcal pharyngitis, and treated in time. Obtaining acute and convalescent sera showing a rise in antibody titer is definitive proof of a preceding streptococcal infection. However, because it is not always easy or feasible to obtain paired sera, it must be emphasized that the occurrence of a single isolated titer that is high is also evidence of a previous streptococcal infection. Streptococcal antibody tests provide evidence only for an antecedent streptococcal infection. Together with the clinical findings, the tests may support the diagnosis of ARF and poststreptococcal glomerulonephritis but are not by themselves diagnostic of these diseases. It cannot be emphasized too strongly that the use of streptococcal antibodies is not indicated in the management of routine uncomplicated streptococcal infections. Prevention of both initial and recurrent attacks of rheumatic fever depends on control of GABHS tonsillopharyngitis (strep throat). Prevention of first attacks (primary prevention) is accomplished by proper identification and adequate antibiotic treatment of streptococcal infections. The individual who has had an attack of rheumatic fever is at high risk of developing recurrences after subsequent GAS pharyngitis and needs continuous antimicrobial prophylaxis for years to prevent such recurrences (secondary prevention).

"As it takes two to make a quarrel, so it takes two to make a disease, the microbe and its host."

—Charles V Chaplin

■ ACKNOWLEDGMENT

Our grateful thanks to the American Heart Association (AHA) for the kind permission. Reproduced with permission. Circulation. 2009;119:1542-51@2009 American Heart Association Inc.

■ REFERENCES

1. Siegel AC, Johnson EE, Stollerman GH. Controlled studies of a streptococcal pharyngitis in a pediatric population, 1: factors related to the attack rate of rheumatic fever. N Engl J Med. 1961;265:559-65.

2. Denny FW, Wannamaker LW, Brink WR, Rammelkamp CH Jr., Custer EA. Prevention of rheumatic fever: treatment of the preceding streptococcal infection. JAMA. 1950;143:151-3.

3. Dajani AS. Current status of nonsuppurative complications of group A streptococci. Pediatr Infect Dis J. 1991;10 (suppl):S25-7.

4. Smith TD, Wilkinson V, Kaplan EL. Group A *Streptococcus*-associated upper respiratory tract infections in a day-care center. Pediatrics. 1989;83:380-4.

5. Falck G, Kjellander J. Outbreak of group A streptococcal infection in a day-care center. Pediatr Infect Dis J. 1992;11:914-9.

6. Stollerman GH, Siegel AC, Johnson EE. Variable epidemiology of streptococcal disease and the changing pattern of rheumatic fever. Mod Concepts Cardiovasc Dis. 1965;34:45-8.

7. Stollerman GH. Nephritogenic and rheumatogenic group A streptococci. J Infect Dis. 1969;120:258-63.

8. Bisno AL. The concept of rheumatogenic and non-rheumatogenic group A streptococci. In: Read SE, Zabriski JB (Eds). Streptococcal diseases and the immune response. New York, NY: Academic Press; 1980. p. 789.

9. Rammelkamp CH, Denny FW, Wannamaker LW. Studies on the epidemiology of rheumatic fever in the armed services. In: Thomas L (Ed). Rheumatic Fever. Minneapolis, Minnesota, United States: University of Minnesota Press Minneapolis; 1952. pp. 72-89.

10. Stetson CA. The relation of antibody response to rheumatic fever. In: McCarty M (Ed). Streptococcal Infections. New York: Columbia University Press; 1954. pp. 208-18.

11. Coburn AF, Pauli RH. Studies on the immune response of the rheumatic subject and its relationship to activity of the rheumatic process. IV. Characteristics of strains of hemolytic streptococci, effective and non-effective in initiating rheumatic activity. J Clin Invest. 1935;14:755-62.

12. Rammelkamp CH Jr, Weaver RS. Acute glomerulonephritis. The significance of the variations in the incidence of the disease. J Clin Invest. 1953;32:345-58.

13. Wannamaker LW. Differences between streptococcal infections of the throat and of the skin. N Engl J Med. 1970;282:23.

14. Bisno AL, Pearce IA, Wall HP, Moody MD, Stollermann GH. Contrasting epidemiology of acute rheumatic fever and acute glomerulonephritis. Nature of the antecedent streptococcal infection. N Engl J Med. 1970;283:561-5.

15. Potter EV, Svartman M, Mohammed I, Cox R, Poon-King T, Earle DP, et al. Tropical acute rheumatic fever and associated streptococcal infections compared with concurrent acute glomerulonephritis. J Pediatr. 1978;92:325-33.

16. Stollerman GH. Rheumatic Fever. Lancet. 1997;349:935-42.

17. Stollerman GH. Can we eradicate rheumatic fever in the 21st century? Indian Heart J. 2001;53(1):25-34.

18. Frank PF, Stollerman GH, Miller LF. Protection of a military population from rheumatic fever. JAMA. 1965;193:775-83.

19. Beachey EH, Stollerman GH, Chiang EY, Chiang TM, Seyer JM, Kang AH. Purification and properties of M protein extracted from group A streptococci with pepsin. Covalent structure of the amino terminal region of type 24 M antigen. J Exp Med. 1977;145:1469-83.

20. Beachey EH, Stollerman GH, Johnson RH, Ofek I, Bisno AL. Human immune response to immunization with a structurally defined polypeptide fragment of streptococcal M protein. J Exp Med. 1979;150:862-77.

21. Bessen DE, Jones KF, Fischetti VA. Evidence for two distinct classes of streptococcal M-protein and their relationship to rheumatic fever. J Exp Med. 1989;169:269-83.

22. Bessen DE, Veasy LG, Hill HR, Augustine NH, Fischetti VA. Serologic evidence for a class I group A streptococcal infection among rheumatic fever patients. J Infect Dis. 1995;172:1608-11.

23. Bessen DE, Sotir CM, Readdy TL, Hollingshead SK. Genetic correlates of throat and skin isolates of group A streptococci. J Infect Dis. 1996;174:896-900.

24. Dale JB, Chiang EC. Intranasal immunization with recombinant group A streptococcal M fragment fused to the B subunit of Escherichia coli labile toxin protects mice against systemic challenge infections. J Infect Dis. 1995;171:1038-41.

25. Federle MJ, McIver KS, Scott JR. A response regulator that represses transcription of several virulence operons in the group A *Streptococcus*. J Bacteriol. 1999;181:3649-57.

26. Stollerman GH, Ekstedt RD, Cohen IR. Natural resistance of germ-free mice and colostrum-deprived piglets to group A streptococci. J Immunol. 1965;95:131-40.

27. Beachey EH, Ofek I. Epithelial cell binding of group A streptococci by lipoteichoic acid on fimbriae denuded of M protein. J Exp Med. 1976;143:759-71.

28. Lancefield RC. Specific relationship of cell composition to biological activity of hemolytic streptococci. Harvey Lectures (1940–1941). 1941;35:251.

29. Wilson AT. The relative importance of the capsule and the M antigen in determining colony form of group A streptococci. J Exp Med. 1959;109:257.

30. Stollerman GH, Ekstedt R. Long chain formation by strains of Group A streptococci in the presence of homologous antiserum: a type-specific reaction. J Exp Med. 1957;106:345-56.

31. Stollerman GH, Rytel M, Ortiz J. Accessory plasma factors involved in the bactericidal test for type-specific antibody to group A streptococci: II. Human plasma cofactors(s) enhancing opsonization of encapsulated organisms. J Exp Med. 1963;117: 1-17.

32. Rothbard S, Watson RF. Variation occurring in group A streptococci during human infection. Progressive loss of M substance correlated with increasing susceptibility to bacteriostasis. J Exp Med. 1948;87:521-33.

33. Ozeri V, Rosenhine I, Mosher DF, Fässler R, Hanski E. Roles of integrins and fibronectin in the entry of *Streptococcus pyogenes* into cells via protein F1. Mol Microbiol. 1998;30:625-37.

34. Neeman R, Keller N, Barzilai A, Korenman Z, Sela S. Prevalence of internalization-associated gene, prtF1, among persisting group-A *Streptococcus* strains isolated from asymptomatic carriers. Lancet. 1998;352:1974-7.

35. Jadoun J, Sela S. Mutation in csrR global regulator reduces Streptococcus pyogenes internalization. Microbiol Pathogen. 2000;29:311-7.

36. Ravins M, Jaffe J, Hanski E, Shetzigovski I, Natanson-Yaron S, Moses AE. Characterization of a mouse-passaged highly encapsulated variant of group A *Streptococcus* in vitro and in vivo studies. J Infect Dis. 2000;182:1702-11.

37. Dougherty BA, van de Rijn I. Molecular characterization of has A from an operon required for hyaluronic acid synthesis in group A streptococci. J Biol Chem. 1994;269:169-75.

38. Ashbaugh CD, Warren HB, Carey VJ, Wessels MR. Molecular analysis of the role of the group A streptococcal cysteine proteinase, hyaluronic acid capsule and M protein in a murine model of human invasive soft tissue infections. J Clin Invest. 1998;102:550-60.

39. Working Group on Pediatric Acute Rheumatic Fever and Cardiology Chapter of Indian Academy of Pediatrics, Saxena A, Kumar RK, Gera RP, Radhakrishnan S, Mishra S, et al. Consensus guidelines on pediatric acute rheumatic fever and rheumatic heart disease. Indian Pediatr. 2008;45(7):565-73.

40. Bisno AL, Gerber AM, Gwaltney JM Jr, Kaplan EL, Schwartz RH. Infectious Diseases Society of America. Practice guidelines for the diagnosis and management of group A streptococcal pharyngitis. Clin Infect Dis. 2002;35:113-25.

41. Kaplan E, Top F Jr, Dudding B, Wannamaker LW. Diagnosis of streptococcal pharyngitis: differentiation of active infection from the carrier state in the symptomatic child. J Infect Dis. 1971;123:490-501.

42. Kaplan E. The group A streptococcal upper respiratory tract carrier state: an enigma. J Pediatr. 1980;97:337-45.

43. Dunlap MB, Bergin JW. Subsequent health of former carriers of hemolytic streptococci. N Y State J Med. 1973;73:1875-80.

44. American Academy of Pediatrics, Committee on Infectious Diseases. Red Book: Report of the Committee on Infectious Diseases, 27th edition. Elk Grove Village, Ill: American Academy of Pediatrics; 2006.

45. Webb KH. Does culture confirmation of high-sensitivity rapid streptococcal tests make sense? A medical decision analysis. Pediatrics. 1998;101:E2.

46. Gerber MA, Tanz RR, Kabat W, Dennis E, Bell GL, Kaplan EL, et al. Optical immunoassay test for group A beta-hemolytic streptococcal pharyngitis: an ice-based, multicenter investigation. JAMA. 1997;277:899-903.

47. Cohen JF, Bertille N, Cohen R, Chalumeau M. Rapid antigen detection test for group A *Streptococcus* in children with pharyngitis. Cochrane Database Syst Rev.2016;7(7):CD010502.

48. Shet A, Kaplan EL. Clinical use and interpretation of group A streptococcal antibody tests: a practical approach for the pediatrician or primary care physician. Pediatr Infect Dis J. 2002;21:420-30.

49. Kaplan E, Anthony B, Chapman S, Ayoub EM, Wannamaker LW. The influence of the site of infection on the immune response to group A streptococci. J Clin Invest. 1970;49:1405-14.

50. Rantz LA, Boisvert PJ, Spink WW. Hemolytic streptococcal sore throat: antibody response following treatment with penicillin, sulfadiazine, and salicylates. Science. 1946:103;352-3.

51. Committee on Rheumatic Fever, Endocarditis and Kawasaki Disease of the Council on Cardiovascular Disease in the Young, the American Heart Association. Treatment of acute streptococcal pharyngitis and prevention of Rheumatic Fever: A Statement for Health Professionals. Pediatrics. 1995;96:758-64.

52. Ayoub E, Wannamaker L. Evaluation of the streptococcal deoxyribonuclease B and diphosphopyridine nucleotidase antibody tests in acute rheumatic fever and acute glomerulonephritis. Pediatrics. 1962;29:527-38.

53. Wannamaker L, Ayoub E. Antibody titers in acute rheumatic fever. Circulation. 1960;21:598-614.

54. McCarty M. The antibody response to streptococcal infections. In: McCarty M (Ed). Streptococcal infections. New York: Columbia University Press; 1954. pp. 130-42.

55. Kaplan E, Ferrieri P, Wannamaker L. Comparison of the antibody response to streptococcal cellular and extracellular antigens in acute pharyngitis. J Pediatr. 1974;84:21-8.

56. Dajani AS. Special writing group of the Committee on Rheumatic fever, Endocarditis and Kawasaki disease of the Council of Cardiovascular disease in the young of the American Heart Association. Guidelines for the diagnosis of rheumatic fever: Jones criteria, 1992 Update. JAMA. 1992;268:2069-73.

57. Wannamaker LW, Yasminch W. Streptococcal nucleases: I. Further studies on the A, B, and C enzymes. J Exp Med. 1967;126:475-96.

58. Wannamaker LW. Immunology of streptococci. In: Good RA, Nahmias AJ, O'Reilly RJ (Eds). Comprehensive immunology: immunology of human infection. New York: Plenum; 1981. pp. 47-91.

59. Klein GC. Immune response to streptococcal infection. In: Rose N, Friedman H (Eds). Manual of clinical immunology. Washington, DC: American Society for Microbiology; 1980. pp. 431-40.

60. Tillett WS. Studies on the enzymatic lysis of fibrin and inflammatory exudates of products of hemolytic streptococci. Harvey Lect. 1952;45:149.

61. Stollerman GH, Lewis AJ, Schultz I, Angelo T. Relationship of immune response to group a streptococci to the course of acute, chronic and recurrent rheumatic fever. Am J Med. 1956;20: 163-9.

62. Dudding BA, Ayoub EM. Persistence of streptococcal group A antibody in patients with rheumatic valvular disease. J Exp Med. 1968;128:1081-98.

63. Fischetti V. Streptococcal M protein. Sci Am. 1991;64:58-65.

64. Wannamaker LW, Rammelkamp CH Jr, Denny FW, Brink WR, Houser HB, Hahn EO, et al. Prophylaxis of acute rheumatic fever by treatment of preceding streptococcal infection with various amounts of depot penicillin. Am J Med. 1951;10:673-95.

65. Shvartzman P, Tabenkin H, Rosentzwaig A, Dolginov F. Treatment of streptococcal pharyngitis with amoxicillin once a day. BMJ. 1993;306:1170-2.

66. Feder HM Jr, Gerber MA, Randolph MF, Stelmach PS, Kaplan EL. Once-daily therapy for streptococcal pharyngitis with amoxicillin. Pediatrics. 1999;103:47-51.

67. Clegg HW, Ryan AG, Dallas SD, Kaplan EL, Johnson DR, Norton HJ, et al. Treatment of streptococcal pharyngitis with once-daily compared with twice-daily amoxicillin: a noninferiority trial. Pediatr Infect Dis J. 2006;25:761-7.

68. Lennon DR, Farrell E, Martin DR, Stewart JM. Once-daily amoxicillin versus twice-daily penicillin V in group A beta-hemolytic streptococcal pharyngitis. Arch Dis Child. 2008;93:474-8.

69. Bass JW, Crast FW, Knowles CR, Onufer CN. Streptococcal pharyngitisin children: a comparison of four treatment schedules with intramuscular penicillin G benzathine. JAMA. 1976;235:1112-6.

70. Tack KJ, Hedrick JA, Rothstein E, Nemeth MA, Keyserling C, Pichichero ME. Cefdinir Pediatric Pharyngitis Study Group. A study of 5-day cefdinir treatment for streptococcal pharyngitis in children. Arch Pediatr Adolesc Med. 1997;151:45-9.

71. Pichichero ME, Gooch WM, Rodriguez W, Blumer JL, Aronoff SC, Jacobs RF, et al. Effective short-course treatment of acute group A beta-hemolytic streptococcal tonsillopharyngitis: ten days of penicillin V vs 5 days or 10 days of cefpodoxime therapy in children. Arch Pediatr Adolesc Med. 1994;148:1053-60.

72. Aujard Y, Boucot I, Brahimi N, Chiche D, Bingen E. Comparative efficacy and safety of four-day cefuroxime axetil and ten-day penicillin treatment of group A beta-hemolytic streptococcal pharyngitis in children. Pediatr Infect Dis J. 1995;14:295-300.

73. Dajani AS. Pharyngitis/tonsillitis: European and United States experience with cefpodoxime proxetil. Pediatr Infect Dis J. 1995;14(suppl):S7-11.

74. Ray WA, Murray KT, Meredith S, Narasimhulu SS, Hall K, Stein CM. Oral erythromycin and the risk of sudden death from cardiac causes. N Engl J Med. 2004;351:1089-96.

75. Huang BH, Wu CH, Hsia CP, Yin Chen C. Azithromycin-induced torsade de pointes. Pacing Clin Electrophysiol. 2007;30:1579-82.

76. Tanz RR, Shulman ST, Shortridge VD, Kabat W, Kabat K, Cederlund E, et al. North American Streptococcal Pharyngitis Surveillance Group. Community-based surveillance in the United States of macrolide-resistant pediatric pharyngeal group A streptococci during 3 respiratory disease seasons. Clin Infect Dis. 2004;39:1794-801.

77. Gerber MA. Antibiotic resistance in group A streptococci. Pediatr Clin North Am. 1995;42:539-51.

78. Wickman PA, Black JA, Moland ES, Thomson KS. In vitro activities of DX-619 and other comparison quinolones against Gram-positive cocci. Antimicrob Agents Chemother. 2006;50:2255-7.

79. Feinstein AR, Wood HF, Epstein JA, Taranta A, Simpson R, Tursky E. A controlled study of three methods of prophylaxis against streptococcal infection in a population of rheumatic children, II: results of the first three years of the study, including methods for evaluating the maintenance of oral prophylaxis. N Engl J Med. 1959;260:697-702.

80. Majeed HA, Yousof AM, Khuffash FA, Yusuf AR, Farwana S, Khan N. The natural history of acute rheumatic fever in Kuwait: a prospective six year follow-up report. J Chronic Dis. 1986;39:361-9.

81. Taranta A, Kleinberg E, Feinstein AR, Wood HF, Simpson R, Stollerman G. Rheumatic fever in children and adolescents: a long-term epidemiologic study of subsequent prophylaxis, streptococcal infections, and clinical sequelae, V: relation of the rheumatic fever recurrence rate per streptococcal infection to pre-existing clinical features of the patients. Ann Intern Med. 1964;60(Suppl 5):58-7.

82. Kuttner AG, Mayer FE. Carditis during second attacks of rheumatic fever: its incidence in patients without clinical evidence of cardiac involvement in their initial rheumatic episode. N Engl J Med. 1963;268:1259-61.

83. Lue HC, Wu MH, Hsieh KH, Lin GJ, Hsieh RP, Chiou JF. Rheumatic fever recurrences: controlled study of a 3-week versus 4-week benzathine penicillin prevention programs. J Pediatr. 1986;108:299-304.

84. Lue HC, Wu MH, Wang JK, Wu FF, Wu YN. Long-term outcome of patients with rheumatic fever receiving benzathine penicillin G prophylaxis every three weeks versus every four weeks. J Pediatr. 1994;125 (pt 1):812-6.

85. Bawazir Y, Towheed T, Anastassiades T. Post-Streptococcal reactive arthritis. Curr Rheumatol Rev. 2020;16(1):2-8.

86. Ahmed S, Ayoub EM, Scornik JC, Wang CY, She JX. Poststreptococcal reactive arthritis: clinical characteristics and association with HLA-DR alleles. Arthritis Rheum. 1998;41:1096-102.

87. Mackie SL, Keat A. Poststreptococcal reactive arthritis: what is it and how to we know? Rheumatology. 2004;43:949-54.

88. Swedo SE, Leonard HL, Garvey M, Mittleman B, Mittleman B, Allen AJ, et al. Pediatric autoimmune neuropsychiatric disorders associated with streptococcal infections: clinical description of the first 50 cases [published correction appears in Am J Psychiatry 1998;155:578]. Am J Psychiatry. 1998;155:264-71.

89. Kurlan R, Kaplan EL. The pediatric autoimmune neuropsychiatric disorders associated with streptococcal infections (PANDAS) etiology for tics and obsessive-compulsive symptoms: hypothesis or entity? Practical considerations for the clinician. Pediatrics. 2004;113:883-6.

90. Prato A, Gulisano M, Scerbo M, Barone R, Vicario CM, Rizzo R. Diagnostic Approach to Pediatric Autoimmune Neuropsychiatric Disorders Associated with Streptococcal Infections (PANDAS): A narrative review of literature data. Front Pediatr. 2021;9:746639.

6

Laboratory Diagnosis of Group A β-hemolytic Streptococcal Infections

Sneha K Chunchanur

■ INTRODUCTION

Group A β-hemolytic *Streptococcus* (GAS), also known as *Streptococcus pyogenes*, is an important cause of acute pharyngitis, a common childhood infection. Streptococcal pharyngitis can affect 20–30% of children worldwide, more so in developing countries such as ours. GAS pharyngitis can lead to suppurative (peritonsillar abscesses, cervical lymphadenitis, and sepsis) and nonsuppurative complications [acute rheumatic fever (ARF) and acute glomerulonephritis]. Rheumatic heart disease (RHD), resulting from immune-inflammatory injury to cardiac valves, is a chronic sequel of ARF.[1]

Group A *Streptococcus* is one of the aggressive pathogens encountered in clinical microbiology laboratories. GAS strains express many virulence factors, viz., surface protein M, streptolysins, streptokinase, hyaluronidase, peptidoglycan, teichoic acid, C5a peptidase, streptolysin O and S. Streptolysin O and S are also of diagnostic importance as they form β-hemolytic pattern on blood agar (BA) plates, which is used as a guide to identify GAS,[2] and determination of antistreptolysin O antibodies (ASOs) is used for confirming a diagnosis of GAS pharyngitis as well as ARF.[3]

After an episode of acute pharyngitis, GAS can lead to autoimmunity by way of molecular mimicry and cause ARF in genetically susceptible individuals.[4] ARF/RHD results from a complex interplay among multiple streptococcal antigens, cross-reactive antibodies, and multipronged immune targets. Streptococcal M protein of GAS is known to share an α-helical coiled structure with cardiac protein such as myosin and antibodies from ARF patients are known to cross-react with both M protein and heart tissue. However, molecular pathways linking GAS to ARF/RHD are yet to be completely delineated.[5]

The major virulence factor in GAS, the M protein, is encoded by *emm* gene. With the advent of molecular techniques, sequence-based emm typing (gold standard for GAS molecular typing) is replacing classical serotyping. Heterogeneity of GAS *emm* types coupled with high burden of ARF/RHD in India highlights the need for looking into their virulence potential. Profiling of superantigen, streptococcal pyrogenic exotoxins (SPEs), serves as alternative molecular typing tool.[6] SPEs are erythrogenic toxins produced by lysogenic strains activating macrophages and T-helper cells inducing the release of powerful immune mediators including interleukin-1 (IL-1), IL-2, IL-6, tumor necrosis factor-alpha (TNF-α), TNF-β, interferons, and cytokines, which induce shock and organ failure. Molecular typing of GAS is crucial for providing information on possible shifts in clone prevalence, as well as for the early detection of clones with enhanced virulence, transmission, or antimicrobial resistance (AMR).[6]

Despite few reports of diminished in-vitro susceptibility to penicillin, GAS continues to be exquisitely susceptible to penicillin. Simultaneously, resistance to other antibiotics such as macrolides is on the rise, which can be monitored by regular AMR testing of GAS strains.[7]

Estimated average prevalence of ARF/RHD in India is 0.5/1,000 children aged 5–15 years and there are expected to be more than 3.6 million patients of RHD as per 2011 census. Almost 44,000 patients are added every year, and expected mortality is 1.5–3.3% per year.[8] Though reports show declining trend in the incidence of ARF/RHD,[8] these two complications continue to affect children and engage cardiologists and cardiac surgeons alike. Associated morbidity/mortality and later cardiac complications necessitating surgical intervention lead to heavy socioeconomic burden on the families of affected children.[3]

"A stitch in time saves nine". RHD diagnosed early with timely institution of secondary prophylaxis can prevent the progression to permanent valve damage due to recurrent episodes of ARF. WHO experts endorse a multilevel approach for the control and/or eradication of RF/RHD ranging from primordial prevention to tertiary prevention.[1] Strong *primary* prevention (active case detection and treatment of streptococcal sore throat) along with *secondary* prevention is the key strategy. This in turn relies on timely microbiological diagnosis of GAS pharyngitis in clinically suspected cases.[3]

Though throat swab culture is considered the gold standard, rapid diagnostic tests (RDTs) for antigen detection are known to be used for diagnosis of GAS pharyngitis in Indian settings. They offer point-of-care diagnostics and thereby reduce the time to initiate treatment and help in improving antibiotic stewardship in pediatrics.[9]

LABORATORY DIAGNOSIS

"Laboratory report can only be as good as the sample collected."

Sample Collection and Transportation[10]

A well-taken throat swab determines the success of isolating GAS in culture.

Samples have to be collected prior to starting antibiotic treatment.

Swabs should be taken from tonsillar areas and posterior pharyngeal wall, taking care not to touch the oral cavity.

They should be transported to the laboratory as soon as possible, preferably using transport media such as Pike's medium and processed in the laboratory without any delay.

Isolation in Culture and Identification[2]

The key for culture is using quality sheep blood agar (SBA) plates. Horse or ox blood can also be used; but in Indian situation, they are more difficult to obtain than sheep blood. Outdated human blood obtained from blood bank should not be used, since human blood often contains antibiotics and other antibacterial substances including antistreptococcal antibodies that inhibit the growth of GAS.

The swabs are inoculated on BA plates and incubated at temperature range of 35–37°C in the presence of 5% CO_2 for 24 hours. To increase detection rates, negative cultures should be re-examined after an additional 24 hours of incubation. The typical appearance of *S. pyogenes* colonies is dome-shaped with a smooth or moist surface and clear margins, white–grayish color, and diameter of >0.5 mm, surrounded by a zone of β-hemolysis.

Microscopically, *S. pyogenes* appears as gram-positive cocci, arranged in chains **(Fig. 1)**.

After the detection of β-hemolytic colonies displaying a typical *S. pyogenes* morphology **(Fig. 2)**, negative catalase test indicates that the isolates are streptococci.

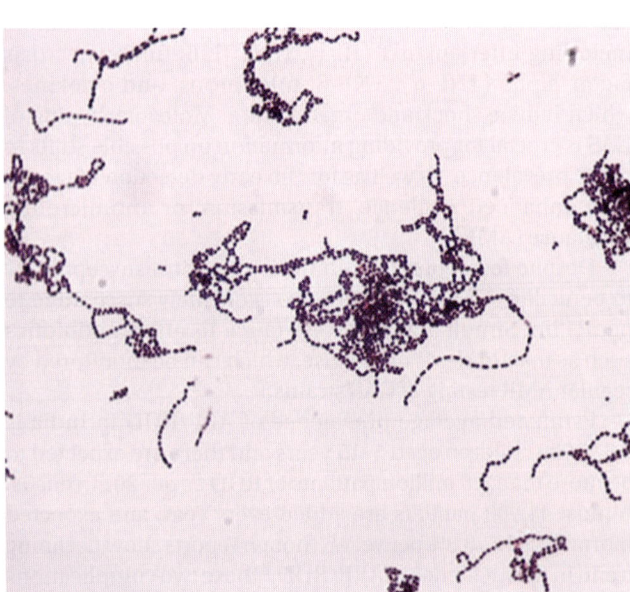

FIG. 1: *Streptococcus pyogenes (S. pyogenes)* appear as gram-positive cocci, arranged in chains.

Source: Donald E. Low *Streptococcus pyogenes.* Infect Dis. 2019.

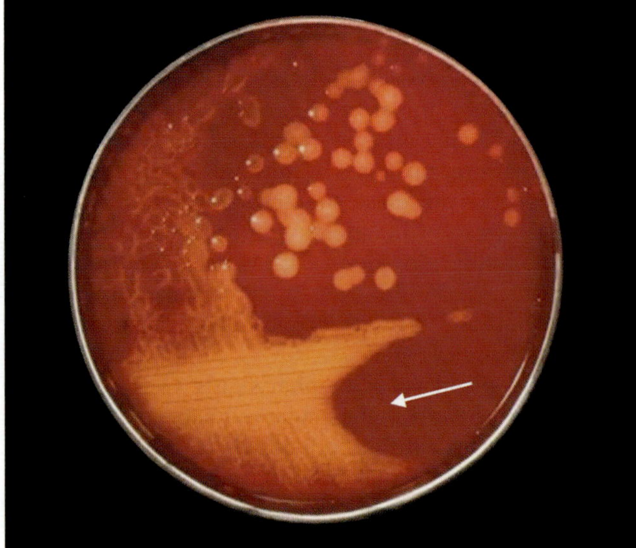

FIG. 2: β-hemolytic colonies displaying a typical *Streptococcus pyogenes (S. pyogenes)* morphology.

Source: Johansson L, Thulin P, Low DE, Norrby-Teglund A. Getting under the skin: the immunopathogenesis of *Streptococcus pyogenes* deep tissue infections. Clin Infect Dis. 2010;51:58-65.

For presumptive identification of *S. pyogenes*, cultures should be tested for bacitracin susceptibility and L-pyrrolidonyl-β-naphthylamide (PYR) activity.

Bacitracin Susceptibility

The strain being tested is streaked with several individual colonies of a pure culture on an SBA plate and a disk containing 0.04 U of bacitracin is placed at the center of SBA plate. After overnight incubation at 35°C in 5% CO_2, a zone of inhibition surrounding the disk indicates the susceptibility of the strain.

L-pyrrolidonyl-β-naphthylamide Test

The PYR test is a rapid colorimetric method often used to test for the presence of the enzyme pyrrolidonyl aminopeptidase to distinguish *S. pyogenes* from other β-hemolytic streptococci with a similar morphology. This enzyme hydrolyzes PYR to β-naphthylamide, which produces a red color when a cinnamaldehyde reagent is added. The test can be performed on paper strips or commercially available spot tests.

Group Identification[3]

The recommended method of GAS identification is by testing β-hemolytic colonies on BA for group A specific carbohydrate antigen. Numerous methods are available in the laboratory for this, of which the time-tested Lancefield's hot-acid extraction technique and Fuller's formamide extraction method are the most widely used. When performed together with the coagglutination reagents, this technique can identify a GAS strain from a BA plate in about 30–45 minutes. Unavailability of grouping antisera used for grouping of BHS is a deterrent for many laboratories to identify GAS. Commercially available antisera are exorbitantly costly.

Antibiotic Susceptibility Testing[10]

The antimicrobial susceptibility testing is performed by the disk diffusion method on Mueller–Hinton agar with 5% sheep blood according to the recommendations of the Clinical and Laboratory Standards Institute (CLSI).

Resistance testing for penicillins or other β-lactams approved for treatment of *S. pyogenes* is not necessary for clinical purposes, in accordance with CLSI recommendations. Since macrolide resistance rates among *S. pyogenes* isolates have been noted, resistance testing is mandatory. It is done by performing antimicrobial susceptibility testing of GAS isolates to erythromycin and extrapolating to azithromycin and clarithromycin. To detect inducible clindamycin resistance in *S. pyogenes*, CLSI recommends D test assay. Similar to the resistance situation for penicillins, a reduced susceptibility to glycopeptides has not yet been found in *S. pyogenes*.

Detection of resistance genes by polymerase chain reaction (PCR), for example, erm(A) and erm(B) for macrolide resistance can also be done.

Automated ID Platforms

Automated bacterial identification systems such as matrix-assisted laser desorption ionization time-of-flight (MALDI-TOF), Vitek 2, Phoenix, and BD system, etc., can identify *S. pyogenes*. They are reliable and offer advantages in terms of rapid turnaround time. However, conventional methods can be considered as cost-effective, practical option in the clinical diagnostics.

Rapid Diagnostic Test[9]

Numerous assays for direct detection of the group A-specific carbohydrate antigen in throat swabs starting with latex agglutination, color immunochromatographic, lateral flow assays (enzyme immunoassays, or EIAs), and optical immunoassays, antibody conjugated to reporter molecules, resulting in a signal indicating a positive test are commercially available. Digital immunoassays (DIAs) incorporate an instrument to analyze the detector particles conjugated with the antigen antibody complex. These systems are based on the principle of using either fluorescence-labeled (such as the Quidel Sofia) or other detector molecule-labeled (such as the BD Veritor) microparticles that are captured in the antigen–antibody complex. They help in rapid diagnosis, prompt treatment, avoiding sequelae, and reducing transmission. However, due to moderate sensitivity of RDT, negative results need to be confirmed with a throat culture in children and because of their cost, use of commercially available kits to identify GAS directly from throat cultures has not become popular in India.[3]

Serological Testing[10]

Antibody detection aids in diagnosis of poststreptococcal sequelae and not that GAS pharyngitis. A fourfold rise in antibody titers is regarded as a definitive proof of antecedent streptococcal infection. ASO starts rising after 1 week of infection and reaches maximum levels at about 3–6 weeks of infection. The classical test for measuring ASO titers is a neutralization assay, where hemolysis through streptolysin O is inhibited by patient serum that harbors ASOs. Results are expressed as Todd units, which are the reciprocal of the highest titer not showing any hemolysis. Newer tests based on latex agglutination and nephelometric measurements are also available.

Molecular Methods

Polymerase Chain Reaction[2,10]

Polymerase chain reaction offers a rapid and increased specificity as compared to traditional identification schemes. Several PCR assays are available for diagnosis of GAS. The GAS direct test is a DNA probe hybridization assay for the detection of group streptococcal RNA from throat swabs. The AccuProbe group B *Streptococcus* assay is a hybridization protection assay that utilizes a DNA probe for the detection of 16S ribosomal RNA sequences. A fully integrated automated real-time PCR-based GeneXpert system has been developed by Cepheid (Sunnyvale, California); this offers a qualitative assay for the detection of group B *Streptococcus* DNA directly from a swab. A commercial PCR method for the direct detection of *S. pyogenes* using the illumigene system (Meridian Bioscience, Inc, 2015) has recently received FDA clearance; test relies on loop-mediated isothermal amplification (LAMP) technology. Cobas Strep A test, running on the Cobas Liat platform (F Hoffmann-La Roche Ltd, 2015), and the Simplexa Group A Strep Direct Test (Focus Diagnostics, Inc, 2013) provide PCR results for individual samples within 20 minutes.

Though molecular techniques have been standardized recently with improved sensitivity, factors such as cost and feasibility have hindered their use in smaller laboratories.[3]

Typing[10]

Typing has no immediate diagnostic or therapeutic consequences, but is important for epidemiologic surveys or in outbreak situations, and may provide important information about the evolutionary relatedness of various strains. A molecular typing system is based on the amplification and subsequent nucleotide sequencing of an *emm* gene fragment by a conserved primer pair. Molecular typing through *emm* sequencing has evolved into the "gold standard".[10]

■ CONCLUSION

Laboratory stewardship for appropriate patient selection and proper method of testing are key to diagnosis of GAS pharyngitis. Though molecular assays may take over conventional testing, differentiating carriage from infection with GAS remains important while employing molecular assays for laboratory diagnosis of GAS pharyngitis, throat swab culture (gold standard) remains crucial. Studies aimed at identifying cutoffs for GAS molecular tests and finding a biomarker specific to bacterial infection in conjunction with GAS to establish its role as a pathogen will be very helpful.

■ REFERENCES

1. Noubiap J, Agbor V, Bigna J, Kaze A, Nyaga U, Mayosi B. Prevalence and progression of rheumatic heart disease: a global systematic review and meta-analysis of population-based echocardiographic studies. Sci Rep. 2019;9(1):53540-4.

2. Tille P. Bailey & Scott's Diagnostic Microbiology, 13th edition, [S.l.]. Amsterdam, Netherlands: Elsevier-Health Science; 2007.

3. Brahmadathan K, Gladstone P. Microbiological diagnosis of streptococcal pharyngitis: Lacunae and their implications. Indian J Med Microbiol. 2006;24(2):92.

4. Leal M, Passos L, Guarçoni F, Aguiar J, Silva R, Paula T, et al. Rheumatic heart disease in the modern era: recent developments and current challenges. Rev Soc Bras Med Trop. 2019;52:e20180041.

5. Zühlke L, Beaton A, Engel M, Hugo-Hamman C, Karthikeyan G, Katzenellenbogen J, et al. Group A *Streptococcus*, Acute Rheumatic Fever and Rheumatic Heart Disease: Epidemiology and Clinical Considerations. Curr Treat Options Cardiovasc Med. 2017;19(2):15.

6. Abraham T, Sistla S. Decoding the molecular epidemiology of group A *Streptococcus*: an Indian perspective. J Med Microbiol. 2019;68(7):1059-71.

7. Mathur P, Bhardwaj N, Behera B, Mathur K, Kapil A, Misra M. Antimicrobial resistance in beta-haemolytic streptococci in India: A four-year study. Indian J Med Res. 2018;147(1):81.

8. Negi P, Sondhi S, Asotra S, Mahajan K, Mehta A. Current status of rheumatic heart disease in India. Indian Heart J. 2019;71(1):85-90.

9. Balasubramanian S, Amperayani S, Dhanalakshmi K, Senthilnathan S, Chandramohan V. Rapid antigen diagnostic testing for the diagnosis of group A beta-haemolytic streptococci pharyngitis. Natl Med J India. 2018;31(1):8.

10. Spellerberg B, Brandt C. (2021). Laboratory Diagnosis of *Streptococcus pyogenes* (group A streptococci) [Internet]. [online] Available from https://pubmed.ncbi.nlm.nih.gov/26866238/. [Last accessed August, 2022].

7

Etiopathogenesis and Pathology of Carditis in Rheumatic Fever

Saroja Bharati, Pradeep Vaideeswar,
Sarasa Bharati

INTRODUCTION

Acute rheumatic fever (ARF) is an acute nonsuppurative systemic inflammation, which results from an immune-mediated granulomatous response to group A hemolytic streptococcal pharyngitis in genetically susceptible patients.

EPIDEMIOLOGY OF ACUTE RHEUMATIC FEVER

Since ARF and rheumatic carditis cannot really be separated from each other from the epidemiological point of view, both will have to be discussed together, though it is relevant to note that ARF without carditis is a relatively benign condition and probably occurs much more commonly. It has a low prevalence in the well-developed countries of about 19 cases per 100,000 populations.[1] However, the estimated prevalence in low-income and middle-income countries (including India) ranges from 2.7 to 51 cases per 1,000 populations, which highlights the disease association with low socioeconomic status, overcrowding, and malnutrition.[2] In India, the prevalence reported varies from very infrequent to very high levels depending upon the source of information.[3] The age of occurrence varies from 5 to 15 years with a peak of around 11 years in India; it is uncommon before the age of 3 years and generally after 21 years.[4] Though both sexes may be affected, males appear more susceptible in the ratio of 4:1.

PATHOGENESIS OF ACUTE RHEUMATIC FEVER

Acute rheumatic fever appears to be an almost exclusive complication of a hemolytic streptococcal infection of the upper respiratory tract, which suggests a site-specific genetic susceptibility. Similar infections at other sites such as the skin do not often lead to the autoimmune inflammation. The exact mechanism involved in the pathogenesis still remains unclear. After the initial streptococcal infection, there is activation of the B-cells and their further maturation to plasma cells with the production of antibodies against the highly antigenic cell wall components of streptococci, particularly M protein and carbohydrate antigen (N-acetyl-β-D-glucosamine).[5] During this phase, the antibodies cross-react with human cardiac proteins (such as myosin and laminin) as well as certain other noncardiac host molecules, resulting in antibody-mediated injury. An additional recruitment of the T-cells induces the characteristic granulomatous response.[5] Despite the antigenic similarity, only 3% of patients develop ARF, indicating the existence of a genetic susceptibility. Implicated in the pathogenesis is not only related to human leukocyte antigen (HLA) (especially *HLA-DQA1* to *HLA-DQB1* region), but also the immunoglobulin heavy chain locus.[6]

The target of the autoimmune inflammation is the interstitial connective and the effects are produced not only in the heart, but also other extracardiac tissues such as the joints, subcutaneous tissue, central nervous system, and also sometimes the lungs. The involvement also is accompanied by constitutional symptoms. The initial attack of ARF may subside or may also be followed by recurrent episodes. The collagen reacts by becoming edematous, later eosinophilic (i.e., necrotic), and gets surrounded by lymphocytes and macrophages. This altered ground substance is described as fibrinoid necrosis and is characteristic of the early phase. In the next proliferative or granulomatous phase, these histiocytes soon enlarge and may develop prominent nuclei with nucleoli—the Anitschkow cells and may become multinucleated—the Aschoff giant cells **(Fig. 1)**. The inflammatory aggregates so formed are ovoid and fairly

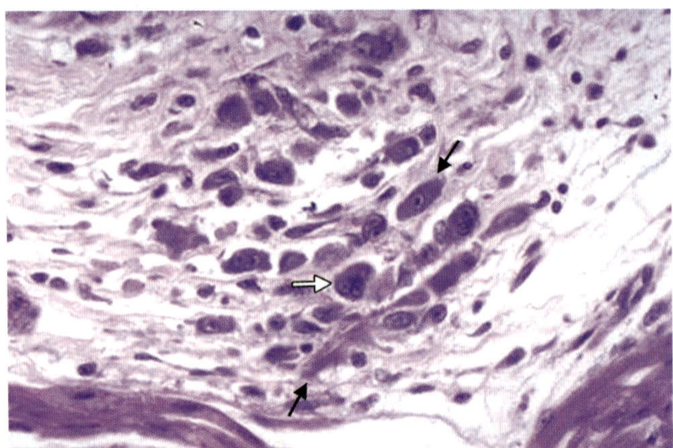

FIG. 1: Well-formed, globoid Aschoff body with Anitschkow cells (black arrow) and Aschoff cells (white arrow), both of which show "owl-eye" nuclei. Thick black arrow points to fibrinoid necrosis (H and E, ×400).

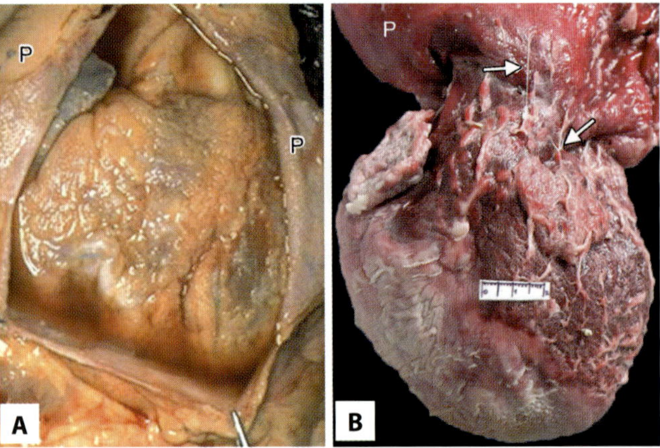

FIGS. 2A AND B: (A) ARF with an effusion, and collection of moderate amount of amber-colored, hazy fluid, as seen on incising the pericardium P; (B) close-up of the anterior surface of the heart in a 12-year-old male. The epicardial surface is remarkably congested with fibrinous/hemorrhagic exudates. Note delicate adhesions (arrows) between parietal (P) and visceral pericardial layers.

(ARF: acute rheumatic fever)

circumscribed, and are termed Aschoff bodies. During the course of the next few weeks, proliferating tissue replaces the areas of fibrinoid necrosis resulting in the presence of fusiform or ovoid perivascular scars.

PATHOLOGY OF ACUTE RHEUMATIC FEVER

The essential tissue reaction seen in acute carditis revolves around the production of a nonsuppurative form of acute inflammation following triggering of the autoimmune mechanism. This tends to involve all layers of the heart—acute pancarditis.

In the pericardium, varying degrees of effusion may be seen, either completely serous **(Fig. 2A)** or generally serofibrinous. The epicardium is covered by whitish or even hemorrhagic exudates, which cause adhesion between the two layers of the pericardium. On separation of these layers, a shaggy appearance is seen (due to the high-fibrin content of the exudates), reminiscent of separated buttered slices of bread, hence the terms "bread and butter" pericarditis or *cor villosum* are used to describe the acute fibrinous pericarditis **(Fig. 2B)**. Aschoff bodies may also be present. Some of the epicardial coronary arterial radicles may also be involved in the inflammatory process.

With *acute rheumatic myocarditis*, the appearance of the heart depends on the severity of the disease. Generally, the heart is enlarged, flabby, and globular in shape **(Fig. 3A)**. The chambers are enlarged, especially the left ventricle with dilatation of the annuli of the mitral and tricuspid valves leading to incompetence. Histologically, in the early 3 weeks, a nonspecific chronic inflammatory reaction in the form of lymphocytic infiltrate occurs, giving rise to electrophysiological changes. Later, submiliary sized Aschoff nodules develop in the myocardium, especially in

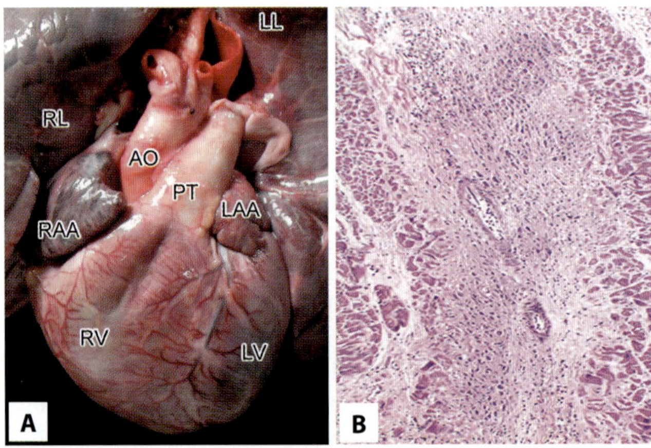

FIGS. 3A AND B: (A) Enlarged globular heart flanked by the lungs. There is moderate biventricular dilatation. Note minimal pericarditis and intense congestion of arborizing epicardial vessels; (B) acute rheumatic myocarditis showing numerous Aschoff bodies in the perivascular connective tissue (H and E, ×100).

(AO: aorta; LAA: left atrial appendage; LL: left lung; LV: left ventricle; RL: right lung; RV: right ventricle; RAA: right atrial appendage; PT: pulmonary trunk)

the basal portions of the interventricular septum, posterior papillary muscle, and left atrial wall in the interstitial and perivascular connective tissue **(Fig. 3B)**. Although the submiliary nodule is primarily in the interstitial tissue, the surrounding muscle fibers are often seen to be involved. Changes in the blood vessels are common, not infrequently one encounters narrowing or occlusion of the lumens with thrombi. The Aschoff bodies in the perivascular space compress one segment of the wall against another. When two or more submiliary nodules are close together but on

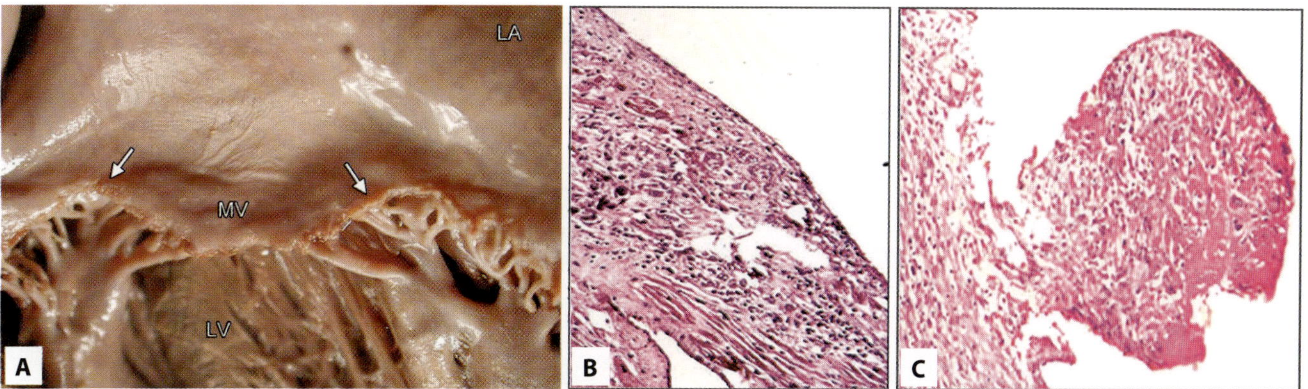

FIGS. 4A TO C: (A) Fine, firm, tan-colored vegetations present at the lines of closure of thickened MV leaflets. There is minimal involvement of commissures and chordae; (B) Aschoff bodies at the basal aspect of valve leaflet (H and E, ×250); (C) Vegetation seen as extruded clump of fibrin and platelets (H and E, ×250).

(MV: mitral valve; LA: left atrium; LV: left ventricle)

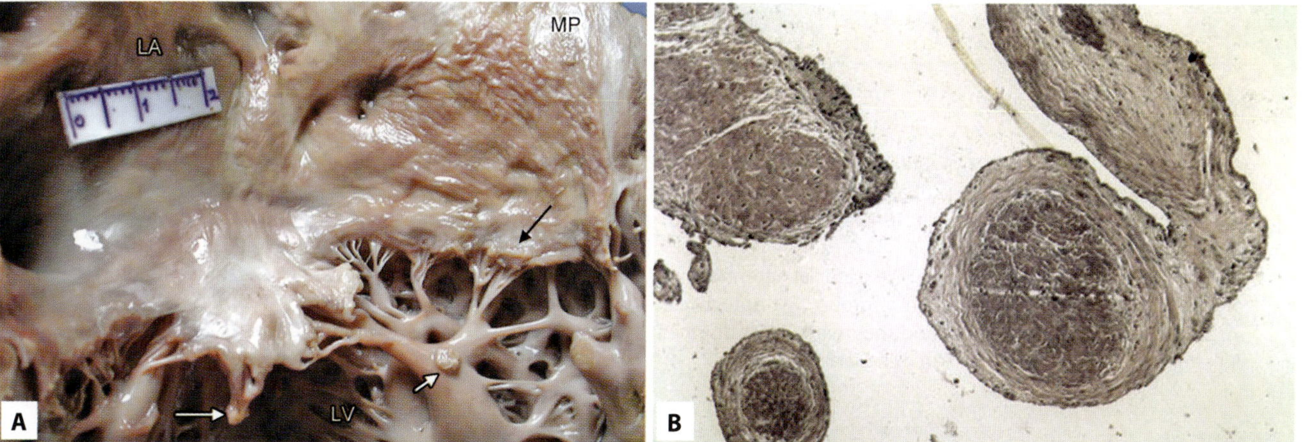

FIGS. 5A AND B: (A) Verrucous endocarditis of the mitral valve (black arrow) has produced chordal rupture (long white arrow). Short white arrow indicates the site of rupture. Note also a corrugated appearance of left atrial posterior wall. It represents mural endocarditis, i.e., MacCallum's patch—MP; (B) Cross-sections of chordae showing layer of inflammation (Elastic van Gieson, ×200).

different sides of a vessel, the edema in the region of such foci probably forms a constricting ring. Endarteritis, with swelling and proliferation of the endothelium as well as of the other intimal cells, is not infrequently encountered in the smaller branches of the coronary arteries.

The *acute rheumatic endocarditis* involves the endocardium over the valves and/or the chambers, especially over the posterior wall of the left atrium. The mitral valve is the one to be predominately involved. Initially, the leaflets are thin and translucent, later become thick, opaque, and leathery, especially in the regions of the annulus and basal areas. If the inflammation is severe, the entire valve may be involved. More severe inflammation results in the production of tiny verrucae **(Fig. 4A)**, i.e., rows of pinhead sized, pale brown, nonfriable translucent vegetations confined to the lines of closure on the flow surfaces. Histologically, these vegetations show Aschoff nodules with an addition,

extrusion of damaged collagen, and deposition of platelets and fibrin on them. These either overlie or are seen adjacent to necrotic foci **(Figs. 1B and C)**. This manifestation of valvular endocarditis is referred to as *verrucous endocarditis*. These verrucae may form continuous ridges or may extend onto the chordae tendineae and papillary muscles. When the reaction is intense, even chordae may rupture **(Figs. 5A and B)**. Aortic valve **(Fig. 6A)** is the second most common valve and, at times, both are involved. Involvement of the tricuspid **(Fig. 6B)** or pulmonary valves may also occur, but is rather rare. Recurrent inflammation results in chronically inflamed valves. When mural endocarditis occurs, it is mainly seen in the posterior wall of the left atrium near the base of the posterior mitral leaflet as a thick, rugose endocardium with a distinct granularity produced by thrombi over endocardial/subendocardial conglomerate of Aschoff. It is designated as MacCallum's patch.

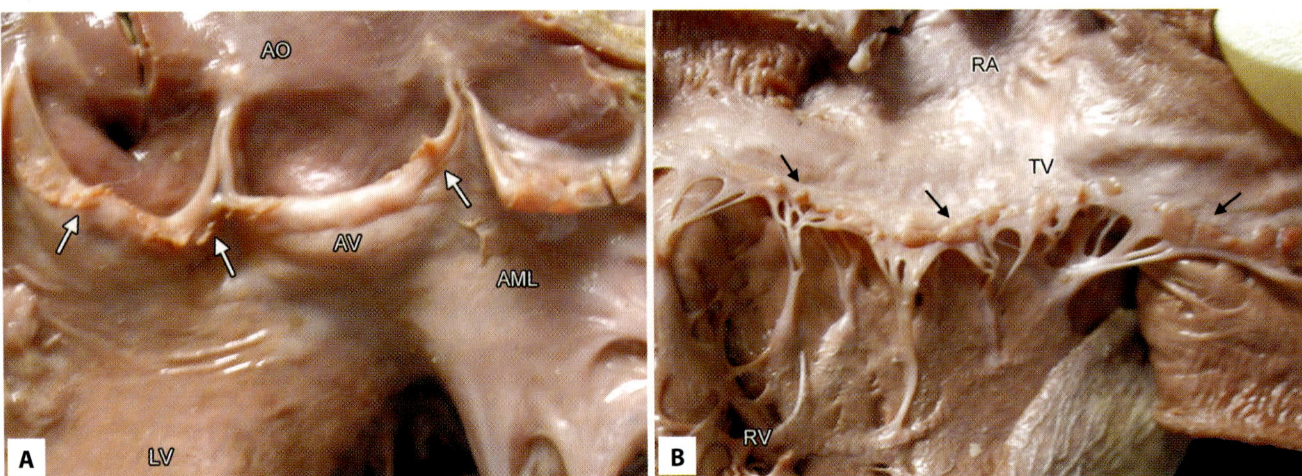

FIGS. 6A AND B: Vegetations (arrows) over lines of closure of: (A) Aortic and (B) Tricuspid, valves.

(AO: aorta; AML: anterior mitral leaflet; AV: aortic valve; LV: left ventricle; RA: right atrium; RV: right ventricle; TV: tricuspid valve)

■ REFERENCES

1. Watkins DA, Johnson CO, Colquhoun SM, Karthikeyan G, Beaton A, Bukhman G, et al. Global, regional, and national burden of rheumatic heart disease, 1990-2015. N Engl J Med. 2017;377:713-22.

2. Coffey PM, Ralph AP, Krause VL. The role of social determinants of health in the risk and prevention of group A streptococcal infection, acute rheumatic fever and rheumatic heart disease: A systematic review. PLoS Negl Trop Dis. 2018;12:e0006577.

3. Karthikeyan G, Guiltherme L. Acute rheumatic fever. Lancet. 2018;392:161-74.

4. Arvind B, Ramakrishnan S. Rheumatic fever and rheumatic heart disease in children. Indian J Pediatr. 2020;87:305-11.

5. Azevedo PM, Pereira RR, Guilherme L. Understanding rheumatic fever. Rheumatol Int. 2012;32:1113-20.

6. Muhamed B, Parks T, Sliwa K. Genetics of rheumatic fever and rheumatic heart disease. Nat Rev Cardiol. 2020;17:145-54.

8

Pathology of Chronic Rheumatic Heart Disease

Pradeep Vaideeswar

INTRODUCTION

Chronic phase of rheumatic heart disease (RHD) is inevitable and the major brunt is borne by the heart valves. It manifests as deforming valvular disease that leads to permanent dysfunction with ensuing significant morbidity and mortality. This has, therefore, given rise to the well-known clinical cliché of "rheumatic fever licks the joints and bites the heart".

PATHOLOGY OF CHRONIC RHD[1,2]

The acute pancardiac lesions largely heal by fibrosis. The inflammatory exudates over the pericardium usually resolves in time, leaving behind flimsy adhesions or milk spots/patches (soldier's spots) that appear as smooth, white, glistening, opaque, single or multiple areas of epicardial fibrosis **(Fig. 1A)**. Rarely, if there had been excessive fibrin, the pericardial cavity is obliterated by fibrous

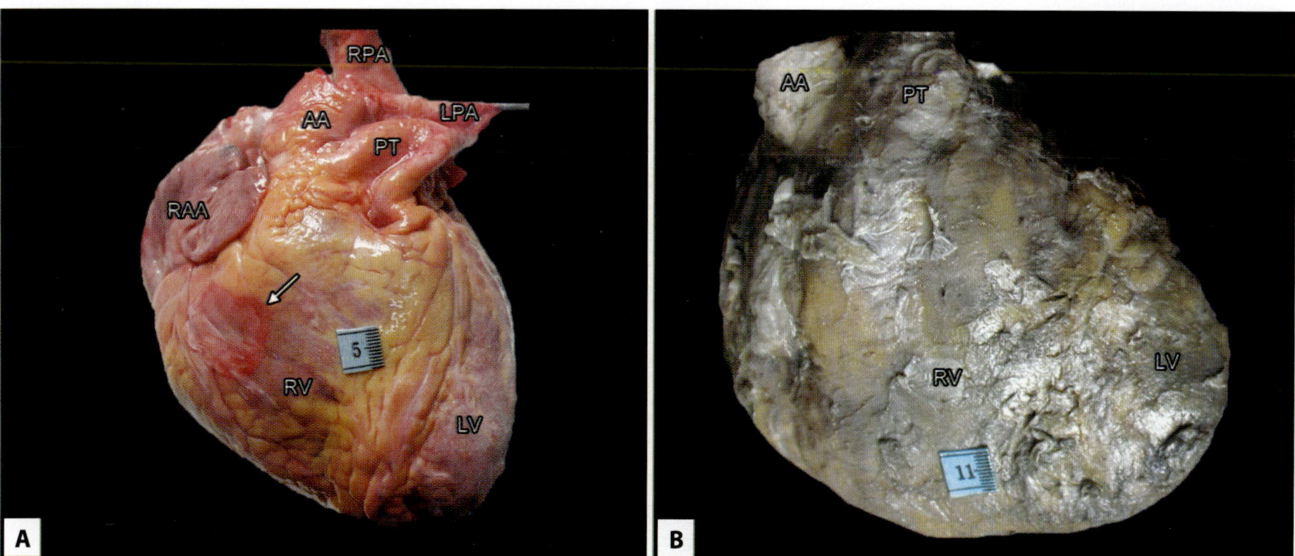

FIGS. 1A AND B: (A) Healing of acute pericarditis has resulted in "milk" patches (arrow) over anterior surface of right ventricle RV. Noted enlargement of the right-sided chambers and the pulmonary trunk PT and its branches; (B) Case of chronic RHD. Extensive thickening and multifocal adhesions between the layers of the pericardium. The apex appears expanded and rounded.

(AA: ascending aorta; LPA: left pulmonary artery; LV: left ventricle; PT: pulmonary trunk; RAA: right atrial appendage; RHD: rheumatic heart disease; RPA: right pulmonary artery; RV: right ventricle)

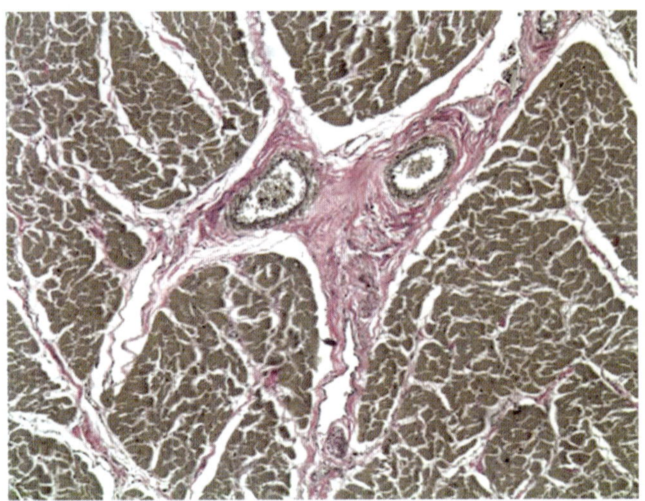

FIG. 2: Stellate perivascular scar in the left ventricular myocardium following healing of myocarditis (Elastic van Geison, ×200).

adhesions. However, such adhesions occur most often after surgical intervention **(Fig. 1B)** or occasionally due to a second pathology such as tuberculous pericarditis. In the nonfatal cases of acute rheumatic myocarditis, healing results in fine perivascular **(Fig. 2)** and interstitial scars, sometimes identified as grossly visible streaky fibrosis in the myocardium. As the recovery starts, the chambers start returning to their normal size, with concomitant correction of valvular insufficiency. The recovery may take several months to a year, depending upon the severity of myocardial damage. By and large, the ventricular function returns to normalcy.

In sharp contrast to minimal side effects of healing of epimyocardial lesions, fibrosis renders discernible alterations in the normal architecture of the valves with heavy collagenization and neovascularization **(Fig. 3A)**. Variable number of chronic inflammatory cells (mainly lymphocytes) may be present **(Fig. 3B)**. Gradually, there is calcific deposition **(Fig. 3C)**, which is now considered as

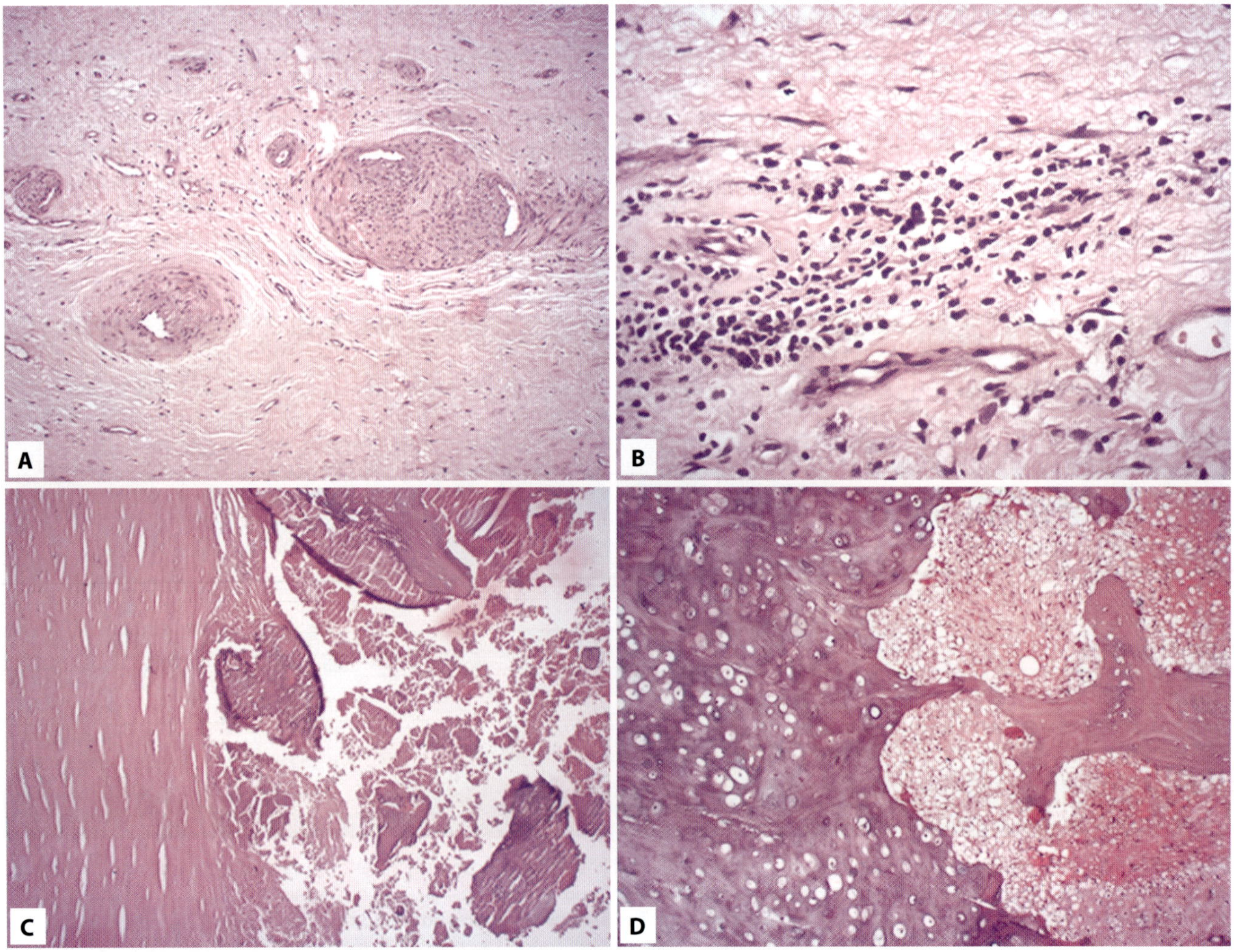

FIGS. 3A TO D: Valvular tissue with: (A) fibrosis with thick-walled vessels (neovascularization, H and E, ×250); (B) Clusters of lymphocytes amidst vascularized fibrous tissue (H and E, ×400); (C) Calcification seen as granular basophilic deposition (H and E, ×250); (D) Osteochondromatous metaplasia (H and E, ×250).

an active process (metaplastic calcification), mediated by cytokines such as osteopontin. These induce myofibroblasts into chondrocytic or osteoblastic differentiation mode with osseous or chondroid metaplasia **(Fig. 3D)**. Occasionally, there can be dystrophic amyloidosis.

Involvement of one or more components of the valve results in subclinical or clinical valvular dysfunction in the form of stenosis, regurgitation or their combination, and in fact, a significant proportion of patients in India seek medical advice at this stage. The valves may be affected singly or in combination; if multivalvular, the combination may be concordant or discordant. The most common is sole involvement of mitral valve (MV), followed by involvement of both MV and aortic valve (AV). All three valves, i.e., MV, AV, and tricuspid valve (TV) are affected in 15% of cases, while all four valves or isolated AV disease is rare. Though the valves are affected in the initial phase of the disease, there is usually a latent period between acute rheumatic fever (ARF) and valvular deformity of about 20–30 years. However, a short latency of 2 or 3 years (juvenile disease) occurs when ARF strikes at an early age, is recurrent, or is of severe degree, which is a common scenario in India.

Mitral stenosis (MS) is considered to be "sine qua non" of chronic RHD. In the early stages of healing of acute mitral valvulitis, there is mild thickening of the leaflets and chordae with loss of scalloping of posterior leaflet. The lines of closure show a ridge or a row of fibrous nodules. Concomitant with these changes, healing of valvular tissue adjoining the commissures produces fibrous adhesions and gradual obliteration, i.e., commissural fusion with resultant orifice stenosis. The degree of stenosis varies with the amount of fusion. The normal MV area is about 4–6 cm^2; when the size is reduced to 1 cm^2, stenosis is considered critical. When viewed from the left atrium (LA) aspect, the orifice appears crescentic, a feature designated as "fish mouth" or "buttonhole" deformity **(Fig. 4A)**. The leaflets too show fibrotic thickening **(Figs. 4B to D)**, especially in their distal third **(Fig. 4E)**, with loss of pliability. Severe subvalvular stenosis occurs when there is thickening, shortening, and fusion of the chordae with each other as well as with leaflets. Consequently, there is obliteration of the interchordal spaces and direct attachment of leaflets to papillary muscles. The MV then assumes a funnel-shaped profile when inspected through the left ventricular aspect; the orifice may be central or eccentric **(Figs. 5A and B)**. Adding insult to injury is the development of nodular commissural/leaflet calcification **(Fig. 6A)**. Larger deposits occur in men; calcification is less common in cases of juvenile MS. The calcific deposits can

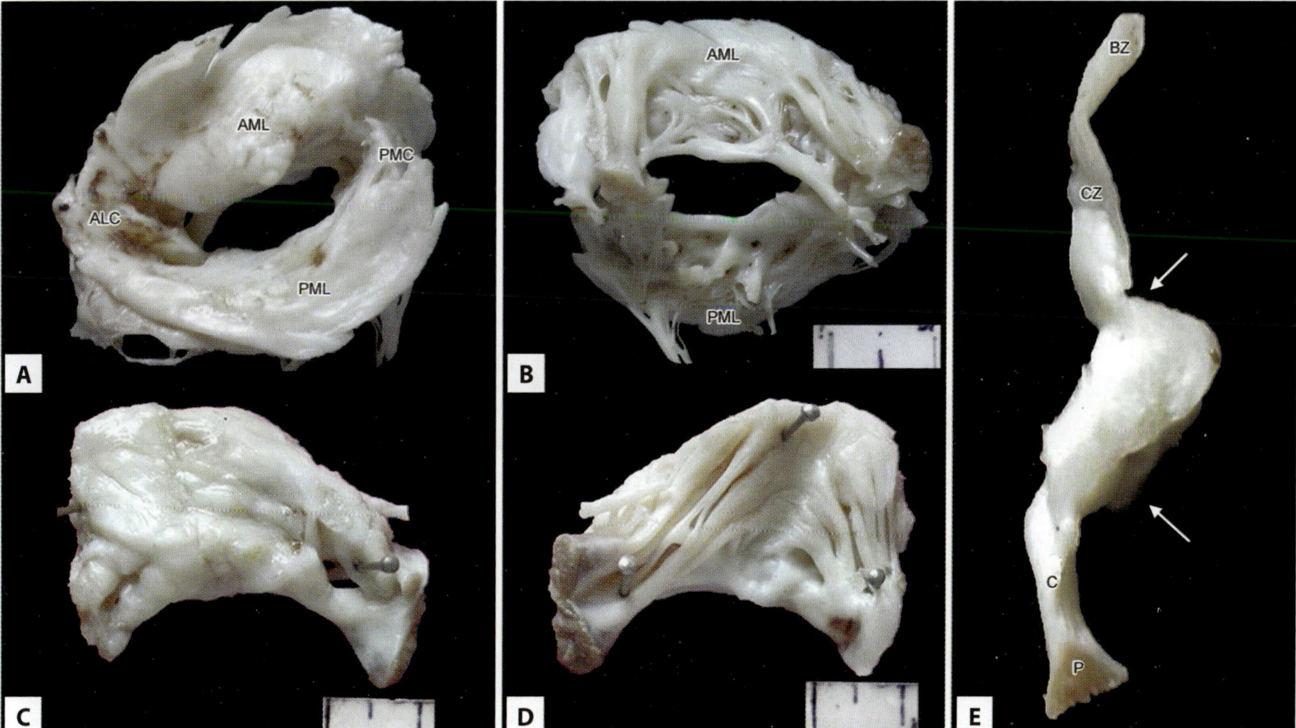

FIGS. 4A TO E: (A) Crescentic appearance of the orifice as inspected from left atrial aspect (flow surface) in a surgically excised specimen of a stenotic MV; (B) Left ventricular aspect or nonflow surface of the same valve; (C) Flow and (D) nonflow surfaces of excised, thickened anterior mitral leaflet. In order to retain the LV geometry, there is an increasing tendency to incompletely excise MV; (E) It is to be noted that the maximal changes are at the rough zone (arrows) with little involvement of clear CZ and basal BZ zones.

(ALC: anterolateral commissure; AML: anterior mitral leaflet; C: fused, thickened chordae; P: stump of papillary muscle; PMC: posteromedial commissure; PML: posterior mitral leaflet)

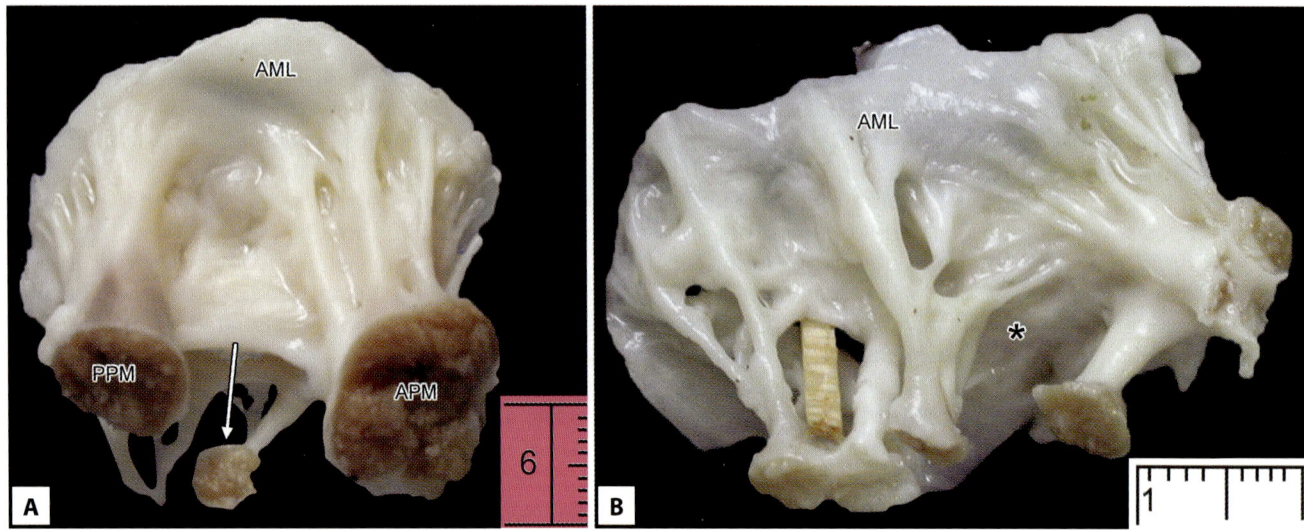

FIGS. 5A AND B: (A) Funnel-shaped appearance of the mitral valve produced by chordal shortening and interchordal fusion. The papillary muscles are directly attached to leaflets. Nearly symmetrical involvement has produced a central slit-like orifice (arrow); (B) A probe has been passed through an eccentric orifice of the valve due to marked fusion of anterolateral commissure(*).

(AML: anterior mitral leaflet; APM: anterior papillary muscle; PPM: posterior papillary muscle)

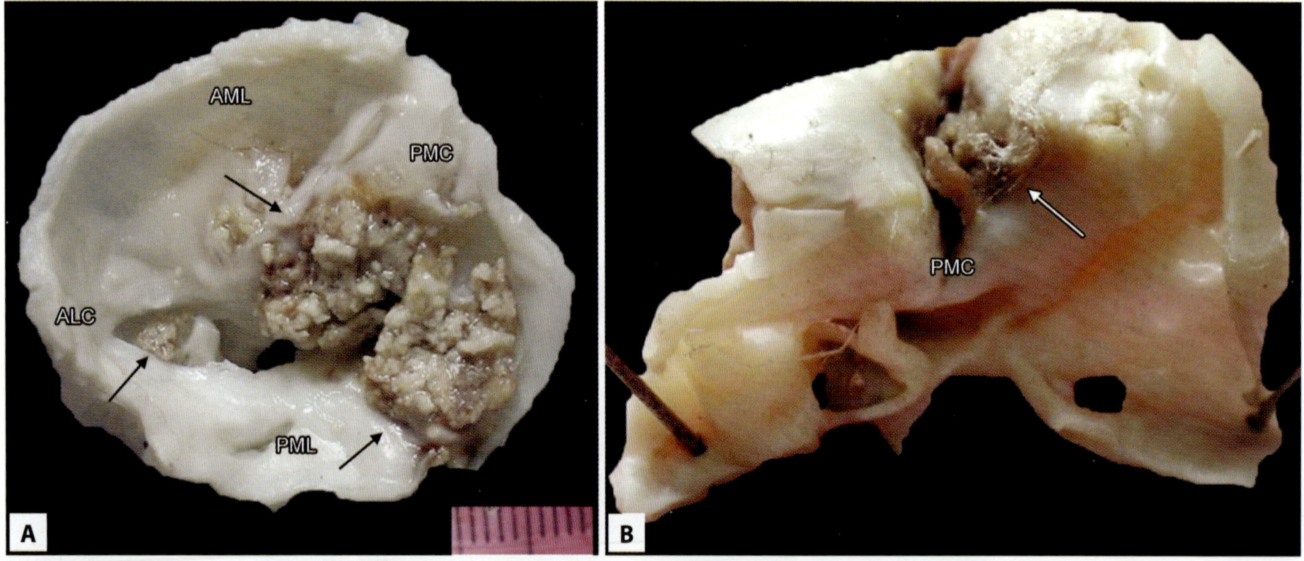

FIGS. 6A AND B: (A) Extensive calcification (arrows) is predominantly present at the fused posteromedial commissure (PMC) with extension into the adjoining leaflets; (B) The fused and calcified PMC in this valve is eroded and covered by granular red–brown thrombus, which was bland on histology.

(ALC: anterolateral commissure; AML: anterior mitral leaflet; PML: posterior mitral leaflet)

erode the overlying endocardium to be sources of calcium emboli or may also have superimposed thrombi **(Fig. 6B)**.

Progressive stenosis outstrips the LA capacity to hypertrophy and the chamber dilates to accommodate residual blood. With tight stenosis, the LA is ballooned out with often a paper-thin wall **(Fig. 7A)** with endocardial thickening and its eggshell-like calcification. The enlarged atrium may compress the surrounding structures. A small volume of blood is ejected into the left ventricle (LV); the chamber is consequently small in size. Blood stasis due to

LA chamber dilatation and atrial fibrillation (a frequent accompaniment of chronic disease) predispose to mural **(Figs. 7A and B)** and/or appendageal thromboses, which are frequent sources of systemic thromboembolism. Aschoff bodies can sometimes be seen in excised left atrial appendages **(Figs. 8A and B)** and even in the papillary muscle stumps. The deformed valves, due to the flow alterations, can predispose to the formation of nonbacterial thrombotic endocarditis, which in turn serves as a nidus for infection **(Fig. 8C)**. Rising LA pressure is reflected on to the

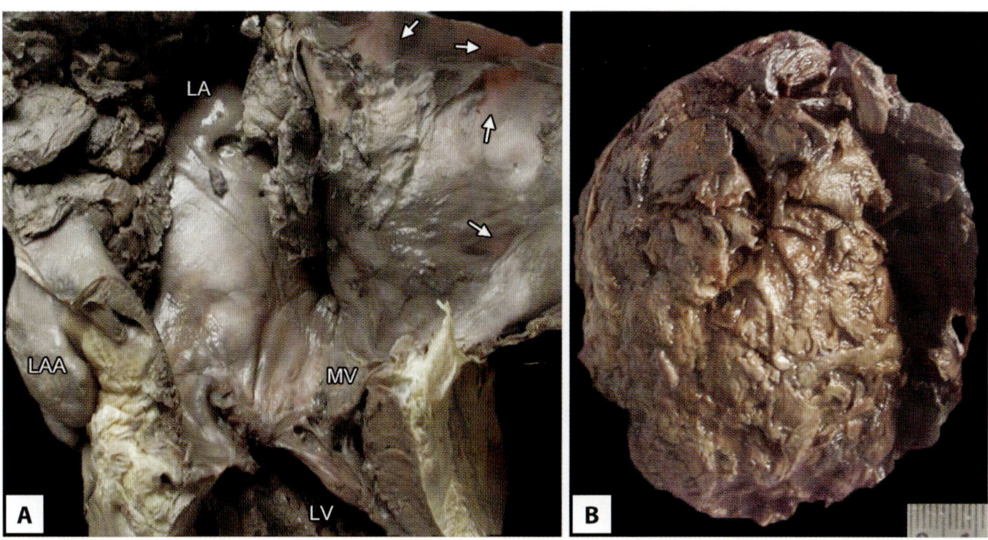

FIGS. 7A AND B: (A) Severe MS has produced left atrial LA dilatation. Note parchment-like wall (arrows) with mural thrombi in the cavity and within the appendage LAA; (B) Surgically excised LA thrombus.

(LA: left atrium; LAA: left atrial appendage; LV: left ventricle; MV: mitral valve)

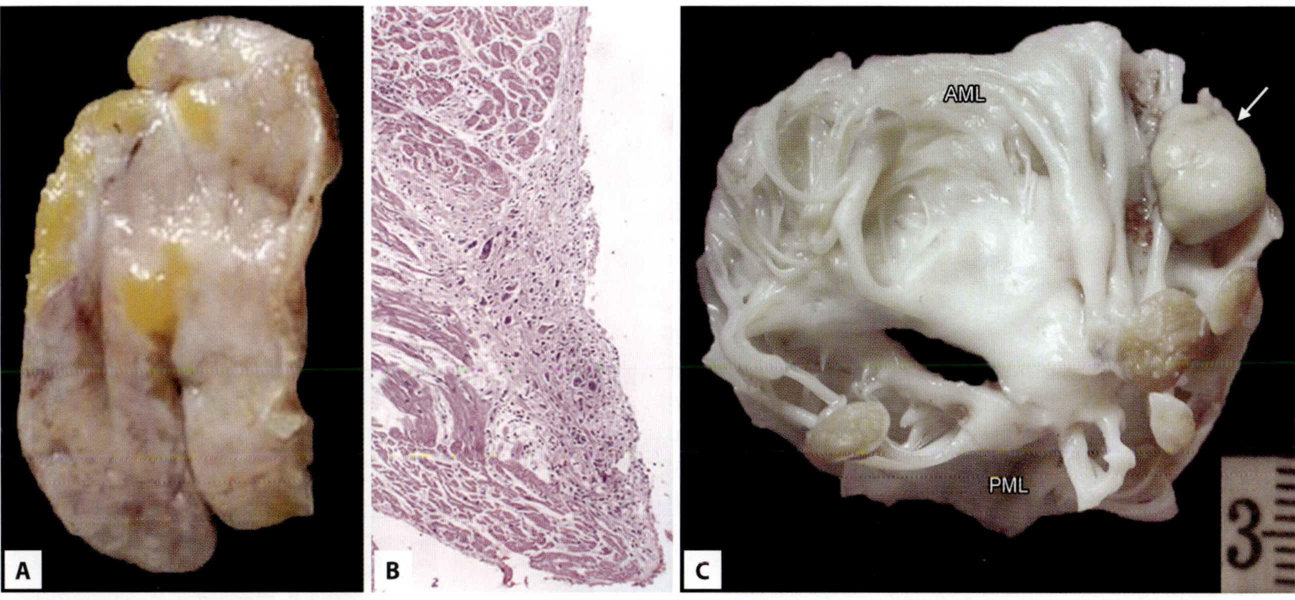

FIGS. 8A TO C: (A) Excised left atrial appendage; (B) Subendocardial Aschoff body seen as an incidental finding (H and E, ×250); (C) Smooth-surfaced pale yellow infective vegetation (arrow) seen on the nonflow aspect of the excised mitral valve.

(AML: anterior mitral leaflet; PML: posterior mitral leaflet)

pulmonary vasculature producing secondary effects in the form of pulmonary venous and then arterial hypertension, brown induration of the lungs, right ventricle (RV)/right atrium (RA) dilatation/hypertrophy and functional tricuspid regurgitation (TR). A high degree of turbulence across the stenotic valve can also cause intravascular hemolysis.

Aortic valve disease is seen in more than half the cases of RHD and is almost always associated with MV deformity, though the latter at times may be minimal. The common manifestation is aortic stenosis (AS). There is fusion of the cusps at the commissures and the narrowed orifice is roughly triangular or round, depending on the extent of commissural fusion **(Figs. 9A and B)**. In some instances, there is more severe involvement of one commissure producing an "acquired bicuspidization". Secondary cuspal and commissural calcification aggravates the stenosis **(Figs. 9C and D)**; superimposed thrombi can also be present. Development of frictional lesions on the valves such as Lambl's excrescences or papillary fibroelastomas **(Figs. 10A and B)** further adds to stenosis (both MV

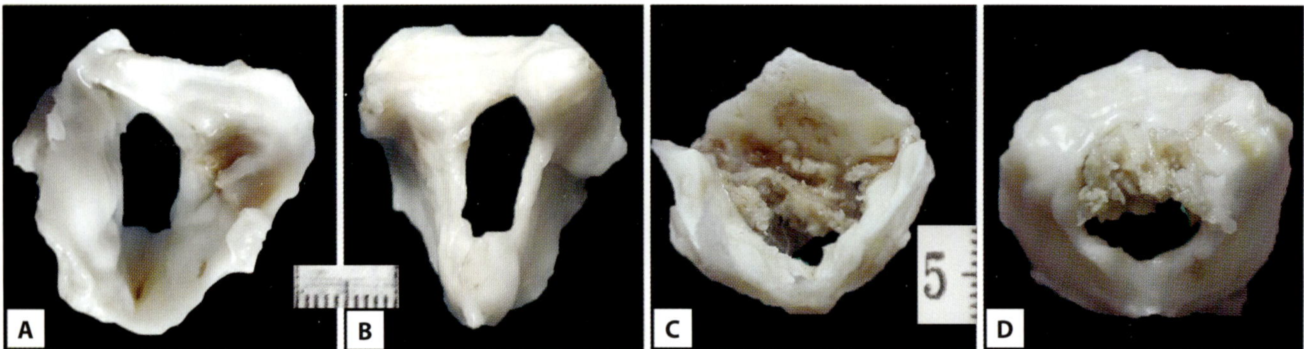

FIGS. 9A TO D: (A) Flow and (B) nonflow surfaces of the aortic valve with marked fusion of all commissures producing a narrow orifice, resembling a dented Mercedes Benz logo. There is extreme cuspal fibrosis; (C) Flow and (D) nonflow surfaces of another stenotic valve accompanied by dystrophic calcification.

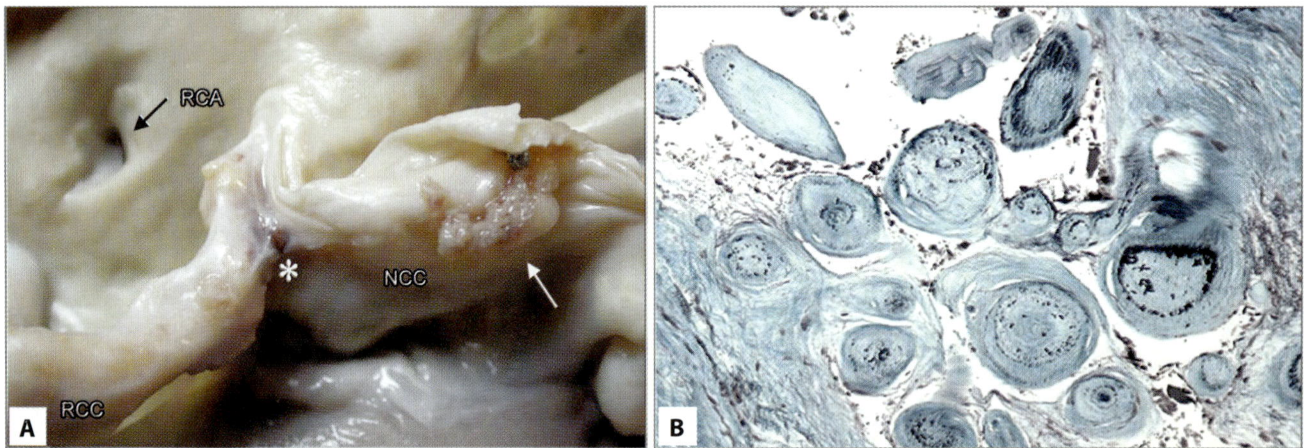

FIGS. 10A AND B: (A) Stenotic aortic valve with fused commissure(*) between right (RCC) and noncoronary (NCC) cusps with a papillary fibroelastoma (white arrow) over the noncoronary cusp (right coronary artery ostium (RCA), black arrow); (B) Cross-sections of the papillae of papillary fibroelastoma (Movat pentachrome, ×250).

and AV) by promoting thrombogenesis and subsequent organization. The heart is moderately or markedly enlarged in size due to LV hypertrophy, which can lead to myocardial ischemia and focal fibrosis. The jet from the stenotic orifice often produces localized jet lesions over the ascending aorta and can lead to weakening of the wall and saccular aneurysms.

Pure rheumatic valvular incompetence is rare and is often seen in children. Commissural fusion and commissural, cuspal, or leaflet calcification are either absent or minimal. With MV involvement, there is annular dilatation with accompanying leaflet or chordal changes, but chordal shortening and fusion are also mild **(Figs. 11A and B)**. The dysfunction results in a jet lesion over the LA posterior wall (not to be confused with the MacCallum's patch), LV dilatation, and hypertrophy. Similarly in AV, with fibrosis and contracture, there is malalignment of the cusps, leading to aortic regurgitation (AR). The cusps have rolled margins **(Figs. 11C and D)** and jet lesions produced by the regurgitant stream are seen in the subaortic region of the interventricular septum or over the ventricular aspect of anterior mitral leaflet (AML). The LV cavity also gets dilated.

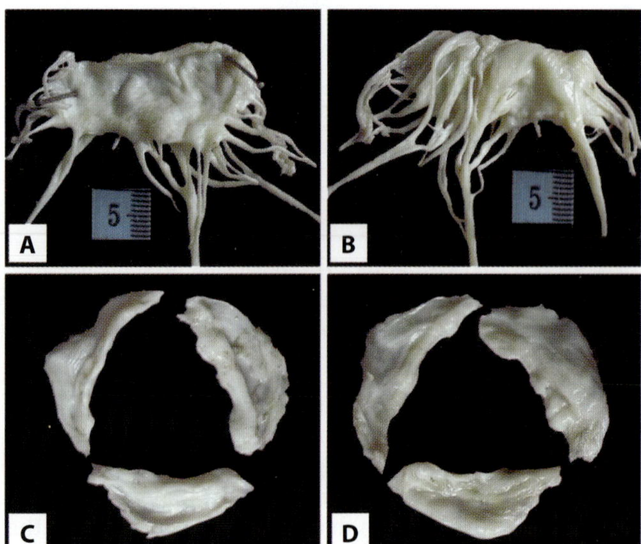

FIGS. 11A TO D: (A) Flow and (B) nonflow surfaces of an excised anterior mitral leaflet in a patient with mitral regurgitation. Note mild leaflet and chordal changes. There is minimal fusion of the chordate tendineae; (C) Flow and (D) nonflow surfaces of separately excised semilunar cusps in a case of aortic regurgitation. There is mild fibrosis with prominent rolling of the free margins.

Tricuspid valve involvement is seen commonly, but is largely subclinical and detected at autopsy **(Fig. 12)** and, at times, only on histology. Functional incompetence is more often than organic disease. Stenosis of significant degree is seen in 10% of cases, with changes similar to those in the MV. Calcification is rare. The same is true for pulmonary valve (PV), though stenosis is vanishingly rare.

Figures 13A to F show the comparative sizes of the heart and its chambers depending on the valve involved and its associated dysfunction. So long as the fibrous tissue is pliable, the result is usually pure valvular stenosis **(Fig. 13A)**. But, with increasing collagen deposition and calcification, there is poor coaptation of the leaflets or cups, leading to an element of regurgitation. This leads to combined stenosis and insufficiency **(Fig. 13B)**. Superimposed infective endocarditis can also increase the extent of regurgitation. Acute incompetence can occur in patients with MS due to tearing of leaflets **(Fig. 14)**, which may be seen a complication during the interventional balloon valvotomy. It is also important to remember that RHD can also occur along with congenital heart diseases, classic example being its occurrence with atrial septal defects.

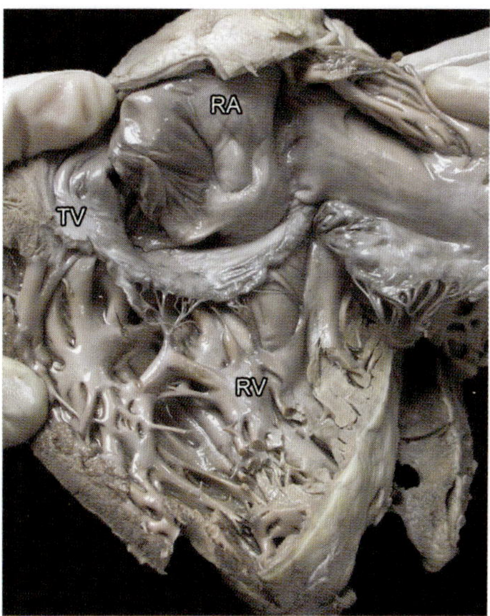

FIG. 12: Subtle involvement of the tricuspid valve TV in chronic RHD with mild thickening of the leaflets and rounding of the free margins.

(RA: right atrium; RHD: rheumatic heart disease; RV: right ventricle; TV: tricuspid valve)

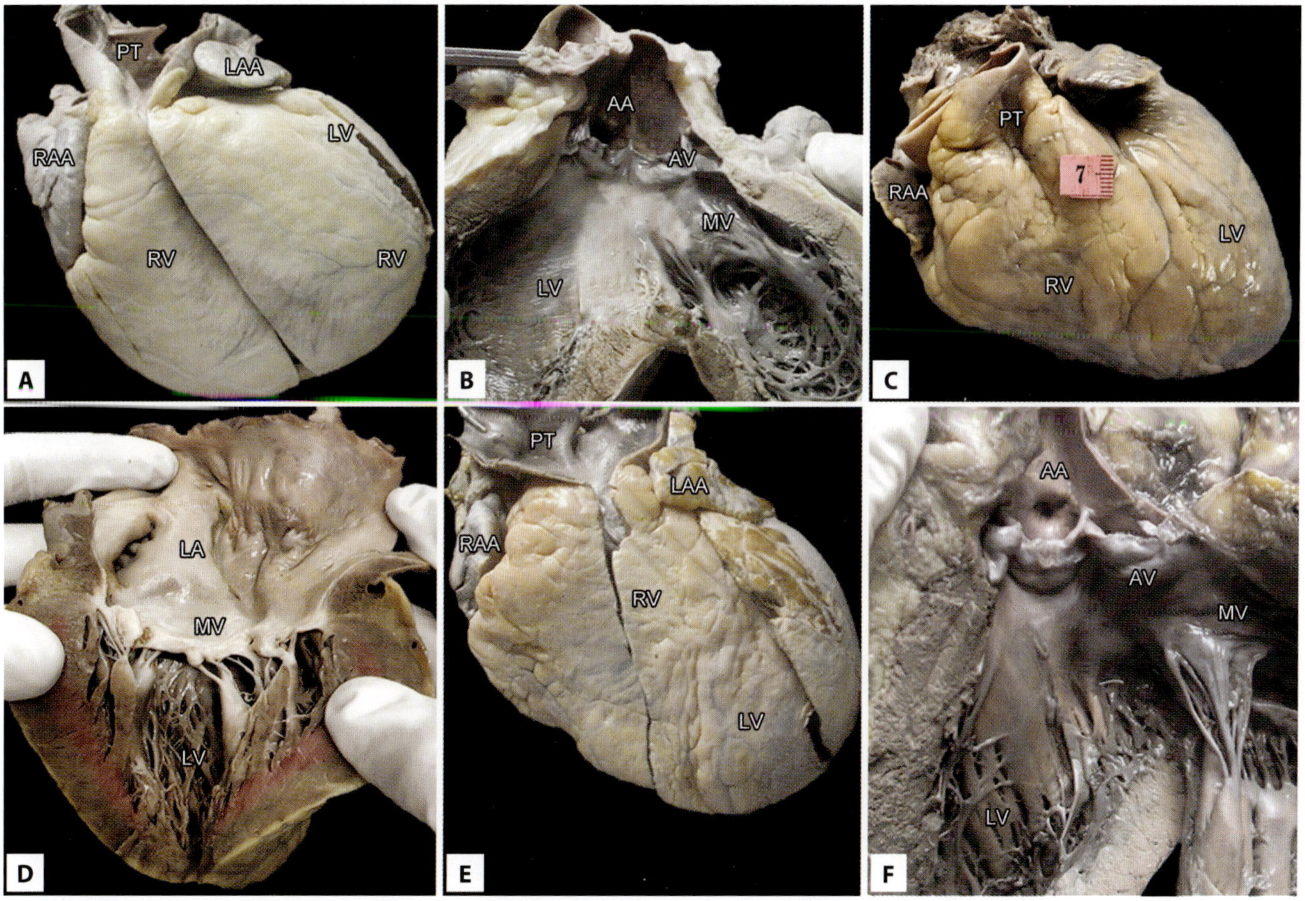

FIGS. 13A TO F: (A and B) the external surface and left ventricular (LV) outflow tract in pure MS. Note that right ventricle (RV) occupies much of the anterior surface and LV is hardly seen. The mitral valve (MV) is funnel shaped, while the aortic valve (AV) is normal; (C and D) the external surface and LV inflow tract in MS with MR. Note the presence of moderate commissural fusion and LV enlargement. The chordae are thickened but not unduly shortened; (E and F) the external surface and LV outflow tract in MS with AS. There is almost equal enlargement of the ventricles and the apex is rounded. The pulmonary trunk (PT) is also dilated with thick intima.

(AML: anterior mitral leaflet; AS: aortic stenosis; MR: mitral regurgitation; MS: mitral stenosis; RAA: right atrial appendage; LAA: left atrial appendage)

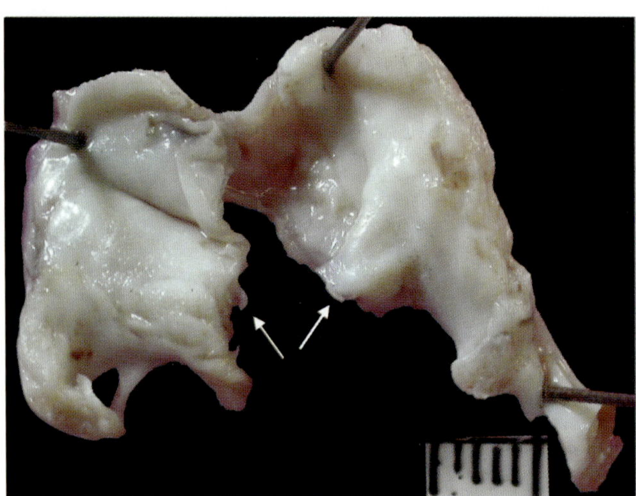

FIG. 14: Surgically excised anterior mitral leaflet. Balloon valvotomy had produced a tear (arrows) in the mid-portion of the leaflet, extending from the free margin to the almost the basal aspect.

■ REFERENCES

1. Remenyi B, ElGuindy A, Smith Jr SC, Yacoub M, Holmes Jr DR. Valvular aspects of rheumatic heart disease. Lancet. 2016;387:1335-46.

2. Ravisha MS, Tullu MS, Kamat JR. Rheumatic fever and rheumatic heart disease: Clinical profile of 550 cases in India. Arch Med Research. 2003;34:382-7.

9

Etiopathogenesis, Clinical Manifestations, and Diagnosis of Acute Rheumatic Fever

IB Vijayalakshmi, Chitra Narasimhan

> *"The most essential part of a student's instruction is obtained, as I believe, not in the lecture room, but at the bedside."*
>
> **—Oliver Wendell Holmes** (1809–1894)
> (US Humorist and Physician)

INTRODUCTION

Acute rheumatic fever (ARF) and its long-term sequelae, rheumatic heart disease (RHD), are a major problem in children, adolescents, and young adults.[1] The morbidity and mortality due to ARF and its consequences RHD remain very high.[2] Despite the tremendous progress made in cardiology, ARF is the leading cause of acquired heart disease in children and young adults worldwide. In many developing countries including India, RHD has remained a burning problem.

It is estimated, according to WHO,[3] that 15.6 million people are affected worldwide by ARF, and 3 lakhs out of 5 lakhs individuals that acquire ARF every year go on to develop RHD in due course. The magnitude of the problem is enormous. Hence, in order to reduce the disease burden, comprehensive knowledge of the etiopathogenesis, clinical manifestations, and diagnosis is very important for any clinician to evaluate and manage the patient properly.

BACKGROUND

Acute rheumatic fever follows 0.3–3% of cases of group A beta-hemolytic streptococcal (GABHS) pharyngitis.[4,5] As many as 39% of persons with ARF may develop varying degrees of pancarditis associated with valve insufficiency, heart failure, and even death in some cases. Annually, about 233,000 deaths are directly attributable to ARF or RHD.[3] India is in the phase of "epidemiological transition". On one hand, there is a substantial burden due to RHD; on the other hand, resources are scarce to treat and prevent the disease.

ETIOPATHOGENESIS OF RHEUMATIC FEVER

Pathogenesis of ARF and RHD is a complex maze of events that are immunologically intricate, pathologically significant, and clinically devastating for the patients.[6] Despite years of intensive investigation, the exact pathogenesis of rheumatic fever and RHD remains unclear. However, it is evident that an abnormal humoral and cellular immune response occurs.

Acute rheumatic fever is generally considered to be an inflammatory disorder of connective tissue. It is an autoimmune response to untreated or inadequately treated GABHS pharyngitis in a genetically predisposed host. Due to an autoimmune reaction, many parts of the body may be affected leading to multisystem disease.

It has been proposed that the triggering factor leading to autoimmunity in individuals is the antigenic mimicry between streptococcal antigens, mainly M protein epitopes, and human tissues, such as heart valves, myosin, and tropomyosin, brain proteins, synovial tissue, and cartilage. This is observed in individuals with a genetic predisposition.[7]

Though several genetic markers of susceptibility have been studied, no consistent association has been found.[8] But in several populations, associations with different human leukocyte antigens (HLAs) class II have been observed.[9-17]

Molecular mimicry was first demonstrated by the humoral immune response. Streptococcal antibodies cross-react with several human tissues including the heart, skin, brain, glomerular basement membrane, and striated and smooth muscles.[18]

There is a suggestion of the direct role of the CD4+ T-cells in the pathogenesis of RHD and this has been proven by the presence of these cells at the lesion sites in the heart.[19,20] Infiltrating T-lymphocytes from heart lesions of severe RHD patients and peripheral T-lymphocytes were capable of recognizing immunodominant myocardium M5 peptides and valve proteins. These results have emphasized the significance of molecular mimicry between beta-hemolytic streptococci and the heart tissue assessing the T-cell repertoire leading to local tissue damage in RHD.[21,22] **Figure 1** illustrates the events that occur during the development of ARF/RHD.

Acute rheumatic fever occurs equally in boys and girls in the age group of 6–15 years. It is rare in children <5 years of age. In families prone to the disorder, it is difficult to distinguish between the heredity factors and the effects of lifestyle factors such as overcrowding and poor medical care. Antibody titers to group A carbohydrate are significantly higher and more persistent in patients who develop RHD than in those who do not.[23] This may be due to a genetic basis. A large proportion of B-lymphocyte cells with a specific alloantigen have been found in 99% of patients with rheumatic fever as opposed to only 14% of controls.[24] A high incidence of class II HLA has also been found in rheumatic fever patients, but the definite association is questionable due to the variability of dominant HLA types in different populations.

Although the genetic pattern of rheumatic fever has not been fully established, it is generally accepted that an immunologic mechanism, either humoral or cellular, is responsible for the injury. During the period of 1–3 weeks after apparent recovery from streptococcal pharyngitis, antibodies to breakdown products from the bacteria cross-react with molecularly similar host tissue in the heart, joints, and central nervous system.[25,26] These cross-reactive antibodies return to a normal level only after several months to years. Rheumatic heart valves have macrophages, mononuclear cells, and fibroblasts. In valve tissue removed from patients, T-cell subpopulations have been identified. T-cells react predominantly with the valve tissue rather than the myocardium. This corresponds to the clinical course of RHD. One theory proposes that the cellular response causes the cardiac effects of the disease, while the humoral response accounts for the other clinical manifestations.

Unfortunately, the affection of all the systems subsides except the heart. The upper respiratory infection by many strains of GABHS can produce ARF. In the past, it was believed that pyoderma caused by GABHS was not responsible for ARF. However, today potential danger of skin infection by group C and group G streptococci are also being investigated. It is believed that repeated sore throat by GABHS is needed to stimulate the immune system to cause an autoimmune reaction in order to cause ARF finally. The four phases of the disease are shown in **Figure 2**.

The manifold clinical signs of rheumatic fever have been the cause of much confusion in our conception of the essential nature of the disease.[27] Another reason for this confusion is the fact that so many diseases at times have

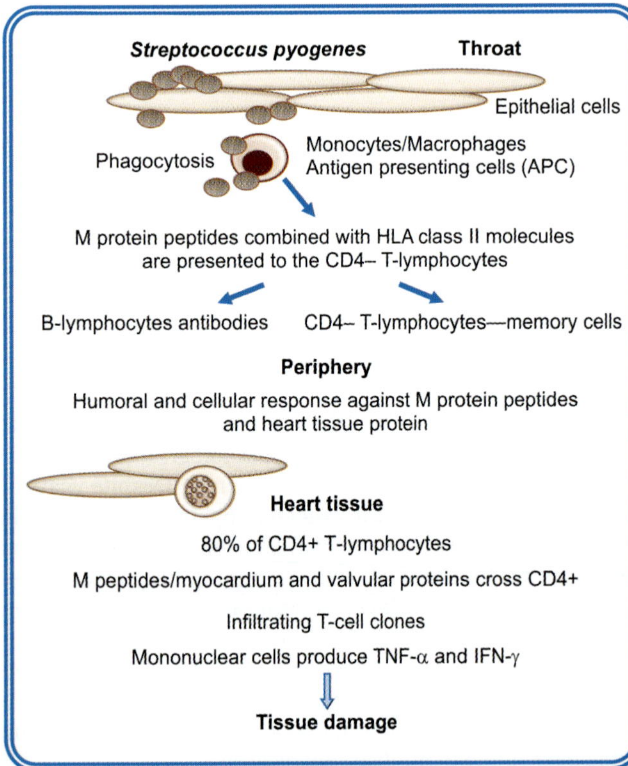

FIG. 1: Schematic representation of the etiopathogenesis sequence occurring during the development of carditis.

(HLA: human leukocyte antigen; IFN-γ: interferon-γ; TNF-α: tumor necrosis factor-alpha)

Source: Reproduced with permission from Binotto MA, Guilherme L, Tanaka AC. Rheumatic Fever. Images Paediatr Cardiol. 2002;11:12-5.

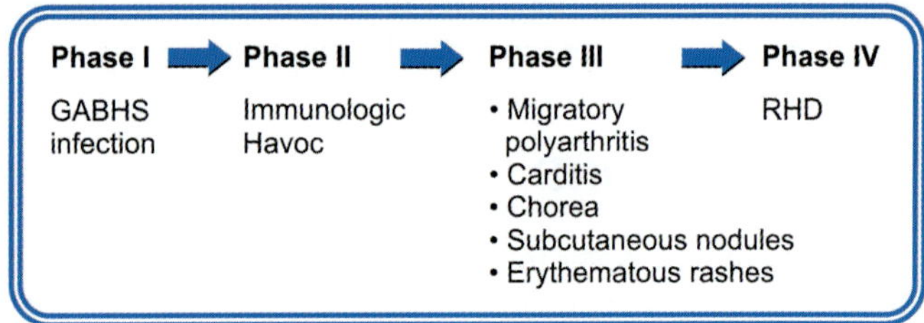

FIG. 2: The four phases of RHD.

(GABHS: group A beta-hemolytic streptococcal infection; RHD: rheumatic heart disease)

joint pains as a part of their symptom complex. Wiesel has stated that no less than 80 different pathological conditions have been included under the term rheumatism. Gradually, as more exact knowledge of various diseases has been acquired, one after another of these numerous conditions has been placed in its proper nosological position and we now realize that inflammation of the joints or muscles is usually a symptom of some general disease. In fact, most specific bacterial infections may occasionally have arthritis as one of their complications.

But, the disease known today as rheumatic fever was generally regarded, until recent years, as having arthritis as its principal manifestation. With auscultatory methods and the application of statistical studies, it became evident a century ago that chronic cardiac valvular disease was frequently preceded by acute arthritis. Endocarditis was then regarded as a complication or sequelae of ARF but we now realize that heart involvement is the most important part of the disease and that the patient is often suffering from active visceral infection with little or no evidence of arthritis. This altered conception of the disease is reflected in changes in the names applied to it from time to time; viz., acute articular rheumatism, acute inflammatory rheumatism, or ARF. The last appellation is probably best because the infection not infrequently passes into a subacute or chronic form.

Generations of medical students have been taught concepts about the pathogenesis of rheumatic fever, which have great appeal. The concept of "molecular mimicry" lays down that, few components of the walls of certain strains of streptococci fortuitously show close molecular similarity with connective tissue components of heart valves and antibodies produced against the bacterial antigen cross-react against the heart, causing damage. The theory always had inconsistencies. The Aschoff body has no histological features that suggest humoral damage and bound gamma globulin is not present in the tissues. The studies show that T-cells from the hearts of subjects who have had rheumatic fever can recognize both cardiac and bacterial wall antigens and the damage to the heart is probably cell-based, a small but important change in thinking. Pathogenesis of rheumatic fever is a delayed complication of pharyngeal infection with group A beta-hemolytic streptococci.

Susceptible individuals develop a diffuse inflammatory disease of the heart, joints, brain, blood vessels, and subcutaneous tissue. Carditis is the most serious manifestation of the disease. It may culminate in chronic valvular disease and can lead to heart failure and ultimately death.

Susceptibility

Every case with GABHS infection does not get ARF. Only 3–6% of the population is susceptible to ARF. The ARF in monozygotic twins and many children in the same family indicate that susceptibility is inherited. The HLA class II allele is strongly associated with susceptibility for ARF. In association, many patients with ARF have a high level of mannose-binding lactin and polymorphisms of

transforming growth factor B1 gene and immunoglobulin genes in circulation.[28-30] High level of a particular alloantigen present on B-cells, D-8 to D-17 has been found in patients with a history of ARF. Intermediate level expression is found in first-degree family members suggesting susceptibility is inherited.

Immune Response

The autoimmune reaction occurs when a susceptible person gets GABHS sore throat. The damage to the connective tissue occurs due to cross-reactivity between epitopes on the cell wall of GABHS and the host.[31,32] The epitopes present in the cell wall, cell membrane, and A, B, and C repeat regions of group A Streptococcal M protein are immunologically similar to molecules in human myosin, tropomyosin, keratin, actin, laminin, vimentin, and N-acetylglucosamine. This molecular similarity is the basis for autoimmune reactions resulting in ARF. It is hypothesized that the molecules particularly epitopes in cardiac myosin sensitize the T-cells. When subsequent GABHS infection occurs, these T-cells are recalled as they are immunologically similar to epitopes. The valvular damage is the hallmark of carditis in ARF. But, myosin cross-reactivity with M protein does not explain the involvement of valves, as the myosin is not present on valve tissue. But, the antibodies to the cardiac valve tissue cross-react with the N-acetylglucosamine of group A streptococcal carbohydrate. There is evidence to show that these antibodies may be responsible for valvular damage in the heart.

Histopathology of Lesions in Acute Rheumatic Fever [27]

Acute rheumatic fever is a self-limited, multisystem disease that can affect the heart, joints, brain, and cutaneous and subcutaneous tissues. The gross clinical manifestations of rheumatic arthritis are pain, tenderness, swelling, redness, and local heat diffusely distributed about the joint. An examination of the synovial fluid reveals many exudative cells, mostly polymorphonuclear leukocytes. Remarkable features of the acute arthritis are: (1) the tendency for the inflammation to migrate or to jump from one joint to another without any apparent involvement of the intervening tissues, (2) the failure of the process to go on to suppuration, and (3) the rapid disappearance of the symptoms and signs of inflammation after the patient has taken such antipyretic drugs as certain derivatives of salicylic acid or phenyl-cinchoninic acid.

Histopathology of Joint Lesions

The inflammation of the joints, a most outstanding feature from the patient's viewpoint, has been the least studied by histopathological methods. The transient nature of arthritis and the fact that patients rarely succumb to acute disease easily explain the apparent gap in our knowledge. Heart failure is practically always accountable for the death of these patients at a time when arthritis has disappeared and hence the chief attention of the pathologist has been directed to this organ.

Nevertheless, Fahr has found changes in the capsule of the knee of patients succumbing to rheumatic fever, which he states are in every way comparable to the myocardial lesions. Coombs makes a similar statement concerning the shoulder joint of one patient. Portions of the capsule of the knee or ankle examined at the acute stages of rheumatic arthritis had focal lesions of the synovia, focal necrosis of the capsule, thrombosis of the smaller arteries, and endothelial and perivascular reactions, comparable with changes found in the heart and in subcutaneous nodules. The presence of many small nerves in the joint capsule and surrounding ligaments easily explains the great pain in rheumatic arthritis. The finding of distinct histological lesions in the joint capsule of a patient fully under the influence of neocinchophen and from whom all clinical signs of arthritis had disappeared indicates that the essential rheumatic process may go on despite these antiphlogistic drugs.

Histopathology of Cardiac Lesions

Cardiac damage is the only potentially chronic debilitating effect. In fatal cases, the longest recognized and most striking gross feature found postmortem is the appearance of rows of small beadlike excrescences along the free margins of the heart valves. On microscopic examination, the verrucae are seen to be made up of coagulated elements derived from the circulating blood, in other words, small globular thrombi deposited on the valvular endocardium at a place where the lining endothelium has disappeared. In older verrucae, there is also definite evidence of a tendency to heal; the verrucae are covered with endothelium and invaded by organizing connective tissues. But even in the young lesions, there is seen in the substance of the heart valve under the endocardium distinct evidence of inflammation, not exudative but proliferative in nature. It is a moot point whether the destruction of the endothelium is primary or subsequent to an injury to the underlying tissue. Of this, however, we are certain that characteristic lesions occur in the mural subendocardial region without primary injury to the endothelium and also are found in the base of the valve leaflets. It is not difficult to conceive, therefore, of the primary injury of the valves occurring in their substance rather than on their surface and if this is true, it would be better to consider the rheumatic disease of these structures as a valvulitis rather than simple endocarditis. If edema and swelling are present in the valves to the same extent as in the joints, it is easy to think of them as being functionally faulty and to see the possibility of the swollen covering endothelium being broken by repeated impacts against an opposing valve leaflet.

When the pericardium is extensively inflamed, there is often a widespread pouring out of serofibrinous exudate with a plastering together of the two layers of the pericardial sac. Upon first glance, this seems an entirely different process than is found in other tissues but the presence in the pericardium of focal lesions similar to Aschoff bodies indicates that the essential or primary pathological process is similar to that found elsewhere, but that the gross appearance is altered by the peculiar anatomical structure of the pericardial sac and the manner in which such large endothelial membranes respond to injury.

Bedside study and electrocardiographic investigation in a series of patients indicate that the myocardium or conduction system was disturbed in about 95% of the cases. While it is conceivable that these functional disturbances may have been merely toxic in origin, it seems more rational to conclude that there is a direct relationship between the histopathological lesions demonstrable postmortem and the disturbed myocardial function found during life. The transitory nature of many of these cardiac disturbances is no argument against their being due to actual focal lesions, for evidence is constantly increasing that focal lesions persist in inflamed joints, even though clinical manifestations of arthritis are present only for a few days.

It is important, on the other hand, to realize that active disease of the heart may be the only demonstrable evidence of continuing rheumatic activity. In two fatal cases, myocardial weakness was the sole clinical picture and in the postmortem, the only distinct lesions were Aschoff bodies widely disseminated throughout the heart muscle. In several patients suffering from chronic cardiac disease, it was observed relapse after relapse with pyrexia and the general features of recurring infection in which all of the symptoms and signs were referable to myocardial and endocardial involvement. Postmortem, these cases have shown widespread rheumatic myocarditis, along with endocarditis and pericarditis. These correlated clinical, physiological, and pathological studies are giving us a clear conception of the chronic or relapsing nature of rheumatic fever.

Histopathology of Subcutaneous Nodules

For many years, English clinicians have called attention to the frequent occurrence of fibroid nodules in the subcutaneous tissue of children with ARF. Anatomically, they are found in the deep fascia over bony prominences and in tendon sheaths and tendons. The essential histological picture is similar to that seen in the Aschoff body. In close apposition to areas of cellular proliferation, there is tissue destruction varying in size from small submiliary areas to long strands of hyaline necrosis affecting connective tissue fibers and combined with necrosis are deposits of fibrin. Surrounding these destroyed foci are found numerous cells similar in appearance and staining reaction to the type of cells found in Aschoff bodies and multinuclear giant cells are also present. In nodules, it is not difficult to demonstrate these endothelioid cells arising from perivascular spaces as well as from the vascular endothelium. In fact, the participation of the blood vessels in the general response is one of the most marked features of the subcutaneous nodules. Many capillaries are seen in which the swollen endothelium has practically obliterated the lumen; in the arterioles, the proliferation of the endothelium at times takes the form of a crescent-shaped mass of cells, appreciably narrowing the vessel. Still, other small arteries are seen obliterated by thrombi and in others, the media are involved, and surrounding many of the smaller vessels, there can often be seen collections of endothelioid cells evidently compressing the walls. The participation of fibroblasts arising from the connective tissue is easy to demonstrate. A few polymorphonuclear cells and lymphocytes invade the diseased tissue and foci of edema are demonstrable. While, grossly, these nodules vary in size from 0.5 to 5 or 10 mm, it is evident upon microscopic examination that the larger nodules are composed of a conglomeration of submiliary nodules. The pathological unity of the myocardial and subcutaneous lesions is, therefore, easily comprehensible.

These subcutaneous nodules attract attention clinically only on account of their mechanical presence. They are usually painless because they are not in close apposition to nerves. Involving only connective tissue, which has no important function except that of a supporting structure, they are not a local source of danger. Their chief significance is that they indicate a similar process going on in such important organs as the heart or brain.

Histopathology of Chorea Minor

The relation of St Vitus' dance, or chorea minor, to rheumatic fever has been discussed for many years. It has been known that valvular heart disease and chorea were frequently concomitant and also that arthritis and chorea occurred together. The relatively few studies of the brains of chorea patients reported in the literature indicate that the chief lesion is vascular in origin. Thrombi, endothelial proliferation, and perivascular collections of round cells together with small focal changes in the nervous tissue contiguous to these vessel lesions have been described. The very small amount of connective tissue in the parenchyma of the brain and the fact that the response of the central nervous system to injury is normally a neuroglia proliferation would naturally cause a different histological picture in the brain than would be seen elsewhere. The finding, however, of typical Aschoff bodies in the hearts of patients dying from chorea and the demonstration of subcutaneous fibroid nodules in others who have recovered, all support the viewpoint that the lesions in the various organs are all evidence of tissue response to a common causative agent of rheumatic fever.

Correlation of Symptoms and Histopathological Lesions of Rheumatic Fever

With this conception of the essential pathology of rheumatic fever, viz., disseminated focal submiliary nodules with edema in the connective tissues during the acute stages, combined with lesions of blood vessels, it is not difficult to reconcile the manifold and apparently unrelated manifestations of the disease. It is apparent that the type of response is an effort on the part of the body to limit the activity of the autoimmune reaction. The edema redness and local heat seen in the

joints with acute arthritis are evidence of intense tissue response to the reaction. These gross clinical signs, however, disappear quickly, both spontaneously and following the consumption of certain drugs. But, small disseminated lesions of a focal character are evidently present in the periarticular tissue and synovia much the same as in other organs and are doubtless slower in undergoing complete resolution than the rapid recession of clinical symptoms would indicate. The pain and tenderness of acute arthritis are probably due to the implication of numerous nerves in the acute exudative process. With the disappearance of extensive edema, these symptoms usually disappear but not infrequently one encounters patients in whom slight pain, stiffness, and tenderness persist in certain joints for weeks or months. These continuing symptoms might easily result from the persistence of focal lesions of a subacute or chronic character. The intensity of the response about the joints is probably an important factor in the complete healing of arthritic lesions. The synovia and perisynovial tissues are rich in blood vessels and, hence, are in a condition to respond quickly and intensely to numerous small focal injuries. In subcutaneous nodules, on the other hand, the tissue involved is less vascular acute exudation is less marked than about joints. Perivascular cellular proliferation is very prominent and the more subacute type of response is made evident by a slower disappearance of the evidence of injury. As already mentioned, the absence of nerves in the tissues implicated by subcutaneous nodules easily explains the lack of pain or tenderness about them. With an understanding of what happens in joints and subcutaneous nodules, it is not difficult to construct a picture of the various cardiac lesions. On pathological examination, the valves are thickened and display rows of small nodules along their apposing surfaces.

The Aschoff body closely reproduces the changes seen in a single vessel in a subcutaneous nodule. In the heart, there is a relatively smaller amount of connective tissue than is present in subcutaneous nodules, and in addition, as the submiliary nodules usually occur in small arteries, their microscopic size is easily understood. Again, a low degree of vascularity compared with the articular tissues explains the comparatively small amount of exudation but transitory exudation is suggested by the rapidity with which electrocardiographic signs of myocardial involvement appear and disappear during the acute stages of rheumatic fever. Partial or complete occlusion of the arterioles would also result in a compromising of the nutrition of the portion of the heart supplied by them. There is also actual destruction of muscle fibers to explain certain symptoms of myocardial disease. It is, therefore, probably not overstressing the point to contend that in rheumatic fever disturbance of cardiac function points to the presence of focal lesions in the myocardium or cardiac blood vessels. Focal lesions of the pericardium, if small, may result in localized pericarditis and on the other hand, if widespread, may be followed by extensive exudation. In fact, the outpouring of a serofibrinous exudate is the usual mode of response to extensive injury of large endothelial lined cavities like the pericardium and pleura, even though the character of lesions produced by the causative organisms in other tissues is usually focal in nature, for example, tuberculosis of the pleura or pericardium is ordinarily accompanied by a serofibrinous exudate. The organization of this exudate with the secondary changes incident to such organization is merely the logical outcome of widespread pericarditis.

The peculiar character of rheumatic valvular endocarditis is more difficult to reconcile with the other focal lesions of this disease. As already mentioned, if we conceive of edema of the valve occurring as an exudative response to focal rheumatic lesions in the valve substance, it is not difficult to see how the endothelium at the line of closure would be injured and small thrombi deposited on the valves at this site of injury. The healing of these thrombi must be necessarily accompanied by the formation of new blood vessels and fibrous tissue and with this process, there is not only the scarring of the valves leading to a disturbance of their function but also the production of a locus minoris resistance in or about which subsequent relapses of rheumatic fever are liable to set up new foci of inflammation. It is only fair to state that we are still uninformed of the exact mechanism by which chronic inflammation of the valves leads to progressive narrowing or funnel-shaped deformities. The manner in which multiple vascular and perivascular lesions in the brain set up the symptoms of chorea is not entirely clear. In chorea, however, there is usually evidence of widespread encephalitis. Sometimes, practically all of the voluntary movements of the body are rendered incoordinate, and at other times, the symptoms point to a less extensive distribution of the pathological process. The symptoms of the implication of the central nervous system by rheumatic fever, therefore, point to the existence of many small foci, probably in the corpus striatum, but also in the cerebral cortex and we may regard these foci as similar in nature to those found in other tissues of the body.

It is evident that there are two distinct types of response on the part of the body to the reaction of rheumatic fever, viz., proliferative and exudative. The perivascular proliferative type of lesion, resembling an infectious granuloma, explains the subacute and chronic character of the clinical symptoms in many patients with this disease. Marked exudation of serum into the periarticular tissues and of serum and cells into the joint cavities are concomitants of acute arthritis occurring with high fever and general intoxication and these acute exudations disappear following the administration of certain drugs. But, their disappearance does not mean necessarily that all lesions of the proliferative type have resolved. In fact, we know that these last-mentioned lesions, when present in the subcutaneous tissues, often continue for months, and from analogy, we may conclude that they have a similar persistent character in other tissues of the body.

CLINICAL MANIFESTATIONS

The signs and symptoms of ARF vary greatly and are determined by the systems involved, the severity of the lesions, their time of appearance in the course of the disease, and the stage of the disease at the time the patient is first observed by the physician. The clinical manifestations that follow streptococcal infections occur simultaneously with a frequency far exceeding chance and may occur in close succession singly or in various combinations in an individual patient. To promote uniformity in diagnosis, Jones proposed a set of criteria based on which he termed, the major and minor clinical and laboratory manifestations of rheumatic fever. The criteria are designed to establish the diagnosis in patients of rheumatic fever. The words "major" and "minor" are related to their importance as diagnostic criteria and do not refer to the severity of the process, its activity, or prognosis. They should not be used for measuring rheumatic activity nor for establishing the diagnosis of inactive RHD.[33,34]

The criteria were revised in 1992 by the American Heart Association's Committee on Rheumatic Fever and Bacterial Endocarditis and Kawasaki Disease of the Council on Cardiovascular Disease in the Young **(Table 1)**[35] and consists of five major criteria, five minor criteria plus supporting features. In the absence of a specific diagnostic test for rheumatic fever, the revised criteria serve as guidelines for making the diagnosis. In 2002–2003, World Health Organization criteria for the diagnosis of rheumatic fever and RHD (based on the 1992 revised Jones criteria) is given in **Table 2**.[36] In 2015, American Heart Association drafted a Scientific Statement revising the Jones criteria to suit the era of Doppler echocardiography, as given in **Table 3**.[37]

TABLE 1: Revised Jones criteria for diagnosis of acute rheumatic fever. [35]	
Major criteria	*Minor criteria*
Carditis: • Polyarthritis • Chorea • Erythema marginatum • Subcutaneous nodules	Clinical findings: • Arthralgia • Fever Laboratory findings: • Elevated acute phase reactant (ESR or CRP) • Prolonged PR interval on ECG
Supporting evidence of antecedent group A streptococcal infection: • Positive throat culture or rapid antigen test • Elevated or rising streptococcal antibody titer	
Diagnosis of ARF requires two major criteria or one major and two minor criteria, plus supporting evidence of antecedent group A streptococcal infection	
(CRP: C-reactive protein; ECG: electrocardiogram; ESR: erythrocyte sedimentation rate)	

TABLE 2: WHO criteria for the diagnosis of rheumatic fever and rheumatic heart disease.[36]

Diagnostic categories	Criteria
The primary episode of rheumatic fever	Two major or one major and two minor manifestations *plus* evidence of preceding group A streptococcal infection
Recurrent attack of rheumatic fever in a patient without established rheumatic heart disease	Two major or one major and two minor manifestations *plus* evidence of preceding group A streptococcal infection
Recurrent attack of rheumatic fever in a patient with established rheumatic heart disease	Two minor manifestations *plus* evidence of preceding group A streptococcal infection
• Rheumatic chorea • Insidious onset rheumatic carditis	Other major manifestations or evidence of group A streptococcal infection not required
Chronic valve lesions of rheumatic heart disease (patient presenting for the first time with pure mitral stenosis or mixed mitral valve disease and/or aortic valve disease)	Do not require any other criteria to be diagnosed as having rheumatic heart disease

TABLE 3: Modified 2015 Jones criteria for the diagnosis of acute rheumatic fever in the era of Doppler echocardiography.[37]

Low-risk population	High-risk population
Major criteria	
• Carditis (clinical or subclinical) • Arthritis—only polyarthritis • Chorea • Erythema marginatum • Subcutaneous nodules	• Carditis (clinical or subclinical) • Arthritis—monoarthritis or polyarthritis • Polyarthralgia • Chorea • Erythema marginatum • Subcutaneous nodules
Minor criteria	
• Polyarthralgia • Hyperpyrexia (≥38.5°C) • ESR ≥ 60 mm/h and/or CRP ≥ 3.0 mg/dL • Prolonged PR interval (after taking into account the differences related to age; if there is no carditis as a major criterion)	• Monoarthralgia • Hyperpyrexia (≥38.0°C) • ESR ≥ 30 mm/h and/or CRP ≥ 3.0 mg/dL • Prolonged PR interval (after taking into account the differences related to age, if there is no carditis as a major criterion)

(ESR: erythrocyte sedimentation rate; CRP: C-reactive protein)

Major Manifestations of Acute Rheumatic Fever

The major manifestations of ARF are: (i) carditis, (ii) polyarthritis, (iii) chorea, (iv) erythema marginatum, and (v) subcutaneous nodules. They are least likely to lead to an improper diagnosis.

Minor Manifestations of ARF

The minor manifestations of ARF may be frequently present but are too nonspecific. They are not sufficient to make the diagnosis of ARF. They include such common clinical findings as fever, arthralgia, elevated acute phase reactants in the blood such as C-reactive protein (CRP) and elevated erythrocyte sedimentation rate (ESR), elevated leukocyte count, prolonged PR interval on electrocardiogram (ECG), and helpful information such as history of previous ARF or RHD. The presence of two major criteria or one major and two minor criteria is considered highly indicative of the diagnosis, if clearly supported by evidence of a recent streptococcal infection such as increased or rising antistreptolysin O (ASLO) titer or the other streptococcal antibodies or a positive GABHS throat culture or rapid antigen test for group A streptococci or recent scarlet fever.

The importance of antecedent streptococcal infection has been emphasized in subsequent revisions of the Jones criteria, in which a diagnosis of ARF required the demonstration of streptococcal etiology.[34] Though the inclusion of this criterion helped to improve diagnostic specificity, it impaired sensitivity, especially in patients with insidious and chronic carditis, where the evidence of antecedent streptococcal infection had already subsided or in cases of chorea where the manifestations of ARF are delayed.[38] Hence, the late manifestations of ARF were subsequently exempted from the requirement to demonstrate streptococcal etiology.[35,39] The antecedent streptococcal infection regularly precedes ARF. This has been demonstrated by antibody studies. More than one-third of patients do not remember having had any illness in the preceding month and even those who recall may report a nondescript respiratory infection and not always clearly a sore throat. Patients who recall sore throat would have seldom consulted a physician for treatment but throat culture would not have been done and adequate antibiotics would not have been prescribed to prevent rheumatic fever. The high frequency of a history of the patient having no sore throat is surprising when one considers the relation of severity of streptococcal pharyngitis to the attack of rheumatic fever. A positive throat culture or rapid streptococcal antigen tests are less adequate than rising antibody titers, as they reflect colonization rather than recent or current infection. If the ASLO titers are not suggestive, antibodies to deoxyribonuclease B, hyaluronidase, or streptokinase may be used.[35]

DIAGNOSIS

Unfortunately, precise diagnosis of ARF has presented problems since Hippocrates, who provided the first written description of arthritis in a man in 400 BC.[40] Lack of specific criteria had led to diagnostic chaos until the publication of the listings of Duckett Jones in 1944.[41] Despite the four revisions and modifications of the Jones criteria,[41-43] ARF remains either underdiagnosed leading to nearly half of the patients with established RHD not receiving prophylaxis or overdiagnosed, leading to unnecessary treatment with penicillin prophylaxis. ARF and RHD occur in almost all the developing countries but are more common in the Indian subcontinent, sub-Saharan Africa, New Zealand, and Pacific nations. The reasons for ARF to remain a burning problem are confusion in diagnosis, confusion in management, poor socioeconomic condition, lack of hygiene and awareness, lack of prophylaxis, lack of vaccine, and no national rheumatic fever control program in India.

The diagnosis of ARF is a clinical challenge. As a result, >50% of ARF/RHD detected in surveys and health check- up camps are unaware of their disease. More than 70% do not receive secondary prophylaxis regularly.[42] The penicillin prophylaxis was mentioned in the history of some 25% of all subjects with active rheumatic fever. The others had either received no prophylaxis at all (35%) or were receiving penicillin only occasionally. In patients with previous rheumatic fever who were followed up prospectively for recurrences, asymptomatic streptococcal infections accounted for 54–70% of rheumatic recurrences. The precise diagnosis of ARF is eluding the clinician because of many pitfalls of Jones criteria. For example, it is difficult to clinically diagnose ARF when carditis is the only manifestation of the disease, particularly in a recurrence or when a patient has subclinical carditis or apparent carditis but supportive noncarditis criteria are not fulfilled. When the previous cardiac status is unknown, it is not possible to know whether the findings are new or old. In cases of polyarthralgia, which is a minor criterion, if the patient is neglected and not evaluated for ARF, underdiagnosis of ARF can occur. Due to these lacunae in Jones criteria though "carditis" is the only presentation of ARF that causes death during the acute stage or leads to permanent damage with long-term morbidity and mortality due to RHD and congestive heart failure (CHF), precise and early diagnosis of "carditis" in ARF is eluding the clinicians.

Overall, 452 consecutive patients, suspected to have ARF, were evaluated in a prospective study.[44] Out of them, 200 were from rural and 252 from an urban background. In this study of ARF, 230 were males and 222 females. ARF usually occurs in children between the age of 5 and 15 years. But in this study, the youngest patient was 1 year 11 months and oldest patient with the first attack of ARF was 51 years and there was one lady with recrudescence of rheumatic activity at the age of 65 years. The mean age was 11.7 ± 5.4 migratory polyarthritis was present in 260 cases (57.12%) polyarthralgia in 239 out of which only 38 cases (15.9%) were clinically suspected of carditis, but 88 cases (36.8%) had ECHO evidence of carditis/

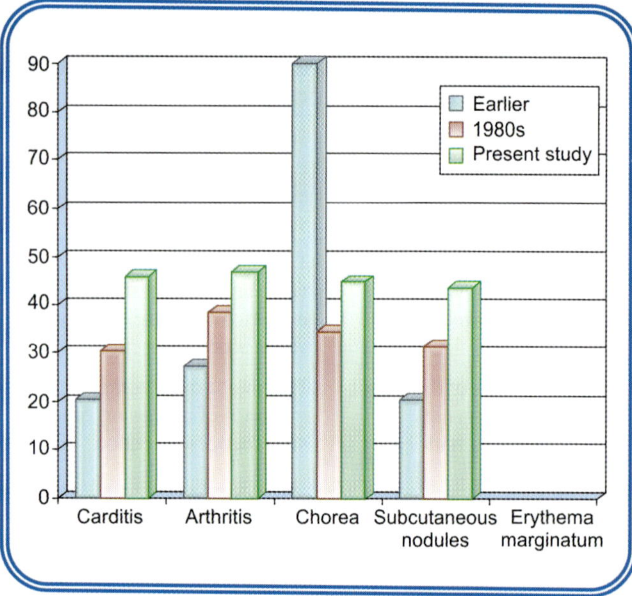

FIG. 3: Changing the clinical profile of acute rheumatic fever.

valvulitis. The incidence of polyarthritis was only 52.8%, carditis 36.28%, chorea 8.8%, subcutaneous nodules 2.4%, and erythema marginatum 0.4%. Interestingly, incidence of polyarthralgia, which is included in minor criteria, is a whopping 47.12%. When compared to previous older studies, probably these numbers of this recent study indicate the changing clinical profile of ARF (**Fig. 3**).

When we look at the changing profile of clinical manifestations of ARF, we realize that the incidence of arthritis is decreasing and the incidence of polyarthralgia with ECHO evidence of carditis is increasing. Therefore, polyarthralgia, which was originally a major criterion in 1944, should be given the same importance as polyarthritis and made a major criterion. Otherwise, it will lead to underdiagnosis in endemic areas. The incidence of erythema marginatum has dwindled to <0.5%, which is very negligible.

CLINICAL FEATURES

The time interval between the onset of symptoms of pharyngitis and the onset of the first symptoms of ARF is called the latent, silent, or lag period of the disease (**Fig. 4**).

There is an absence of evidence of the disease during this interval. Following streptococcal infection, temperature and pulse return to normal but ESR may remain higher in patients who subsequently develop rheumatic fever than those who do not. Streptococci often continue to be carried in the throat but frequently in small numbers and this may require special techniques of a throat culture to demonstrate them.

Clinical manifestations usually show up 1–5 weeks after the onset of pharyngitis and the average interval was 18.6 days in one of the best prospective studies. The average

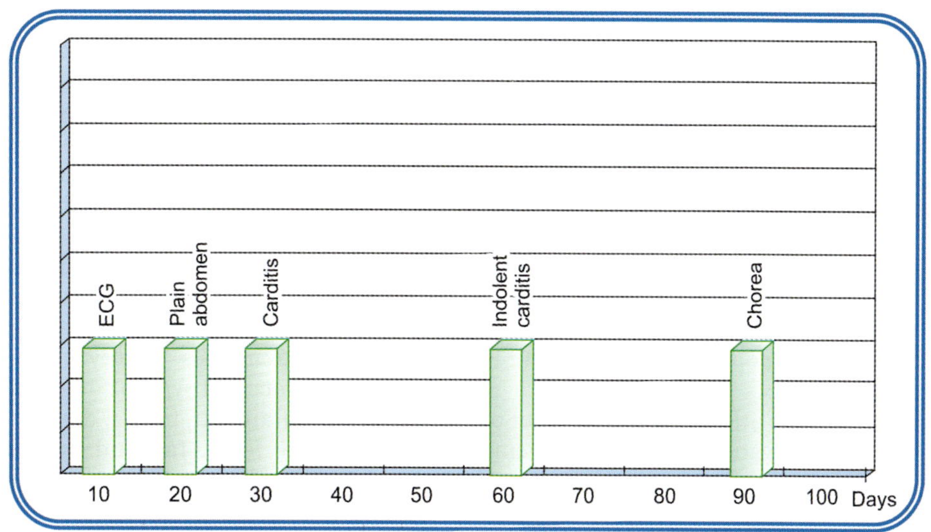

FIG. 4: The latent period between "Strep throat" and onset of symptoms. (ECG: electrocardiography)

latent period is the same for recurrent attacks as for initial episodes.[45] Electrocardiographic evidence of delayed AV conduction with inverted T waves may appear within 9 days after streptococcal infection and as early as 7 days before the onset of arthritis.[35] Chorea and indolent carditis may occur after a long latent period of 3–6 months.

The onset of rheumatic fever may be very variable depending on the manifestations of the disease expressed, the toxicity of the disease, the time at which the patient is brought to the physician, and the thoroughness with which he perceives its manifestations. Onset may be acute or insidious. Acute attacks are usually associated with arthritis or carditis with pericardial effusion. Insidious onset of rheumatic fever is seen in some cases of carditis and chorea, in which early behavior changes may be misinterpreted. Many a time, the patient may present with a high fever and a toxic state or with only mild and prolonged constitutional symptoms such as fatigue and anorexia. The physician on examination may identify the high-pitched soft blowing murmur of mitral regurgitation (MR), as well as laboratory evidence of an obvious systemic inflammatory process.[35]

Arthritis

Rheumatic fever owes its name to its most common major manifestation which is the involvement of the joints "rheumatism", even though carditis is a far more serious and important manifestation. Though migratory polyarthritis is the most common major criterion, it is the least specific criterion. Arthritis frequency increases with age, being seen in up to three-quarters of patients as an isolated presentation, or in association with other manifestations of the disease.[46] Perhaps in no other disease, joints are more painful than in ARF. The inability to change the posture without agonizing pain, the drenching sweats, the prostration, and utter

helplessness combine to make it one of the most distressing of febrile afflictions. A special feature of the disease is the tendency of the inflammation to subside in one joint while developing with great intensity in another. Sir William Osler's vivid description of acute polyarthritis a century ago[47] referred to rheumatic fever.

Arthritis typically is nonsuppurative, asymmetrical, migratory or fleeting, self-limited, nondeforming, large joint polyarthritis, especially of the knees, ankles, elbows, and wrists. Characteristically, arthritis begins in the large joints of the lower extremities and migrates to other large joints in the lower or upper extremities. Hip joints and smaller joints of hands and feet are less commonly involved and the spine and temporomandibular joints are only rarely involved. Joint involvement becomes more common with the increasing age of the patient, which is related to the concomitant decrease in the incidence of carditis and chorea.

The diagnosis of arthritis is made when the signs of active joint inflammation are present. The "hot joint" is typically red, hot, swollen and extremely tender, and limited in its range of movement.[48] The migratory nature is very characteristic of this disease. The term "migratory" reflects the sequential involvement of joints, with each completing a cycle of inflammation and resolution, so that some joint inflammation may be resolving while others are beginning.[6] By the time, another joint is involved the pain and swelling in the previous joints subsides. Usually, one or two joints are affected at any given time with each being only involved for between a few hours and a few days. Overlap of multiple joints may occur. When the disease is allowed to express itself fully without antirheumatic treatment, as many as 16 joints may be involved and at least six in half of the patients.[35]

In a large series of patients with ARF and associated arthritis, most of whom had been treated, involvement of only a single large joint was common in 25%, one or both knees were affected in 76% and one or both ankles were affected in 50%. Elbows, wrists, hips, or small joints of the feet were involved in 12–15% of patients, and shoulders or small joints of the hand were affected in 7–8%. Rarely, affected joints included the lumbosacral (2%), cervical (1%), sternoclavicular (0.5%), and temporomandibular (0.5%). Involvement of the small joints of the hands or feet alone occurred in only 1% of these patients.[49]

Monoarthritis can occur and its frequency increases when anti-inflammatory therapy is initiated before ARF is considered or confirmed.[6] Monoarticular arthritis is recognized to be important in populations where ARF is common.

The pain associated with the arthritis is typically out of proportion to the objective findings of inflammation. Patients may experience severe discomfort even due to the presence of clothing, blankets, or bedsheets covering the affected joints due to their extreme tenderness. There is a rapid relief of both objective and subjective joint findings with salicylate therapy, usually within 48–72 hours. This is very characteristic of arthritis and is often considered diagnostic of rheumatic fever. If a patient treated for ARF does not respond promptly to salicylate therapy, an alternative diagnosis should be considered.[50] The pain occurs in both active and passive movements and is usually diffuse. The pain may radiate to periarticular areas and is associated with limitation of motion. Other characteristics of inflammation, such as heat, redness, and swelling, although present, are usually less marked. Without treatment, the inflammatory findings last from 1 to 5 days in each joint, reaching maximum severity in the first 2 days, with the entire process subsiding over 2 to 4 weeks.[46] The course of the entire bout of polyarthritis is usually severe for a week in two-thirds of patients, for an additional week or two in the remainder and by the end of 4 weeks, it will have subsided, with rare exceptions. In a small percentage of cases treated with antirheumatic therapy for 4–6 weeks, flare-ups may occur but rarely after a second 6 weeks course of treatment is received.[35]

Synovial fluid analysis in rheumatic arthritis reveals a sterile, inflammatory fluid. There are 10,000 to 100,000 white blood cells/mm^3 with a predominance of neutrophils, a normal glucose level, a protein concentration of about 4 g/dL, and a good mucin clot.[51] There may be a decrease of the complement components C1q, C3, and C4 in synovial fluid indicating their consumption by immune complexes in the joint fluid.[51]

Acute rheumatic fever never causes permanent joint damage, unlike rheumatoid arthritis and the persistence of arthritis or arthralgia beyond the acute phase casts doubt on the diagnosis. A very rare exception may be the so-called Jaccoud type of deformity (**Fig. 5**) of the metacarpophalangeal joints described in a patient with rheumatic fever. Jaccoud first described chronic arthritis appearing after frequent and severe attacks of rheumatic fever, which he named chronic fibrous rheumatism.[52] Jaccoud's arthropathy is suggested to arise due to connective tissue dysplasia resulting in soft tissue impairment in different rheumatic and nonrheumatic diseases.[53] Bywaters[54] suggested criteria for diagnosis of Jaccoud's arthritis, which were later modified by Zvaifler and Murphy, and Staple. The list of features is:

- There is a history of recurrent, prolonged, severe attacks of rheumatic fever.
- Recovery is delayed with joint stiffness in the metacarpophalangeal joints, which later results in the appearance of joint deformity.
- Pathology reveals that the lesion appears to be fibrosis of the periarticular tissues, fascia, and tendons and not due to synovitis.
- The deformity consists of flexion at the metacarpophalangeal joint with some associated periarticular soft tissue swelling and ulnar deviation most marked in the fifth finger. These deformities are characteristically correctable. There may be slight soft-tissue swelling and associated hyperextension of the proximal interphalangeal joints.

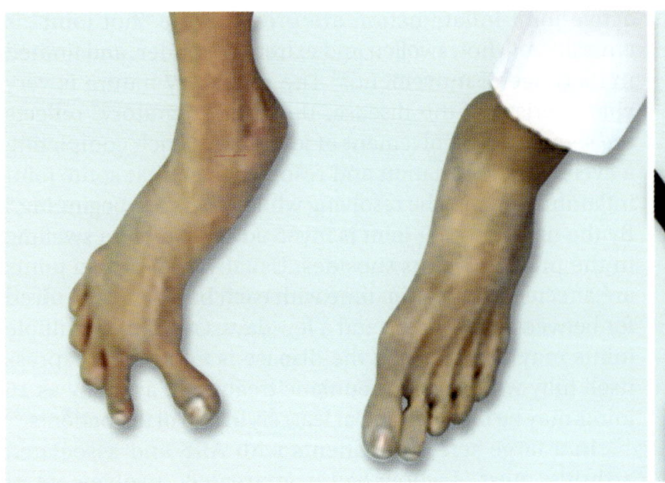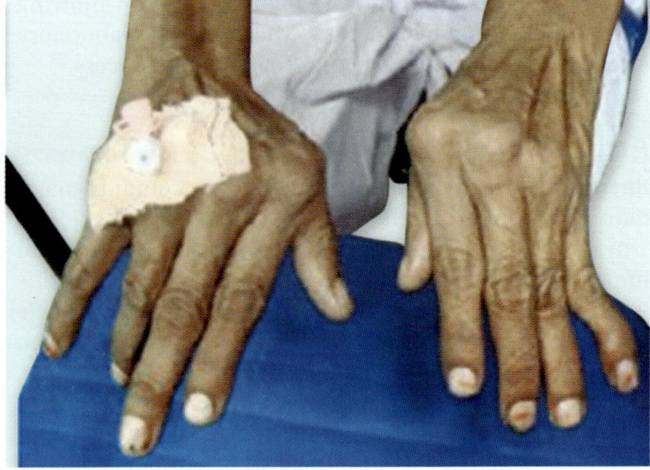

FIG. 5: Jaccoud's arthritis.

- Tendon crepitus may be elicited.
- Joint disease is usually inactive with little or no symptoms and good functional capacity. ESR is normal.
- Radiologically, there is little or no bone damage, which is often in striking contrast to the degree of deformity. In some cases, characteristic hook lesions may be seen on the radial and palmar aspects of the metacarpal heads.
- Tests for rheumatoid factor should be negative.

The incidence and severity of cardiac involvement are lower in patients with severe polyarthritis than in those with milder joint manifestations. Carditis was observed in 26% of patients with red, hot, or swollen joints, in 40% of those with tender joints, and in 96% with arthralgia.[48] The prognosis in patients with red, hot, swollen joints is generally better than in patients with mild arthritis. Thus, the severity of the articular symptoms and signs are inversely proportional to the degree of carditis. Polyarthritis is rarely seen simultaneously with active chorea, mainly due to disparity in the latency period following the antecedent streptococcal infection.[6,25]

Poststreptococcal Reactive Arthritis

Poststreptococcal reactive arthritis (PSRA) is a homogeneous clinical entity distinct from ARF and other forms of reactive arthritis.[55] Goldsmith and Long are credited with the first description of the entity and defined it as arthritis of at least one joint or more joints, associated with a recent group A streptococcal infection in a patient who does not fulfill the Jones criteria for the diagnosis of ARF.[56] Some authors consider PSRA to be part of the spectrum of ARF, whereas other authors consider it to be a different entity. The arthritis of ARF occurs 14–21 days after an episode of GABHS pharyngitis and responds rapidly. Whereas PSRA occurs within 10 days after the GABHS pharyngitis and does not respond readily to anti-inflammatory agents. Arthritis of rheumatic fever is migratory, transient, and usually involves only the large joints, whereas the arthritis of PSRA is persistent or relapsing and can involve large joints, small joints, or the axial skeleton. Arthritis in PSRA can last for weeks or months (average, 2 months) whereas in ARF arthritis lasts for 1–5 days and resolves in an average of 3 weeks. PSRA patients are not associated with other major manifestations of ARF.

It still remains unclear whether it represents a form of reactive arthritis distinct from ARF. This may have important implications regarding prognosis and the need for antistreptococcal prophylaxis. PSRA patients have serological evidence of a recent GABHS infection but not more than half of these patients have GABHS isolated on throat culture.[57]

Deighton[58] proposed the following as distinguishing features of PSRA: (1) onset within 10 days of group A streptococcal infection, as opposed to 2–3 weeks in ARF, (2) prolonged or recurrent arthritis, in contrast to ARF, in which arthritis lasts a few days to 3 weeks, (3) slow and partial response to aspirin, whereas in ARF, the response to aspirin is usually dramatic.

Ayoub and Ahmed[59] proposed the following diagnostic criteria for PSRA based on these clinical features: (1)

arthritis of acute onset, symmetric or asymmetric, usually nonmigratory, can affect any joint, persistent or recurrent. The arthritis is at best only poorly responsive to salicylates or nonsteroidal anti-inflammatory drugs, (2) evidence of antecedent group A streptococcal infection, and (3) failure to fulfill the modified Jones criteria for the diagnosis of ARF. A number of patients presenting initially as post-streptococcal arthritis have later manifested RHD.[60] 5–7% of patients with PSRA have been reported to subsequently develop valvular heart disease.[58] Hence, these patients should be followed up carefully for several months for clinical evidence of carditis. Some experts recommend that these patients receive secondary prophylaxis for up to 1 year after the onset of their symptoms, but its effectiveness is not well established. If clinical evidence of carditis is not observed, the prophylaxis can be discontinued. If the valvular disease is detected, the patient should be classified as having had ARF and should continue to receive secondary prophylaxis.[61]

■ DIFFERENTIAL DIAGNOSIS (TABLE 4)

Polyarthritis unaccompanied by other major manifestations of ARF should be differentiated from many clinical entities. Some differential diagnoses in ARF are other autoimmune diseases, septic arthritis, reactive arthritis, infective endocarditis, Lyme disease, lymphoma/leukemia, viral arthropathy, and sickle cell disease.

Polyarthritis in ARF is almost always associated with a rising or a peak titer of streptococcal antibodies. This helps in identifying isolated bout of polyarthritis as rheumatic or more accurately, in excluding rheumatic fever as an etiology for a given episode of polyarthritis when streptococcal antibodies are not increased in titer.[35]

Arthralgia is defined as pain in the joint without objective signs of inflammation and without limitation of movement or tenderness to touch or swelling or redness of the joints. It may be vague or extensive and impressive. The fleeting joint pain without swelling that is polyarthralgia is considered a minor criterion. Although the difference between arthralgia and arthritis may be only tentative, the distinction is important in establishing the diagnosis of rheumatic fever, especially when arthritis is the only major manifestation.

Arthralgia is a less specific symptom and it is more difficult to be sure of the presence of true joint inflammation when objective signs are lacking. But, polyarthralgia is common. Approximately, one-third of patients with joint involvement reported in a large series of cases of ARF presented with "atypical" articular manifestations, considered by some as a separate entity, i.e., poststreptococcal reactive arthritis. It seems reasonable to include these manifestations as part of the spectrum of ARF. In our study,[44] out of 213 cases of arthralgia (42.88%.), 38 patients (17.84%) had clinical evidence of carditis. Echocardiographic evidence of subclinical carditis or valvulitis, such as thickening and beaded appearance of the valvular leaflets, was present in 88 cases (41.3%). Probably, these polyarthralgia patients

TABLE 4: Differential diagnosis of polyarthritis and fever.[63]

Diagnosis	Confirmatory study
Infectious arthritis	
Bacterial infections: • Septic arthritis • Bacterial endocarditis • Lyme disease • Mycobacterial and fungal arthritis	• Synovial fluid and blood culture • Blood culture • Serological studies • Culture or biopsy
Viral arthritis	Serological studies
Postinfectious or reactive arthritis	
Enteric infection	Culture or serological studies
Urogenital infection (Reiter's syndrome)	Culture
Rheumatic fever	Clinical findings
Inflammatory bowel disease	Clinical findings
Rheumatoid arthritis and Still's disease	Clinical findings
Systemic rheumatic illnesses	Biopsy or angiography
Systemic vasculitis	Serological studies
Systemic lupus erythematosus	
Crystal-induced arthritis	
Gout and pseudogout	Polarizing microscopy of synovial fluid or tophi
Other diseases	
Familial Mediterranean fever	Clinical findings
Cancers	Biopsy
Sarcoidosis	Biopsy
Mucocutaneous disorders dermatomyositis	Biopsy or clinical findings
• Behçet's disease • Henoch–Schönlein purpura • Kawasaki's disease (mucocutaneous lymph node syndrome) • Erythema nodosum • Erythema multiforme • Pyoderma gangrenosum	

go undiagnosed and present as RHD later without a past history of ARF. Therefore, patients with arthralgia must be evaluated for ARF, and secondary prophylaxis should be recommended in these situations to prevent further damage to the heart with recurrent attacks of ARF.

The mechanism or the reason for migratory polyarthritis, which is so characteristic of ARF, is not known.

◼ CLINICAL DIAGNOSIS OF CARDITIS

Carditis is a major clinical manifestation of ARF. It is the most important and serious manifestation of ARF as it will result in death or subsequent disability from its sequel RHD. In its most severe form, carditis causes death from acute CHF. Carditis often implies a severe form of rheumatic fever because of the actual or potential seriousness of the condition. But, cardiac involvement in ARF may often occur in the clinically mildest form of the disease. As noted in the discussion of arthritis, there is actually an inverse correlation between the most toxic forms of arthritis and the frequency of cardiac involvement.[35] Three decades ago, this form of the disease made ARF the leading medical cause of death in school-age children (6–19 years of age), but fulminating rheumatic carditis has now become relatively rare.

Though traditionally acute rheumatic cardiac involvement is described as pancarditis with the endocardium, myocardium, and pericardium all affected to varying degrees, the dominant and most important abnormality is valvulitis. The most common degree of cardiac inflammation, however, is less intense and the predominant effect is scarring of the heart valves. Hence, myocarditis and pericarditis, by themselves, should not be labeled as rheumatic in origin and other etiologies must be considered.[6] The most common involved valve is the mitral, frequently associated with the aortic valve and rarely with tricuspid valve involvement.

Rheumatic carditis most often causes no symptoms of its own and is most often diagnosed in the course of the clinical examination of the patient with arthritis or chorea, due to the organic murmur. Carditis, therefore, is not diagnosed, if other symptoms of rheumatic fever are absent or if the carditis is not severe enough to cause heart failure, prolonged or severe fever, or the pain of pericarditis. Although such patients with undiagnosed carditis may later prove to have RHD, they will give no previous history of a rheumatic attack.

The clinical presentation is quite variable, ranging from the asymptomatic patient with a characteristic heart murmur to the critically ill patient presenting with heart failure. Acute carditis was present in 50% of patients, although it has been reported in some studies as high as 75%.[42,50,63] Some of the variability is likely related to the fact that some patients present only after more than one episode of ARF and carditis when the patient is much more likely to have significant valvular disease and heart failure. About 80% of patients who develop carditis do so within the first 2 weeks of the ARF. If no cardiac involvement is detected in the first 2 weeks, the likelihood of subsequent cardiac involvement during the acute phase is low.[64] The severity of carditis and valvular regurgitation often decreases as the inflammation subsides. If the cardiac involvement is mild, patients may show complete resolution of cardiac findings, but patients with moderate-to-severe carditis are more likely to develop persistent and/or evolving RHD.[63,65]

The four major criteria for the clinical diagnosis of rheumatic carditis are as follows:[33]

1. Organic murmur(s) not previously present
2. Enlargement of the heart
3. Congestive heart failure
4. Pericardial friction rubs or signs of effusion

Signs of carditis[66] include some or all of the following:

- Tachycardia (out of proportion to the degree of fever) is common and its absence makes the diagnosis of myocarditis unlikely.
- A heart murmur of MR or aortic regurgitation (AR), or both, is almost always present. The American Heart Association's Jones criteria recommend not making the diagnosis of acute rheumatic carditis without audible murmurs of MR and/or AR, but this is debatable. Significant ECHO abnormalities may be present in the absence of heart murmur and ECHO findings can determine the severity of cardiac enlargement, the presence and degree of MR and AR, and the presence of pericardial effusion more objectively. Inclusion of ECHO abnormalities may enhance the correct diagnosis of acute rheumatic carditis (Vijayalakshmi et al. 2005).[44] However, a hemodynamically insignificant ECHO finding of MR alone is considered not sufficient to diagnose myocarditis. Gross prolapse of the mitral valve or the presence of a posterolateral (not central) MR jet by color flow mapping may be significant. With chronic rheumatic MR, a fusion of the leaflets and chordae and contracture of these structures occur and the regurgitation jets tend to become more central. Other abnormal ECHO findings may include pericardial effusion, increased left ventricular (LV) dimension, or impaired LV function.
- Pericarditis (friction rub, pericardial effusion, chest pain, and ECG changes) may be present. Pericarditis does not occur without mitral valve involvement in rheumatic fever. Pericardial effusion is usually of a small amount and almost never causes cardiac tamponade.
- Cardiomegaly on chest X-ray films is indicative of the severity of rheumatic carditis or CHF.
- Signs of CHF (gallop rhythm, distant heart sounds, and cardiomegaly) are indications of severe cardiac dysfunction.

Pericarditis is the least common finding in rheumatic carditis. It is not seen as a sole manifestation and occurs in 4–11% of patients with acute rheumatic carditis.[67-70] Clinicians should always look carefully for pericarditis. It may manifest itself in several ways.

Chest pain: It occurs during the course of ARF, typically precordial, and sometimes with radiation to the shoulders, usually the left. Chest pain and fever may be the presenting features of a rheumatic attack. The patient may sit forward in the bed with his arms stretched across the bed table and his forehead pressed on his arms in a characteristic posture to relieve pain and sometimes the dyspnea and tamponade.

Pericardial friction rubs: They are pathognomonic of acute pericarditis when unmistakably present and may be heard when no other features of pericarditis are detected. The characteristic superficial scratching or creaking sound is picked up most often along the left sternal border but also at the base and apex. It is characteristically evanescent and usually heard in both phases of the cardiac cycle but can

be confused with murmurs when heard in either systole or diastole.

Pericardial involvement is diagnosed by the presence of a pericardial friction rub, effusion, distant heart sounds, and typical positional chest pain. The rub is heard as a scratching or grating sound over the precordium, especially along the sternal border, and is heard in both phases of the cardiac cycle, having a to and fro character. It is less transient in rheumatic fever than in pyogenic infections. In the early stages, the friction rub may obscure the murmur of underlying valvular dysfunction and the murmur becomes apparent only when the rub subsides. In mild cases, it can be seen only as an echocardiographic finding.

Pericardial effusion: It frequently presents as a sudden widening of the cardiac shadow on chest X-ray or widening of percussion dullness of the heart waist when the effusion is very large. In rheumatic carditis, however, very large effusions are rare so the signs of this complication are usually absent. One rarely sees symptoms of tamponade without severe heart failure as well and the myocardial failure then dominates the clinical picture. Paradoxical pulse is also rare. The effusion, therefore, is best detected by chest X-ray, which should be taken serially, weekly to avoid being completely overlooked, and even then, it is difficult to comment on the relative contribution to the enlarged heart shadow of pericardial effusion versus myocardial dilatation. Significant effusion and tamponade are rarely found and the rheumatic pericarditis does not result in constriction. Despite its low frequency, pericarditis has diagnostic value by providing evidence of active disease.[46]

Myocarditis manifests as tachycardia that is disproportionate to the patient's fever and which persists during sleep.

Myocarditis may cause rhythm disturbances, cardiomegaly, and CHF.[50] During the first attack, valvulitis is suspected in the presence of a new apical systolic murmur of MR (associated or not with an apical mid diastolic murmur) and/or a basal diastolic murmur of AR. Cardiomegaly is noted on chest X-ray and on echocardiogram. It is contentious if myocardial dysfunction in ARF is valvular or myocardial in origin.[71] Myocarditis is confined to the interstitium and does not usually result in significant myocyte damage, consistent with the preserved LV ejection phase indices seen in patients with active rheumatic activity.[72] Biopsy and autopsy pathologic specimens show evidence of myocardial involvement but unlike other types of myocarditis, myocyte necrosis associated with lymphocytic infiltration does not occur[73] and troponin I levels are not elevated.[74,75] Heart failure does not occur in acute or chronic RHD in the absence of significant valvular dysfunction. In a subset of patients, the initial presentation may be quite severe, with overt heart failure, fever, and toxemia, making the differential diagnosis with infective endocarditis very difficult, in particular in patients with recurrent RHD.

Cardiac involvement is found in nearly 60% of all patients with ARF who eventually develop chronic RHD.[76] In about

40% of patients with ARF with carditis, the changes revert to normal with timely management. The valvular involvement is the hallmark of carditis in ARF. Clinically manifest MR or AR is still considered the diagnostic hallmark of acute rheumatic carditis.[67,77] The most common valve affected is the mitral valve. Sometimes along with the mitral valve, the aortic valve is also affected. But, isolated involvement of the aortic valve is extremely rare. So much so that if an isolated aortic valve is involved it is unlikely to be due to ARF. Rarely tricuspid valve also can be involved along with the mitral and aortic valves. But, the pulmonary valve is rarely involved in ARF. The valvular lesions in ARF often result in residual damage. In milder forms of rheumatic carditis, patients may recover from valvulitis without sequelae.[78] In the first attack, the lesions are predominantly regurgitant, due to ring dilatation, swollen cusps, chordal rupture, or papillary muscle dysfunction. In the chronic phase, obstructive lesions are more frequent.[79]

Murmurs of Acute Rheumatic Fever

The three most important and characteristic murmurs of acute carditis are the apical systolic, the apical mid-diastolic, and the aortic diastolic, in order of frequency. They do not represent definitive valvular dysfunction.[33,34]

Murmurs indicative of carditis are usually present during the 1st week of the illness, in about three-fourths of all the patients whose disease is eventually diagnosed as carditis. By the 2nd or 3rd week, murmurs will become manifest in 85% and <15% of patients with carditis will develop murmurs after the 4th week.[62] The apical systolic murmur of MR is pansystolic, beginning with the first sound, blowing in quality, high pitched, and is heard maximally at the apex with the patient in the left lateral decubitus position. It is transmitted to the left axilla. The intensity of the murmur is variable, especially in the early stages of illness, but is at least grade two on a scale of six. It does not change substantially with position or respiration. The intensity of the murmur is variable, especially in the early stages of illness, but is at least grade two on a scale of six. It does not change substantially with position or respiration. The murmur of MR must be differentiated from functional (innocent) murmurs, which frequently occur in normal individuals, especially children. Functional murmurs usually occupy only a portion of systole. They may be quite loud, particularly in anxious or febrile patients, and are rather widely transmitted in thin chest wall patients. These murmurs are heard at times only intermittently and tend to vary with position and respiration. They are usually of two types: an ejection type murmur heard best over the pulmonic area and a low-pitched, vibratory, groaning or musical murmur heard best along the lower left sternal border. The former is frequently transmitted to the neck and may be mistaken for aortic stenosis. The latter is frequently transmitted to the apex and is most likely to be confused with MR by those unfamiliar with its characteristic quality.

The apical mid-diastolic or Carey Coombs murmur is a low-pitched mid-diastolic murmur, beginning immediately after the third sound and ending before the first sound. The mid-diastolic murmur is often transient, very low pitched, low intensity, and easily missed. The murmur is best heard at the apex or just above it, by using the bell portion of the stethoscope applied lightly against the chest wall with the patient again lying in left lateral decubitus. This apical mid-diastolic murmur occurs when there is MR, is transient, and tends to disappear during the recovery from the acute episode. It may be caused by the increased tautness of the mitral cusps and chordae coupled with a large inflow of blood into the left ventricle in early diastole. This murmur makes the diagnosis of mitral valvulitis more definite and its presence confirms the significance of the apical systolic murmur and adds to the seriousness of the prognosis for permanent valve damage. The mid-diastolic murmur is easily confused with a normal third heart sound, heard so commonly in children, especially during increased cardiac output. In fact, it seems to be an extension and exaggeration of the third heard sound into a murmur. In addition, it should not be mistaken for the rumbling murmur of mitral stenosis which is harsher and longer, has presystolic accentuation (in absence of atrial fibrillation), and merges into the first heart sound. Mitral stenosis is also differentiated by the presence of an opening snap and an accentuated first heart sound and pulmonic second sound. Carey Coombs murmur, although described first in rheumatic carditis, is also heard in severe anemia, thyrotoxicosis, established MR of inactive RHD, other forms of myocarditis with acutely dilated hearts, and in general in situations associated with increased flow through the mitral valve. But, the severity of MR has prognostic significance. If MR is mild to moderate then the mechanism of MR valvulitis is valve prolapse, annulitis, ventricular enlargement, and rarely chordal rupture. In our study,[44] out of 164 patients diagnosed clinically with carditis, only 141 had supporting echocardiographic findings (85.97%), with the remaining 23 patients (14%) having functional murmurs, tachycardia, anemia, fever of some other etiology or congenitally malformed hearts, the latter found in patients with an atrial septal defect and a subaortic fibrous shelf, respectively. We found four patients with severe MR due to chordal tears and flail valvular leaflets.

The basal diastolic murmur of AR has a soft, high-pitched, decrescendo quality and may be found early in the course of the disease as an expression of aortic valvulitis. It is difficult to detect and sometimes has an intermittent character. It is an early diastolic murmur, best heard with the diaphragm of the stethoscope, and is usually loudest at the third space on the left border of the sternum with the patient in the upright position, leaning forward, and after deep expiration. It is important because it always indicates significant carditis when it appears abruptly in ARF. It may occur alone or with mitral valvulitis. As the degree of regurgitation increases, the murmur becomes louder and longer. A diastolic cooing or crying "seagull" murmur is rarely heard but can be present transiently in the aortic valvulitis of acute carditis.

The dominant cardiac abnormality in patients with ARF is MR and occurs in approximately 95% of cases with acute rheumatic carditis. AR occurs in approximately 20–25% of cases with acute rheumatic carditis, usually in combination with MR. Isolated AR occurs in approximately 5% of patients with acute rheumatic carditis.[67,70] Rapid development of mitral stenosis with severe pulmonary hypertension within 6–12 months after the first attack of ARF is reported to be more common among Indian children.[80,81] In an Indian study,[2] mitral insufficiency was the most common valvular lesion, occurring in 91%, whereas mitral stenosis developed in 18%. The more frequent occurrence of juvenile mitral stenosis in previous reports from India is in sharp contrast to this study and may be related to several factors. The mechanism of this MR is due to a combination of annular dilation and chordal elongation that results in abnormal coaptation and in some cases, prolapse of the tip of the anterior mitral leaflet.[82-84] Rarely, mitral valve chordae rupture occurs resulting in a flail mitral leaflet and severe MR.[85] Most patients with acute mild MR are asymptomatic. In patients with acute moderate to severe MR due to LV myocardium volume overload, left heart filling pressures rise, leading to pulmonary venous congestion and pulmonary edema. Such patients usually present with features of left heart failure, including dyspnea, orthopnea, paroxysmal nocturnal dyspnea, cough, and very rarely even hemoptysis. Secondary pulmonary hypertension may develop, resulting in right ventricular dysfunction, tricuspid regurgitation, and right heart failure. Children <5 years of age with ARF and carditis may present with insidious fever, decreased appetite, lethargy, fatigue, and vague pains. Because of these subtle and nonspecific symptoms, the diagnosis may be delayed and presentation with heart failure is more common than in older children.[86,87] Tachycardia is often one of the earliest signs of carditis. Significant MR may result in increased precordial activity, tachypnea, and increased work of breathing. A high-pitched, regurgitant, holosystolic murmur of MR is heard best at the apex, usually radiating into the left axilla. This murmur is best heard at the end-expiration with the patient in the left lateral decubitus position. Although mitral stenosis does not occur with the initial episode of acute ARF and carditis, a low-pitched mid-diastolic apical murmur may be heard in the setting of significant MR due to increased diastolic flow across the mitral valve or the Carey Coombs murmur.

Aortic regurgitation occurs due to leaflet prolapse and this seems one of the mechanisms of this acute valvular dysfunction. Patients with acute mild AR are usually asymptomatic. Moderate to severe acute AR is less well tolerated and may result in heart failure. The large regurgitant volume imposed on a left ventricle that has not had time to compensate for the significant volume load results in decreased forward stroke volume in conjunction with significant elevation of ventricular end-diastolic pressure, leading to a combination of low cardiac output and pulmonary edema.[88] Patients with acute severe AR are tachypneic and have tachycardia. Pulse pressure is often narrow and the pulses are not increased or bounding. Precordial activity is often increased, but the apical impulse may not be significantly displaced. On auscultation, the decrescendo diastolic murmur is softer, lower-pitched, and shorter than the murmur heard with chronic regurgitation. In some patients, this murmur can be easily missed, especially with the tachycardia commonly present during the acute phase of the illness. A short systolic ejection murmur may be heard over the LV outflow tract because of increased flow. A low-pitched mid- to late-diastolic rumbling murmur with presystolic accentuation may be heard at the apex, even with a nonstenotic mitral valve. If present, this Austin Flint murmur is softer and shorter in the setting of acute as compared with chronic severe AR. Acute rheumatic AR is less likely than MR to disappear with the resolution of the acute inflammatory stage of the illness.[2,63,65]

Unfortunately, there is no single laboratory test that definitely establishes the diagnosis of ARF. Recent surveys show that clinical auscultation is a dying art. Edward Kaplan in his article says "detection of active rheumatic carditis is of great prognostic and therapeutic importance and is currently based on the Jones criteria" and the fact that penicillin has failed to eradicate this disease process is irrefutable proof of the need for more laboratory, epidemiological, and clinical research.[89] Classification of rheumatic carditis according to the magnitude of clinical manifestations and electrocardiographic, radiographic, and Doppler echocardiographic findings are described in **Table 5**.

Adults who do not seek medical attention until late in life, when they finally develop symptoms of valvular deformity, surprise some cardiologists by their lack of rheumatic fever history.

They may represent a select population of rheumatic subjects with very mild initial rheumatic carditis, which may have produced subclinical valvular deformity and the latter may have undergone progressive fibrosis from factors other than the rheumatic fever process itself.

Recurrent Carditis[46]

Carditis is rarely present for the first time in recurrences. The term mimetic carditis was proposed, considering that the heart is almost always involved in the subsequent attacks in patients exhibiting carditis in the primary episode. The diagnosis of recurrent carditis in patients with an established rheumatic valvular disease is often difficult. The clinical presentation includes changes in the character of the murmur, the reappearance of a previous murmur, or detection of a new one as the result of the involvement of an additional valve. In addition, detection of a pericardial friction rub or effusion and a significant increase in the size of the heart may also be present. CHF is more common in recurrent carditis. Although the heart is invariably involved in recurrences of patients suffering carditis in the first attack, cardiac failure in the chronic phase could also reflect mechanical stress due to valvular dysfunction, being related

TABLE 5: Classification of rheumatic carditis according to the magnitude of clinical manifestations and electrocardiographic, radiographic, and Doppler echocardiographic findings.[46]*

Type	*Findings*
Subclinical carditis	Absence of auscultatory evidence of carditis associated with normal radiographic and electrocardiological examinations, except for the presence of first-degree heart block. Doppler echocardiographical features show mild regurgitation of mitral and/or aortic valves with different characteristics from physiological regurgitation
Mild carditis	Rapid sleeping pulse, tachycardia out of proportion to fever, possible decrease in the intensity of the first sound, the systolic murmur of mild mitral regurgitation, no cardiac enlargement on chest radiography, possible prolongation of the PR interval in the electrocardiographical examination, mild or mild-to-moderate mitral insufficiency, isolated or associated with mild aortic regurgitation and normal chamber size on echocardiography
Moderate carditis	Clinical signs are more evident than for mild carditis with persistent tachycardia and a more intense murmur of mitral regurgitation, but without a thrill, coming as an isolated lesion or associated with an aortic diastolic murmur. The mitral regurgitation can be accompanied by a Carey Coombs murmur, besides findings of incipient heart failure; a mild or mild to moderate degree of cardiac enlargement in the chest radiography due to left-sided chamber hypertrophy and, if present, the pulmonary congestion is discreet; premature beats, ST-segment, and T wave changes, low-voltage, prolongation of QTc or PR intervals may be observed on the electrocardiogram; mild-to-moderate mitral regurgitation, isolated or associated with aortic valve incompetence of mild or moderate degree, mild-to-moderate enlargement of the left side chambers is seen on echocardiography.
Severe carditis	In addition to the findings of moderate carditis, symptoms and signs of congestive heart failure are found; valvulitis is expressed by murmurs related to more severe degrees of mitral and/or aortic regurgitation and can be associated with pericarditis and arrhythmias. There is evident cardiomegaly with prominent vascular markings on chest radiography; a more severe degree of the electrocardiographic changes of left ventricular hypertrophy is sometimes associated with right ventricular hypertrophy. Moderate-to-severe or severe mitral and/or aortic insufficiency are observed on echocardiography and the left cardiac chambers show at least moderate enlargement.

*According to the protocol of the Rheumatic Fever Clinic, Department of Pediatrics, Division of Pediatric Cardiology, Hospital das Clínicas/Federal University of Minas Gerais, Brazil.

to the extent of hemodynamic effects. The epidemiological and clinical context, as well as the evidence of a recent streptococcal infection, therefore, must be considered in the diagnosis of recurrent carditis.

Chorea

Sydenham's chorea (St Vitus' dance) may be the sole manifestation of rheumatic fever and commonly occurs in the absence of other manifestations. It occurs in about 10–15% of cases of ARF.[90] Chorea has a prolonged latent period after GABHS infection developing 1–6 months after the initial illness. It is not seen simultaneously with arthritis, as it is generally a late manifestation of ARF. It is more common in females. Sydenham's chorea must be differentiated from other hyperkinetic movement disorders such as essential tremors, hereditary chorea, or drug-induced and toxic forms **(Table 6)**.[91]

Chorea is a neurological disorder characterized by rapid involuntary, quasi-purposive purposeless movements of facial and skeletal muscles associated with generalized muscular weakness and emotional lability. The movements are neither purposeful nor repetitive but abrupt and erratic. The abnormal movements disappear during sleep.

The child may initially become fretful, irritable, inattentive to schoolwork, fidgety, or even severely disturbed. Physical discoordination manifests as clumsiness and a tendency to drop objects. Facial movements include grimaces, grins, and frowns.

When the tongue is protruded, it resembles a "bag of worms" and speech is jerky and staccato. Handwriting becomes illegible. When the hands are extended, the dorsum assumes a "spoon" or "dish" configuration due to flexion of the wrist and hyperextension of the metacarpophalangeal joints. When raising the hands above the head, the patient may pronate one or both hands (pronator sign). When asked to grip the examiner's hand, their irregular, repetitive squeezes have been termed "milkmaid grip". Although the choreiform movements are usually bilateral, they may be unilateral (hemichorea).

There may be "hung up" reflexes. Chorea is a self-limiting illness and the duration is quite variable, ranging from 1 week to >2 years. Three-quarters of the patients recover within 6 months. The manifestations of chorea may wax and wane during its course. Long-term neurological and psychological sequelae have been described, including convulsions, decreased learning ability, behavior problems, and psychosis. The exact relationship, if any, of these conditions to chorea

TABLE 6: Differential diagnosis of chorea.

Diagnosis	Diagnostic clues
Atypical seizures	• Electroencephalographic abnormalities • Change in level of consciousness
Cerebrovascular accidents	MRI or CT evidence of lesion
Collagen vascular disease (e.g., SLE, periarteritis nodosa)	• History and physical examination • Laboratory evidence (e.g., decreased complement levels, possible ANA titers) (*Note*: ANA can be elevated following infection and, therefore, may be positive in acute rheumatic fever)
Drug intoxication	Drug screen, especially for phenytoin, amitriptyline, metoclopramide, and fluphenazine
Familial chorea	The prototype is Huntington's disease, but the diagnosis also includes benign familial chorea, familial paroxysmal dystonic choreoathetosis, familial paroxysmal kinesigenic choreoathetosis, familial chorea with acanthocytosis (check blood smear for acanthocytes), familial calcification of basal ganglia (MRI or CT scan may be helpful) ataxia–telangiectasia, and Hallervorden–Spatz disease
Hormonally induced chorea	• Use of oral contraceptives • Pregnancy (chorea gravidarum)
Hyperthyroidism	Abnormal thyroid function test results
Hypoparathyroidism	• Low serum calcium and magnesium levels • High serum phosphorus level
Lyme disease	• History and accompanying symptoms • Physical examination findings (e.g., rash) • Titers against *Borrelia burgdorferi*
Sydenham chorea	• Other signs of rheumatic fever • Evidence of preceding streptococcal infection
Wilson's disease	• Decreased serum ceruloplasmin level • Increased urinary copper excretion • Kayser–Fleischer rings • Anemia, hepatitis • Family history

(ANA: antinuclear antibody; CT: computed tomography; MRI: magnetic resonance imaging; SLE: systemic lupus erythematosus)

may help to make the diagnosis.[48] Follow-up of patients with pure rheumatic chorea has shown RHD in 23% in a 20-year-old period.[92]

In our study,[44] nearly 70% of rheumatic chorea had associated ECHO evidence of carditis/valvulitis. In our study, rheumatic chorea was found in 40 (8.85%) patients, with eight having bilateral chorea. In one patient, the chorea lasted for 1 year, and in another, it recurred after 2 years. Two other screened siblings of one child with chorea showed no evidence of ARF at the time of screening but developed rheumatic chorea after 3 months. The titers of ASLO were negative in 17 cases (42.5%), but ranged from 400 to 800 international units in the remaining 23 cases (57.5%). That means the traditional saying that other manifestations of ARF are absent is not true in more than half the cases.

Skin Manifestations

Subcutaneous nodules also occur rarely, in fewer than 5% of cases. They appear as small (5–10 mm), nontender, firm, movable masses, usually palpable over the extensor surfaces of the elbows, wrists, and knees. They also may be found over the spinous processes of the thoracic or lumbar vertebrae and over the suboccipital area. They almost always appear in association with a severe form of carditis.[48] These nodules appear 2 –3 weeks after the onset of ARF. They persist from day 1 to 2 weeks to, rarely, more than a month without long-term sequelae. In our study,[44] subcutaneous nodules **(Figs. 6A and B)** were seen in only seven cases (2.4%). All these patients had high titers of ASLO, ranging between 800 and 1,600 international units, but CRP was positive in only four cases. All seven patients had both clinical and echocardiographic evidence of carditis.

Subcutaneous nodules were artificially induced,[93] by first injecting the region of the olecranon process with 1 cc of local anesthesia. From the antecubital vein of the opposite arm, 2–3 cc of blood was removed and immediately injected into the subcutaneous and deep tissues of the anesthetized area. During the next 10 days, frictional pressure was applied by having the patient rub the injected elbow on the bedclothes for several minutes (or until the skin became warm), six times a day. The injection of the patients' own blood into the subcutaneous tissues of subjects with rheumatic fever frequently results in the appearance of subcutaneous nodules in the area injected.

They are clinically indistinguishable from nodules occurring spontaneously. The appearance of nodules in 90% of those patients with clinically active rheumatic fever and in 50% of those with only laboratory evidence of active rheumatic fever (67% of the combined groups) was in striking contrast to their appearance in only 14% of rheumatic fever subjects without evidence of active rheumatic fever and in 14% of those subjects with chorea. From the above, it was evident that these artificially induced nodules occurred more frequently in the patient with active rheumatic fever, as is the case with spontaneous nodules.[93]

is uncertain. Rarely, symptoms may recur over a period of years, exacerbated by stress, pregnancy, oral contraceptives, and intercurrent illnesses.[6,50] Because it is often a late finding, the acute phase reactants may not be elevated. In such cases, echocardiographic evidence of mitral or aortic insufficiency

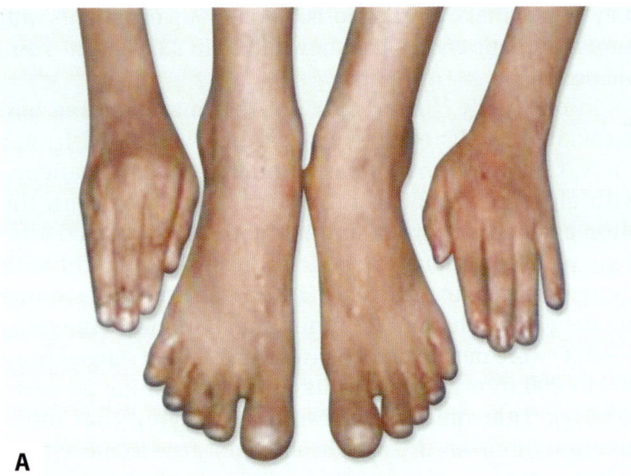

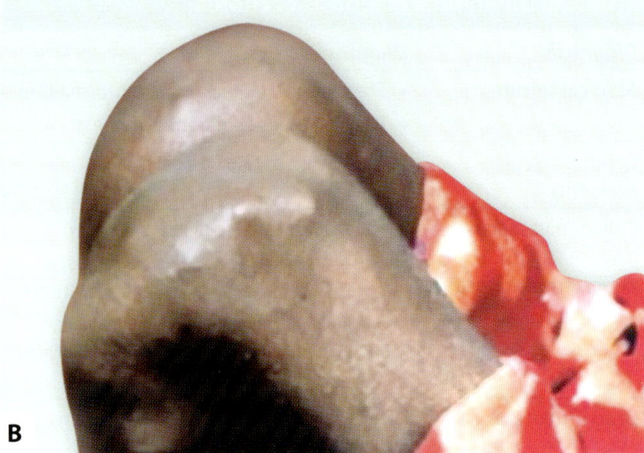

FIGS. 6A AND B: Subcutaneous nodules.

Erythema marginatum is rare, occurring in only 4% of the cases. This is an evanescent, erythematous, nonpruritic rash with pale centers and rounded or serpiginous margins. Lesions occur mainly on the trunk and proximal extremities and may be induced by the application of heat. The rash, which appears on the trunk and proximal extremities, is red with serpiginous margins and central clearing and spreads centrifugally. It is neither raised nor pruritic. The rashes are evanescent appearing and disappearing within hours right in front of the doctors' eyes. A warm bath or contact with hot towels characteristically accentuates it. It is difficult to detect in dark-skinned patients.[48] Lesions occur mainly on the trunk and proximal extremities and never on the face. In our study,[44] erythema marginatum was seen in only 2 (0.4%) of our patients **(Figs. 7A and B)**. The youngest child was 1 year 11 months old. Both of our patients had clinical evidence of carditis, confirmed by the echocardiogram. Erythema marginatum is not unique to ARF and may be seen during sepsis, drug reactions, glomerulonephritis, the rash of juvenile rheumatoid arthritis, and the circinate rash of Lyme disease (erythema chronicum migrans). It can occur in children in whom no etiology is evident.[6]

Minor Manifestations

- Arthralgia refers to joint pain without the objective changes of arthritis. Arthralgia must not be considered a minor manifestation when arthritis is present.
- Fever [usually with a temperature of at least 102°F (38.8°C)] is present early in the course of untreated rheumatic fever.
- In laboratory findings, elevated acute phase reactants (elevated CRP levels and elevated ESR) are objective evidence of an inflammatory process.
- A prolonged PR interval on the ECG is neither specific for ARF nor an indication of active carditis.

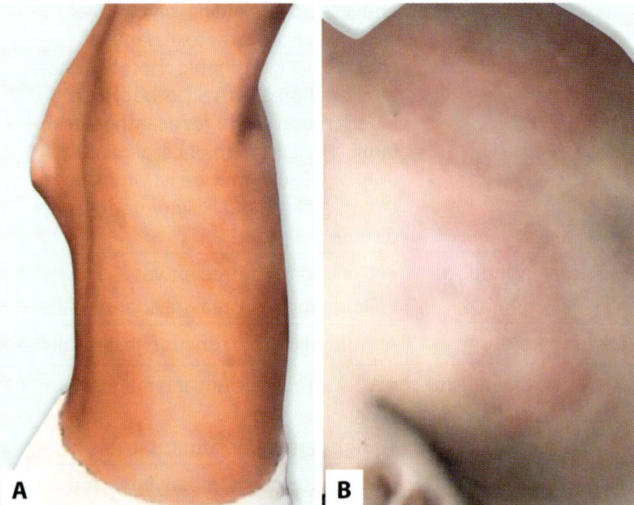

FIGS. 7A AND B: (A) Erythema marginatum in a 7-year-old girl and (B) in a 1-year 11-month-old boy with acute rheumatic fever.

■ CLINICAL FINDINGS

The two clinical features included in the minor manifestations are fever and arthralgia. Both are termed as minor criteria not necessarily because they occur less frequently than the major criteria, but rather because they lack diagnostic specificity.

Fever is very commonly present at the onset of illness, usually ranging from 101° to 104°F (38.4–40.0°C). There is no characteristic pattern. Children with mild carditis without arthritis may have a low-grade fever and patients with pure chorea are afebrile. Fever generally resolves within several weeks, even without treatment. Usually, fever is low grade, associated with elevated CRP and ESR. Occasionally, leukocyte count is mildly elevated.

Arthralgia may be used as a minor manifestation, only in the absence of polyarthritis as a major manifestation. There is joint pain, usually of the large joints, without objective signs of arthritis. Arthralgia may be migratory and varies in severity; it may be present for days to weeks.

Abdominal pain and epistaxis may occur in only about 5% of patients with ARF. Due to the lack of specificity of these symptoms, they have not been considered a part of the Jones criteria. However, they may be of considerable clinical importance because they often appear hours or days before major manifestations of the disease and may mimic a variety of other acute abdominal conditions.

LABORATORY FINDINGS

The two laboratory minor criteria are elevation of acute phase reactants and prolongation of the PR interval on ECG. These are nonspecific findings. When a patient has only one major manifestation, these minor criteria may be useful.

Erythrocyte sedimentation rate and CRP are the most commonly used acute phase reactants. They are elevated in most inflammatory states and are almost always highly abnormal in ARF. The exceptions are when chorea is present as an isolated manifestation or when a patient presents with indolent carditis, as the acute phase reactant levels may have normalized by the time medical attention is sought. In addition, the ESR may be decreased in the presence of cerebrospinal fluid (CSF), whereas the CRP may be elevated. Typically, the ESR may remain elevated for 6 weeks to 3 months.[94]

Prolongation of the PR interval on ECG (first-degree heart block) is the most common ECG abnormality in ARF patients. Atrioventricular conduction delay is unrelated to carditis and it has no prognostic value in terms of cardiac sequelae. It is present in about 35% of patients with ARF[51] and in 60% of the patients who show ECG abnormalities. The second most frequent abnormality is the inversion of T1, T2, or T4, alone or in combination. It is found in 35% of patients in whom ECG abnormalities are present. Serial records are of value in determining the significance of borderline T changes. ST–T wave changes and major arrhythmias occur in ARF. Significant serial changes of these minor abnormalities can be taken as evidence of cardiac involvement rather than an abnormal finding in a single tracing. ECG may reveal the polycyclic nature of the course of a patient with ARF in the absence of clinical evidence of such polycyclic activity. Carditis may be obvious clinically in the absence of abnormalities in the ECG despite early and frequent tracings.[95]

LABORATORY EVIDENCE OF A PRECEDING STREPTOCOCCAL INFECTION

It is well established that every episode of ARF is preceded by a pharyngeal infection. Approximately one-third of the patients diagnosed with ARF will have no history of recent throat pain or illness. Thus, it is necessary to demonstrate evidence of recent infection in making the diagnosis of ARF. This can be established in one of three ways: (a) positive throat culture, (b) positive group A streptococcal antigen test from throat swab, or (c) elevated or rising serum antistreptococcal antibody titer. Positive throat cultures or rapid streptococcal antigen tests for group A streptococci are less reliable than antibody tests because they do not distinguish between recent infection and chronic pharyngeal carriage. Positive throat culture for GABHS as evidence of recent streptococcal infection is uncommon and up to 50% of culture-positive patients may be chronic pharyngeal carriers.[90,96] Similarly, a rapid streptococcal antigen test is positive in only 10–20% of cases.[90] Specific antibodies are more important diagnostically, as they reach a peak after the onset of ARF and confirm preceding infection rather than the transient carriage of streptococci. If the onset of rheumatic fever can be clearly defined, raised ASLO titers are invariable. The ASLO titer is a commonly used streptococcal antibody test in establishing the diagnosis of ARF. The peak ASLO titers occur 3–4 weeks after the acute infection and usually are maintained for 2–3 months before declining.[97] The peak titers usually coincide with the most active phase of the polyarthritis. Serum antibody is judged to be elevated if the titer exceeds the upper limit of the normal titer range for a community, where the upper limit is defined as the titer exceeded by no >20% of the population. The range of normal values for each test is variable and depends upon the age of the patient, geographical locale, and the season of the year.[6] In the absence of specific information regarding the appropriate range of such values in a given geographic area, a single ASLO titer is generally considered to be modestly elevated if it is at least 240 Todd units in adults and 320 Todd units in children. To document a recent streptococcal infection by rising antibody titers, acute and convalescent serum samples should be obtained at 2–4-week intervals and all samples should be tested simultaneously. Patients, especially children, with other diseases may have increased streptococcal antibody titers without rheumatic fever.[35]

The ASLO titers can be normal in up to 20% of ARF patients.[98] Other antibody tests should be assessed. Other useful streptococcal antibodies include anti-deoxyribonuclease-B (anti-DNase-B), antistreptokinase, and anti-hyaluronidase. These are especially useful when the ASLO titer is normal or borderline. Anti-DNase titers of 240 Todd units or greater in a school-aged patient and 120 Todd units or greater in an adult patient are viewed as elevated.[35]

If three antistreptococcal antibody tests (ASLO, anti-DNase-B, and antihyaluronidase tests) are obtained, a titer for at least one antibody test is elevated in over 95% of patients.[66]

The Streptozyme test, which detects antibodies, is a relatively simple slide agglutination test, but it is less standardized and less reproducible than the other antibody tests. It should not be used as a diagnostic test for evidence of antecedent group A streptococcal infection.[66]

Among the minor criteria, a raised ESR was the most common, found in 314 cases (69.46%). The highest ESR was 140 mm in the 1st hour. The ASLO titer was elevated in 311 cases (68.8%). Fever was present in 224 cases (49.55%). CRP was positive in only 181 cases (40%). Culture for beta-hemolytic *Streptococcus* was positive in 79 cases (17.47%) and these children showed marked rising titers of ASLO, with neither the ESR nor symptoms subsiding subsequent to treatment with aspirin. In this study, there was no history of scarlet fever, a preceding beta-hemolytic streptococcal infection, in any of our patients.[44]

Electrocardiographic changes include PR prolongation, which may have an earlier onset should not be regarded as evidence of carditis. ECG and radiograph abnormalities may be present in as few as 30% of patients with carditis.[99]

NEW DIAGNOSTIC TECHNIQUES FOR RHEUMATIC CARDITIS

Echocardiography

The use of echocardiography to detect rheumatic carditis is discussed in Chapter 11.

Endomyocardial Biopsy[6]

Since myocarditis is an obligatory component of cardiac involvement in ARF, the value of endomyocardial biopsy has been investigated for diagnosing rheumatic carditis. To establish the histological characteristics of carditis, endomyocardial biopsies from patients presenting with the first episode of ARF were compared to biopsies from patients with quiescent chronic RHD. The results demonstrated that myocarditis was virtually absent (defined by the Dallas criteria to be focal or diffuse myocytic necrosis associated with cellular infiltration of mononuclear lymphocytes). Instead, there was evidence of interstitial inflammation that ranged from perivascular mononuclear cellular infiltration to histiocytic aggregates and Aschoff nodule formation. Histiocytic aggregates and Aschoff nodules were identified in only 30% of patients. On the other hand, Aschoff nodules were seen in 40% of the endomyocardial biopsies taken from patients with preexisting RHD and who developed a possible recurrence of rheumatic carditis with CHF. These results suggested that an endomyocardial biopsy is not likely to provide additional diagnostic information for patients with clinical carditis in a primary episode of ARF. The results also suggested that an onset of unexplained CHF in patients with established RHD and who presented with only minor manifestations of ARF and elevated ASLO titers would indicate a high probability of rheumatic carditis and that an invasive test may not be needed for the diagnosis.

Radionuclide Imaging[6]

Radionuclide techniques are simple, noninvasive modalities that have been commonly used to evaluate a variety of cardiovascular disorders. The pathology of rheumatic myocarditis is characterized predominantly by the presence of myocardial inflammation, with some damage to myocardial cells. Gallium-67, radiolabeled leukocytes, and radiolabeled antimyosin antibodies have all been used to image myocardial inflammation. Although radionuclide imaging has been used successfully to identify rheumatic carditis by noninvasive means, there is not enough experience with such methods to allow them to be used for the routine diagnosis of ARF. However, the results of these studies have revealed that Gallium-67 imaging has better diagnostic characteristics than antimyosin scintigraphy and the results also confirmed that rheumatic carditis is predominantly infiltrative, rather than degenerative in nature.

CONCLUSION

- Acute rheumatic fever occurs as a result of a complex interaction between GABHS, a susceptible host, and the environment.
- An abnormal immune response to GABHS infection leads to an acute inflammatory illness that most commonly affects the joints, brain, heart, or skin. Although the other manifestations are self-limiting and resolve without sequelae, carditis may result in significant morbidity and mortality.
- The degree of cardiac involvement is quite variable, ranging from mild, asymptomatic valvulitis to severe carditis with significant acute mitral and/or AR resulting in heart failure.
- The acute rheumatic cardiac involvement may resolve or persist and evolve into chronic rheumatic valvular disease, with cardiac symptoms developing years after the initial episode.
- Carditis and subsequent RHD are responsible for long-term morbidity and mortality and it is true that *"rheumatic fever licks the joints but bites the heart"*.
- Since there is no pathognomonic test, the diagnosis of an initial episode of ARF is made using the modified Jones criteria. Diagnostic criteria (updated Jones criteria and World Health Organization) should serve as guidelines to assist in the diagnosis of both initial and recurrent attacks of ARF.
- The clinical profile of ARF is changing and adherence to revised Jones criteria may lead to underdiagnosis among Indian children with polyarthralgia and overdiagnosis in clinically diagnosed carditis.

Treatment for ARF is only symptomatic. There is no specific laboratory test for diagnosis or drug, in particular, that can either cure or alter the course. However, timely diagnosis and penicillin prophylaxis can prevent the repeated GABHS infection and reduce the recrudescence of rheumatic activity and further damage to the heart valves.

ACKNOWLEDGMENTS

Our grateful thanks to Rockefeller University Press for granting permission to use the article from the Journal of Experimental Medicine. 1924;39:497-508. Also, our grateful thanks to Binotto MA, Guilherme L, Tanaka AC for permission to utilize their figure from their article Rheumatic Fever. Images Paediatr Cardiol. 2002;11:12-25.

Our grateful thanks to Dr S Kiran of Narayana Hrudayalay.

REFERENCES

1. Sanyal SK, Thapar MK, Ahmed SH, Hooja V, Tewari P. The initial attack of acute rheumatic fever during childhood in North India; a prospective study of the clinical profile. Circulation. 1974;49:7-12.

2. Sanyal SK, Berry AM, Duggal S, Hooja V, Ghosh S. Sequel of the initial attack of acute rheumatic fever in children from North India. A prospective 5-year follow-up study. Circulation. 1982;65:375-9.

3. Carapetis JR. The current evidence for the burden of group A streptococcal diseases. WHO/FCH/CAH/05·07., Geneva: World Health Organization; 2004. pp. 1-57.

4. Rammelkamp CH, Denny FW, Wannamaker LW. Studies in the epidemiology of rheumatic fever in the armed services. In: Thomas L (Ed). Rheumatic Fever. Minneapolis: University of Minnesota Press; 1952. pp. 72.

5. Siegel AC, Johnson EE, Stollerman GH. Controlled studies of streptococcal pharyngitis in a pediatric population: Factors related to the attack rate of rheumatic fever. N Engl J Med. 1961;265:559.

6. WHO. Rheumatic fever and rheumatic heart disease: report of a WHO Expert Consultation, Geneva 29 October – 1 November 2001. WHO technical report series; 923. Geneva: World Health Organisation; 2004.

7. da Silva NA, Pereira BA. Acute rheumatic fever. Still a challenge. Rheum Dis Clin North Am. 1997;23:545-68.

8. Gibofsky A, Khanna A, Suh E, Zabriskie JB. The genetics of rheumatic fever: relationship to streptococcal infection and autoimmune disease. J Rheumatol Suppl. 1991;30:1-5.

9. Ayoub EM, Barrett DJ, Maclaren NK, Krischer JP. Association of class II human histocompatibility leukocyte antigens with rheumatic fever. J Clin Invest. 1986;77:2019-26.

10. Anastasiou-Nana MI, Anderson JL, Carlquist JF, Nanas JN. HLA-DR typing and lymphocyte subset evaluation in rheumatic heart disease: a search for immune response factors. Am Heart J. 1986;112:992-7.

11. Rajapakse CN, Halim K, Al Orainey I, Al Nozha M, Al Aska AK, A genetic marker for rheumatic heart disease. Br Heart J. 1987;58:659-62.

12. Jhinghan B, Mehra NK, Reddy KS, Taneja V, Vaidya MC, Bhatia ML. HLA, blood groups and secretor status in patients with established rheumatic fever and rheumatic heart disease. Tissue Antigens. 1986;27:172-8.

13. Guilherme L, Weidebach W, Kiss MH, Snitcowsky R, Kalil J. Association of human leukocyte class II antigens with rheumatic fever or rheumatic heart disease in a Brazilian population. Circulation. 1991;83:1995-8.

14. Weidebach W, Goldberg AC, Chiarella JM, Guilherme L, Snitcowsky R, Pileggi F, et al. HLA class II antigens in rheumatic fever. Analysis of the DR locus by restriction fragment-length polymorphism and oligotyping. Hum Immunol. 1994;40:253-8.

15. Maharaj B, Hammond MG, Appadoo B, Leary WP, Pudifin DJ. HLA-A, B, DR, and DQ antigens in black patients with severe chronic rheumatic heart disease. Circulation. 1987;76:259-61.

16. Olmez U, Turgay M, Ozenirler S, Tutkak H, Duzgun N, Duman M, et al. Association of HLA class I and class II antigens with rheumatic fever in a Turkish population. Scand J Rheumatol. 1993;22:49-52.

17. Guedez Y, Kotby A, El Demellawy M, Galal A, Thomson G, Zaher S, et al. HLA class II associations with rheumatic heart disease are more evident and consistent among clinically homogeneous patients. Circulation. 1999;99:2784-90.

18. Stollerman GH. Rheumatogenic streptococci and autoimmunity. Clin Immunol Immunopathol. 1991;61:131-42.

19. Raizada V, Williams RC Jr, Chopra P, Gopinath N, Prakash K, Sharma KB, et al. Tissue distribution of lymphocytes in rheumatic heart valves as defined by monoclonal anti-T cell antibodies. Am J Med. 1983;74:90-6.

20. Kemeny E, Grieve T, Marcus R, Sareli P, Zabriskie JB. Identification of mononuclear cells and T cell subsets in rheumatic valvulitis. Clin Immunol Immunopathol. 1989;52:225-37.

21. Guilherme L, Cunha-Neto E, Coelho V, Snitcowsky R, Pomerantzeff PM, Assis RV, et al. Human heart-infiltrating T-cell clones from rheumatic heart disease patients recognize both streptococcal and cardiac proteins. Circulation. 1995;92:415-20.

22. Guilherme L, Oshiro SE, Fae KC, Cunha-Neto E, Renesto G, Goldberg AC, et al. T-cell reactivity against streptococcal antigens in the periphery mirrors reactivity of heart-infiltrating T lymphocytes in rheumatic heart disease patients. Infect Immun. 2001;69:5345-51.

23. Dudding BA, Ayoub EM. Persistence of group A antibody in patients with rheumatic valvular disease. J Exp Med. 1968;128:1081.

24. Khanna AK, Buskirk DR, Williams RC Jr, Gibofsky A, Crow MK, Menon A, et al. Presence of a non-HLA B cell antigen in rheumatic fever patients and their families as defined by a monoclonal antibody. J Clin Invest. 1989;83:1710.

25. Bronze MS, Dale JB. The re-emergence of serious group A streptococcal infections and acute rheumatic fever. Am J Med Sci. 1996;311:41.

26. Husby G, Van de Rijn I, Zabriskie JB, Abdin ZH, Williams RC Jr. Antibodies reacting with cytoplasm of the subthalamic and caudate nuclei neurons in chorea and acute rheumatic fever. J Exp Med. 1976;144:1904.

27. Swift HM. The pathogenesis of rheumatic fever. J Exp Med. 1924;39(4):497-508.

28. Schafranski MD, Stier A, Nisihara R, Messias-Reason IJ. Significantly increased levels of mannose-binding lectin (MBL) in rheumatic heart disease: a beneficial role for MBL deficiency. Clin Exp Immunol. 2004;138:521-5.

29. Chou HT, Chen CH, Tsai CH, Tsai FJ. Association between transforming growth factor-beta1 gene *C-509T* and *T869C* polymorphisms and rheumatic heart disease. Am Heart J. 2004;148:181-6.

30. Berdeli A, Celik HA, Ozyurek R, Aydin HH. Involvement of immunoglobulin *FcgammaRIIA* and *FcgammaRIIIB* gene polymorphisms in susceptibility to rheumatic fever. Clin Biochem. 2004;37:925-9.

31. Cunningham MW. Pathogenesis of group A streptococcal infections. Clin Microbiol Rev. 2000;13:470-511.

32. Cunningham MW. Autoimmunity and molecular mimicry in the pathogenesis of post-streptococcal heart disease. Front Biosci. 2003;8:s533-43.

33. Stollerman GH, Markowitz M, Taranta A, Wannamaker LW, Whittemore R. Report of the ad hoc Committee on Rheumatic Fever and Congenital Heart Disease of American Heart Association: Jones Criteria (Revised) for guidance in the diagnosis of rheumatic fever. Circulation. 1965;32:664-8.

34. Stollerman GH. Rheumatic fever and streptococcal infection. New York: Grune and Stratton; 1975.

35. Special Writing Group of the Committee on Rheumatic Fever. Endocarditis, and Kawasaki Disease of the Council on Cardiovascular Disease in the Young, American Heart Association: Guidelines for the diagnosis of rheumatic fever: Jones criteria, updated 1992. JAMA. 1992;268:2069-73.

36. World Health Organization. Rheumatic fever and rheumatic heart disease. World Health Organ Tech Rep Ser. 2004;923:1-122.

37. Gewitz M, Baltimore R, Tani L, Sable CA, Shulman ST, Carapetis J, et al. Revision of the Jones Criteria for the Diagnosis of Acute Rheumatic Fever in the Era of Doppler Echocardiography: A Scientific Statement from the American Heart Association. Circulation. 2015;131:1806-18.

38. Okuni M. Problems in clinical application of revised Jones diagnostic criteria for rheumatic fever. Jpn Heart J. 1971;12:436-41.

39. Committee on Rheumatic Fever and Bacterial Endocarditis of the American Heart Association. Jones criteria (revised) for guidance in the diagnosis of rheumatic fever. Circulation. 1984;69:203A-8A.

40. Hippocrates. The genuine works of Hippocrates (translated from Greek by Francis Adams). New York: Wood; 1986. pp. 192-273.

41. Jones TD. Diagnosis of rheumatic fever. JAMA. 1944;126:481-4.

42. Adhoc Committee on Rheumatic Fever and Bacterial Endocarditis of the American Heart Association. Jones criteria (revised) for guidance in the diagnosis of rheumatic fever. Circulation. 1965;32:664-8.

43. Strasser T, Dondog N, El Kholy A, Gharagozloo R, Kalbian VV, Ogunbi O, et al. The community control of rheumatic fever and rheumatic heart disease: report of a WHO international cooperative project. Bull WHO. 1981;59:285-94.

44. Vijayalakshmi IB, Mithravinda J, Deva AN. The role of echocardiography in diagnosing carditis in the setting of acute rheumatic fever. Cardiol Young. 2005;15:583-8.

45. Rammelkamp CH Jr, Stolzer BL. The latent period before the onset of acute rheumatic fever. Yale J Biol Med. 1961-1962;34:386-98.

46. Cleonice Coelho Mota C, Demarc hi Aiello V, Anderson RH. Rheumatic Fever. In: Pediatric Cardiology, 3rd edition. London: Churchill Livingstone; 2010. pp. 1091-114.

47. Osler W. The principles and practice of medicine: designed for the use of practitioners and students of medicine. New York: D. Appleton; 1892. p. 272.

48. Steeg C, Walsh C, Glickstein J. Rheumatic fever: No cause for complacence. Contemp Pediatr. 2000;1:128.

49. Feinstein AR, Spagnulo M. The clinical patterns of rheumatic fever: A reappraisal. Medicine. 1962;41:279-305.

50. Guzman-Cottrill JA, Jaggi P, Shulman ST. Acute rheumatic fever: Clinical aspects and insights into pathogenesis and prevention. Clin Appl Immunol Rev. 2004;4:263-76.

51. Svartman M, Potter EV, Poon-King T. Immunoglobulin components in synovial fluids of patients with acute rheumatic fever. J Clin Invest. 1975;56:111-7.

52. Jaccoud S. Lerons de clinique medicale faites a l'Hospital de la Charite, 2nd edition. , Paris: Delahaye; 1869.

53. Shostak NA. Jaccoud's arthropathy. Ter Arkh. 1995;67(11):80-3.

54. Bywaters EGL. The relation between heart and joint disease including "rheumatoid heart disease" and chronic post rheumatic arthritis type Jaccoud. B Heart J. 1950;12:101.

55. Mackie SL, Keat A. Poststreptococcal reactive arthritis: what is it and how do we know? Rheumatology. 2004;43:949-54.

56. Goldsmith DP, Long SS. Post streptococcal disease of childhood: a changing syndrome. Arthritis Rheum. 1982;25(Suppl 4):S18.

57. Ahmed S, Ayoub EM, Scornik JC, Wang CY, She JX. Poststreptococcal reactive arthritis: clinical characteristics and association with HLA-DR alleles. Arthritis Rheum. 1998;41:1096-102.

58. Deighton C. Beta haemolytic streptococci and reactive arthritis in adults. Ann Rheum Dis. 1993;52:475-82.

59. Ayoub EM, Ahmed S. Update on complications of group A streptococcal infections. Curr Prob Pediatr. 1997;27:90-101.

60. Schaffer FM, Agarwal R, Helm J, Gingell RL, Roland JM, O'Neil KM. Poststreptococcal reactive arthritis and silent carditis: a case report and review of the literature. Pediatrics. 1994;93:837-9.

61. Gerber MA, Baltimore RS, Eaton CB, Gewitz M, Rowley AH, Shulman ST, et al. Prevention of rheumatic fever and diagnosis and treatment of acute Streptococcal pharyngitis: a scientific statement from the American Heart Association Rheumatic Fever, Endocarditis, and Kawasaki Disease Committee of the Council on Cardiovascular Disease in the Young, the Interdisciplinary Council on Functional Genomics and Translational Biology, and the Interdisciplinary Council on Quality of Care and Outcomes Research: endorsed by the American Academy of Pediatrics. Circulation. 2009;119(11):1541-51.

62. Pinals RS. Polyarthritis and fever. N Eng J Med. 1994;330:769-74.

63. Bland EF, Jones TD. Rheumatic fever and rheumatic heart disease: A twenty year report on 1,000 patients followed since childhood. Circulation. 1951;4:836-43.

64. Massell BF. The diagnosis and treatment of rheumatic fever and rheumatic carditis. Med Clin North Am. 1958;42:1343-60.

65. Feinstein AR, Stern EK, Spagnuolo M. The prognosis of acute rheumatic fever. Am Heart J. 1964;68:817-34.

66. Park MK. Acute Rheumatic Fever. In: Park MK (Edn). Pediatric Cardiology for Practitioners, 5th edition. Philadelphia: Mosby; 2007. p. 383.

67. Veasy LG, Tani LY, Hill HR. Persistence of acute rheumatic fever in the intermountain area of the United States. J Pediatr. 1994;124:9-16.

68. Bitar FF, Hayek P, Obeid M, Gharzeddine W, Mikati M, Dbaibo GS. Rheumatic fever in children: A 15-year experience in a developing country." Pediatr Cardiol. 2000;21:119-22.

69. Chagani HS, Aziz K. Clinical profile of acute rheumatic fever in Pakistan. Cardiol Young. 2003;13:28-35.

70. Arora R, Subramanyam G, Khalilullah M, Gupta MP. Clinical profile of rheumatic fever and rheumatic heart disease: A study of 2,500 cases. Indian Heart J. 1981;33:264-9.

71. Essop MR, Wisenbaugh T, Sareli P. Evidence against a myocardial factor as the cause of left ventricular dilation in active rheumatic carditis. J Am Coll Cardiol. 1993;22:826-9.

72. de Oliveira SKF, Ribeiro M. Review for the primary care physician: Rheumatic fever. Pediatr Rheumatol Online J. Estados Unidos, v. July, 2004.

73. Narula J, Chopra P, Talwar KK, Reddy KS, Vasan RS, Tandon R, et al. Does endomyocardial biopsy aid in the diagnosis of active rheumatic carditis? Circulation. 1993;88:2198-205.

74. Kamblock J, Payot L, Iung B, Costes P, Gillet T, Le Goanvic C, et al. Does rheumatic myocarditis really exists? Systematic study with echocardiography and cardiac troponin I blood levels. Eur Heart J. 2003;24:855-62.

75. Williams RV, Minich LL, Shaddy RE, Veasy LG, Tani LY. Evidence for lack of myocardial injury in children with acute rheumatic carditis. Cardiol Young. 2002;12:519-23.

76. Carapetis JR, Steer AC, Mulholland EK, Weber M. The global burden of group A streptococcal diseases. Lancet Infect Dis. 2005;5:685-94.

77. Dajani AS, Allen HD, Taubert KA. Echocardiography for diagnosis and management of rheumatic fever (letter). JAMA. 1993;269:2084.

78. Sollerman GH. Rheumatic fever. Lancet. 1997;349:935-42.

79. Binotto MA, Guilherme L, Tanaka AC. Rheumatic Fever. Images Paediatr Cardiol. 2002;11:12-25.

80. Roy SB, Bhatia ML, Lazaro EJ, Ramaligaswami V. Juvenile mitral stenosis in India. Lancet. 1963;2:1193.

81. Vaishnava S, Webb JKG, Cherian J. Juvenile rheumatism in South India. A clinical study of 166 cases. Indian J Child Health. 1960;9:290.

82. Marcus RH, Sareli P, Pocock WA, Meyer TE, Magalhaes MP, Grieve T, et al. Functional anatomy of severe mitral regurgitation in active rheumatic carditis. Am J Cardiol. 1989;63:577-84.

83. Barlow JB, Marcus RH, Pocock WA, Barlow CW, Essop R, Sareli P. Mechanisms and management of heart failure in active rheumatic carditis. S Afr Med J. 1990;78:181-6.

84. Zhou LY, Lu K. Inflammatory valvular prolapse produced by acute rheumatic carditis: Echocardiographic analysis of 66 cases of acute rheumatic carditis. Int J Cardiol. 1997;58:175-8.

85. de Moor MM, Lachman PI, Human DG. Rupture of tendinous chords during acute rheumatic carditis in young children. Int J Cardiol. 1986;12:353-7.

86. Tani LY, Veasy LG, Minich LL, Shaddy RE. Rheumatic fever in children younger than 5 years: Is the presentation different? Pediatrics. 2003;112:1065-8.

87. Rosenthal A, Czoniczer G, Massell BF. Rheumatic fever under 3 years of age. A report of 10 cases. Pediatrics. 1968;41:612-9.

88. Bonow RO, Carabello B, de Leon AC Jr, Carabello BA, Erwin JP 3rd, Gentile F, et al. Guidelines for the management of patients with valvular heart disease: Executive summary. A report of the American College of Cardiology/American Heart Association Task Force on Practice Guidelines (Committee on Management of Patients with Valvular Heart Disease). Circulation. 1998;98: 1949-84.

89. Kaplan EL. Pathogenesis of acute rheumatic fever and rheumatic heart disease: evasive after half a century of clinical, epidemiological and laboratory investigation. Heart. 2005;91:34.

90. Homer C, Shulman ST. Clinical aspects of acute rheumatic fever. J Rheumatol. 1991;18(Suppl 29):2-13.

91. Swedo SE. Sydenham's chorea. A model for childhood auto-immune neuropsychiatric disorders. JAMA. 1994;272:1788-91.

92. Bland EF. Chorea as a manifestation of rheumatic fever. A long term perspective. Trans Am Clin Climatol Assoc. 1961;73: 209-13.

93. Massell BF, Mote JR, Jones TD. The artificial induction of subcutaneous nodules in patients with rheumatic fever. J Clin Invest. 1937;16:125.

94. Lennon D. Acute Rheumatic Fever in Children. Pediatr Drugs. 2004;6(6):363-73.

95. Sokolow M. Significance of electrocardiographic changes in rheumatic fever. Am J Med. 1948;5(3):365-78.

96. Kaplan EL, Top FH, Dudding BA, Wannamaker LW. Diagnosis of streptococcal pharyngitis: Differentiation of acute infection from the carrier state in the symptomatic child. J Infect Dis. 1971;123:490-501.

97. Ayoub EM. Streptococcal antibody tests in rheumatic fever. Clin Immunol News. 1982;3:107-11.

98. Stollerman GH, Lewis AJ, Schultz I, Taranta A. Relationship of immune response to group A streptococci to the course of acute, chronic, and recurrent rheumatic fever. Am J Med. 1956;20:163-9.

99. Swenson JM, Fischer DR, Miller SA, Boyle GJ, Ettedgui JA, Beerman LB. Are chest radiographs and electrocardiograms still valuable in evaluating new pediatric patients with heart murmurs or chest pain? Pediatrics. 1997;99:1-3.

10

Cardiac Complications of Acute Rheumatic Fever

IB Vijaylakshmi, Shibba Takkar Chhabra

> *"A clinician is complex. He is part craftsman, part practical scientist, and part historian."*
>
> —**Thomas Addis** (1881–1949)
> US Physician

INTRODUCTION

Acute rheumatic fever (ARF) results from an autoimmune response to infection with Group A beta-hemolytic streptococci (GABHS). Acute illness causes significant morbidity and mortality, but the major impact is because of valvular involvement. With improvement in living conditions, nutrition, hygiene and availability of better antibiotics, the incidence and prevalence of disease have considerably decreased. But, still it remains a major problem in developing countries such as India, South Africa, and indigenous population of developed countries. According to WHO,[1] at least 15.6 million people have rheumatic heart disease (RHD), 60% of 0.5 million individuals who acquire ARF/RHD go on to develop RHD and 233,000 deaths annually are attributable to ARF or carditis. According to Padmavati,[2] the incidence of ARF in India was 54 per lakh per year as in 2001. The epidemiological trends of ARF/RHD as per population-based survey studies revealed prevalence of 1.8/1,000 to 4.58/1,000. The school-based surveys reported prevalence of 1–11/1,000, 1.3–6.4/1,000 and less than 1/1,000 in clinical screening methods of 1960s to 1990s, clinical screening confirmed by echocardiography in 1990s to 2000 and clinical screening confirmed by echocardiography after 2000, respectively.[3] However, Ramakrishnan et al. in 2009 reported a high cumulative disease burden in India with similar high RHD burden reported by systematic review by Dixit et al. in 2022.[4,5] Hence, reduction in RHD burden is probably just among the privileged population and the socioeconomically poor and underprivileged continue to be the victims of this preventable disease.[6]

Acute rheumatic fever is a multisystem disease involving many organ systems, but none of its manifestation except carditis leaves behind significant residual deformity. Carditis is predominantly responsible for morbidity and mortality related with ARF. Carditis was seen in around 72% of patients of ARF studied in USA in 1987.[7] The prevalence of subclinical carditis ranged from 0 to 53% in a meta-analysis with weighted pool persistence or worsening of carditis in patients with subclinical carditis reported as 44.7%.[8]

MECHANISM OF INJURY

The autoimmune response that causes rheumatic fever might be triggered by molecular mimicry between epitope on pathogen (GABHS) and specific human tissue. The structural and immunological similarity between M protein and myosin, with both alpha helical and coiled molecules, seems essential for development of rheumatic carditis. M protein epitope causes sensitization of CD4+ T-cells, which cross-react with host's own cardiac myosin.[9,10] The initial damage to heart valves may be due to presence of laminin, another alpha helical coiled molecule present in the valvular basement membrane and endothelium which are recognized by T cells as similar to myosin and M protein.[11]

Antibodies against N-acetylglucosamine of group A *Streptococcus* cross-react with cardiac valve tissue and lead to valvulitis.[12,13]

Carditis in rheumatic fever is an early manifestation of the disease. About 80% of patients who develop carditis manifest it within first 2 weeks. Cardiac complications of ARF can present in a number of ways, including subclinical cardiac involvement, indolent, subacute or acute or even fulminant congestive cardiac failure, mitral and aortic regurgitation (MR and AR), and less frequently tricuspid valve involvement. Pulmonary valve involvement is a rarity. Rheumatic carditis is a pan carditis involving all the three layers—pericardium, myocardium, and endocardium. Although involvement of all layers is responsible for the whole clinical picture, significant valvular involvement is responsible for unfavorable prognosis. Severe carditis and heart failure occur in 13-64% of rheumatic fever and represent 15-50% of patients with carditis.[14] If the cardiac involvement is less, chances of resolution of cardiac findings are very likely. Pathological changes in cardiac involvement of rheumatic fever show fibrinous pericarditis, pinhead vegetations in valve leaflets with edema and hemorrhage in leaflet tissue, fibrinoid necrosis in the valve leaflet, cellular infiltrate and revascularization of the valve. Myocardial interstitial infiltrate and myocardial necrosis are a rarity.

Subendocardial Aschoff granuloma is a pathological hallmark of rheumatic carditis. McCallum patch is basically a scar because of the regurgitant lesion. Aschoff bodies are seen in 30–40% of patients with proven or suspected carditis.

ENDOCARDITIS

Clinically, endocarditis manifests as valvulitis. Mitral valve involvement is seen in 70–75% of patients of ARF, whereas aortic valve involvement is seen in 20-25% of patients. Isolated aortic valve involvement is seen in 5–8% of patients. Tricuspid valve involvement is a rarity and pulmonary valve involvement is almost never reported. Pathological studies report tricuspid valve involvement in 30–50% of patients, but clinical tricuspid valve involvement is rare in first attack of rheumatic fever.[15] MR is dominant cardiac abnormality in patients with rheumatic fever, occurring in approximately 95% of patients with acute rheumatic carditis.[9] Both echocardiographic and surgical observation studies have demonstrated that the mechanism of mitral regurgitation is a combination of annular dilatation and chordal elongation, which result in abnormal coaptation and, in some cases, prolapse of the tip of mitral leaflet.[16-18] Rarely, mitral chordae ruptures resulting in flail mitral leaflet and severe mitral regurgitation.[19-22] Patients with acute mild MR are usually asymptomatic, but in moderate-to-severe MR, left ventricle (LV) myocardium may not be able to handle the volume overload and left heart filling pressures rise leading to pulmonary venous congestion and pulmonary edema. Such patients usually present with left ventricular failure

(LVF), dyspnea, orthopnea, paroxysmal nocturnal dyspnea, cough, or hemoptysis. Secondary PAH may develop leading to right ventricle (RV) dysfunction, tricuspid regurgitation (TR), and right-sided heart failure. Tachycardia is often the earliest sign of carditis. Auscultatory sign is characterized by holosystolic murmur grades II to IV of MR, best heard at apex in left lateral decubitus position at the end of expiration.

Valvular stenoses [mitral stenosis (MS) and aortic stenosis (AS)] do not occur in acute setting of first episode of rheumatic fever, but mid-diastolic low-pitch murmur may be heard at apex because of combination of valvulitis and increased diastolic flow across mitral valve (Carey Coombs murmur).

Aortic valve can be involved in approximately 25–40% of patients[23] diagnosed by presence of early diastolic murmur of AR, best heard along the base in the left parasternal area. Isolated AR is seen in around 5% of patients. These patients of acute AR have no time for evolving compensatory mechanisms and, therefore, develop decreased stroke volume and elevation of LV end diastolic pressure leading to a condition of low-cardiac output and pulmonary edema. Therefore, these patients usually have a narrow pulse pressure aortic regurgitation. Clinically there is low-pitch mid- to late-diastolic rumbling murmur with presystolic accentuation, in absence of MS known as Austin Flint murmur, along with early diastolic murmur of AR as mentioned above. Usually, AR disappears with resolution of inflammation.

MYOCARDITIS

Severity of LV dysfunction, even in acute setting of carditis, correlates with extent of valvulitis rather than with any myocardial injury. Rheumatic myocarditis in the setting of preserved LV function is not associated with troponin level elevation as seen in viral myocarditis.[24] Both echocardiography and postmortem pathology reveal that severe heart failure in ARF is because of altered myocardial mechanics caused by MR and AR rather than secondary to myocarditis. Traditionally, the diagnosis of myocarditis has been made on the basis of auscultation of mitral or aortic regurgitation in the setting of heart failure.

PERICARDITIS

Rheumatic pericarditis occurs in approximately 4–11% of patients with rheumatic carditis. When it occurs, it is usually associated with significant left-sided valvular lesions. In the absence of significant AR/MR, pericardial effusion is usually due to another cause than rheumatic fever. It, therefore, must be evaluated thoroughly for other etiology. This is clinically characterized by pericardial friction rub, which may obscure murmurs and rub may be intermittent or evanescent. Rheumatic pericarditis is often associated with serosanguinous or hemorrhagic effusion that usually resolves without any residual.

■ INAPPARENT OR SILENT CARDITIS

Patients with chorea without any evidence of carditis may develop mitral stenosis on long-term follow-up suggesting multiple subclinical attacks of carditis. Histopathological form of carditis in absence of any clinical evidence of carditis has also been reported. This presentation is termed as silent carditis.[25-28] Doppler echocardiography has been proposed for identifying subclinical carditis in patients with rheumatic fever, who do not have audible murmurs, although American Heart Association (AHA) presently does not favor using Doppler echocardiography in absence of clinical criteria to support diagnosis of rheumatic carditis.

■ DIAGNOSIS[29]

- The revised Jones criteria identify the individuals at low risk of ARF/RHD as incidence <2 per 100,000 school-aged children (5–14 years old) per year, or an all-age prevalence of RHD of ≤1 per 1,000 population per year (Class IIa, level of evidence C). Children not clearly from a low-risk population are conserved as moderate-to-high risk depending on their reference population (Class I, level of evidence C).
- *Clinical manifestations of ARF*: The major clinical manifestations of ARF are carditis and arthritis, followed in descending frequency by chorea (with a female predominance), subcutaneous nodules, and erythema marginatum (uncommon but specific of ARF).
- *Carditis diagnosis in present era of echocardiography*: Over 25 studies reported echocardiographic evidence of mitral or aortic valve regurgitation in ARF patients even when no classical auscultatory findings were present.
- It is recommended that 2D echocardiography with Doppler should be performed in all cases of confirmed and suspected ARF (Class I, level of evidence B).
- In any patient with diagnosed or suspected ARF, serial echocardiography/Doppler studies can be considered even if documented carditis is not present on diagnosis (Class IIa, level of evidence C).
- In moderate-to-high-risk populations and when ARF is considered likely echocardiography/Doppler testing should be done to look for any subclinical carditis in absence of auscultatory findings (Class I, level of evidence B).
- Moreover, when echocardiographic findings are not consistent with carditis, it is imperative to exclude the diagnosis of ARF in patients with a heart murmur otherwise thought to be due to rheumatic carditis (Class I, level of evidence B).
- *Rheumatic valvulitis (specific echocardiography/Doppler criteria)*:
  - *Mitral regurgitation (all four)*—seen in ≥2 views, jet length ≥2 cm, peak velocity >3 m/s, and pan systolic
  - *Aortic regurgitation (all four)*—seen in ≥2 views, jet length ≥1 cm, peak velocity >3 m/s, pan diastolic

- *Evidence of preceding Streptococcal infection*: Laboratory evidence of antecedent group A streptococcal infection is needed to exclude diseases mimicking ARF whenever possible and in doubtful diagnosis.
  Markers of preceding infection (anyone):
  - Increased or rising anti-streptolysin O titer or other streptococcal antibodies (anti-DNase B) (Class I, level of evidence B) (rising titer better evidence)
  - Throat culture positive for GABHS (Class I, level of evidence B)
  - Rapid group A streptococcal carbohydrate antigen test positive in children with clinical presentation highly suggestive of streptococcal pharyngitis (Class I, level of evidence B).

Modified Jones criteria for diagnosis of rheumatic fever (2015) are presented in **Box 1**.

Electrocardiography (ECG) features: PR prolongation (25–40% patients due to increased vagal activity, Mobitz types I and II, even high-grade atrioventricular (AV) block, atrial fibrillation, supraventricular arrhythmias and rarely sudden death (VT). These conduction abnormalities bear a low sensitivity and specificity for the diagnosis of carditis.

Although an Aschoff's granuloma is considered as pathological hallmark of rheumatic carditis (seen in only 30–40% of patients), biopsy does not contribute much to the diagnosis of rheumatic carditis. McCallum patch visible as a scar in left atrium probably reflects a regurgitant lesion. The typical biopsy findings of rheumatic carditis are fibrinoid

BOX 1	Modified Jones criteria for diagnosis of rheumatic fever (2015).

Major criteria:
- *Low-risk population*: Carditis (clinical or subclinical), arthritis—only polyarthritis, chorea, erythema marginatum, subcutaneous nodules
- *High-risk population*: Carditis (clinical or subclinical), arthritis—monoarthritis or polyarthritis, polyarthralgia, chorea, erythema marginatum, subcutaneous nodules

Minor criteria:
- *Low-risk population*: Polyarthralgia, hyperpyrexia (≥38.5°C), ESR ≥ 60 mm/h and/or CRP ≥ 3.0 mg/dL, prolonged PR interval (after taking into account the differences related to age; if there is no carditis as a major criterion)
- *High-risk population*: Monoarthralgia, hyperpyrexia (≥38.0°C), ESR ≥ 30 mm/h and/or CRP ≥ 3.0 mg/dL, prolonged PR interval (after taking into account the differences related to age if there is no carditis as a major criterion)

Diagnosis of initial episode of ARF—two major or one major + two minor criteria

Diagnosis of subsequent ARF episode: Reliable past history of ARF/RHD in presence of documented group A streptococci infection, two major/one major and two minor/three minor manifestations suffice for presumptive diagnosis (Class IIb level of evidence C)

(ARF: acute rheumatic fever; CRP: C-reactive protein; ESR: erythrocyte sedimentation rate; RHD: rheumatic heart disease)

necrosis, cellular infiltrate and neovascularization of valve with pinhead vegetations and hemorrhage in leaflet.

PROGNOSIS

The prognosis of patient with rheumatic carditis depends upon the severity of first attack and number of recurrences. Assessment of severity is important regarding decision of therapy and use of steroid. The increasing severity implies poor prognosis and greater need for prophylaxis. In the absence of anemia and other complicating factors, cardiomegaly indicates severe carditis, the larger the heart more severe is the carditis. Patients with severe acute carditis seem to have greater incidence of chronic carditis.

MANAGEMENT

The aim of acute management of proven attack of rheumatic carditis is to suppress inflammatory response and to minimize the effect on the heart, to eradicate GABHS from the pharynx and provide symptomatic relief. Appropriate dose of anti-inflammatory agents, e.g., aspirin 100 mg/kg/day in 4/5 divided doses and prednisolone 1–2 mg/kg/day can be given. Patient with carditis improves rapidly with corticosteroids especially in setting of heart failure, but meta-analysis of eight randomized controlled trials has failed to show superiority of steroids, intravenous (IV) immunoglobulin or salicylates in progression of RHD.

For treatment of acute rheumatic carditis, follow established guidelines for management of congestive cardiac failure (CCF) and severe valvular regurgitation. Unless regurgitation and heart failure are refractory to drug therapy, surgery is avoided during acute episodes. Surgical morbidity and mortality have been significant and failed repair leading to valve replacement is frequent if operated in acute phase, although postoperative ventricular function improved significantly. Secondary prevention is recommended as per guidelines for prevention of recurrence of rheumatic fever and thus rheumatic carditis, leading to decrease in the sequelae of recurrent carditis.

REFERENCES

1. Carapetis JR. The current evidence for the burden of group A streptococcal disease. WHO/FCH/CAH/05-07 Geneva WHO Technical Report Series, No. 923/2004/1. [online] Available from http://apps.who.int/iris/bitstream/handle/10665/69063/WHO_FCH_CAH_05.07.pdf;jsessionid=55C6E1DF093F9C8650C15564D65FAD6B?sequence=1. [Last accessed October, 2022].

2. Padmavati S. Rheumatic fever and rheumatic heart disease in India at the turn of century. Indian Heart J. 2001;53:35-7.

3. Negi PC, Sondhi S, Asotra S, Mahajan K, Mehta A. Current status of rheumatic heart disease in India. Indian Heart J. 2019;71(1):85-90.

4. Dixit J, Brar S, Prinja S. Burden of Group A Streptococcal Pharyngitis, Rheumatic Fever, and Rheumatic Heart Disease in India: A Systematic Review and Meta-Analysis. Indian J Pediatr. 2022;89(7):641-50

5. Ramakrishnan S, Kothari SS, Juneja R, Bhargava B, Saxena A, Bahl VK, et al. Prevalence of rheumatic heart disease: has it declined in India? Natl Med J India. 2009;22(2):72-4.

6. Arvind B, Saxena A. Rheumatic Heart Disease in India: Has It Declined or been Forgotten? Indian J Pediatr. 2022;89(7):637-8.

7. Veasy LG, Wiedmeier SE, Orsmond GS, Ruttenberg HD, Boucek MM, Roth SJ, et al. Resurgence of acute rheumatic fever in the intermountain area of the United States. N Engl J Med. 1987;316(8):421-7.

8. Tubridy-Clark M, Carapetis JR. Subclinical carditis in rheumatic fever: a systematic review. Int J Cardiol. 2007;119(1):54-8.

9. Cunningham MW. T cell mimicry in inflammatory heart disease. Mol Immuno. 2004;40:1121-7.

10. Smith SC, Allen PM. Expression of myosin class II major histocompatibility complex in the normal myocardium occurs before induction of auto-immune myocarditis. Proc Nati Acad Sci USA. 1992;89:9131-5.

11. Galvin JE, Hemric ME, Ward K, Cunningham MW. Cytotoxic mAb from rheumatic carditis recognizes heart valves and laminin. J Clin Invest. 2000;106:217-24.

12. Cunningham MW. Autoimmunity and molecular mimicry in the pathogenesis of post-streptococcal heart disease. Front Biosci. 2003;8:s533-43.

13. Goldstein I, Halpern B, Robert L. Immunological relationship between *Streptococcus* A polysaccharide and the structural glycoproteins of heart valve. Nature. 1967;213:44-7.

14. Tani YL. Rheumatic fever and rheumatic heart disease. In: Allen HD, Driscoll DJ. Shaddy RE, Feltes TF (Eds). Moss and Adams Heart disease in infants, children and adolescent including fetus and young adults, 7th edition. Philadelphia (PA): Lippincott Williams & Wilkins; 2008. p. 1256.

15. Kinare SG. Chronic rheumatic valvular heart disease. Ann Indian Acad Med Sci. 1972;8:47-52.

16. Marcus RH, Sareli P, Pocock WA, Meyer TE, Magalhaes MP, Grieve T, et al. Functional anatomy of severe mitral regurgitation in active rheumatic carditis. Am J Cardiol. 1989;63:577-84.

17. Barlow JB, Marcus RH, Pocock WA. Mechanism and management of heart failure in active rheumatic carditis. S Afri Med J. 1990;78:181-6.

18. Zhon LY, Lu K. Inflammatory valvular prolapse produced by acute rheumatic carditis: Echocardiographic analysis of 66 cases of acute rheumatic carditis. Int J Cardiol. 1997;58;175-8.

19. Aron AM, Freeman JM, Carter S. The natural history of Sydenham's chorea. Review of the literature, long-term evaluation with emphasis on cardiac sequelae. Am J Med. 1965;38:83-95.

20. de Moor MM, Lachman PI, Human DG. Rupture of tendinuous chords during acute rheumatic carditis in young children. Int J Cardiol. 1986;12:353-7.

21. Oliveira DB, Dawkin KD, Kay PH, Paneth M. Chordal rupture 1: aetiology and natural history. Br Heart J. 1983;50:312-7.

22. Kalangos A, Beghetti M, Vala D, Jaeggi E, Kaya G, Karpuz V, et al. Anterior mitral leaflet prolapse as a primary cause of pure rheumatic mitral insufficiency. Ann Thorac Surg. 2000;69:755-61.

23. Raju BS, Turi ZG. Rheumatic Fever. In: Libby P, Bonow RO, Mann DL, Zipes DP, Braunwald E (Eds). Braunwald's Heart Disease: Textbook of Cardiovascular Medicine, 8th edition. Philadelphia: Saunders; 2008. p. 2079.

24. Kamblock J, Payot L, Lung B, Costes P, Gillet T, Le Goanvic C, et al. Does rheumatic myocarditis really exist? Systematic study with Echocardiography and cardiac troponin I blood levels. Eur Heart J. 2003;24:855-62.

25. Bland EF. Chorea as a manifestation of rheumatic fever: A long-term perspecptive. Trans Am Clin Assoc. 1961;73:209-13.

26. Edwards WD, Peterson K, Edwards JE. Active valvulitis associated with chronic rheumatic valvular disease and active myocarditis. Circulation. 1978;57:181-5.

27. Veasy LG. Myocardial dysfunction in active rheumatic carditis. J Am Coll Cardiol. 1994;24:581-82.

28. Chandrasekhar Y, Narula J. Rheumatic fever. In: Alpert JS, Dalen JE, Rahimtoola SH (Eds). Valvular heart disease, 3rd edition. Philadelphia: Lippincott Williams & Wilkins; 2000. p. 4.

29. Gewitz MH, Baltimore RS, Tani LY, Sable CA, Shulman ST, Carapetis J, et al. American Heart Association Committee on Rheumatic Fever, Endocarditis, and Kawasaki Disease of the Council on Cardiovascular Disease in the Young. Revision of the Jones Criteria for the diagnosis of acute rheumatic fever in the era of Doppler echocardiography: a scientific statement from the American Heart Association. Circulation. 2015;131(20): 1806-18.

Role of Echocardiography in Diagnosis of Carditis in Acute Rheumatic Fever

IB Vijayalakshmi

"Declare the past, diagnose the present, foretell the future."

—Hippocrates, 460–357 BC
Greek Physician

INTRODUCTION

The acute rheumatic fever (ARF) and its long-term sequel, chronic rheumatic heart disease (RHD), are major burning problems in children, adolescents, and young adults in India.[1] The varying degrees of carditis associated with valve insufficiency, heart failure, pericarditis, and even death may occur in 39% of patients with ARF.[2] Unless carditis is detected in time and treated appropriately and put on secondary penicillin prophylaxis, further recrudescence of rheumatic activity can damage valves, causing RHD and consequently atrial dilation, atrial fibrillation, ventricular dilation, ventricular dysfunction, heart failure, and ultimately untimely death.

BACKGROUND

Two-dimensional (2D) transthoracic echocardiography (TTE) is a noninvasive, essential key tool for the diagnosis and evaluation of carditis in ARF.[3] The etiology, severity, hemodynamic consequences, and ventricular dilatation to grade of valvular regurgitation can be assessed with appropriate echocardiographic techniques. Echo can assess severity of mitral regurgitation (MR), aortic regurgitation (AR), tricuspid regurgitation (TR), and grade it as mild, moderate, and severe. This assessment has both diagnostic and prognostic significance. Echo can detect mechanism of MR. For example, whether MR is due to valvulitis, valve prolapse, annulitis, ventricular enlargement, or chordal rupture (rarely) can be made out only by Echo. But, all these pathophysiologies causing MR cannot be distinguished by clinical examination. It is essential to make an accurate diagnosis of carditis and put patient on secondary prophylaxis, as in 35–40% of the cases, timely management can make the heart almost normal and prevent recrudescence of rheumatic activity. The TTE also has an important role in therapeutic decision making and providing prognostic information. Hence, for the first time, recent revised Jones criteria of 2015 by American Heart Association (AHA) have included "echocardiography" as a major criterion for the diagnosis of carditis in ARF.[4]

CHANGES IN JONES CRITERIA

In view of the heterogeneity in global disease burden, a single set of diagnostic criteria may no longer be sufficient for all population groups and in all geographic regions. The addition of echocardiography and Doppler to the armamentarium of tests in the diagnosis of ARF will lead to detection of more cases of carditis in ARF. Hence, recent revised Jones criteria include technology-driven Echo and also focus on epidemiological differences seen in high-risk and low-risk populations so that more ARF patients are detected in time. The introduction of especially subclinical

TABLE 1: Changes in the original Jones criteria.

Symptoms	1944	1956	1965	1984	1992	2002	2015
Carditis	Major	Major	Major	Major	Major	Major	Major subclinical
Polyarthritis	Major	Major	Major	Major	Major	Major	Major
Polyarthralgia	Major	Minor	Minor	Minor	Minor	Minor	Major
Chorea	Major	Major	Major	Major	Major	Major	Major
Subcutaneous nodules	Major	Major	Major	Major	Major	Major	Major
Erythema marginatum	Major	Major	Major	Major	Major	Major	Major
Echocardiography							Major

carditis and polyarthralgia as major criteria in high-risk populations, such as in some parts of India, will bring more patients into the net of secondary prophylaxis. Revision of the Jones criteria for the diagnosis of ARF in the era of echocardiography with Doppler should be performed in all cases of confirmed and suspected ARF. The changes in original Jones criteria made from time to time are shown chronologically in **Table 1**.

Duckett Jones established diagnostic criteria in 1944. They were first modified in 1955, then revised in 1965, edited in 1984, then updated in 1992, and later revised by WHO in 1988 and then again in 2003.[5-8] Despite these modifications, revision, and re-revision of the Jones criteria several times, "carditis" in ARF is either underdiagnosed or overdiagnosed,[9] and still worse, many patients go undiagnosed! The WHO bulletin (1981) showed that in ARF/RHD detected in surveys and health check-up camps, >50% of patients were unaware of the disease and >70% were not receiving regular secondary prophylaxis.[10] Diagnosis of carditis based only on traditional characteristic auscultatory findings can lead to overdiagnosis in many patients.[10-12] Echocardiography has become widely available and evolved over the past two decades and several papers documenting utility of early diagnosis of carditis, even in the absence of apparent clinical findings (subclinical carditis), have been published.[10,12] Therefore, the sixth revision of the Jones criteria in 2015 is historic as it has included subclinical carditis, which is echocardiographic valvulitis as a major criterion. For the first time, TTE is included as a major criterion in Jones criteria.[4,5]

◼ CARDITIS

Traditionally, clinical diagnosis of carditis is based on the auscultation of classical murmurs that indicate either regurgitation of the mitral or aortic or rarely tricuspid valves.[13,14] Until 2015, echocardiographic findings were always considered secondary to other clinical findings of carditis. More studies substantiate "subclinical carditis" which is missed by clinical examination. A review of 23 articles showed that the prevalence of subclinical carditis

ranged from 0 to 53%, emphasizing the high variability of the finding. Pooled evidence puts the prevalence of subclinical carditis at 16.8% of ARF.[4] Newer evidence suggests that by including echocardiographic evidence of subclinical carditis, an additional 15–20% of ARF patients can be identified and secondary prophylaxis can be extended.[15,16]

Echocardiography versus Clinical Examination

The MR in ARF is usually mild to moderate and assessment of its mechanism and severity has prognostic significance. The various mechanisms of MR are: (a) valvulitis, (b) valve prolapse, (c) annulitis with annular dilatation, (d) ventricular enlargement, and (e) rarely, chordal tear and papillary rupture. On clinical examination, only MR can be diagnosed and not its mechanism. In our prospective study, 492 consecutive clinically diagnosed ARF patients (according to Jones criteria) were examined thoroughly by pediatricians, who had used appropriate laboratory tests. The TTE was done by a well-trained and experienced echocardiographer who was unaware of the clinical diagnosis (double-blind). Echo evidence of carditis was observed in only 59.4% of Jones criteria fulfilled cases, i.e., clinically diagnosed as carditis by well-qualified pediatricians.[9] On analysis, of these patients who had overdiagnosis of carditis (40.6%), they actually had fever, anemia, tachycardia, functional murmurs, and congenital heart diseases! Echo evidence of carditis/valvulitis was observed in 46.9% of patients with polyarthralgia, though it was a minor criterion then. Thus, in endemic areas of ARF, if arthralgia is taken as a minor criterion and Echo is not done, it leads to gross underdiagnosis. Hence, in the 2015 new revised Jones criteria, polyarthralgia is considered as major criteria and TTE is recommended for all the suspected cases of ARF.[5]

Goals of Echo Interrogation

It is very pertinent to realize that Echo is the only investigating modality by which we can assess, both clinical and subclinical carditis, and formulate the management strategies. Hence, the goals of Echo interrogation are:

- To make a precise and early diagnosis of carditis in ARF. As timely management can make the heart normal in 35–40% of cases of ARF and in remaining children, the secondary prophylaxis can further prevent the recrudescence of rheumatic activity.
- To prevent both "overdiagnosis" and "underdiagnosis" of carditis by depending on the traditional clinical auscultatory findings,[9] which could be fallacious and lead to unnecessary drugging and psychological impact on the children and their parents or miss the subclinical carditis and not get the secondary prophylaxis.

Echo Features of Carditis in ARF

It is very important to know the common various Echo features of carditis in ARF and also their incidence. The details of incidence of various Echo features of carditis in our study[9] are given in order of occurrence in **Table 2**.

M-mode

In patients with carditis, M-mode shows a dilated left atrium (LA) and left ventricle (LV). Normally, LA and aorta (AO)

TABLE 2: The incidence of various echocardiographic features.[9]

Type of involvement	Number of cases	Percentage
Mitral thickness > 4 mm	132	93.62%
Mitral regurgitation grades I–II	118	83.69%
Mitral valve prolapse (MVP)	80	56.74%
Rheumatic nodules	38	26.95%
Aortic regurgitation (AR)	31	21.99%
Tricuspid regurgitation (TR)	31	21.99%
Pancarditis	13	9.22%
Pericardial effusion (PF)	13	9.22%
Chordal tear	4	2.84%

have almost the same dimension. But, in carditis of ARF, LA is dilated with alteration in the LA to AO ratio.

Two-dimensional Echo

The thickened mitral and aortic leaflets >4 mm (normal <3 mm) is seen very often **(Figs. 1A and B)**. Sometimes, valve thickening could be 9–10 mm. Rarely, tricuspid valve also could be thickened.

In the regions where ARF is endemic if arthralgia is taken as minor criteria and Echo is not done, then it leads to gross underdiagnosis and many children go undiagnosed as they have subclinical carditis. The tricuspid valve thickening, beading with regurgitation was detected by Echo in 60 patients.[16] All these patients had other features of rheumatic carditis,[16] such as thickened mitral valves, beaded appearance, and hyperechogenic submitral structures. This shows that the carditis cannot be reliably clinically diagnosed in the absence of clinical signs of valve regurgitation, especially in subclinical carditis. This may lead to significant underdetection of carditis in ARF. Echo with Doppler can diagnose carditis precisely and accurately, especially subclinical carditis/valvulitis. The TTE also shows that increased end-diastolic volume (EDV) and end systolic volume (ESV) and the ejection fraction (EF) are reduced marginally. In ARF with carditis, the mitral valve is the most commonly affected valve. The inflamed edematous valve is seen on Echo as thickened >4 mm in 93.6% of cases with reduced mobility and hyperechogenicity of submitral structures.[9]

Beaded Appearance

The ridge or row of small pink aphthous ulcer-like lesions on the rims of mitral valve on autopsy **(Fig. 2A)** is seen as beaded appearance on Echo in short-axis **(Fig. 2B)**. The beaded appearance of mitral valve on Echo is nothing but the Echo images of small thrombi that form on the valve at the edge. Rarely, beaded appearance is seen on submitral structures **(Fig. 2C)**. Similarly, the autopsy specimen of

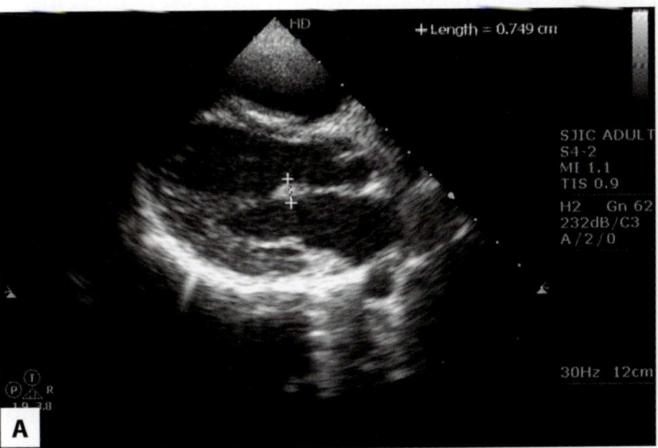

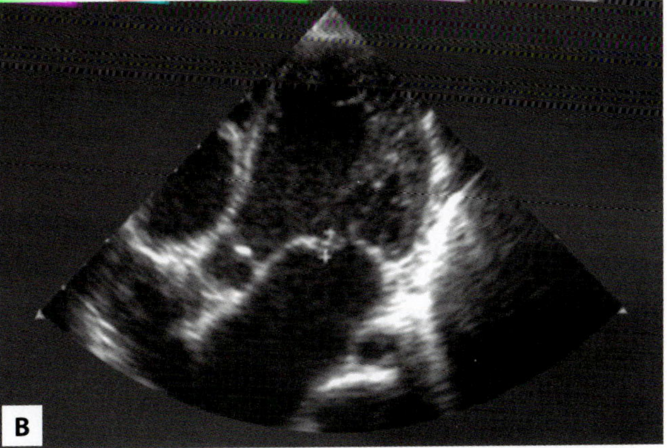

FIGS. 1A AND B: (A) Parasternal long axis shows 7-mm thick anterior mitral leaflet (AML), (B): Apical 5-chamber view shows along with thickened AML, the thickening of aortic valve, and hyperechogenic submitral structure such as chordae and papillary muscles are seen in 8-year-old boy with ARF.

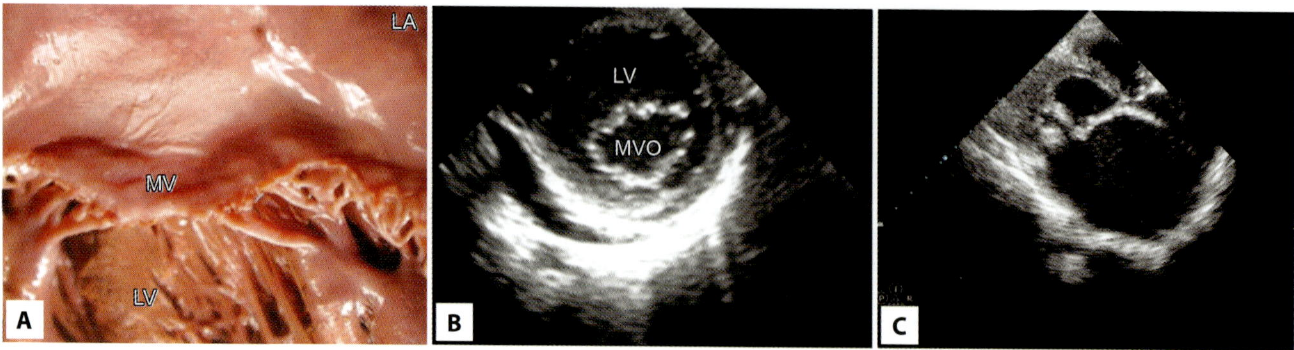

FIGS. 2A TO C: (A) Row of small pink thrombi at the edge of the valve at autopsy, and compared to (B) Echo in parasternal short-axis view showing beaded appearance of the valve. (C) Parasternal long-axis view shows beaded appearance of AML, PML, submitral structures, and aortic valve with dilated left atrium in 16-year-old boy with ARF with carditis.

(AML: anterior mitral leaflet; LA: left atrium; LV: left ventricle; MV: mitral valve; MVO: mitral valve orifice; PML: posterior mitral leaflet)

Source: Autopsy image courtesy of Dr Pradeep Vaideeswar.

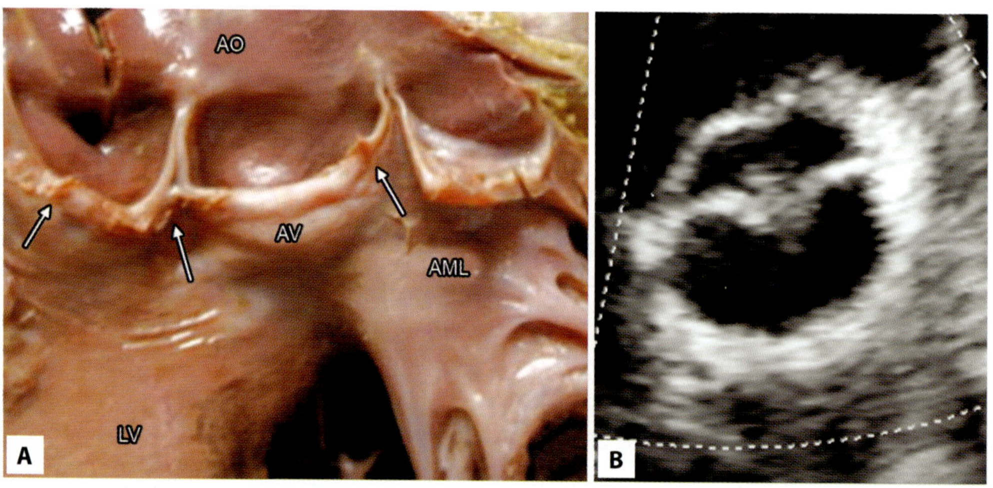

FIGS. 3A AND B: (A) Autopsy specimen of aortic valve showing active valvulitis. The valve is slightly thickened and displays small "verrucae" on the edge of valve; (B) Transthoracic echocardiography in short axis shows thickened AV valve with beaded appearance.

aortic valve showing active valvulitis in the form of inflamed thickened aortic cups with small "verrucae" on the edge of valve **(Fig. 3A)**. The TTE in short axis shows thickened AV valve with irregular beaded appearance of aortic valve **(Fig. 3B)** and tricuspid valve too.

Echo criteria have been evolved in our study for the diagnosis of carditis by giving two points for each of eight echocardiographic features of carditis. The cases with an echo score of ≥6 out of 16 were taken as Echo positive, so as to avoid overdiagnosis of MR, and its efficacy was tested in a prospective double-blind study.[17] On review of literature, there are no studies that have come out with Echo criteria for the diagnosis of carditis in ARF. As regurgitation lesions are common in ARF, most of the studies have suggested that it be included in Jones criteria.[17-22]

In ARF, clinically rheumatic nodules looked for on knees and elbows **(Fig. 4A)**. Similar to these rheumatic nodules, small irregular thickening seen on the free edge of valve cusp, indicating inflammation in autopsy **(Fig. 4B)**, are seen as thickened irregular nodular leaflets on Echo **(Figs. 4C and D)**. These nodules are seen just proximal to the free edge of mitral valves, where the cusps come into apposition, at the site of maximum natural trauma. These nodules on the body and tip of mitral leaflets do not have chaotic motion like vegetation in bacterial endocarditis, which are attached to the valve and not embedded. They may disappear on follow-up. It is thought that these nodules may be equivalents of verrucae seen at autopsy in patients who died of ARF.[17,23]

Application of Vijaya's Echo Criteria

Our own prospective, double-blind study clearly showed that Echo can prevent both underdiagnosis and overdiagnosis. Our two studies titled "role of echocardiography in diagnosing carditis in setting of ARF"[9] and "efficacy of echocardiographic criteria for diagnosis of carditis in ARF"[16] are quoted in the

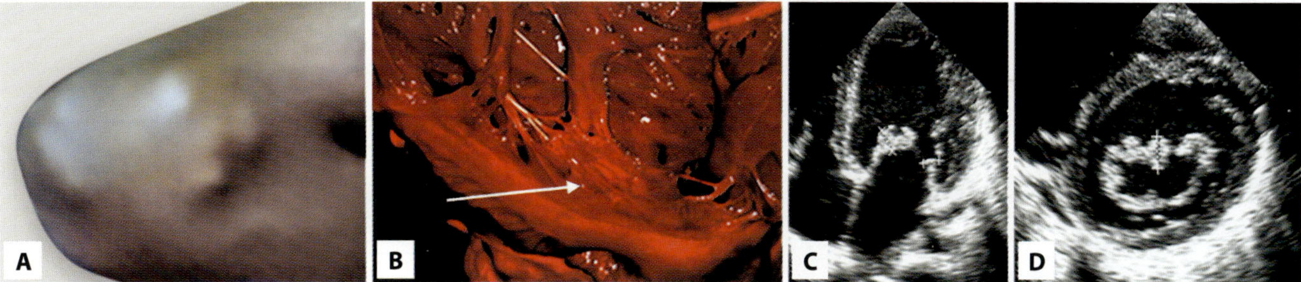

FIGS. 4A TO D: (A) Rheumatic nodules on the extensor aspect of elbow. (B) Autopsy picture of mitral valve shows thickened irregular nodules on the free edge of MV. (C) Transthoracic echocardiography in apical four-chamber view shows the club-like nodules on the body and tip of mitral leaflets do not have chaotic motion like vegetations, thickened anterior mitral leaflet (9 mm), posterior mitral leaflet (6 mm); (D) Parasternal short axis shows beaded appearance of mitral valve (MV); thickness of anterior mitral leaflet is 9 mm nodular irregular mitral valve akin to nodules seen in autopsy and on clinical examination in a 9-year-old girl with acute rheumatic fever (ARF).

2015 article of revised Jones criteria.[4] Any patient getting less than 6 scores is unlikely to be of rheumatic etiology as shown in **Figure 5** in a child with mucopolysaccharidosis with severe MR due to grade-III MVP (Echo score is only 4). Hence, only if valvular regurgitation is associated with other features such as thickened valves, reduced mobility, beaded appearance, hyperechogenic submitral structures, and chordal tear, with an Echo score of more than 6, it is taken as carditis of rheumatic etiology. Vijaya's Echo criteria have 81% sensitivity with 93% specificity.[16] Vijaya's Echo criteria are for the precise diagnosis of carditis/subclinical valvulitis by giving 2 points for each of the eight Echo features of carditis as shown in **Table 3**. The cases with an Echo score of more than 6 out of 16 are taken as Echo positive, so as to avoid overdiagnosis of MR **(Fig. 4)** in nonrheumatic case. Whereas TTE in apical four-chamber view shows mitral valve prolapse (MVP) with chordal tear of both anterior mitral leaflet and posterior mitral leaflet. And apical four-chamber view with color Doppler shows severe MR and TR in 10-year-old girl in heart failure with ARF as shown in **Figures 6A and B**.

The remaining "subauscultatory" cases are those with the mild degree of mitral/tricuspid/AR. If rheumatic in origin, >80% of these valvular lesions are likely to heal without scarring when put on appropriate secondary prophylaxis to avoid recrudescence of rheumatic activity and further damage to the valves. Although the previous Jones criteria specify clinical auscultatory evidence for the diagnosis of mitral and aortic insufficiency, like our study,[16] more and more reports discuss subclinical carditis, in which MR is noticeable only on Echo and not detected by auscultating the murmur. Several investigators have concluded that 2D echocardiography using color and pulsed Doppler imaging is useful in identifying subclinical lesions.[24,25] But, if Echo features of ARF are used in support then regurgitant lesion of ARF can be distinguished from functional as well as regurgitation of other conditions.[8,16] Therefore, Echo is the

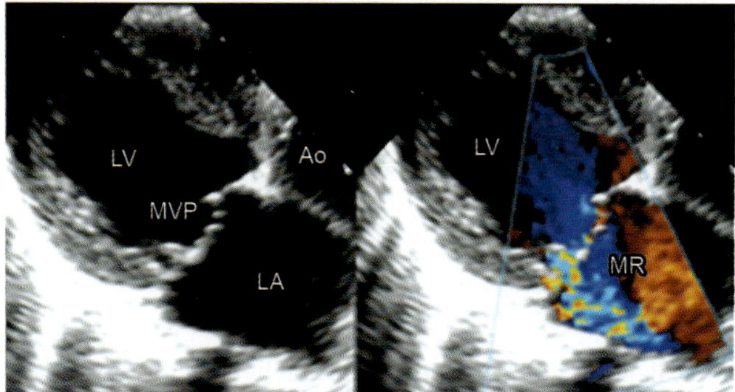

FIG. 5: Parasternal long axis with Color Doppler compare shows myxomatous redundant mitral valve (MV) with grade III mitral valve prolapse (MVP) with moderate mitral regurgitation (MVP—2, MR—2, and Echo score—4) in a 10-year-old boy with mucopolysaccharidosis.

TABLE 3: Vijaya's Echo criteria.[16]	
Echo feature	*Score*
Mitral valve and aortic valve thickness > 4 mm	2
Increased echogenicity of submitral structures	2
Rheumatic nodules (beaded appearance)	2
Mitral valve prolapse/aortic valve prolapse/tricuspid valve prolapse	2
Mitral regurgitation and aortic regurgitation/tricuspid regurgitation	2
Reduced mobility of valves	2
Chordal tear	2
Pericardial effusion	2
Total score	16
Score of ≥6 is diagnostic of rheumatic carditis.	

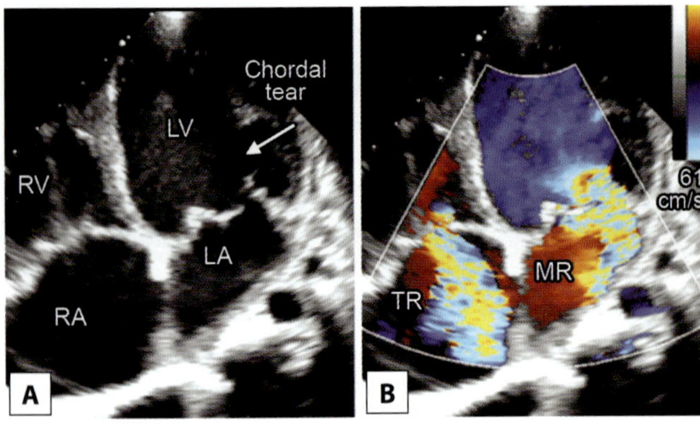

FIGS. 6A AND B: (A) Transthoracic echocardiography in apical four-chamber view shows mitral valve prolapse with chordal tear of both anterior mitral leaflet and posterior mitral leaflet. (B) Apical four-chamber view with color Doppler shows severe MR and TR in a 10-year-old girl in heart failure with ARF.

(RA: right atrium; RV: right ventricle; TR: tricuspid regurgitation; MR: mitral regurgitation; TR: tricuspid regurgitation)

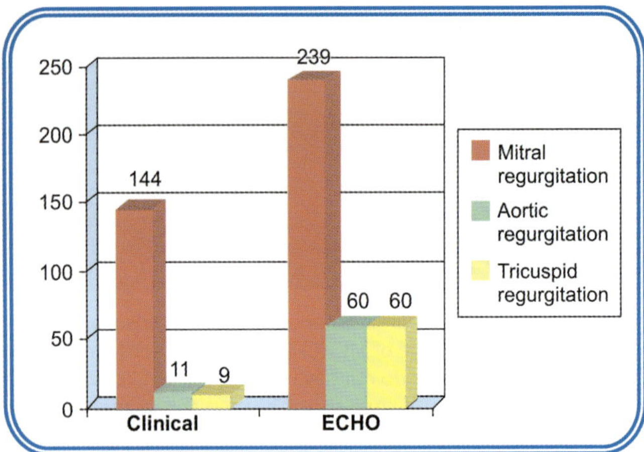

FIG. 7: Comparison of detection of mitral, aortic, and tricuspid valve regurgitation by clinical examination and by echocardiography.[16]

key for precise diagnosis of carditis in ARF and hence rightly made as a major criterion for diagnosis of ARF.[4]

REGURGITATION

The diagnosis of MR is usually done by auscultating a soft, blowing, high-pitched, pansystolic murmur at the apex conducted to the axilla. AR is detected by auscultating a soft, high-pitched, early diastolic murmur in new aortic or Erb's area. Studies have shown that clinical auscultation is a dying art, especially in countries where ARF is declining and residents only diagnose significant MR in less than half of the cases.[15,16] In our study, regurgitation of mitral, aortic, and tricuspid valves was more often diagnosed by TTE than clinically **(Fig. 7)**.[16] Hence, the clinical diagnosis of carditis in ARF may not be made with sufficient confidence which was very well shown. Moreover, it is very important to detect the valve damage and put them on both penicillin prophylaxis and subacute bacterial endocarditis (SBE) prophylaxis otherwise further damage can occur with recrudescence of rheumatic activity or SBE on the damaged valve **(Fig. 8)**.

Rheumatic versus Nonrheumatic Regurgitation

The mitral or aortic valve regurgitation can occur in many other conditions. The Echo allows visualization of valve structure, and allows detection of nonrheumatic causes of valve regurgitation, such as myxomatous mitral valve with grade III prolapse and moderate degree of MR **(Fig. 4)**. In contrast, in a 12-year-old girl who presented with palpitation and acute breathlessness, Echo showed severe MR with chordal tear and pericardial effusion (PE) **(Fig. 5)**. Though clinical diagnosis of AR is easy, Echo alone can differentiate nonrheumatic AR of aortic valve prolapse from rheumatic AR **(Figs. 9A and B)**.

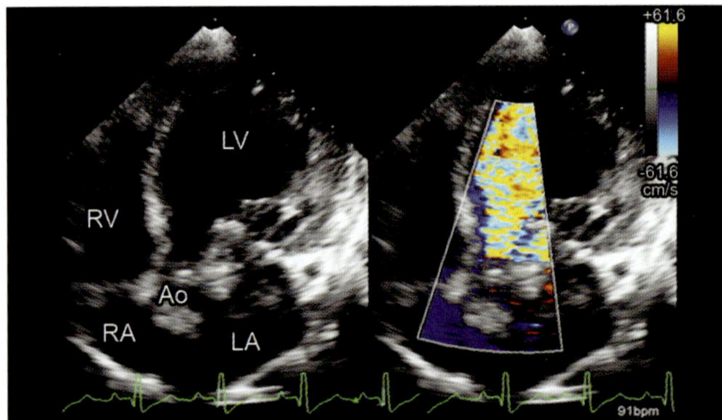

FIG. 8: TTE in apical four-chamber view with color compare shows thickened mitral and aortic valve with beaded appearance with hyperechogenic submitral structure indicating RF with fuzzy Echo on aortic valve, indicating SBE with severe aortic regurgitation in a 14-year-old boy who presented with fever for 3 weeks. He was neither on penicillin prophylaxis nor SBE prophylaxis.

(SBE: subacute bacterial endocarditis; TTE: transthoracic echocardiography)

In many Echo and Doppler studies,[9,17-20] most cases of rheumatic carditis are not severe enough to be symptomatic and the diagnosis of isolated carditis previously depended on auscultation alone. 80% or more cases of MR that are detected by Echo are also readily diagnosed by experienced physicians by auscultation alone. But today, auscultation has become a dying art and many youngsters miss the murmurs.

Physiological versus Pathological Regurgitation

It is very important to distinguish the physiological/functional MR from pathological regurgitation. The pathological valvular regurgitation can be easily differentiated from physiological regurgitation by demonstrating:

- Substantial color jet in two planes extending well beyond valve leaflets (extending >1 cm beyond coaptation point).

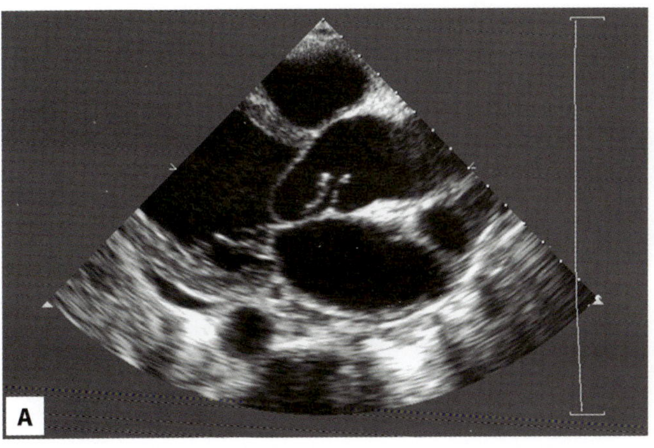 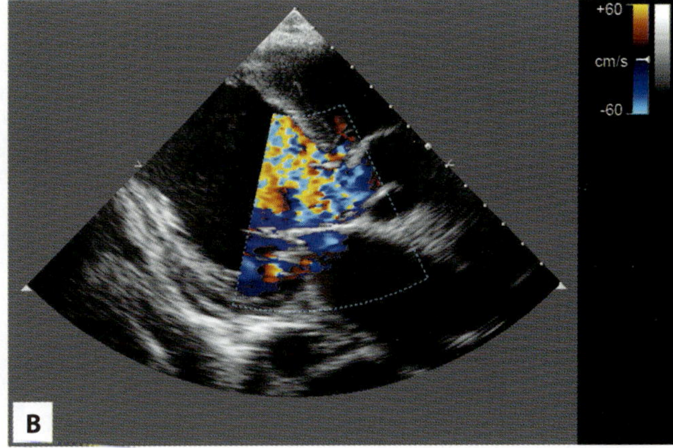

FIGS. 9A AND B: Parasternal long axis with color Doppler shows aortic valve prolapse with severe aortic regurgitation in a 22-year-old man with nonrheumatic aortic regurgitation (AR) (Echo score: AVP—2, AR—2, Echo score—4).

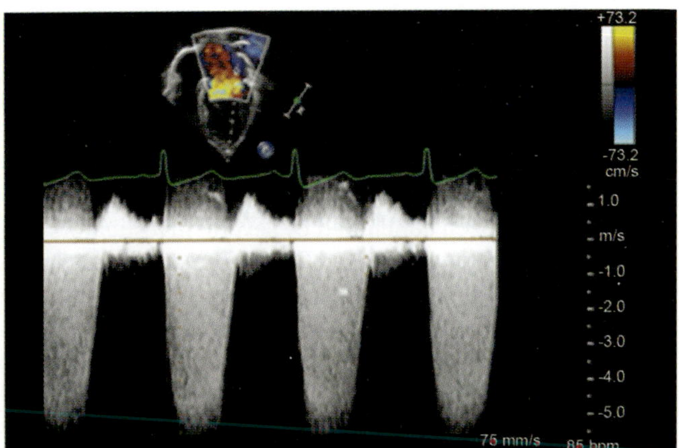

FIG. 10: Color Doppler shows well-defined, dense, high-velocity, holosystolic spectral envelope in pathological MR in a 12-year-old girl.

- Color jet of MR passes over the posterior wall of LA, it is a high-velocity signal in pulse Doppler, with a well-defined, dense, high-velocity spectral envelope and it is holosystolic **(Fig. 10)**.
- The pathological MR is graded as trivial, grades I, II, and III. Mitral regurgitation can be demonstrated by color flow mapping even in the absence of cardiac murmur.

Moreover unless valve regurgitation is associated with other features such as "thickened valves, beaded appearance, hyperechogenic submitral structures", with an Echo score of more than 6, it is not taken as significant and pathological **(Fig. 11A)**. It is important to differentiate torn chordae, with MR, from vegetations on mitral valve **(Fig. 11B)**. Vegetations are more likely on LA side and torn chordae are on LV side. However, one has to interpret the Echo with the clinical background. Pancarditis with PE, dilated LV, chordal tear of both anterior mitral leaflets and posterior mitral leaflet with MVP, and MR with chordal tear are shown in **Figures 12A and B**.

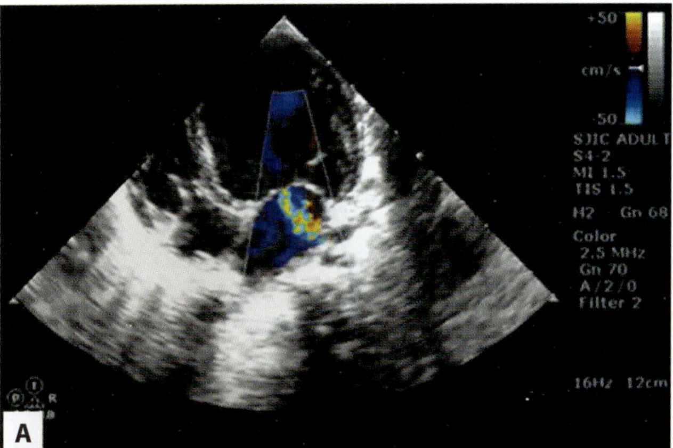

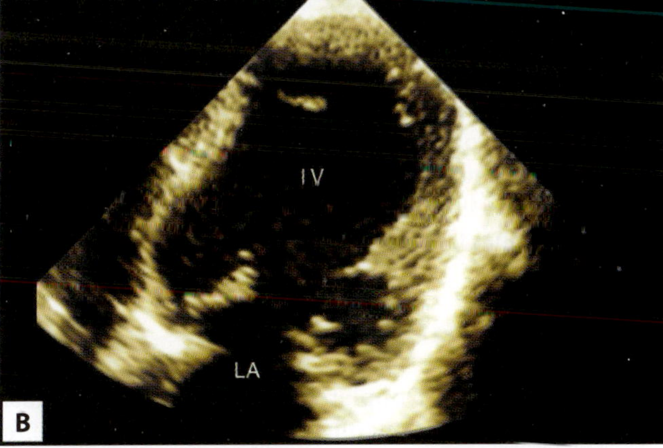

FIGS. 11A AND B: (A) Transthoracic echocardiography in apical four-chamber view shows grossly dilated left ventricle with central jet of mitral regurgitation in a 10-year-old boy with dilated cardiomyopathy. Echo score is only 2 for functional mitral regurgitation. (B) Transthoracic echocardiography in modified two-chamber view shows the torn rolled up chordae at the tip of both anterior mitral leaflet and posterior mitral leaflet with flail mitral valve in a case of ARF with severe MR in a 10-year-old boy.

(ARF: acute rheumatic fever; LA: left atrium; LV: left ventricle)

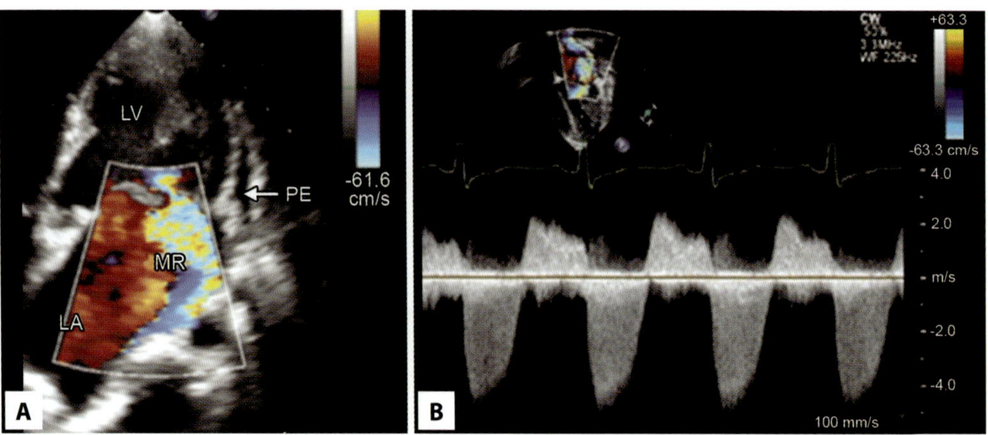

FIGS. 12A AND B: Apical four-chamber view with color compare shows chordal tear—2, severe MR—2, thickened beaded valve—2, pericardial effusion—2. Echo score is 8 in a 12-year-old girl with ARF. (B) CW Doppler shows well-defined, dense, high velocity holosystolic spectral envelope of MR indicating pathological MR.

(CW: continuous wave; MR: mitral regurgitation)

BOX 1	Criteria for pathological regurgitation.

Pathological mitral regurgitation (all four criteria met):
1. Seen in at least 2 views
2. Jet length ≥2 cm in at least 1 view
3. Peak velocity >3 m/s
4. Pansystolic jet in at least 1 envelope

Pathological aortic regurgitation (all four criteria met):
1. Seen in at least 2 views
2. Jet length ≥1 cm in at least 1 view
3. Peak velocity >3 m/s
4. Pandiastolic jet in at least 1 envelope

The severity of MR depends on the severity of carditis. TTE and Doppler have prognostic significance. MR in carditis in ARF is mild to moderate. Rarely, MR could be severe in which case it could be due to chordal tear and that can be detected precisely with Echo. Doppler findings in rheumatic valvulitis—Jones Criteria—2015 is shown in **Box 1**.

ECHO IS THE KEY

In many echo and Doppler studies,[12,20-22] the diagnosis of isolated carditis depended on auscultation alone, as most cases of carditis in ARF were not severe enough to be symptomatic. More than 80% of the MR cases detected by Echo are also readily diagnosed by auscultation alone by experienced physicians. The cases with mild degree of MR, AR, or TR are the "subauscultatory" cases or "subclinical cases". >80% of the valvular lesions are likely to heal without scarring, if rheumatic in origin. In children and in very thin, active individuals with highly elastic valve leaflets and rings, sensitivity of echo may detect degrees of valvular regurgitation within the physiologic range, which are not functionally significant. Though Jones criteria specify clinical auscultatory evidence for the diagnosis of mitral and aortic insufficiency, like in our study,[16] more and more reports discuss subclinical carditis in which MR is noticeable only on Echo. It has been concluded by several investigators that 2D Echo using color and pulsed Doppler imaging is useful in identifying subclinical lesions. And Echo findings improve the detection of subclinical carditis and do not signify an increase in ARF incidence. Hence, valve regurgitation alone is not enough to call it as carditis of ARF.[9,22] The additional supportive evidence of Echo features of ARF helps in differentiating a regurgitant lesion of ARF from functional as well as regurgitation due to other conditions.[10] Hence, Echo is the key for the precise and early diagnosis of carditis. The patients with isolated manifestations of ARF such as arthritis/chorea may have "subclinical" carditis, stretching of chordae tendineae with prolapse of the anterior mitral leaflet.[17,24]

APPLICATION OF REVISED JONES CRITERIA, 2015

It is a historic revision of the Jones criteria for the sixth time in 2015. The diagnosis of carditis, which is a major manifestation of ARF, is mainly by Doppler echocardiography. The guidelines have recommended that echocardiography with Doppler should be performed in all cases of confirmed or suspected ARF. This is in similarity with other international guidelines for the diagnosis of ARF. Even if clinical diagnosis does not document carditis, particularly in moderate-to-high-risk populations, it is reasonable to consider performing serial echocardiography or Doppler studies in any patient with diagnosed or suspected ARF. In patients with a heart murmur, the diagnosis of rheumatic carditis

BOX 2	**Morphological findings on Echo in rheumatic valvulitis.**

- *Acute mitral valve changes*:
  - Annular dilation
  - Chordal elongation
  - Chordal rupture resulting in flail leaflet with severe mitral regurgitation
  - Anterior (or less commonly posterior) leaflet tip prolapse
  - Beading/nodularity of leaflet tips
- *Chronic mitral valve changes: not seen in acute carditis*:
  - Leaflet thickening
  - Chordal thickening and fusion
  - Restricted leaflet motion
  - Calcification
- *Aortic valve changes in either acute or chronic carditis*:
  - Irregular or focal leaflet thickening
  - Coaptation defect
  - Restricted leaflet motion
  - Leaflet prolapse

should be excluded if echocardiography or Doppler findings are not consistent with carditis. The specific Doppler and morphological echocardiography findings in rheumatic valvulitis are distinctly defined in the guidelines. The suggested morphological echocardiographic and Doppler findings are given in **Box 2**. These findings can also be seen in chronic RHD.[5,23]

Can new Jones criteria change the epidemiological face of RF and RHD?

What is the impact of Echo?

Yes. The patients with both clinical and subclinical carditis are more likely to be detected during their first attacks of ARF. Detecting subclinical carditis will prevent from a more relaxed and inappropriate secondary prophylaxis. There is a significant prognostic implication of finding a normal heart or finding unrelated causes of murmurs in this population. Dr Edward Kaplan in his editorial in Laboratory diagnosis of group A streptococcal infection, WHO, Geneva, 1998 states—"detection of active rheumatic carditis is of great prognostic and therapeutic importance and is currently based on the Jones criteria. The fact that penicillin has failed to eradicate this disease process is irrefutable proof of the need for more laboratory, epidemiological, and clinical research". Large chunk of patients in our study,[9] i.e., 32.5%, with subclinical carditis, could be put on adequate duration of secondary prophylaxis that can probably prevent the recrudescence of rheumatic activity and further damage to the valves. Hence, it is the lack of penicillin prophylaxis

rather than failure of penicillin. Echo can be used with gratifying result for risk stratification of the patient once afflicted with ARF. The presence of carditis in first attacks makes these patients more prone to recurrent attacks and frequent carditis in subsequent attacks. Repeated attacks of recurrences of rheumatic activity are harmful and constitute the most important prognostic factor. Recurrences increase cardiovascular mortality and residual heart disease. New Jones criteria with Echo as a major criterion will take the teeth from ARF. The impact of this historic modification of Jones criteria—2015 is going to be tremendous. The old sayings "50% of RHD patients do not have past history of ARF" and "RF lick the joints and bites the heart" will no longer hold good in future. In other words, adding echocardiography with Doppler to the armamentarium of tests in the diagnosis of ARF will definitely change the epidemiological face of ARF in India.

■ CONCLUSION

The early and precise diagnosis of carditis in ARF is very essential to prevent morbidity and mortality in the young, and unnecessary expenditure on sophisticated treatment on RHD in future. It is possible only by Echo interrogation. Using Echo as a major criterion in Jones criteria is likely to detect carditis during their first attack of ARF. The TTE is a very simple, noninvasive, reproducible, and a useful tool for making such an early and precise diagnosis of carditis and will prevent further damage to the valves during recrudescence of rheumatic activity. Detecting subclinical carditis will prevent from a more relaxed and inappropriate secondary prophylaxis. Hence, new Revised Jones Criteria, 2015 should be followed strictly. The precise, early, and accurate diagnosis of carditis in ARF is possible only by Echo. By incorporating Echo criteria as a major criterion, more patients, especially with subclinical carditis, can be brought into the net of secondary prophylaxis. This will prevent further damage to the valves during recrudescence of rheumatic activity. Impact of this historic modification of Jones Criteria, 2015 is going to be tremendous in India. Adding echocardiography and Doppler to the armamentarium of tests in the diagnosis of carditis will definitely change the epidemiological face of ARF in India.

My prayer is-

Dawn is nowhere in the sight, yet I am waiting for the light!!!

Oh, God grant me the serenity to accept what I cannot change (poor hygiene and socioeconomical condition).

Courage to change the things I can—diagnostic criteria, awareness. The wisdom to know the difference

Echo has given the new missile to shoot the RF.

REFERENCES

1. Sanyal SK, Thapar MK, Ahmed SH, Hooja V, Tewari P. "The initial attack of acute rheumatic fever during childhood in North India; a prospective study of the clinical profile." Circulation. 1974;49:7-12.
2. Ralph A, Jacups S, McGough K, McDonald M, Currie BJ. The challenge of acute rheumatic fever diagnosis in a high-incidence population: a prospective study and proposed guidelines for diagnosis in Australia's Northern Territory. Heart Lung Circ. 2006;15:113-8.
3. Vijayalakshmi IB. Echocardiography in acute rheumatic fever and chronic rheumatic heart disease. In: Nanda NC (Ed). Comprehensive textbook of echocardiography. New Delhi: Jaypee Brothers Medical Publishers; 2014. pp. 765-825.
4. Gewitz MH, Baltimore RS, Tani LY, Sable CA, Shulman ST, Carapetis J, et al. Revision of the Jones criteria for the diagnosis of acute rheumatic fever in the era of Doppler echocardiography: a scientific statement from the American Heart Association Committee on Rheumatic fever, endocarditis, and Kawasaki disease of the Council on Cardiovascular Disease in the Young. Circulation. 2015;131:1806-18.
5. Jones TD. Diagnosis of rheumatic fever. JAMA.1944;126:481-4.
6. Gewitz MH, Baltimore RS, Tani LY, Sable CA, Shulman ST, Carapetis J, et al. Jones Criteria (revised) for guidance in the diagnosis of rheumatic fever. Circulation. 1965;32:664-8.
7. Rutstein DD, Bauer W, Dorfman A, Gross RE, Lichty JA, Taussig HB, et al. Report of the committee on standards and criteria for programs of care. Jones Criteria (revised) for guidance in the diagnosis of rheumatic fever. Circulation. 1984;70:204A-8A.
8. Special Writing Group of the Committee on Rheumatic Fever, Endocarditis, and Kawasaki Disease of the Council on Cardiovascular Disease in the Young of the American Heart Association. Guidelines for the diagnosis of rheumatic fever. Jones Criteria, 1992 update. Special Writing Group of the Committee on Rheumatic Fever, Endocarditis, and Kawasaki Disease of the Council on Cardiovascular Disease in the Young of the American Heart Association. JAMA. 1992;268:2069-73.
9. Vijayalakshmi IB, Mithravinda J, Deva AN. The role of echocardiography in diagnosing carditis in the setting of acute rheumatic fever. Cardiol Young. 2005;15:583-8.
10. Strasser T, Dondog N, El Kholy A, Gharagozloo R, Kalbian VV, Ogunbi O, et al. The community control of rheumatic fever and rheumatic heart disease: report of a WHO international cooperative project. Bull World Health Organ. 1981;59: 285-94.
11. Narula J, Chandrasekhar Y, Rahimtoola S. Diagnosis of active rheumatic carditis. The echoes of change. Circulation. 1999;100:1576-81.
12. Beg A, Sadiq M. Subclinical valvulitis in children with acute rheumatic fever. Pediatr Cardiol. 2008;29:619-23.
13. Caldas AM, Terreri MT, Moises VA, Silva CM, Len CA, Carvalho AC, et al. What is the true frequency of carditis in acute rheumatic fever? A prospective clinical and Doppler blind study of 56 children with up to 60 months of follow-up evaluation. Pediatr Cardiol. 2008;29:1048-53.
14. St Clair EW, Oddone EZ, Waugh RA, Corey GR, Feussner JR. Assessing house staff diagnostic skills using a cardiology patient simulator. Ann Intern Med. 1992;117:751-6.
15. Mangione S, Nieman LZ, Gracely E, Kaye D. The teaching and practice of cardiac auscultation during internal medicine and cardiology training. A nationwide survey. Ann Intern Med.1993;119:47-54.
16. Vijayalakshmi IB, Vishnuprabhu RO, Chitra N, Rajasri R, Anuradha TV. The efficacy of echocardiographic criterions for the diagnosis of carditis in acute rheumatic fever. Cardiol Young. 2008;18:586-92.
17. Elevli M, Celebi A, Tombul T, Gökalp AS. "Cardiac involvement in Sydenham's chorea: Clinical and Doppler echocardiographic findings." Acta Paediatr. 1999;88:1074-7.
18. Veasy LG, Wiedmeier SE, Orsmond GS, Ruttenberg HD, Boucek MM, Roth SJ, et al. Resurgence of acute rheumatic fever in the intermountain area of the United States. N Engl J Med.1987;316:421-7.
19. Veasy LG, Tani LY, Hill HR. Persistence of acute rheumatic fever in the intermountain area of the United States. J Pediatr. 1994;125:673-4.
20. da Silva CH. Rheumatic fever: a multicenter study in the state of São Paulo. Pediatric Committee–São Paulo Pediatric Rheumatology Society. Rev Hosp Clin Fac Med Sao Paulo. 1999;54:85-90.
21. Feinstein AR, Stern EK, Spagnuolo M. The prognosis of acute rheumatic fever. Am Heart J. 1964;68:817-34.
22. Minich LL, Tani LY, Pagotto LT, Shaddy RE, Veasy LG. Doppler echocardiography distinguishes between physiologic and pathologic "silent" mitral regurgitation in patients with rheumatic fever. Clin Cardiol. 1997;20:924-6.
23. Reményi B, Wilson N, Steer A, Ferreira B, Kado J, Kumar K, et al. World Heart Federation criteria for echocardiographic diagnosis of rheumatic heart disease: an evidence-based guideline. Nat Rev Cardiol. 2012;9:297-309.
24. Figueroa FE, Fernández MS, Valdés P, Wilson C, Lanas F, Carrión F, et al. Prospective comparison of clinical and echocardiographic diagnosis of rheumatic carditis: long-term follow-up of patients with subclinical disease. Heart. 2001;85:407-10.
25. Ozkutlu S, Ayabakan C, Saraçlar M. Can subclinical valvitis detected by echocardiography be accepted as evidence of carditis in the diagnosis of acute rheumatic fever? Cardiol Young. 2001;11:255-60.

Clinical Profile of Rheumatic Heart Disease

AS Chandrasekhara Rao, N Sudhayakumar

> *"There is no short cut, nor 'royal road' to the attainment of medical knowledge".*
>
> **—John Abernethy** (1764–1831),
> English Surgeon,
> St Bartholomew's Hospital, London

INTRODUCTION

The importance of clinical examination as a first step in the assessment of valvular disease is stressed by both the American Heart Association (AHA)/American College Cardiology and the European Society of Cardiology guidelines.[1,2] By integrating examination findings with imaging results, the clinician may improve the diagnostic skills and understand the underlying pathophysiology. Furthermore, employing a carefully methodical approach to physical examination provides information concerning the severity of the hemodynamic consequences of any given valvular lesion.[3,4] With a clinical assessment of severity, the patient may be followed up for disease progression with serial examinations. Based on severity and progression, valvular heart diseases are staged as follows **(Table 1)**.

CARDITIS IN ACUTE RHEUMATIC FEVER

The clinical profile of acute rheumatic fever (ARF) is discussed in Chapter 9 in this book. A brief review of carditis in ARF is done here. In general, rheumatic carditis involves all three layers of the heart: the endocardium, myocardium, and pericardium—predominantly the valvular

Stage	Definition	Description
		TABLE 1: Stages of valvular heart disease.
A	At risk	Patients with risk factors for development of VHD
B	Progressive	Patients with progressive VHD (mild-to-moderate severity and asymptomatic)
C	Asymptomatic severe	Asymptomatic patients who have the criteria for severe VHD: C1: Asymptomatic patients with severe VHD in whom the left or right ventricle remains compensated C2: Asymptomatic patients with severe VHD, with decompensation of the left or right ventricle
D	Symptomatic severe	Patients who have developed symptoms as a result of VHD

(VHD: valvular heart disease)

endocardium. The most common manifestation is mitral regurgitation (MR). Clinical examination of the heart may reveal normal heart size or mild left ventricular dilatation. First heart sound (S_1) may be normal or decreased in intensity particularly when there is prolonged PR interval in the electrocardiogram (ECG). Second heart sound (S_2) may be normal or split depending on the degree of MR. Third heart sound (S_3) is commonly heard especially if there is significant MR. S_3 in children can be a normal physiological one and can be exaggerated in presence of hyperdynamic circulations such as fever; physiological S_3 decreases or disappears on standing. The three typical murmurs of rheumatic carditis are the apical soft pansystolic murmur of MR (most common), soft blowing early diastolic murmur (EDM) of aortic regurgitation (AR) and the soft mid-diastolic murmur over apex (Carey Coombs murmur) which is contributed by the excess mitral flow secondary to MR and the mitral valvulitis due to endocarditis. When severe heart failure develops, tricuspid regurgitation (TR) with typical systolic murmur may be heard along with signs of pulmonary hypertension (PH). Pericardium may be involved in <15% of cases causing pericardial rub (scratchy systolic-diastolic triphasic event) and is always associated with severe carditis and MR. Concept of myocarditis in ARF is debated now—cardiac troponin is not significantly elevated and systolic function remains normal in majority of cases with carditis; cardiac failure in ARF is mainly contributed by valvular regurgitation due to endocarditis. Declining auscultatory skill has been cited as one of the reasons for the clinical and echocardiographic discrepancy in the diagnosis of carditis. Recent studies have highlighted the role of echocardiography in detecting subclinical carditis; hence, echocardiographic findings are also included in the revision of Jones criteria released in the AHA Scientific Statement 2015.[5] Based on echocardiographic findings, rheumatic heart disease (RHD) has been recently classified as subclinical RHD (clinically normal; echo abnormal), asymptomatic clinical RHD (clinical + echo), symptomatic established RHD, and advanced RHD.[6-9]

Symptomatology

The common symptoms in RHD include dyspnea, palpitation, chest pain, and edema legs; less common ones are syncope and hemoptysis.

Dyspnea

Progressive exertional dyspnea is the most common symptom of mitral valve disease, which produces progressive elevation of the left atrial pressure and consequently pulmonary venous, capillary, and arterial hypertension. Pulmonary venous and capillary hypertension leads to pulmonary congestion and transudation of fluid into interstitium and alveoli resulting in reduction in lung compliance, which produces the symptom of dyspnea. Juxtacapillary receptors (J-receptors) located in the alveolar interstitium and supplied by unmyelinated fibers of the vagus nerve are stimulated by pulmonary congestion. This activates the Hering–Breuer reflex whereby inspiratory effort is terminated before full inspiration is achieved, resulting in rapid and shallow breathing. Transudation of fluid into pleural spaces also contributes to dyspnea. Left atrial pressure is determined by six factors—volume of blood coming to left atrium (LA), volume leaving LA to left ventricle (LV), LA compliance, rate of mitral flow, LV diastolic pressure, and LV–LA gradient. As the pulmonary capillary pressure progressively rises, the symptoms worsen from New York Heart Association (NYHA) Class I to IV. When the pulmonary capillary pressure goes above 25 mm Hg, they may develop orthopnea (dyspnea on lying down and relieved on sitting up) and paroxysmal nocturnal dyspnea (PND). Acute rise in LA pressure due to fever, infections, tachyarrhythmias, undue exercise, withdrawal of drugs, etc., can result in occurrence of acute pulmonary edema, which if not treated promptly can be fatal. Any hyperdynamic circulatory states such as anemia, pregnancy, and thyrotoxicosis worsen the symptom of dyspnea due to further rise in LA pressure (high LA volume, reduced diastolic emptying time due to fast heart rate and increased mitral flow rate).

Paroxysmal nocturnal dyspnea: Patient goes to bed comfortably; about 2 hours into sleep, he/she develops acute onset severe dyspnea, wakes up, sits with legs hanging down, may even goes to the open windows and gasps for breath; may have associated cough with pink frothy sputum; dyspnea gradually subsides over 15–30 minutes and will have a comfortable sleep after that with no recurrence in same night.

Mechanisms: Gradual increase in venous return due to shift of fluid from extravascular to the intravascular compartment, increase in venous return in supine position, and fluid-retaining effect of antidiuretic hormone released during sleep lead to increase in LA volume and pressure resulting in high pulmonary capillary pressure and transudation of fluid into interstitium and alveoli. Fluctuations in heart rate with increase in the rate during REM sleep contribute to the problem in patients with mitral stenosis (MS). In left ventricular failure (LVF), reduction in sympathetic tone during certain phases of sleep takes away the compensatory LV inotropic support, which further raises the LV diastolic and consequently the LA pressure. Reduced tidal volume of recumbency (elevated diaphragm and reduced chest expansion) also contributes to the symptom.

Palpitation: It is a common symptom but is very nonspecific. It could be due to change in heart rate, regularity, and/or force of ventricular contraction. Irregular palpitation in mitral valve disease indicates atrial fibrillation (AF). In ventricular volume overload as in AR, force of contraction increases (Frank–Starling mechanism) and can produce strong thuddy palpitation.

Chest pain: Chest pain in valvular heart disease is not common. But, severe aortic stenosis (AS) can produce effort angina; in severe AR, they can have nocturnal angina. Dilated dynamic aorta putting pressure effect on thoracic vertebra also could be a cause for somatic chest pain. Right ventricular ischemia due to severe PH can occasionally produce effort angina.

Hemoptysis: It is not uncommon in severe MS; it is commonly secondary to pulmonary infection or associated with acute pulmonary edema and PND. Rarely, acute rise in LA pressure as in pregnancy can rupture the pulmonary/bronchial vasculature leading to massive hemoptysis (pulmonary apoplexy) which usually settles down as the left atrial pressure drops with the blood loss. Pulmonary embolism, which can occur in any valvular heart disease with congestive heart failure (CHF), is also a cause for hemoptysis.

Edema legs, puffiness of face, and abdominal distention manifest when they go in for CHF. Exertional syncope/presyncope is an ominous sign of severe AS.

Physical Signs

Pulse (Fig. 1)

Careful assessment of pulse gives valuable contributions to diagnosis and management. Irregularly irregular pulse with varying pulse volume suggests AF. In AF with fast heart rate, many cycles will be very short resulting in poor diastolic filling of the ventricles. In such cycles, the stroke volume may not be adequate enough to produce a *palpable* pulse resulting in apex-pulse deficit of >10 per minute. High-volume collapsing pulse (rapid upstroke, ill sustained peak, rapid downstroke in systole, and low dicrotic notch) indicates severe AR, in the absence of other conditions such as hyperdynamic circulations. Bisferiens pulse (high volume, rapid upstroke, second peak in latter part of systole, and low dicrotic notch) occurs in severe AR with or without associated stenosis. Typical low-volume slow rising pulse (pulsus parvus et tardus/anacrotic pulse) is diagnostic of severe AS. Low/normal volume pulse with a collapsing-like character may be seen in severe MR. Absence of peripheral pulses may be a clue for embolic manifestation especially in presence of AF.

Blood Pressure

Low systolic pressure with narrow pulse pressure indicates low stroke volume; in the absence of hypovolemia, this occurs in severe MS/regurgitation, severe AS and in presence of PH or CHF. Wide pulse pressure with low diastolic pressure <60 mm Hg in valvular heart disease indicates severe AR. Normally, the systolic pressure in lower limb is higher than that in upper limb by up to 20 mm Hg; value more than this (Hill's sign) occurs in AR and in severe cases, it can be even >60 mm Hg.

Jugular Venous Pulse

It gives valuable information in evaluation of heart diseases. Internal jugular vein is assessed in 45° position with abdominal clothes loosened (can also be assessed in sitting position with legs hanging down). It can be confused with carotid artery pulsations; but the following points help us:

- *Surface anatomy*—internal jugular vein lies from a point between the two heads of sternocleidomastoid to the angle of mandible; in the lower third, it is behind the muscle, middle third underneath, and upper third anterior to the muscle. Carotid artery lies anterior to the muscle throughout.
- Jugular venous pulse (JVP) is better seen than felt; carotid artery is better felt.
- Venous pulse is wavy; arterial pulse is jerky.
- JVP has a definite upper level, which varies with posture, respiration, and abdominal compression; arterial pulse goes into the skull and hence upper level will not be identified.
- Venous pulse can be obliterated by pressure, not the arterial pulse.

Normally, the venous column is seen at the root of the neck in 45° position; hence, we can assess the waveform also. Internal jugular vein is in line with superior vena cava (SVC) and has no valves; hence, it faithfully reflects the right atrial events—the pressure and waveforms. Pressure is measured as the vertical height in centimeters from the sternal angle + 5 [angle of Louis is 5 cm from the center of right atrium (RA)]; normally, the column can rise for 3–5 cm from the sternal angle. Recent recommendation is to assess the venous column in sitting position with legs hanging down and reference point is root of neck; normally, it does not go above

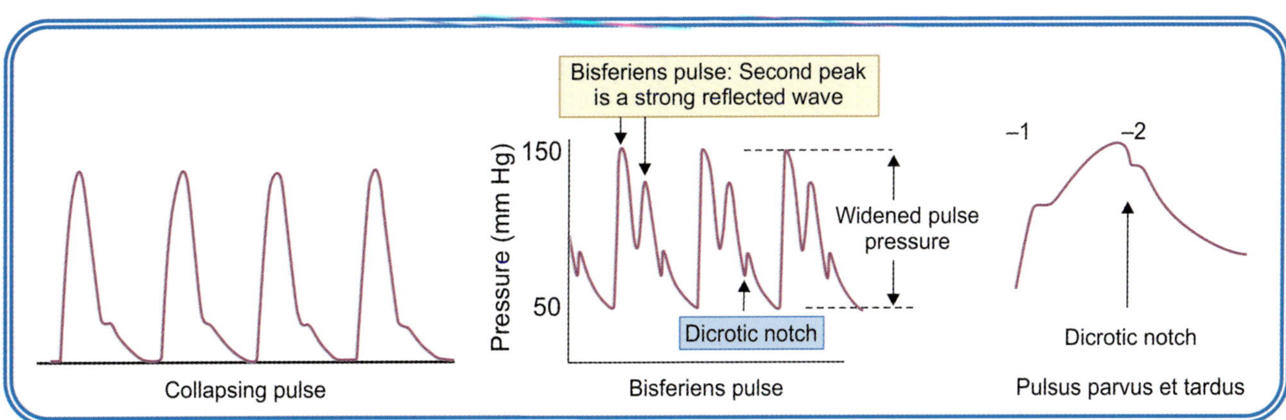

FIG. 1: Typical arterial pulse patterns.

the medial end of clavicle. In borderline elevation, look for the abdominojugular reflux; on sustained periumbilical compression, the venous column normally rises but falls to basal levels within few cardiac cycles. The splanchnic venous blood is squeezed into RA and ventricle; normal right ventricle (RV) empties the extra volume by increasing the force of contraction (Frank–Starling principle). Sustained elevation for >15 seconds indicate abnormality [right ventricular failure, tricuspid stenosis (TS), or constrictive pericarditis]. Absence of the reflux indicates hypovolemia or vena cava obstruction.

Elevation of jugular venous pressure indicates systemic venous congestion commonly due to right heart failure; but, it can be elevated in hyperdynamic circulatory states and pericardial and tricuspid valve diseases also. Normal venous column falls with inspiration as the negative intrathoracic pressure is transmitted to RA; rise of the pressure during inspiration (Kussmaul sign) is typical of constrictive pericarditis, but can occur in tricuspid valve obstructions and in any condition with severe CHF. Waveforms give us an idea about the underlying valvular disease. Normally, there are three waves—A, C, and V with their descends labeled as X, X', and Y **(Fig. 2)**. With slow heart rate, an additional small H wave before A wave may be recorded. A is an active wave due to atrial contraction and its relaxation produces the initial part of X descent; following this, isovolumetric contraction pushes the tricuspid valve apparatus into the floor of RA with resultant marginal rise in right atrial pressure producing the small C wave, which interrupts the X descent. During the rapid ejection phase, the tricuspid valve apparatus descends resulting in the rapid fall of right atrial pressure producing the second part of the X descent—X'; rapid ejection of blood from both ventricles to great arteries reduces the intracardiac volume and thus the intrapericardial pressure, which also contributes to the X'. During the latter part of systole, continued venous return to RA results in gradual rise in the atrial pressure producing the V wave. After systole and isovolumetric relaxation, tricuspid valve opens and atrium empties its blood to the ventricle resulting in rapid drop in atrial pressure producing the Y descent. A wave corresponds to fourth heart sound (S_4), onset of C to S_1 and peak of V to S_2.

Prominent A wave occurs in conditions with RV inflow obstructions (TS) or reduced RV compliance [right ventricular hypertrophy (RVH) as in severe PH or pulmonary stenosis and RV myocardial diseases such as ischemic heart disease or cardiomyopathy]; it is absent in AF. Prominent V wave occurs in TR. In TR, the V wave encroaches the X' and in severe TR, the V wave merges with the C wave to produce the CV or S wave. V waves are prominent in other conditions where large volume or pressure reaches RA as in atrial septal defect with MR, LV to RA shunt (Gerbode type ventricular septal defect), and ruptured sinus of Valsalva aneurysm to RA. Sharp Y descent is a feature of severe TR (also typical in constrictive pericarditis); slow Y descent is diagnostic for TS.

Precordial Examination

Active precordium indicates volume-loaded ventricles. Normal heart size with tapping apex is typical of MS. Presence of left parasternal heave and epigastric pulsations suggest RVH due to PH, which may produce systolic pulsations in second left intercostal space with palpable S_2. RV dilatation due to severe TR and RV failure can also contribute to left parasternal heave. Systolic expansion of large LA in severe MR produces a systolic pulsation near left sternal border, but more laterally and superiorly. Forcible/hyperdynamic apex, which is displaced down and out, indicates volume-overloaded LV as in severe AR/MR. In severe AS, apex will be of heaving character but enlargement is minimal. Diastolic thrill over apex is diagnostic for MS; AS may produce systolic thrill over aortic area, which when transmitted to carotids produces the carotid shudder. Thrill is less common in MR and extremely rare in AR. Auscultatory findings are described in detail with each lesion.

Innocent Murmurs

A murmur audible in the absence of any underlying cardiac structural abnormality is considered as a functional or an innocent murmur. They are almost always systolic, soft, and relatively less loud (no thrill); it is commonly seen in hyperdynamic conditions as midsystolic murmur in pulmonary and aortic areas. It is very common in children and adolescents (Still's murmur—may be present in up to 60% of children). Flat chest (straight back syndrome) compresses the chest producing prominent midsystolic murmur over pulmonary area mimicking pulmonary stenosis, but this murmur almost completely disappears with full inspiration. Venous hum heard at the root of neck in children and mammary soufflé over breast in pregnant women are examples of innocent continuous murmurs.

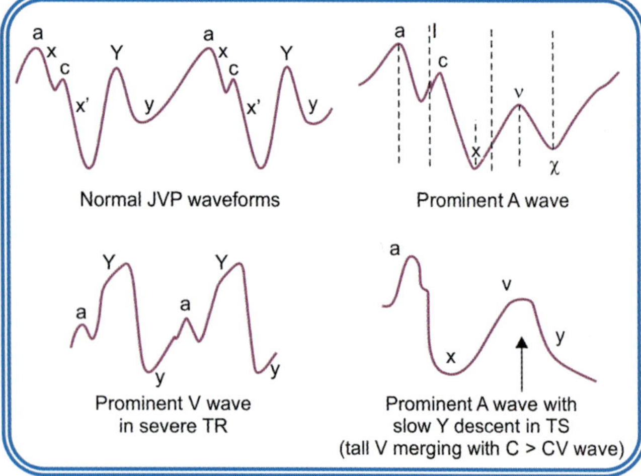

FIG. 2: Venous pulse patterns.
(JVP: jugular venous pulse; TS: tricuspid stenosis; TR: tricuspid regurgitation)

CHRONIC RHEUMATIC HEART DISEASE

Mitral Stenosis[10]

Mitral valve is the most commonly affected one in chronic RHD and 25% of patients have isolated MS. Additional 40% have combined MS and MR. Multivalvular involvement is seen in 38% of MS patients—aortic valve involvement in 35% and tricuspid valve in about 5%. However, TS has been reported to be about 15–33% in autopsy series.[11] Pulmonary valve involvement is extremely rare and is usually associated with all other valve lesions. Almost all cases of MS are of rheumatic etiology with the classical pathology being commissural, cuspal, and chordal fusion. Rare causes of mitral obstruction include congenital MS, mitral annular calcification, left atrial myxoma, carcinoid syndrome, mucopolysaccharidoses, systemic lupus erythematosus, rheumatoid arthritis, Fabry's disease, Whipple's disease, and methysergide toxicity.[12] Nearly, two-thirds of patients with MS are female. Clinical profile of patients with MS in India has been shown to be different from those in the West and this has been reported since over four decades. MS occurs in younger age (<20 years) in India, with significant PH and has been labeled as juvenile MS[13] and is attributed to smouldering rheumatic activity or multiple episodes of severe rheumatic fever.

Pathophysiology

Normal mitral valve area in adults is 4–6 cm^2 (4 cm^2/m^2 body surface area); no hemodynamic change occurs till the valve area is reduced to about 2.5 cm^2. Impedance to blood flow from LA to LV results in progressive increase in transmitral gradient with proportionate rise in left atrial, pulmonary venous, pulmonary capillary, and pulmonary artery diastolic pressures (passive postcapillary PH). Later, reactive pulmonary vasoconstriction results in progressive rise in pulmonary artery pressure leading to severe precapillary PH, RVH, and CHF; rarely obstructive changes in pulmonary vasculature may occur but seldom it exceeds Heath Edwards stage III pathology. In severe cases, cardiac output also starts falling (**Fig. 3**). Stasis of blood in LA contributes to thrombus formation and systemic embolism, the risk of which increases many fold with onset of AF.

Transmitral gradient for a given mitral valve area is influenced by many factors—volume of blood coming to LA, volume going out of LA (related to the duration of diastole which is inversely proportional to the heart rate), LA compliance, LV diastolic pressure, and the mitral flow rate. The gradient is proportional to the square of diastolic flow rate; doubling of flow rate quadruples the gradient. Any condition, which increases the heart rate, increases the mitral flow rate and the transmitral gradient significantly and hence is deleterious.

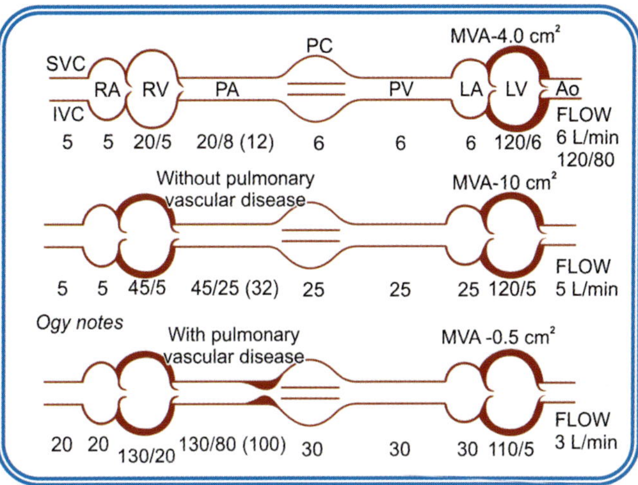

FIG. 3: Hemodynamics in normal versus MS—top is normal; middle is MS with postcapillary PH, lower is with precapillary PH.

(Ao: aorta; IVC: inferior vena cava; LA: left atrium; LV: left ventricle; MVA: mitral valve area; MS: mitral stenosis; PA: pulmonary artery; PC: pulmonary capillary; PV: pulmonary vein; PH: pulmonary hypertension; RA: superior vena cava; RV: right ventricle; SVC: superior vena cava)

Clinical Features

The typical patient is a young female of 20–30 years of age. In about 50% of patients, there is no past history of rheumatic fever. The common symptoms are dyspnea, palpitation, cough, and hemoptysis; when they develop CHF edema, abdominal distention, and puffiness of face occur. MS is a slowly progressive disease. Many patients appear asymptomatic by adjusting their lifestyles to a more sedentary level. Symptoms are generally precipitated by effort, emotional stress, respiratory infection, fever, pregnancy, or arrhythmias such as AF with fast ventricular rate.[14] Dyspnea is the most common presenting symptom associated with fatigue and decreased effort tolerance.[15] In MS, impaired emptying of blood from LA to LV results in stasis of blood in LA with increase in pressure which is transmitted to pulmonary vasculature. Any situation, which increases the heart rate, reduces the duration of diastole with consequent reduction in LA emptying, which augments the LA pressure with worsening of symptoms; high heart rate raises the mitral flow rate also augmenting the mitral gradient. Conditions, which increase the venous return, raise the LA volume and thus the pressure, e.g., fluid overload and supine position (responsible for orthopnea and PND). In hyperdynamic situations such as pregnancy, anemia, and thyrotoxicosis, heart rate, volume status, and flow rate are high and hence patients become more symptomatic. Acute change in these parameters results in acute elevation of LA pressure precipitating pulmonary edema as in AF with fast heart rate, fever, infections, etc. LA compliance is another factor, which modifies LA pressure; reduced LA compliance as seen in relatively young people results in disproportionate rise in LA pressure and in such situations, patients with even moderate MS will have severe symptoms and high pulmonary artery pressures. As the severity of stenosis increases, patient develops progressive worsening of symptoms from NYHA Class I to IV with orthopnea and PND. In a typical case in the natural history, pulmonary edema occurs relatively early followed by PND and orthopnea.

Palpitation is a common symptom in patients with MS. It is exertional and may be present at rest also (due to the loud S_1 and tapping apex). Episodic palpitation occurs when they go in for paroxysmal AF; later when permanent AF settles, they may have irregular palpitation at rest aggravated by exertion due to increase in heart rate caused by enhanced atrioventricular (AV) conduction.

Cough is another important symptom in patients with MS due to transudation of fluid into alveoli secondary to elevated pulmonary capillary pressure. It tends to be dry, irritating, and spasmodic with frothy sputum, more in supine position and hence frequently with nocturnal exacerbation. Patients with MS are prone for frequent respiratory infections due to the fluid in alveoli and compression of left bronchus by the dilated LA. Dilated hypertensive pulmonary artery consequent to development of PH compresses the left recurrent laryngeal nerve resulting in hoarseness of voice (Ortner's syndrome). Rarely, they can have dysphagia due to the pressure effect of dilated hypertensive LA on esophagus.

Hemoptysis is also not uncommon. Pink frothy sputum is classical for acute pulmonary edema and can occur during PND also. More commonly, it may be due to respiratory infection. Communications of pulmonary veins to bronchial veins open up to decompress the pulmonary venous pressure. Acute rise in the LA pressure as in conditions such as new onset AF with fast heart rate, infections, and pregnancy with consequent rise in pressure in the pulmonary and bronchial veins can lead to rupture of these vessels resulting in massive hemoptysis (pulmonary apoplexy). To a certain extent, this is a protective mechanism as with the loss of blood the pulmonary venous pressure drops preventing pulmonary edema. Hemoptysis could also be secondary to pulmonary embolism to which they are prone especially when they go in for CHF and AF.

About 15% of patients with MS may complain of chest pain, sometimes indistinguishable from that of angina pectoris. RVH secondary to PH is another cause of chest pain in MS—right ventricular angina. It can also occur due to associated atherosclerotic coronary artery disease and rarely due to coronary embolism. Pulmonary infarction due to venous thromboembolism produces pleuritic-type chest pain. Dilated hypertensive pulmonary artery may also contribute to nonspecific chest pain. In patients with severe MS and PH, fatigue manifests due to reduction in cardiac output. Syncope is uncommon except in cases with severe PH or those with ball valve thrombus producing intermittent severe obstruction. In later stages when CHF develops, patient may complain of puffiness of face, distention of abdomen, edema legs, and decreased appetite. Severe splanchnic congestion can produce multiple gastrointestinal symptoms and in chronic cases, they may develop protein losing enteropathy and cardiac cirrhosis. Arterial embolism such as stroke is common after development of AF, though it can occur even in sinus rhythm.

Physical Signs

The characteristic mitral facies, pink purple patches on cheeks, is uncommon in Indian patients, whose complexion is dark. The arterial pulse is usually normal; but in severe cases, it can be of low volume (pulsus parvus). It becomes irregularly irregular with varying volume in presence of AF. Systemic embolism of clots from LA especially in those with AF can result in loss of peripheral arterial pulses. Blood pressure is usually normal in isolated MS; severe PH and CHF result in low volume pulse with narrow pulse pressure. Wide pulse pressure with high volume pulse is a clue for associated AR. JVP is normal but may exhibit prominent A waves when severe PH develops. With the onset of AF, A wave disappears. Prominent V waves indicate significant TR and slow Y descent suggests associated TS.

Cardiomegaly is unusual but occurs with development of RV enlargement secondary to PH and TR. Apex is typically of tapping nature (due to the palpable loud S_1) with or without a diastolic thrill. With development of PH, the pulmonary artery pulsation and S_2 could be palpable in second left intercostal space; RVH secondary to PH results in left parasternal heave and epigastric pulsation. The auscultatory findings in isolated MS are:

- Loud sharp S_1 with prolongation of Q-S_1 interval (in view of the high LA pressure). It takes a longer time for the ventricular pressure to rise from the onset of systole (Q wave in ECG) to the LV–LA pressure cross over which times with S_1 (theoretically this can delay M_1 resulting in $T_1 M_1$ sequence for S_1). Loud sharp S_1 signifies that the mitral valve leaflets are flexible. Normally, the leaflets floats back after atrial contraction; the high LA pressure prevents this keeping them fully open throughout diastole resulting in a wider closing excursion at onset of systole, which contributes to the loudness of S_1. Though varying S_1 intensity is described in presence of AF, it is unlikely with severe MS as the high LA pressure keeps the valve fully open in all cycles. S_1 becomes soft and dull when the leaflets get grossly fibrosed and/or calcified.

- The pulmonary component (P_2) of S_2 becomes accentuated as pulmonary artery pressure rises and when loud is heard all over the precordium. The splitting of S_2 narrows with further elevation of pulmonary artery pressure as P_2 occurs earlier due to reduction in the pulmonary hang out interval because of the reduced compliance of the pulmonary vascular bed. With development of severe RV systolic dysfunction P_2 gets delayed.

- *Opening snap (Potain's sound)*: Mitral valve opening causes a sharp sound, the opening snap (OS), which is due to sudden tensing of the domed valve leaflets.

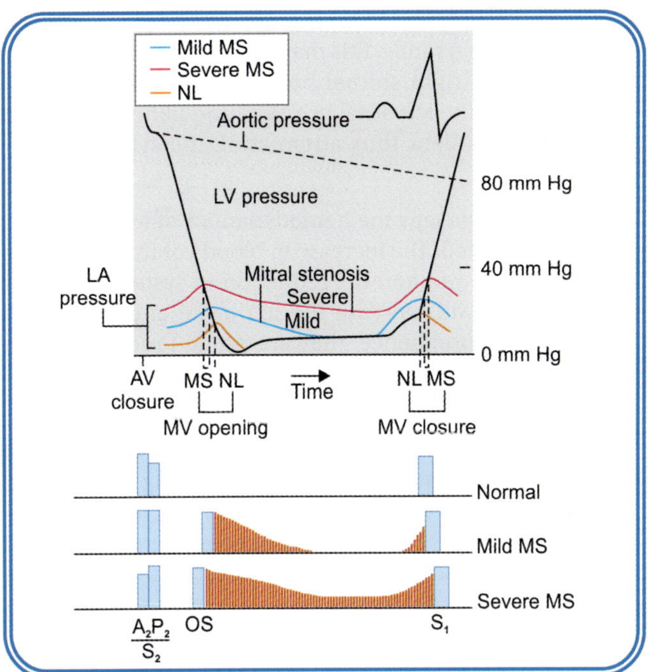

FIG. 4: Murmur in mild versus severe MS and hemodynamics to explain the A_2–OS interval, gradient versus shape of murmur and explanation for the possible presystolic accentuation in presence of AF. From A_2 to LV–LA pressure crossover is the isovolumetric relaxation (A_2–MO interval) and from the pressure crossover to the LV diastolic dip pressure is the MO–OS interval. From the onset of isovolumetric contraction to closure of mitral valve is the clinical presystole versus physiological systole which contributes to the presystolic accentuation in atrial fibrillation.

(AV: aortic valve; LA: left atrium; LV: left ventricle; MS: mitral stenosis; MV: mitral valve; MO: mitral valve opening; NL: normal; OS: opening snap)

OS signifies that the valve leaflets are pliable. The A_2-OS interval has two components **(Fig. 4)**—A_2 to mitral valve opening interval (A_2–MO) which represents the isovolumetric relaxation time and the MO–OS interval (as the OS occurs at the end of the opening excursion). As the LA pressure rises, the isovolumetric relaxation time (A_2-MO) gets shortened; rapid opening excursion of mitral leaflets due to high LA pressure shortens the MO–OS interval also. Thus, the A_2-OS interval is inversely proportional to the LA pressure; shorter the interval more severe is the MS (value ranges from 40 to 120 ms; <60 ms indicates severe MS). However, this interval will not be reliable indicator of severity of MS in the following situations:

- Prolonged isovolumetric relaxation as in hypertension, AS and LV myocardial diseases; A_2-MO interval lengthens resulting in long A_2-OS despite severe MS
- Nonpliable valve can result in long MO–OS interval
- Low output situations such as severe PH, RV failure, and tricuspid valve lesions decompress the LA thereby reducing the transmitral gradient, which prolongs the A_2-MO interval.

- In AF, the S_2-OS interval varies depending on cycle length; in the cycles following short R-R interval, the LA pressure will be high resulting in early OS and vice versa.

At bedside, we have to differentiate OS from S_3. OS is higher pitched, heard medial to apex and along left sternal border; S_3 is soft and localized to apex (LV S_3). On standing, OS gets delayed due to reduced venous return reducing the LA pressure whereas the timing of S_3 does not change but its intensity comes down. Cycle length variation modifies the timing of OS but not of S_3.

- Vascular constant pulmonary ejection click due to dilated pulmonary artery may be audible in the presence of severe PH.
- RV S_4 may be heard in presence of severe PH in sinus rhythm.
- *Diastolic murmur of MS*: The classical mid-diastolic murmur (MDM) in MS is a low-pitched, rough, rumbling murmur with presystolic accentuation best heard with the bell of stethoscope at the apex during expiration, with the patient in left lateral recumbent position. Usually, it is localized to the apex, but when loud, it may be heard in the axilla and lower left sternal border also. The intensity of the murmur is not related to the severity of MS, but the duration of the murmur is proportional to the severity of MS. The murmur commences with the OS and is limited to earlier part of diastole and presystole in mild MS; as the severity increases, the murmur becomes long and starts with an early OS followed by a decrescendo-crescendo pattern extending up to S_1. Shape of the murmur correlates with the LV–LA gradient in diastole, high in the early phase, then gradually falls with LA emptying and further rise during atrial contraction. The presystolic accentuation of the MS murmur is due to atrial contraction which augments the LA pressure and transmitral gradient and this presystolic accentuation usually disappears with onset of AF. It has been shown that it requires a gradient of at least 10 mm Hg at the onset of LV contraction to create a presystolic crescendo. The presystolic murmur extends to the early part of LV isovolumetric contraction also when the LA pressure is still higher than LV pressure. Mitral annular narrowing due to ventricular contraction contributes to the higher gradient during this period which also contributes to the presystolic accentuation (Q-S_1 interval—Q corresponds to the onset of systole and S_1 occurs at the LV–LA pressure crossover; hence, Q-S_1 interval is physiologically systole but clinically presystole. In MS, the Q-S_1 interval gets prolonged due to the high LA pressure). This mechanism is preserved even in presence of AF, which can explain theoretically the presystolic accentuation in AF especially with fast rate—better in short cycles as LA pressure will be higher due to short LA emptying time.[16] Hemodynamic trace of **Figure 4** illustrates this phenomenon.

The murmur may be masked in patients with thick chest wall, pulmonary emphysema, and low cardiac output states. In the so-called "silent MS", the RV may occupy the cardiac apex and the murmur may be inaudible or heard in the mid or posterior axillary line and particularly heard after mild exertion; calcified valve also attenuates it. Mitral MDM can occur in other conditions also—LV inflow obstructions such as LA myxoma, supravalvular mitral ring, and cor triatriatum and due to increased mitral diastolic flow as in post-tricuspid conditions such as ventricular septal defect, patent ductus arteriosus, and ruptured aneurysm of Valsalva to right heart; Austin Flint murmur in AR and Carey Coombs murmur of acute rheumatic carditis are also causes for mitral diastolic murmur.

When significant PH develops, secondary pulmonary regurgitation (PR) and TR occur. TR murmur is a high-pitched soft pansystolic murmur best heard along lower left sternal border, which increases with inspiration (Rivero–Carvallo sign) and passive leg raising and attenuates on standing. PR murmur due to PH (Graham–Steell murmur) is a soft high-pitched decrescendo EDM confined to pulmonary area. It can be confused with the murmur of AR; but the following points are useful:

- Statistically in MS, presence of EDM favors AR.
- PR murmur is localized; AR murmur is widely transmitted along the left sternal border.
- PR murmur is better heard in supine position during inspiration and augmented with passive leg raising; AR murmur is better heard with patient sitting up, leaning forward, and breath held in expiration.
- Presence of other signs of PH (loud P_2, pulmonary ejection click) for PR versus wide pulse pressure and peripheral signs for AR

Juvenile MS:[12,13] Severe MS in young with male pre-ponderance. They have tight stenosis with severe PH due to reactive and obstructive pulmonary vascular changes. However, the incidence of AF and systemic embolism is relatively less.

Lutembacher syndrome (ostium secundum atrial septal defect with rheumatic MS): MS causes resistance to blood flow from LA to LV and hence augments left to right shunt across the defect; rarely, this may produce a soft continuous murmur along right sternal border.[17] Atrial septal defect decompresses the left atrial pressure and hence diminishes transmitral gradient thus attenuating the symptoms and findings of MS.

Pregnancy: It worsens the hemodynamics of MS and hence is poorly tolerated. The increase in blood volume, heart rate, and cardiac output and the reduction in systemic vascular resistance all will increase the left atrial and pulmonary capillary pressure; hence, they are prone for development of pulmonary edema and pulmonary apoplexy during mid-trimester and labor.

Clinical assessment of severity of MS: NYHA Class III/IV symptoms, orthopnea, PND, heart failure, long murmur with short A_2–OS interval, long Q–S_1 interval, and features of PH indicate severe MS. Though AF occurs more frequently with severe MS, it is also related to the duration of the disease and age of the patient.

Complications: Major complications of MS are acute pulmonary edema, AF, thromboembolism, PH, and CHF. Acute rise in LA pressure due to sudden increase in blood volume, heart rate, or cardiac output as in fever, infections, tachyarrhythmias such as AF, pregnancy, undue exercise, and fluid overload results in acute rise in pulmonary capillary pressure leading to massive transudation of fluid into lung alveoli leading to acute pulmonary edema which if not promptly treated could be fatal. AF is the major arrhythmia in MS; LA fibrosis due to rheumatic pathology and long-standing LA hypertension and dilatation are the substrates for development of AF. Loss of atrial kick and the fast heart rate contributes to impaired LA emptying resulting in further rise in LA pressure and aggravation of symptoms. Stasis of blood leads to formation of thrombus in LA (mainly in the appendage) with systemic embolism; quite often, this occurs in presence of AF, but 20% of patients may be in sinus rhythm (probably had paroxysmal AF). Sometimes, thrombus may

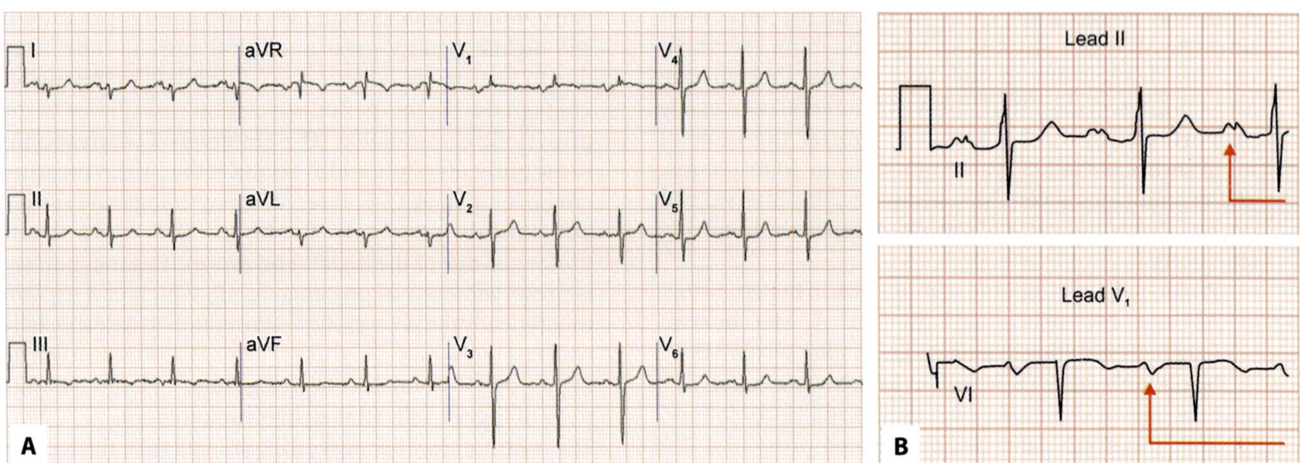

FIGS. 5A AND B: ECG showing right axis of QRS, right ventricular hypertrophy, and left atrial enlargement (P-mitrale and Morris index) in a patient with severe mitral stenosis.

form in the LA body and remains free-floating ball valve thrombus. Infective endocarditis is infrequent in MS.

Electrocardiogram

In patients with mild MS, the ECG may be within normal limits. In moderate and severe MS, characteristic ECG changes occur **(Fig. 5)**. The ECG findings include:

- *Evidence of LA enlargement*: Left atrial activation time is prolonged resulting in the typical P mitrale—wide bifid P wave better seen in lead II and left chest leads, >100 ms duration, second hump taller than first, and separated from first by ≥40 ms. P wave axis of +45° to –30° in the frontal plane is found in about 90% of patients with significant MS. The negative P terminal force in V_1 becomes prominent—wide and deep; area ≥1 mm^2 (≥0.004 mv/s or ≥0.04 mm/s) indicates left atrial abnormality (Morris index). Prolonged left atrial activation results in encroachment of the P wave into PR segment of the PR interval; thus, the P width by PR segment length ratio gets prolonged to >1.5 (Macruz index).

- *RVH pattern*: The development of RVH depends on the magnitude of the RV systolic pressure. The important ECG criteria of RVH include right axis deviation, R/S in lead V_1 > 1, qR pattern in lead V_1, deep S in V_6 and ST–T changes in right chest leads. Generally, when RV systolic pressure is between 70 and 100 mm Hg, ECG evidence of RVH is present and when RV pressure is 100 mm Hg, ECG evidence of RVH is consistently present. The frontal plane QRS axis correlates better with the degree of pulmonary vascular resistance and severity of MS. Mean QRS axis between 0° and +60° suggests that mitral valve area is >1.3 cm^2, when the axis is > +60° the mitral valve area is < 1.3 cm^2 and axis >110° indicates significant PH; when pulmonary artery systolic pressure approaches systemic arterial pressure levels, the mean QRS axis in frontal plane averages +150°.

- *Arrhythmias*: Major arrhythmia in MS is AF, which may be preceded by atrial ectopics, atrial tachycardia, or atrial flutter. Initially, it could be paroxysmal. Development of AF depends on the age of the patient, left atrial size, and pressure and fibrosis of left atrial myocardium. Normal organized P waves are replaced by fast irregular nonorganized fibrillary waves—fine or coarse **(Fig. 6)**. It was thought that coarse fibrillary waves represent rheumatic etiology; it is also related to LA size and pressure. But, as time passes because of atrial fibrosis, the waves may become finer. Atrial depolarization is very fast and chaotic; the lazy AV node cannot conduct that much impulses. Hence, it transmits the impulses irregularly to the ventricle resulting in grossly irregular R-R interval (corresponding to the irregular pulse). Initially, the ventricular rate is relatively fast; as time passes, the rate comes down due to chronic AV node fatigue and also due to the effect of the drugs given.

Radiological Findings

The utility of routine chest X-ray in the diagnosis and assessment of MS is declining since the introduction of echocardiography. However, the X-ray may show typical features as follows **(Figs. 7 and 8)**.

- The classical straightening of left border due to prominent main pulmonary artery, bulging left atrial appendage, and underfilled LV.

- *Evidence of LA enlargement*: Double shadow along right border, lifting up of left bronchus with widening of carinal angle, prominent left atrial appendage shadow along left border below the pulmonary artery and indentation

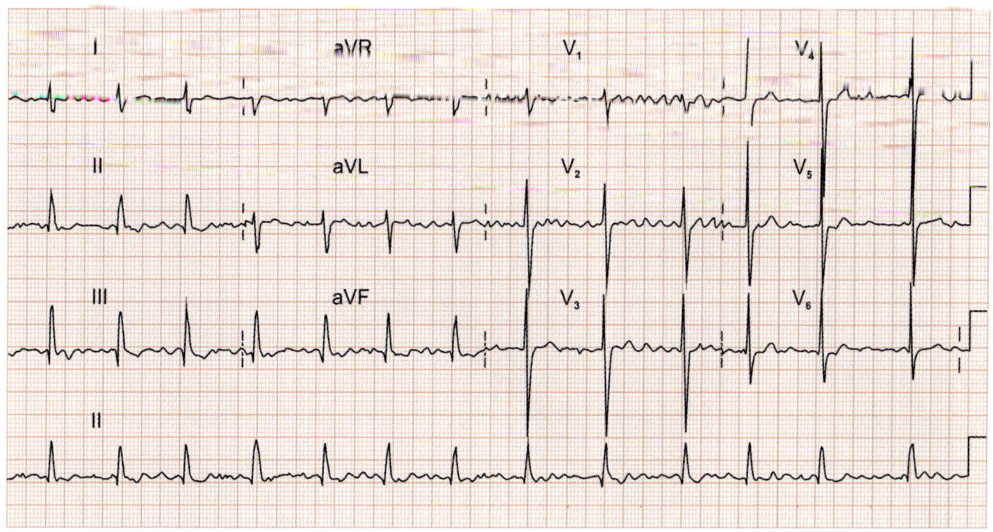

FIG. 6: ECG showing atrial fibrillation—fast irregular fibrillary waves best seen in lead V_1 and irregular RR interval.

of the lower third of barium-filled esophagus in RAO view
- *Evidence of pulmonary venous congestion*: Cephalization of pulmonary vasculature (to decompress the capillary pressure in the major lower lobe, pulmonary arterial resistance of lower lobe vessels increases resulting in diversion of flow to upper lobe), Kerley B lines (dense, short, thick horizontal lines near the costophrenic angles due to dilated lymphatics), Kerley A lines (straight, dense lines up to 4 cm in length running towards hilum), peribronchial cuffing, and pleural effusion (in free space or in fissures). Acute elevation of LA pressure producing pulmonary edema has the classical batwing appearance. Miliary mottling due to pulmonary hemosiderosis following recurrent hemoptysis is rare now. Radiological findings have some hemodynamic correlation also—cephalization occurs with pulmonary capillary pressure of 15–18 mm Hg, Kerley lines with pressures >20 mm; evidence of transudation suggests that the pressure has gone above 25 mm Hg.

- Enlargement of pulmonary arteries, RV, and RA occurs in severe cases with PH and TR. In those with severe cardiac failure and elevated jugular venous pressure, images of dilated SVC and entry of azygos vein to SVC also become prominent.
- Calcification of mitral valve may be seen in chest X-ray, but fluoroscopic examination is better for visualizing calcification.

Echocardiography

Echocardiography is the most accurate tool for diagnosis and evaluation of MS. M-mode, real time two-dimensional, Doppler, and color flow imaging give adequate information in majority of cases for decision making. Occasionally, transesophageal echo evaluation is needed in selected cases. The typical findings in M-mode echo are thickened leaflet traces, flattening of EF slope, blunted A wave, and paradoxical anterior motion of posterior leaflet **(Fig. 9)**. LA dilates, the magnitude of which depends on the severity of the stenosis. 2D real-time imaging findings are illustrated in **Box 1 and Figure 10**.

Based on the morphological features of the leaflets and subvalvular apparatus, Wilkins score can be generated to assess the suitability for mitral commissurotomy **(Table 2)**.

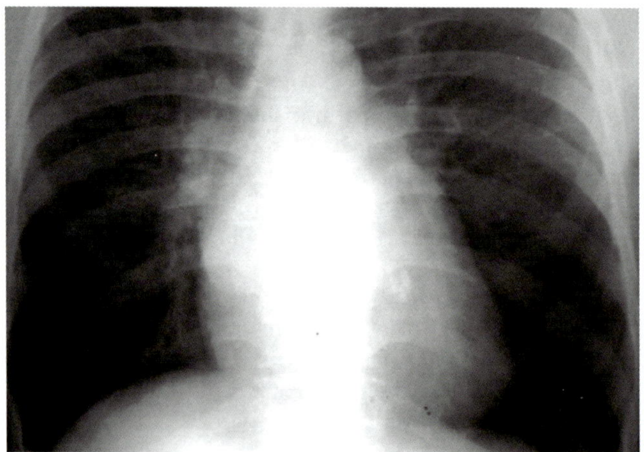

FIG. 7: X-ray chest in mitral stenosis shows straightening of left border, dilated left atrium, prominent upper lobe vessels, and mitral valve calcium.

BOX 1	**2D echo findings in mitral stenosis.**

- Thickening of mitral valve leaflets
- Restricted mobility of the valve leaflets and diastolic doming due to fusion of commissures
- Thickening and shortening of the chordae tendineae
- Calcification of valve apparatus
- Calculation of valve area by planimetry
- Dilated left atrium
- Left atrial thrombus especially in the appendage
- Dilated pulmonary artery in presence of PH
- Right ventricular dilatation in cases with PH, TR, and CHF

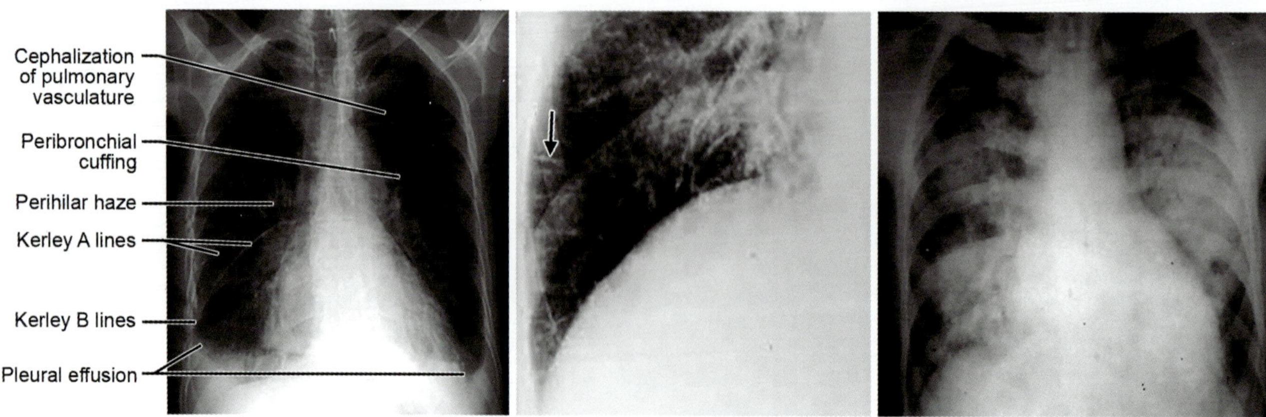

FIG. 8: Radiological features of pulmonary capillary hypertension.

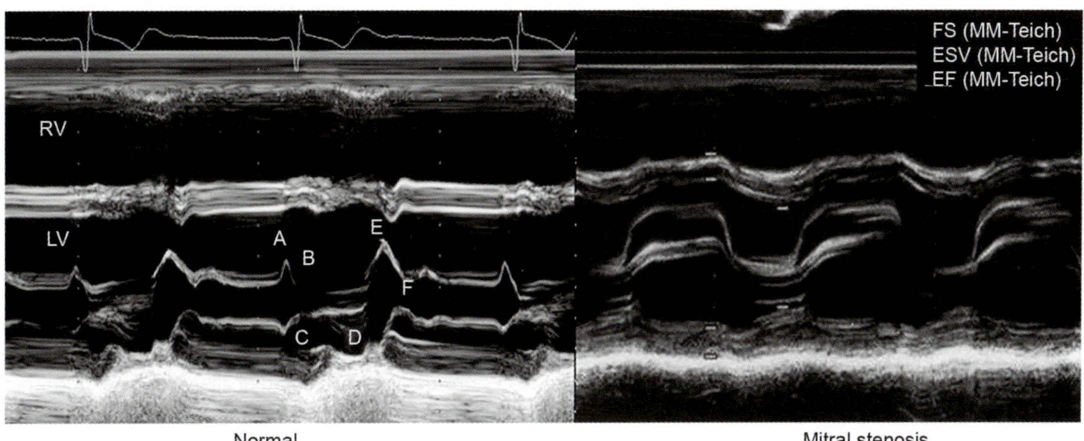

FIG. 9: M-mode echo—MS versus normal; thickened leaflets, flat EF, blunted A, anterior motion of posterior leaflet.

(EF: ejection fraction; LV: left ventricle; MS: mitral stenosis; RV: right ventricle)

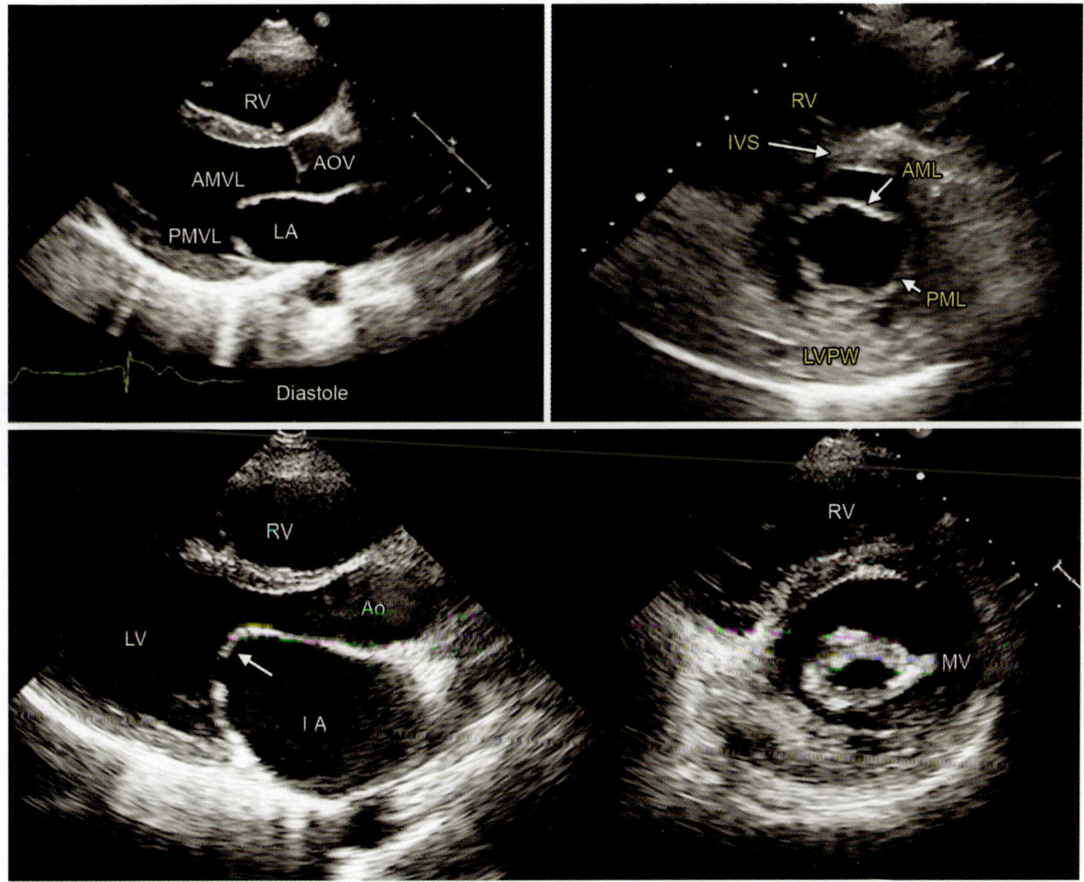

FIG. 10: 2D image—normal versus mitral stenosis.

(AML: anterior mitral leaflet; AMVL: anterior mitral valve leaflet; Ao: aorta; AOV: aortic valve; Ao: aorta; IVC: interventricular septum; LA: left atrium; LV: left ventricle; LVPW: left ventricular posterior wall; PML: posterior mitral leaflet; PMVL: posterior mitral valve leaflet; RV: right ventricle)

Doppler study: Pulse Doppler interrogation of the transmitral flow provides information regarding the gradient and valve area **(Fig. 11)**. Normal mitral flow has two flow velocities: early diastolic (E) and presystolic (A). In MS, the flow velocities increase and the deceleration slope of E becomes shallow. From the E deceleration slope pressure half time in millisecond is automatically derived; mitral valve area is calculated by the formula, 220/pressure half time (pressure

TABLE 2: Wilkins score.

Grade	Mobility	Subvalvular thickening	Leaflet thickening	Calcification
1	Highly mobile with only leaflet tips restricted	Minimal thickening just below the mitral leaflets	Leaflets near normal in thickness (4–5 mm)	A single area of increased echo brightness
2	Leaflet mid and base portions have normal mobility	Thickening of chordal structures extending to one-third of the chordal length	Mid-leaflets normal, considerable thickening of margins (5–8 mm)	Scattered areas of brightness confined to leaflet margins
3	Valve continues to move forward in diastole, mainly from the base	Thickening extended to distal third of the chords	Thickening extending through the entire leaflet (5–8 mm)	Brightness extending into the mid-portions of the leaflets
4	No or minimal forward movement of the leaflets in diastole	Extension thickening and shortening of all chordal structures extending down to the papillary muscles	Considerable thickening of all leaflet tissue (>8 mm)	Extensive brightness throughout much of the leaflet tissue

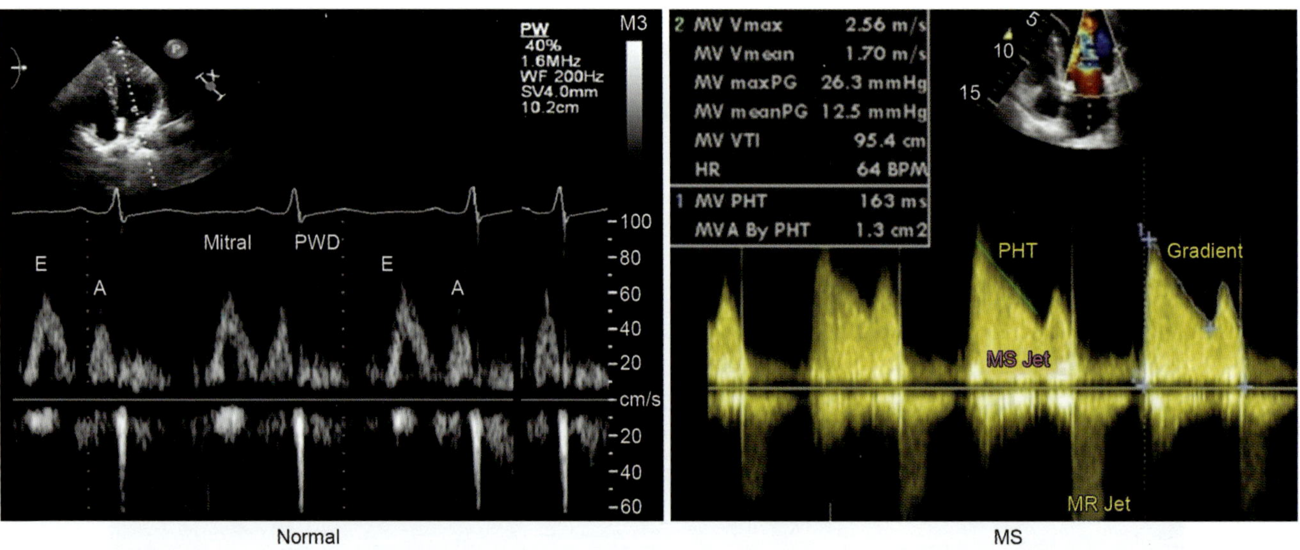

FIG. 11: Mitral flow Doppler—normal versus MS; gradient and calculation of mitral area by pressure half time method.
(MR: mitral regurgitation; MS: mitral stenosis; PHT: pulmonary hypertension; PWD: pulsed-wave Doppler)

TABLE 3: Echocardiographic grading of severity of mitral stenosis.

	Mild	Moderate	Severe
Specific			
Valve area (cm^2)	>1.5	1–1.5	<1
Nonspecific			
Mean gradient (mm Hg)	<5	5–10	>10
PASP (mm Hg)	<30	30–50	>50

(PASP: pulmonary artery systolic pressure)

mean gradient can also be calculated from the spectral trace. Pulmonary artery pressure can be derived from the analysis of spectral trace of TR and PR.

Based on the echocardiographic parameters, severity of MS can be graded as in **Table 3** (normal mitral valve area is 4–6 cm^2; 4 cm^2/m^2 body surface area)

General criteria for severe MS are taken as valve area of <1 cm^2 (<0.6 cm^2/m^2); recent western literature considers valve area <1.5 cm^2 as severe or significant MS and <1 cm^2 as very severe MS.

Transesophageal echo may be indicated in selected situations such as:
- Poor transthoracic window
- Evaluation of left atrial thrombi in patients presenting with systemic embolism features
- Prior to percutaneous transmitral commissurotomy

half time is the time taken for the LA pressure to drop to half its maximal value).[12] Mitral valve area can also be calculated by planimetry, continuity equation, and proximal isovelocity surface area (PISA) method. The maximum and

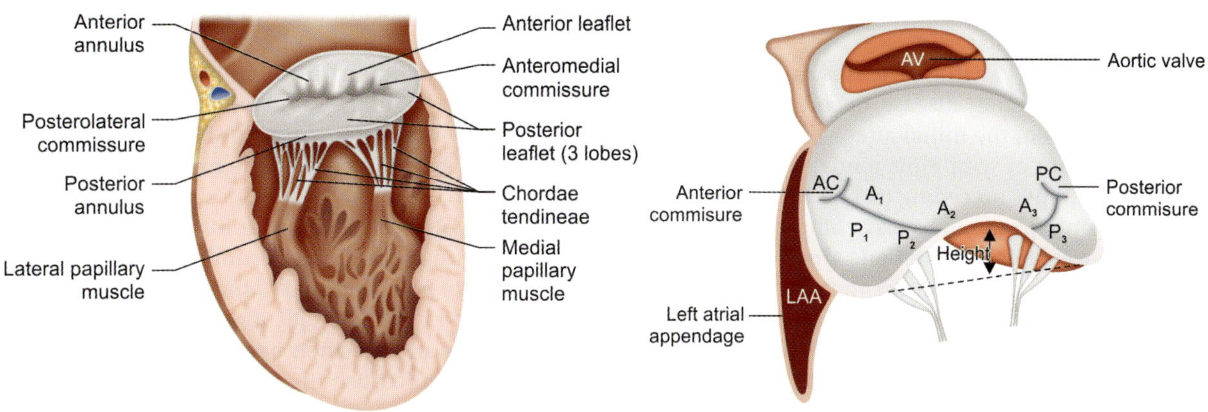

FIG. 12: The complex mitral valve apparatus.

Mitral restenosis: Following successful mitral commissurotomy, the mitral valve area comes down in due course as the rheumatic pathology is a progressive one. Reduction in valve area to <1.5 cm^2 and/or loss of >50% of the gain in area achieved by the procedure is the criteria for diagnosing restenosis. This has to be differentiated from residual stenosis where the procedure did not produce satisfactory result—valve area >1.8 cm and/or gain of area by >50%. Prevalence of restenosis varies in different series; on an average, it is 20–30% over 10-year follow-up. Clinical diagnosis of restenosis is made by the following points:

- Sustained improvement in symptoms by at least two NYHA class
- OS gets delayed and the murmur becomes short
- Clinical findings of PH will take longer time to regress
- Radiological findings of pulmonary venous congestion regress (but chamber enlargement may persist)
- Reduction in the magnitude of the QRS axis
- Regression of the left atrial abnormality pattern in ECG over time
- Serial echocardiographic evaluation

Mitral Regurgitation

Mitral valve apparatus is a complex structure composed of the two leaflets, annulus, chordae tendineae, papillary muscle, LV myocardium, and floor of LA (**Fig. 12**).

Pathophysiology

Structural and/or functional abnormality of any of these components in isolation or combination produces MR. MR is basically classified as primary or secondary—primary being structural abnormality of the mitral valve apparatus and secondary is MR due to other causes such as LV dilatation, ischemic heart disease, and cardiomyopathy.[12] Rheumatic fever is one of the common causes of primary MR especially in the underdeveloped countries; quite often associated with varying degrees of stenosis. Other causes for primary MR include myxomatous degeneration (mitral valve prolapse syndrome), infective endocarditis, congenital, trauma, inflammatory diseases (systemic lupus erythematosus, aortoarteritis, rheumatoid arthritis, etc.), mucopolysaccharidoses, and iatrogenic (postballoon mitral valvotomy, drugs such as ergots). In rheumatic MR, there will be shortening, rigid deformity, and retraction of one or both the leaflets of mitral valve and is associated with shortening and fusion of chordae tendineae and papillary muscles. Unlike rheumatic MS, MR is more common in men. During systole, blood from LV is emptied to both LA and aorta; this in addition to the normal pulmonary venous return increases the LA volume and the diastolic blood flow across the mitral valve. The high LV preload enhances the force of LV contraction by the Starling's principle; the afterload in MR is low as the LV has two outlets—aorta and the highly compliant LA. Both these factors contribute to the enhanced ejection fraction (EF), which maintains forward stroke volume to aorta despite the regurgitation. Hence in chronic MR, EF is more than normal; even a normal EF value in severe MR is considered as LV systolic dysfunction (EF < 60% indicates LV dysfunction in MR) Phasic distention of the very compliant LA during systole followed by free emptying to LV in diastole decompresses the LA and hence the mean LA pressure and pulmonary capillary pressure does not rise much compared to that in MS. This is the reason why patients with severe MR remain asymptomatic or minimally symptomatic for a long time till they develop LV systolic dysfunction. PH is also relatively mild and late in occurrence in isolated MR. Dilated LA and fibrosis of atrial myocardium due to rheumatic pathology results in the development of AF. Dilated LV, LA, and mitral annulus alter the geometry of papillary muscles and MR further aggravates—MR begets MR.

Symptoms

Rheumatic MR patients may remain asymptomatic for a long time despite significant MR and symptoms depend on several factors:

- Severity of MR
- Rate of progression of MR

- LV function
- Atrial tachyarrhythmias
- Associated other valvular diseases, systemic hypertension, coronary artery disease, or cardiomyopathy

The duration from the initial attack of rheumatic fever to the development of symptoms tends to be longer than that in MS, sometimes exceeding two decades. Hemoptysis and systemic embolization are less common than in MS. Symptoms of weakness and fatigue due to low cardiac output are more common than dyspnea in MR. Generally, these patients with MR have only mild disability unless rapid progression of MR occurs as a result of recurrent rheumatic activity, infective endocarditis, or rupture of chordae tendineae. However, many patients may develop serious or irreversible LV dysfunction by the time symptoms of low cardiac output or pulmonary congestion occur. Severe PH and right-sided heart failure features such as hepatomegaly, edema, and ascites are usually late features.

Physical Signs

The arterial pulse may be normal, could be of low volume with brisk upstroke mimicking a collapsing character. AF causes irregularly irregular pulse. Jugular venous pressure is usually normal until right-sided heart failure occurs. Cardiac apical impulse is brisk and hyperdynamic; cardiomegaly is less impressive as the EF is supernormal. However, severe MR especially with systolic dysfunction can produce significant cardiomegaly displacing the apex down and left. Early diastolic rapid LV inflow produces a palpable early diastolic filling impulse corresponding to a prominent S_3. Systolic expansion of the enlarged LA may produce a late systolic thrust in the left parasternal region (little higher up and laterally compared to the typical left parasternal heave of RVH).

S_1 in rheumatic MR is usually diminished in intensity. S_2 is split due to shortening of LV ejection and an earlier A_2 as a result of reduced resistance to LV ejection. When PH develops, P_2 becomes louder. In severe MR, LV S_3 may be heard at the apex, which is a low-pitched, early diastolic sound related to rapid early diastolic ventricular filling. This S_3 should not be interpreted as a sign of LV failure, because it is due to increased flow across mitral valve during rapid filling phase; the same physiology produces an audible mid diastolic rumble over apex. The prominent auscultatory finding is the systolic murmur of MR heard at the apex—soft, blowing, high-pitched, pansystolic murmur, which starts with S_1 and ends with S_2 (may continue beyond A_2, obscuring it because of persistent pressure gradient between LV and LA during the isovolumetric relaxation phase). As the anterior mitral leaflet is predominantly involved in rheumatic MR, the murmur is conducted usually to the left axilla; in posterior leaflet pathology, the murmur will be conducted to upper left sternal border and neck. When there is rupture of chordae tendineae of anterior leaflet of mitral valve, the jet of MR is directed to the posterior wall of LA and the murmur may be transmitted toward the spine.[18] MR

murmur is better heard during expiration and increases in supine position, with isometric handgrip and on squatting, decreases on standing, during the straining phase (phase II) of Valsalva maneuver and with amyl nitrite inhalation (maneuvers, which increase the LV preload or systemic vascular resistance increases the murmur and vice versa). The intensity of the murmur does not correlate with the severity of MR. The MR murmur of rheumatic origin needs to be differentiated from other conditions.

- *MR due to mitral valve prolapse syndrome*: The murmur is preceded by a nonejection click. It is a mid and late systolic murmur which behaves in opposite direction with dynamic auscultation; click occurs earlier and murmur becomes longer in situations which reduce LV volume as on standing, during phase II of Valsalva maneuver and with amyl nitrite inhalation (prolapse starts early when the LV size is small).
- *Tricuspid regurgitation murmur*: It is heard more medially, increases in intensity during inspiration, and is accompanied by a prominent V wave and sharp Y descent in the JVP and systolic hepatic pulsation.
- *Ventricular septal defect*: Small defects produce a harsh loud murmur along the left sternal border usually with a thrill. The murmur becomes less loud as they develop PH.
- In posterior mitral leaflet abnormality, MR murmur may be well heard over apex and upper sternal border and hence can be confused with the murmur of AS. However, the aortic stenotic murmur is harsh, midsystolic, crescendo-decrescendo, and gets conducted to carotids; beat-to-beat variation in length and intensity occurs when there is cardiac irregularity as in ectopics. Normally, the LV systolic pressure does not rise after the ectopic; hence, MR murmur does not change significantly. In presence of LV outflow obstruction, LV systolic pressure rises significantly resulting in augmentation of the murmur of AS; increased stroke volume following the long diastole also contributes.
- MR in hypertrophic obstructive cardiomyopathy becomes louder when the LV cavity size reduces as on standing, during inspiration and during straining phase of Valsalva
- Other causes of MR such as coronary artery disease, cardiomyopathy, and infective endocarditis etc., can be differentiated on clinical grounds and echocardiography helps in such situations.

Electrocardiography

The main ECG findings are features of LA enlargement and left ventricular hypertrophy (LVH) as shown in **Figure 13**. ECG evidence of LVH is seen in only one-third of patients with severe MR as the ventricular cavity size remains normal (Brody's effect—voltage is proportional to the cavity size as blood is a good conductor of electricity). When severe PH develops, ECG evidence of RVH may be present in about 15% of patients, counterbalancing the LVH pattern due to

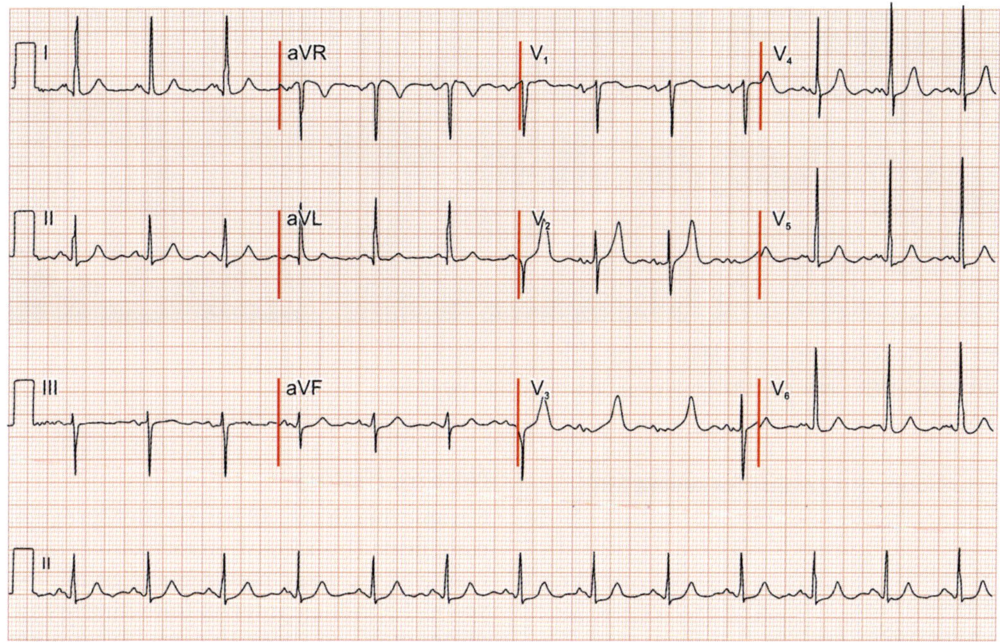

FIG. 13: ECG in severe MR—LVH and left atrial abnormality pattern.

(LVH: left ventricular hypertrophy; MR: mitral regurgitation)

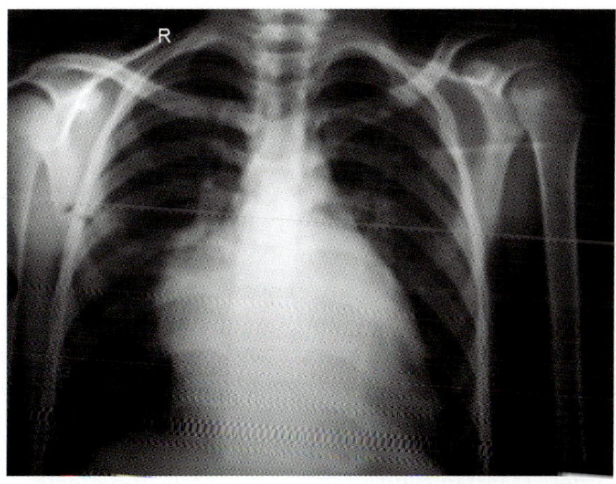

FIG. 14: X-ray in severe MR. Giant LA border is seen extending beyond the RA border; RA touches the diaphragm, LA does not.

(LA: left atrium; MR: mitral regurgitation; RA: right atrium)

MR (please refer elsewhere for the various ECG criteria for LVH and RVH).

Radiological Findings

Cardiac enlargement mainly due to enlargement of LV and LA is the main feature in severe MR. Left atrial enlargement may be massive and aneurysmal; rarely, giant LA can extend beyond the right atrial shadow **(Fig. 14)**. Mitral annular calcification may be seen in chest X-ray, but it is better visualized on fluoroscopy. Long-standing severe MR with left ventricular dysfunction produces radiological features of pulmonary venous and arterial hypertension similar to that in MS but less often.

Echocardiography

Echocardiography plays a pivotal role in the diagnosis and quantification of MR, timing of intervention, assessing the feasibility for repair versus replacement and in determining the etiology of MR **(Fig. 15)**. Two-dimensional real-time imaging may show evidence of enlargement of LA and LV and underlying mechanism of MR such as rheumatic pathology, rupture of chordae, mitral valve prolapse, a flail leaflet or noncoapting valve, and calcification of annulus. In rheumatic MR, the leaflets and subvalvular apparatus will be thickened with restricted mobility of posterior leaflet; in presence of associated MS, doming of the leaflets is diagnostic for rheumatic etiology. Echo also gives diagnostic information regarding LV function and pulmonary artery pressure. Color Doppler study helps in estimating degree of MR, which correlates with angiographic studies. Quantitative assessment of regurgitant fraction, regurgitant volume, and effective regurgitant orifice area (EROA) is quite accurate compared to angiography.[19] The vena contracta defined as the narrowest cross-sectional area of regurgitant jet mapped by color Doppler method predicts the severity of MR.[20] The PISA method, reversal of flow in pulmonary vein during systole, and a high-peak inflow E velocity are other parameters for assessing the severity of MR **(Box 2)**. Transesophageal echo is superior to transthoracic echo in assessing the severity of MR and finer details of mitral

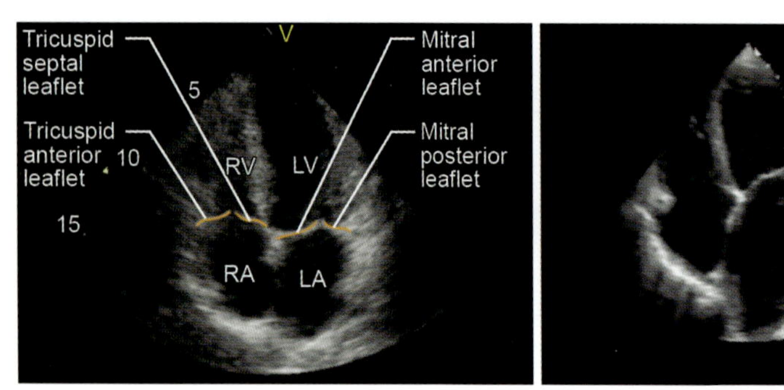

FIG. 15: Echocardiographic findings in severe MR.

(LA: left atrium; LV: left ventricle; MR: mitral regurgitation; RA: right atrium; RV: right ventricle)

BOX 2	Echocardiographic criteria for severe MR

- Flail leaflets
- Vena contracta ≥ 7 mm
- Effective regurgitant orifice area ≥ 0.40 cm^2 (≥40 mm^2)
- Regurgitant volume > 60 mL per cycle
- Regurgitant fraction ≥ 50%
- Pulmonary vein systolic flow reversal
- Color flow area ≥ 40% of LA size
- Eccentric mitral regurgitant jet reaching the superior posterior wall
- LVESV ≥ 40 mm
- Dilated LA—dimension ≥ 55 mm or LA volume index ≥ 60 mL/m^2

(LA: left atrium; LVESV: left ventricular end systolic volume; MR: mitral regurgitation)

BOX 3	Angiographic grading of severity of mitral regurgitation.

- *Grade 1*: Regurgitant contrast does not fill the full LA; it gets cleared with each cycle
- *Grade 2*: Opacifies the full LA after multiple cycles; opacification is less than that of LV; does not clear with one cycle
- *Grade 3*: Complete opacification of LA which equals to that of LV
- *Grade 4*: LA completes opacification with the first cycle itself; it becomes progressively dense; contrast enters LA appendage and pulmonary veins

(LA: left atrium; LV: left ventricle)

valve apparatus to plan intervention. Three-dimensional echo has added value. Cardiac MRI has revolutionized the assessment of MR.

Angiographic grading of MR: Quantitative assessment of MR by Sellers grading in contrast ventriculogram as given in **Box 3** is seldom needed nowadays.

Natural History[12]

Chronic rheumatic MR has a gradual progression only unless complicated by infective endocarditis or recurrent rheumatic reactivation. They may remain asymptomatic for many years; the average interval from diagnosis to development of symptoms is about 16 years. Asymptomatic severe MR in sinus rhythm with normal LV function has an annual mortality of about 1–3%; they may require intervention over the next 5–10 years. On medical follow-up, 30% develop chronic AF and >60% develop CHF by 10 years. Compared with patients having EROA <20 mm^2, those with EROA of ≥40 mm^2 had an increased risk of death from any cause, cardiac death, and sudden death. Asymptomatic severe MR with EF <60% had a 5-year survival of only 55%.

Aortic Regurgitation

Basically, AR could be due to valvular pathology, root dilatation, hypertension, or combined. Rheumatic etiology is one of the common causes for AR when the valve is involved primarily.[21] The aortic cusps become infiltrated with fibrous tissue and retract and cause AR. Fusion of commissures may cause combined AS and AR. Other causes of AR are—congenital aortic valve abnormalities, infective endocarditis, severe hypertension, trauma, connective tissue disorders (Marfan syndrome, osteogenesis imperfecta, and Ehlers–Danlos syndrome), autoimmune diseases (systemic lupus erythematosus, rheumatoid arthritis, ankylosing spondylitis, and Behçet's syndrome), various forms of arteritis (Takayasu's aortoarteritis and giant cell arteritis), mucopolysaccharidoses (Hunter/Hurler syndrome), and aortic aneurysms due to any cause.

Pathophysiology

Regurgitation of blood from aorta to LV leads to LV volume overload enhancing the force of contraction as per Starling principle; to enhance peripheral circulation, the systemic vascular resistance decreases. Both these factors result in increased stroke volume. The basic hemodynamic abnormalities in chronic severe AR are elevated LV diastolic volume, high cardiac output, and low systemic vascular resistance. These contribute to the wide pulse pressure in aorta due to low diastolic pressure (aortic run off) and relatively higher systolic pressure (high stroke volume). Chronic severe AR has the largest LV diastolic volume resulting in a very large heart—"cor bovinum". When they develop LV dysfunction, the cardiac output comes down; still, it will be above normal value resulting in high-output heart failure state. The low-aortic diastolic pressure reduces the coronary perfusion (which is mainly in diastole); this along with the increased oxygen demand due to high myocardial mass and afterload sets the stage for development of myocardial ischemia which manifests as nocturnal angina (during sleep the slow heart rate prolongs the diastole aggravating the regurgitation). With exercise, peripheral resistance decreases and heart rate rises with resultant decrease in diastole, both contributing to a favorable reduction in regurgitant volume; hence, they have a good effort tolerance till LV dysfunction sets in.

Symptoms

Many patients with severe AR may remain asymptomatic for several years and are usually picked up on routine examination.[22] The main symptom is palpitation due to the increased force of contraction of the dilated ventricle. With the development of LV dysfunction, patients start experiencing exertional dyspnea; orthopnea and PND indicate severe LV dysfunction or associated mitral valve disease. Myocardial ischemia may occur due to the mechanisms described earlier.

Physical Findings

General examination reveals features of the etiological background such as Marfan syndrome. Pulse is quite characteristic and gives clue to the diagnosis and more importantly the severity. High-stroke volume, increased force of LV ejection, and the aortic run off to LV and periphery (due to low-vascular resistance) form the basis for all the peripheral signs in severe chronic AR. Wide pulse pressure due to low-diastolic and high-systolic pressure is characteristic; lower the diastolic pressure, severe the AR. Typical pulse of severe AR is the high volume collapsing one—rapid upstroke (due to increased force of ejection), ill-sustained peak and rapid downstroke in systole (due to peripheral run off), and low-dicrotic notch. Some of the peripheral signs are:

- *De Musset's sign*: Head nodding due to increased carotid arterial pulsations striking the angles of the mandible (patients with TR can have lateral movements of head corresponding to the prominent V wave)
- *Lighthouse sign*—flushing and blanching of face with each pulse
- *Landolfi's sign*—contraction and dilation of pupil
- *Becker's sign*—pulsation of retinal arteries
- *Müller's sign*—dancing uvula
- Dancing carotid and brachial arteries (locomotor brachialis)

- *Water hammer or Corrigan's or collapsing pulse*: Sharp upstroke of radial pulse followed by rapid down stroke; this is exaggerated by elevating the wrist.
- *Bisferiens pulse*: It is characterized by two systolic peaks—the percussion and tidal waves separated by a distinct mid-systolic dip; the peaks may be equal or either one may be larger; commonly seen in isolated severe AR; also in combined AR and AS (AR dominant); better felt over carotid and brachial arteries.
- *Mayne's sign*—decreases in diastolic blood pressure by ≥15 mm Hg on raising the arm above head
- *Quincke's sign*—capillary pulsations seen on light compression of nail bed or lips
- *Rosenbach's sign*—hepatic pulsations
- *Gerhardt's sign*—splenic pulsation
- *Traube's sign or pistol shot sounds*: Booming systolic and diastolic sounds heard over femoral arteries. Palfrey's sign is pistol shot sound over radial artery.
- *Duroziez's sign*: Systolic murmur heard over femoral artery when it is compressed proximally (proximal to the stethoscope) and a diastolic murmur heard when it is compressed distally due to the reversal of flow in the aorta.
- *Hill's sign*: Systolic blood pressure in lower limb is higher than that in upper limb by >20 mm Hg (normal < 20 mm Hg). If the difference is >60 mm Hg, it indicates severe AR (40–60 moderate AR, 20–40 mild AR).

Uncommon Signs

- Ashrafian sign is pulsatile pseudoproptosis.
- Bozzolo sign is pulsatile nasal mucosa.
- Drummond sign is systolic expulsion of air from nose when mouth is closed.
- Minervini's sign is strong lingual pulsations.
- Palmar click is pulsating palm.
- Dennison sign/Shelley sign is pulsatile cervix.
- *Lincoln sign*—jerking leg with each pulse when legs are kept crossed in sitting position
- *Sherman sign*—dorsalis pedis pulse is quickly located and unexpectedly prominent in patients >75 years.

Examination of the precordium will reveal cardiac enlargement in severe cases; the apical impulse will be hyperdynamic and displaced laterally and inferiorly. Systolic retraction may be present in left parasternal region. Prominent suprasternal and neck arterial pulsations are seen in severe cases. The augmented systolic volume may cause a systolic thrill at the base of the heart and over carotid arteries, which should not be mistaken for associated AS. S_1 is usually normal or soft but may be loud if associated with MS. It becomes soft in presence of LV dysfunction or due to prolonged PR interval. A_2 will be soft since valve is involved pathologically (but when AR is due to aortic root dilation or hypertension A_2 will be loud). The P_2 may be obscured by the AR murmur, which starts with A_2. Prolonged LV ejection and low aortic hangout interval due to the reduced systemic vascular resistance delays A_2 resulting in single or even paradoxically split S_2. A systolic ejection click is absent in rheumatic AR (heard in AR due to dilated aorta or bicuspid aortic valve). Presence of LV S_3 correlates with high LV end-systolic volume[23] and hence is a sign of LV dysfunction. The AR murmur is a high-pitched soft blowing decrescendo EDM best heard in the third left intercostal space close to sternum (second aortic, neoaortic, or Erb's area), conducted down along the left sternal border, and is better heard with diaphragm; as the murmur is soft and relatively faint, it is best heard with patient sitting up, leaning forward and breath held during end expiration. In AR due to root dilatation, A_2 is loud and murmur gets conducted better down along right sternal border. When the AR is due to avulsion or perforation of the leaflets as in infective endocarditis or due to trauma, the murmur has a musical cooing of dove pattern—the seagull murmur. Rarely, AR murmur can be heard over axilla also where it is called Cole–Cecil murmur (asymmetric jet directed posteriorly). Severity of AR correlates with the duration rather than the intensity of the murmur. As the severity of AR increases, murmur becomes longer; but this relation gets offset in presence of LV dysfunction and in acute severe AR. Rarely, in cusp perforation, we may get a long murmur despite a relatively low regurgitant volume.[23] A mid- and late-diastolic rumble heard at the apex, the Austin Flint murmur, is an additional feature of significant AR. Mechanism is premature partial closure of the mitral valve due to the impinging effect of the regurgitant jet on anterior mitral leaflet and also due to the rising LV diastolic pressure which in severe cases (especially in acute AR) may exceed the left atrial pressure producing diastolic MR. Points to assess whether the apical mid-diastolic murmur is Austin Flint murmur or that of MS is given in **Table 4**. The AR murmur needs to be differentiated from Graham Steell murmur of PR due to PH which is localized to 2nd and 3rd left intercostals space, starts with P_2 rather than A_2, and increases with inspiration; features of PH will be dominant. In patients with chronic severe AR, a harsh midsystolic murmur caused by increased stroke volume and increased ejection rate is heard over the aortic area often radiating to carotids. This has to be differentiated from the presence of organic AS; slow rising pulse, heaving type apex, systolic thrill and long murmur with late systolic peaking suggest associated significant AS.

Electrocardiography

Electrocardiogram in severe AR may show LVH with diastolic overload pattern characterized by increase in initial septal forces (deep narrow q waves in leads I, aVL, V_3–V_6) with upright and relatively tall T waves and mild elevation of ST segment in these leads **(Fig. 16)**. In later stages with LV dysfunction, strain pattern may develop—ST-segment depression and T-wave inversion. QRS axis moves toward left and later intraventricular conduction delay may occur.

TABLE 4: Clinical points to differentiate Austin Flint murmur from MS murmur.		
	MS murmur	**Austin Flint murmur**
S_1	Loud	Normal or soft
OS	+	–
Thrill	+	–
AF	Common	Rare
Severe PAH	+	–
Long history of orthopnea and PND	+	–

(AF: atrial fibrillation; PAH: pulmonary arterial hypertension; PND: paroxysmal nocturnal dyspnea; MS: mitral stenosis)

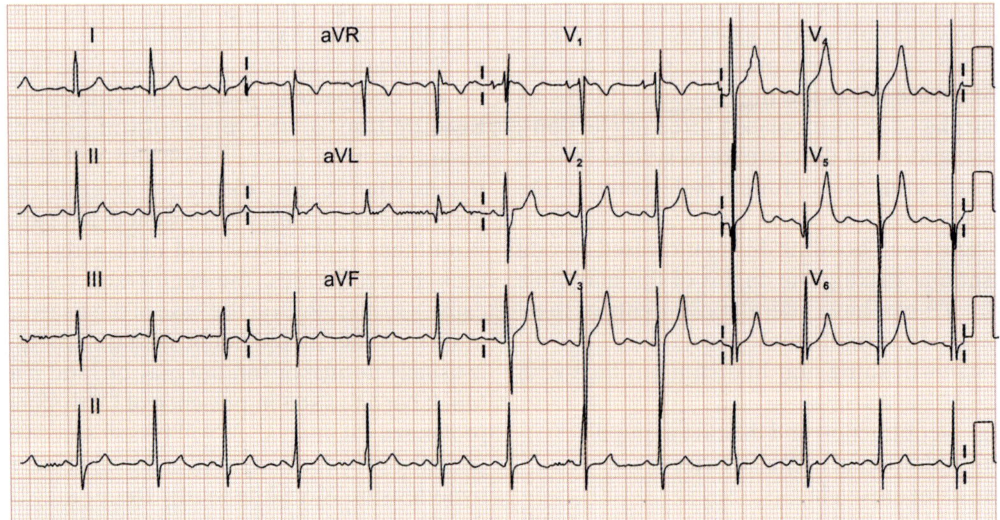

FIG. 16: ECG showing left ventricular hypertrophy with diastolic overload pattern in severe aortic regurgitation.

Radiological Findings

Cardiomegaly is seen, if AR is significant **(Fig. 17)**. As the LV can enlarge posteriorly and inferiorly, the apex dips down the diaphragm and the magnitude of transverse enlargement in X-ray can be attenuated; hence, lateral view is a better indicator of the degree of LV enlargement. Uniform dilatation of aorta is seen in chronic severe AR; selective dilatation of aortic root and ascending aorta gives the clue for aortic pathology as the etiology. Calcification of aortic valve is uncommon in isolated AR. Enlarged LA and radiological features of pulmonary venous congestion indicate LV dysfunction or associated mitral valve disease.

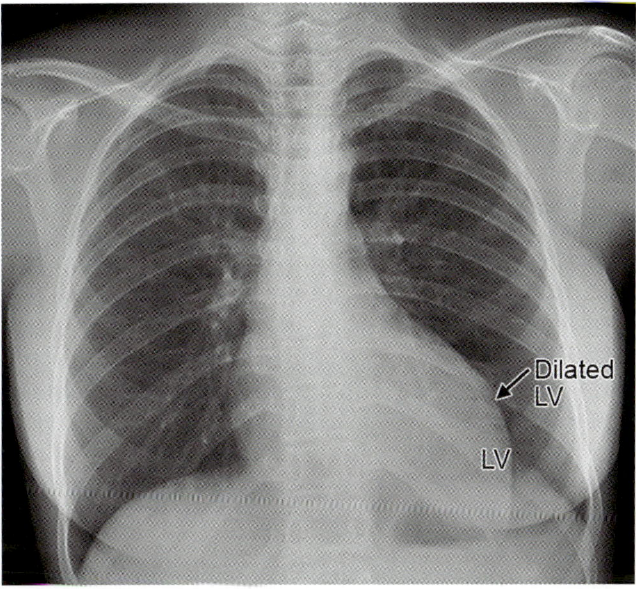

FIG. 17: X-ray chest PA view in AR showing LV type cardiomegaly and dilated aorta.

(AR: aortic regurgitation; LV: left ventricle; PA: posteroanterior)

Echocardiography

The diagnosis, etiology and severity of AR, myocardial function, hemodynamics, and associated other valvular lesions can all be assessed by echocardiography. The thickening and retraction of valve cusps, calcification, and size and shape of the aortic root can be evaluated. The LV end-diastolic and end-systolic dimensions, volume, left ventricular ejection fraction (LVEF), and LV mass can be obtained by transthoracic echo.[23] Fluttering of the anterior leaflet of mitral valve during diastole is an important finding in AR, which can occur even in mild AR. However, if there is associated involvement of mitral valve by rheumatic process, this may not be seen. The degree of AR can be assessed by Doppler and color Doppler studies. Features of severe AR are: dilated LV–end-systolic dimension $\geq$ 50 mm ($\geq$ 25 mm/m^2), pressure half time of AR Doppler trace $\leq$ 200 ms, AR jet width $\geq$ 65% of LV outflow tract (LVOT) width, vena contracta $\geq$ 0.6 cm, regurgitant volume $\geq$ 60 mL/beat, regurgitant fraction $\geq$ 50%, EROA $\geq$ 0.3 cm^2, and holodiastolic flow reversal in proximal abdominal aorta **(Figs. 18A and B)**. Grading of severity of AR by echocardiography is given in **Table 5**.

Indicators of severe AR—clinically wide pulse pressure with low-diastolic pressure < 60 mm Hg, associated peripheral signs, cardiomegaly due to LV dilatation, delayed

TABLE 5: Doppler grading of severity of aortic regurgitation.			
	Mild	*Moderate*	*Severe*
Jet width (% of LVOT)	<25	25–64	≥65
Vena contracta (cm)	<0.3	0.3–0.6	>0.6
Regurgitant volume (ml /beat)	<30	30–59	≥60
Regurgitant fraction (%)	<30	30–49	≥50
Effective regurgitant orifice area (cm^2)	<0.1	0.1–0.29	≥0.3

(LVOT: left ventricular outflow tract)

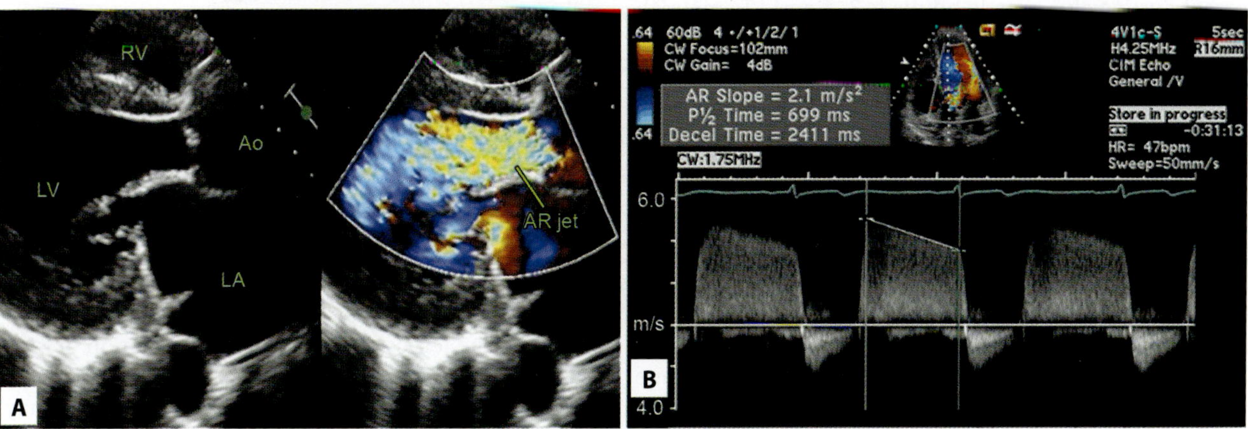

FIGS. 18A AND B: (A) AR color jet, jet to LVOT width > 65%; (B) AR spectral trace showing measurement of pressure half time.

(Ao: aorta; AR: aortic regurgitation; LA: left atrium; LV: left ventricle; LVOT: left ventricular outflow tract; RV: right ventricle)

BOX 4 **Angiographic grading of severity of aortic regurgitation.**

- *Grade 1*: Only small contrast opacifies part of LV which is rapidly cleared with each beat
- *Grade 2*: More contrast enters LV with faint filling of entire LV
- *Grade 3*: Fully opacified LV with density equal to that of aorta
- *Grade 4*: Complete opacification of full LV in the first cycle itself; density in LV more than in aorta

(LV: left ventricle)

A2, long EDM, and Austin Flint murmur; radiologically LV type cardiomegaly; LVH with volume overload pattern in ECG; and echocardiographic parameters as discussed above.

Cardiac MRI gives precise noninvasive quantification of all the important parameters needed to evaluate and plan the management protocol in AR as in MR. Invasive contrast aortography is seldom needed, unless there are other indications for cardiac catheterization. Similar to MR, AR severity is also graded by contrast ventriculography **(Box 4)**.

Aortic Stenosis

Rheumatic fever is one of the less common causes for valvular AS, commonly seen with other lesions such as AR and mitral valve disease; isolated AS of rheumatic etiology is rare. Common causes of AS are congenital bicuspid aortic valve in young people and calcific AS of the elderly; rare causes include homozygous type II hyperlipoproteinemia, ochronosis (alkaptonuria), rheumatoid arthritis, systemic lupus erythematosus, Paget's disease of bone, and irradiation. Rheumatic AS results from adhesions and fusion of commissures and cusps with vascularization of the cusps and the annulus leading to retraction and stiffening of the free borders of the cusps. Later, calcification may occur and the aortic orifice is reduced to small round or triangular opening. Because of this, there is frequent association of AR.

Pathophysiology

Normal aortic valve area in adults is 3-4 cm² (2 cm²/m²); depending on the orifice size, AS is graded as mild (>1.5–2.0 cm²), moderate (1–1.5 cm²), and severe (<1.0 cm² or <0.6 cm²/m²). AS produces chronic systolic pressure overload to LV resulting in concentric LVH (increased LV mass without dilatation). LVH is a compensatory mechanism to reduce wall tension to preserve contractile function (law of Laplace); however, the increased muscle mass and interstitial fibrosis result in diastolic dysfunction, which may persist even after relief of stenosis. The LV systolic function is maintained till late in the natural history of the disease but diastolic dysfunction sets in early. LV systolic pressure rises proportional to the degree of narrowing; ejection time is prolonged but isovolumetric contraction is preserved till systolic dysfunction develops. Diastolic dysfunction results in prolongation of the isovolumetric relaxation period. As LV systolic dysfunction sets in LV starts enlarging. Reduced LV compliance and relaxation reduce the early diastolic filling, which is compensated by a late diastolic atrial kick, which may contribute up to 50% of the ventricular filling. Increase in myocardial oxygen demand coupled with the elevation of LV diastolic pressure, which compromises the subendocardial flow, leads to myocardial ischemia, which also contributes to the development of LV dysfunction. Associated systemic hypertension augments the afterload, thus putting extra myocardial oxygen demand; it also modifies the parameters of assessment of severity of AS.

Symptoms

The principal symptoms of severe AS are exertional dyspnea, exertional *Angina*, exertional *Syncope* and ultimately symptoms of *Heart* failure[24]—*A, S, and H*—in that sequence in the natural history of progressive stenosis. LV diastolic dysfunction resulting in high left atrial pressure and the inability of LV to increase the cardiac output adequately are the factors contributing to the symptoms.[25] With exercise, the cardiac output does not rise proportionately; the available output is diverted to the low-resistance systemic vasculature leading to reduced cerebral blood flow resulting in exertional syncope; however, ischemia and ventricular fibrosis with acute increase in LV systolic pressure during exercise trigger ventricular arrhythmias, which can lead to arrhythmic syncope or even sudden cardiac death. New-onset AF and AV blocks due to extension of calcium into the infrahisian conduction system and malfunctioning baroreceptor mechanisms are other causes for syncope in severe AS. There is a prolonged asymptomatic period even in severe AS followed by rapid deterioration. Orthopnea, nocturnal dyspnea, and right heart failure are relatively late features.

Atrial fibrillation is relatively less frequent in AS occurring in 10–15% of cases; it results in rapid deterioration of the clinical status in view of the loss of atrial kick and also the fast rate impairing the diastolic function. Significant PH is also unusual; if present, look for associated mitral valve disease. Some patients may present with gastrointestinal bleed from associated angiodysplasia of colon (Heyde syndrome).

Physical Findings

Low-volume slow rising pulse—pulsus parvus et tardus or anacrotic pulse—is quite specific for severe valvular AS. But, many patients may have associated AR, systemic hypertension, or other valvular disease, which may alter the pulse character. Pulse pressure is narrow in severe AS; but in elderly or in presence of AR or other hyperdynamic circulatory states, it may be wide. Carotid shudder (jerky thrill) may be felt over carotids due to radiation of systolic murmur of severe AS to carotid arteries. The jugular venous pressure is usually normal but prominent A wave may be seen in severe AS due to Bernheim effect; bulging of the hypertrophied interventricular septum to the RV cavity restricts the RV filling, which is compensated by strong atrial contraction. Other features of RV failure such as elevated jugular venous pressure, hepatomegaly, and edema of legs occur only in late stages. Cardiomegaly is minimal unless there is associated AR or LV dysfunction. The apical impulse is sustained (heaving) with a presystolic impulse (corresponding to S_4) due to strong atrial kick. A systolic thrill is generally felt in the aortic area and left sternal border, which may be transmitted to carotid arteries.

S_1 is usually normal; soft S_1 indicates LV dysfunction or prolonged PR interval due to extension of calcium into the conduction system. Prolonged LV ejection results in delayed closure of aortic valve; hence, the A_2 gets delayed resulting in single or even paradoxically split S_2 (difficult to appreciate as A_2 will be soft in severe rheumatic AS). Paradoxical splitting of S_2 becomes more obvious in presence of LV dysfunction or associated left bundle branch block. Prominent atrial kick to improve the ventricular filling produces a left ventricular S_4, which indicates severe stenosis in the absence of other causes for S_4. Presence of LV S_3 indicates LV systolic dysfunction. Constant aortic ejection click, common in congenital AS, is unusual in AS of rheumatic etiology. The typical murmur of AS is a loud medium-pitched harsh mid-systolic crescendo-decrescendo one conducted to the carotids. Long murmur with late systolic peaking indicates severe AS. When LV failure occurs, the murmur becomes softer and shorter and may even disappear. In elderly patients with calcified valve, the high-frequency component of the murmur tends to radiate toward the apex and may become musical mimicking MR murmur (Gallavardin phenomenon).[26] With variation in cycle length as in AF or presence of ectopics, the intensity of murmur varies in AS but not in MR.[27] Timing of the murmur is also useful—MR murmur usually starts with S_1 whereas the murmur of AS starts after S_1.

Electrocardiography

The main feature in ECG is the presence of LVH, which is seen in majority (85%) of patients with severe AS **(Fig. 19)**. The serial ECG changes as the severity increases are secondary ST–T changes in lateral leads (strain pattern), loss of septal vector (q in lateral leads) due to myocardial fibrosis, and widening of QRS with left axis; left atrial abnormality pattern is an additional finding. However, absence of LVH does not rule out severe AS. Calcification of aortic valve may extend into conduction system and various forms of conduction abnormalities may be seen—left bundle branch block, first degree AV heart block, or even complete AV block. AF is less common (10–15%) in isolated AS, but is more often seen when associated with mitral valve disease.

Radiological Findings

The chest X-ray may reveal normal or mildly enlarged heart size in general. Dilatation of ascending aorta may be seen. Calcification of aortic valve is better seen by fluoroscopy than in chest X-ray film. Left atrial enlargement and pulmonary venous hypertension features may be seen, but if these features are prominent, consider associated mitral valve disease. **Figure 20** shows the landmarks of the cardiac valves in X-ray.

Echocardiography

Echocardiography is the most useful noninvasive investigation for diagnosis, assessment of severity, evaluation for intervention, and follow-up of patients with AS. Accurate anatomical definition, etiology and severity of AS, presence and extent of calcification, annular dimension, associated valvular disease, and LV function all can be

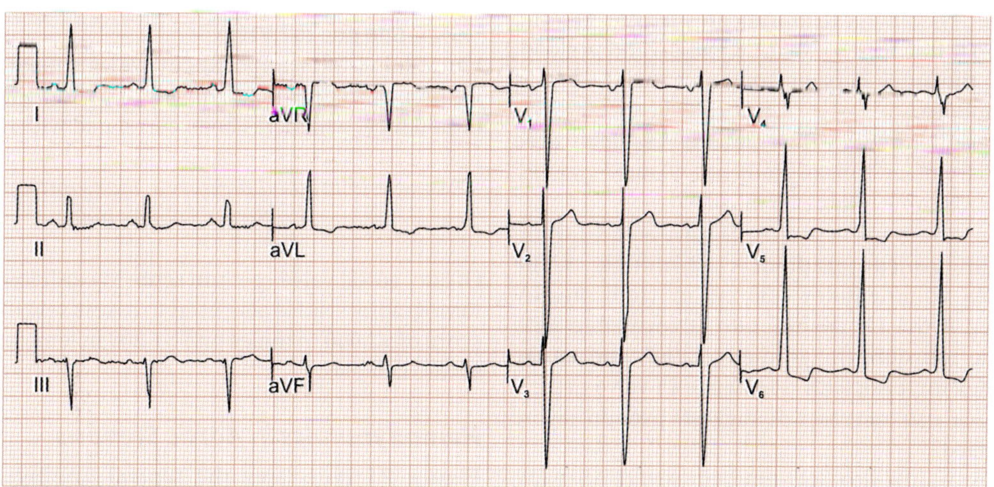

FIG. 19: ECG showing left ventricular hypertrophy with strain pattern in severe aortic stenosis; voltage criteria of LVH, ST–T changes of strain pattern, leftward QRS axis, loss of septal q in V_6, and left atrial abnormality of P wave in V_1.

(LVH: left ventricular hypertrophy)

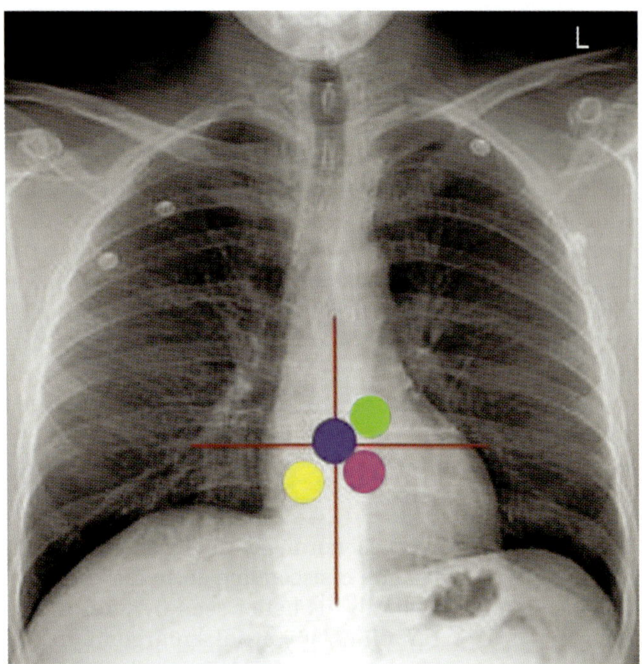

FIG. 20: Valve positions in X-ray. Draw two lines—horizontal line to bisect the cardiac chamber area and vertical midline. Purple is mitral valve, blue aortic valve, yellow tricuspid, and green pulmonary valve anatomy.

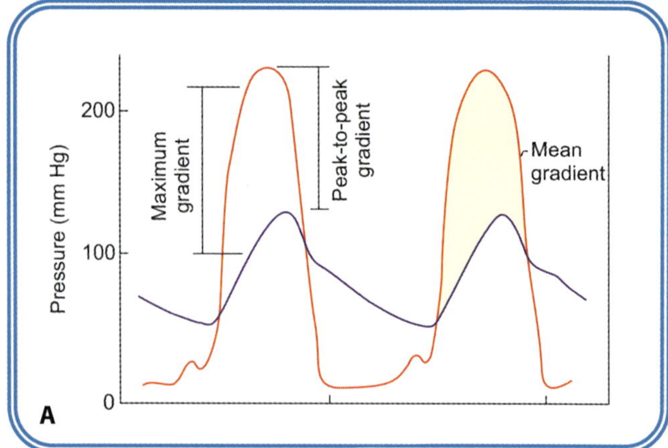

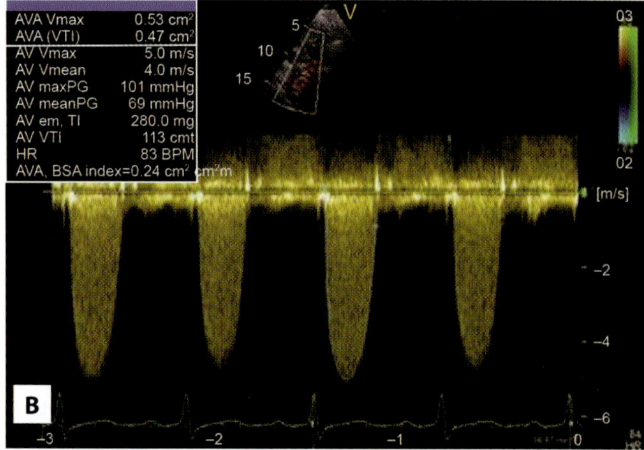

FIGS. 21A AND B: Pressure recordings and Doppler spectral trace in severe aortic stenosis

obtained by echocardiography. Doppler with color flow mapping is crucial in assessing the severity of the lesion—to plan the timing of intervention and to predict the prognosis. Echo parameters of severe AS are aortic valve peak velocity (V_{max}) ≥ 4 m/s, mean gradient ≥ 40 mm Hg, and valve area ≤ 1.0 cm^2 (≤0.6 cm^2/m^2); V_{max} ≥ 5 m/s and mean gradient ≥ 60 mm Hg indicate very severe AS. As the gradient can be influenced by flow, a ratio of LVOT velocity to aortic valve velocity (dimensionless index) is also a good parameter to assess the severity, value < 0.25 indicates severe AS. The gradient in AS is influenced by the LV function and preload. Based on this, the stage D (symptomatic severe) of AS is subdivided as follows:

- *D1*: High-gradient, high-flow severe AS–valve area ≤1.0 cm^2 (≤0.6 cm^2/m^2), mean gradient ≥ 40 mm Hg, LVEF ≥ 50%, stroke volume index ≥ 35 mL/m^2
- *D2*: Low-flow low-gradient severe AS–valve area ≤ 1.0 cm^2 (≤0.6 cm^2/m^2), mean gradient < 40 mm Hg, LVEF < 50%, stroke volume index < 35 mL/m^2 (indicates LV dysfunction; if the LV dysfunction is reversible with dobutamine infusion, the gradient, LVEF, and stroke volume index increase with no change in valve area. If the valve area also increases, it suggests pseudo severe aortic stenosis)
- *D3*: Paradoxical low-flow low-gradient severe AS–valve area ≤ 1.0 cm^2 (≤0.6 cm^2/m^2), mean gradient < 40 mm Hg, stroke volume index <35 mL/m^2, but LVEF ≥ 50% (reduced LV preload as in mitral valve disease, severe PH and right ventricular outflow obstruction, ventricular

septal defect or small LV cavity due to severe LVH reduce the stroke volume with preserved EF; in hypertension, gradient also decreases in addition to the low-stroke volume due to LVH)

Ventriculoarterial impedance (Zva) is a measure of the global LV hemodynamic load considering the valvular and aortic impedance, which has been correlated with prognosis:

Zva = Systolic blood pressure + Transaortic peak gradient/ Stroke volume index

Of late, aortic valve calcium score in cardiac computerized tomography scan is also used to assess severity; Agatson score of >2,000 in males and >1,200 in females indicate severe stenosis.

Hemodynamics in Aortic Stenosis

Figure 21 illustrates the typical findings—aortic valve gradient, slow rising aortic pulse, and prominent presystolic wave in LV pressure trace; pressure gradient across aortic valve is the hallmark of AS. Three types of gradient—peak to peak, peak instantaneous, and mean—are illustrated in the figure. Doppler echo picks up the peak instantaneous gradient and hence overestimates the value a little.

Indicators of Severe Aortic Stenosis

- *Clinical*: Typical symptoms, low-volume slow rising pulse, narrow pulse pressure, heaving apex, LV S_4 in the absence of other causes, delayed A_2, and long late peaking murmur
- *ECG*: LVH with strain pattern
- Echo Doppler parameters as discussed above

Natural history: Aortic stenosis even severe will remain asymptomatic for a long period. Once they develop symptoms, the deterioration is rapid; *average survival* after occurrence of angina is 5 years, syncope 3 years, and heart failure 1½ to 2 years. The rate of progression of stenosis is a reduction in valve area by 0.1 cm²/year, an increase in mean aortic gradient by 7 mm Hg/year and an increase in aortic valve velocity by 0.32 m/s/year.

TRICUSPID VALVE DISEASE

Tricuspid valve is the largest among the four cardiac valves, area ranging from 7 to 9 cm² in adults. Tricuspid valve disease of rheumatic etiology is relatively rare, occurs almost always with mitral valve disease and quite often with aortic valve involvement also. It is reported in about 15% of patients with RHD in autopsy series, but clinically diagnosed in only about 5% of patients.[10] A higher frequency of up to 33% in autopsy series has been reported from India.[29] Isolated pathologic involvement of tricuspid valve is unlikely to be of rheumatic etiology; consider other rare causes such as myxomatous degeneration, congenital, carcinoid syndrome, right ventricular endomyocardial fibrosis, infective endocarditis, Whipple's disease, atrial tumors, and pacemaker leads.

Tricuspid Stenosis

All patients with rheumatic TS will have associated TR and almost always mitral and aortic valve involvement. The valve pathology resembles that of MS with fusion of leaflets at their edges and fusion and shortening of chordae;[28] however, calcification is rare. Obstruction to RV inflow results in transtricuspid diastolic gradient with resultant rise in RA and systemic venous pressure. As TS is always associated with mitral valve disease, they have the symptoms such as dyspnea and orthopnea, but features of systemic venous congestion dominate—puffy face, abdominal distention, edema legs, and gastrointestinal symptoms. With tricuspid valve involvement, either stenosis or regurgitation, the forward flow to pulmonary circulation decreases leading to LA decompression thus attenuating the symptoms of mitral valve disease and AR (but aggravates the symptoms of AS); physical findings of mitral and aortic lesions will also be attenuated.

The physical findings are mostly of associated mitral and aortic lesions and hence the diagnosis of TS is often missed. Jugular venous pressure remains elevated with slow Y descend which is diagnostic for TS. Prominent A wave is seen if patient is in sinus rhythm, but often they will be in AF. Mid-diastolic murmur preceded by a sharp opening snap best heard along the lower left sternal border is the auscultatory hallmark. Compared to MS, the tricuspid diastolic murmur is relatively short, soft and higher pitched, and gets augmented by maneuvers, which increase venous return such as inspiration, passive leg raising, squatting, and Müller's maneuver. The lung fields will be clear despite engorged neck veins. Hepatomegaly with presystolic pulsation and ascites occur in later stages.

Electrocardiography may not be contributory as findings of mitral and aortic valve lesion dominate; however, in sinus rhythm, a disproportionate right atrial P wave is a clue. Huge RA enlargement can produce a qR pattern in lead V_1. Radiologically, huge RA and prominent superior vena cava shadow with less impressive pulmonary vasculature are the clues for tricuspid valve involvement **(Fig. 22)**.

Echocardiography

The echocardiographic features of TS resemble those of MS; thickening of tricuspid valve leaflets, doming motion of the valve, commissural fusion, and chordal thickening are all well delineated by echocardiography. Transesophageal echocardiography gives better delineation of the valve structure. Doppler findings are helpful. Normal diastolic

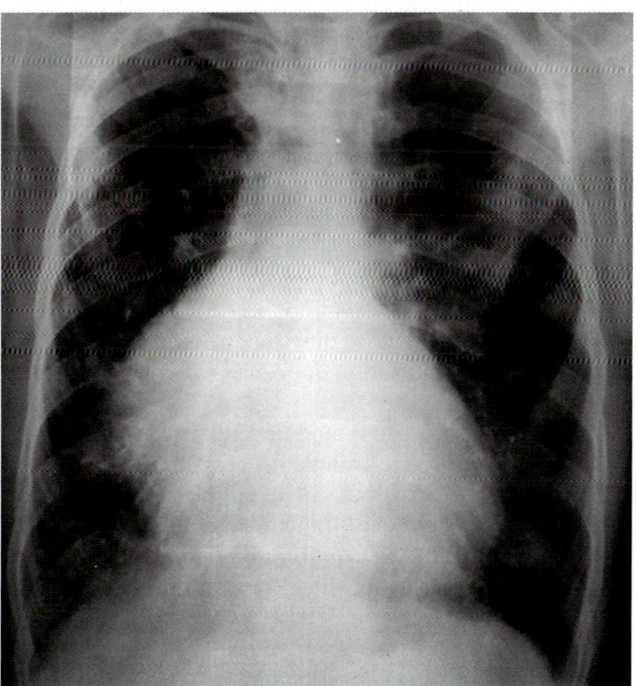

FIG. 22: Huge right atrium in tricuspid valve lesion.

velocity across tricuspid valve is <1 m/s. A mean diastolic gradient of as low as 2 mm Hg is enough to diagnose TS. No generally accepted grading of severity of TS is available; mean gradient of >5 mm Hg is accepted as significant TS.[2]

Tricuspid Regurgitation

Rheumatic TR could be primary (organic) due to structural abnormality of tricuspid valve apparatus or more often secondary (functional) due to dilatation of RV and annulus in patients with PH and RV dysfunction. Generally, if RV systolic pressure is >55 mm Hg, it will cause functional TR. Rheumatic fever affects tricuspid valve directly[30] causing scarring of valve leaflets and chordae tendineae resulting in restricted leaflet mobility leading to TR, or combined TS and TR and usually this will be associated with mitral valve disease.

Symptoms

Since in most patients with rheumatic TR, mitral valve disease is associated, the symptoms of mitral valve disease dominate with symptom of varying degrees of dyspnea; features of systemic venous congestion are striking as in TS. As in TS, the reduced forward flow to pulmonary circulation can decompress the LA. Some patients may complain of throbbing sensation in the neck due to jugular venous distention and prominent systolic V waves in the jugular veins.

Physical Findings

Loss of weight, jaundice, and cyanosis may be present in chronic severe TR. AF is quite frequent. Jugular veins are distended with tall V wave and prominent Y descend. As the degree of TR increases, the V wave encroaches the X′ descend and in severe cases, X′ descent is obliterated; V wave merges with the C wave to produce the CV wave (or S wave). A venous systolic thrill and a murmur may be present over jugular veins. RV dilatation displaces the apex laterally along with prominent left parasternal heave and RV epigastric pulsations. Systolic expansion of RA may rarely produce a right parasternal heave. Tender hepatomegaly with systolic pulsation is common in early phases, but may disappear in chronic cases due to development of cardiac cirrhosis. Systolic pulsation of eyeballs and head nodding have also been described.

S_1 is unremarkable; it is modified by various factors such as associated left heart lesions, PA pressure, RV function, and bundle branch block. Isolated TR (unlikely to be rheumatic) with normal RV function results in reduced RV ejection time and hence can produce early P_2 (mechanism similar to the early A_2 in MR). RV S_3 indicates severe TR or RV systolic dysfunction. The characteristic auscultatory finding of TR is the soft systolic murmur along left sternal border, which increases with inspiration due to the increase in venous return and more importantly due to the annular dilatation. Based on RV systolic pressure, TR can be

BOX 5	Echocardiographic parameters of severe tricuspid regurgitation.

- Color regurgitant jet area ≥ 50% of right atrium area
- Vena contracta ≥ 0.7 cm
- Effective regurgitant orifice ≥ 0.4 cm^2
- Regurgitant volume ≥ 45 mL/beat
- Systolic wave flow reversal in hepatic vein
- Dense full continuous triangular-shaped spectral trace

divided as hypertensive (with PS or PH) or normotensive. Hypertensive TR murmur is a high-pitched pansystolic one, whereas the normotensive is soft and early systolic (as RA pressure rises in the latter part of systole reducing the RV > RA systolic gradient). Maneuvers, which increase the venous return, augment the TR murmur; this is better appreciated in normotensive TR. When the RV is dilated greatly and occupies apical position, the murmur may be head at the apex also and can be mistaken for MR murmur.

Electrocardiogram

Atrial fibrillation is quite frequent; features of RV volume overload such as incomplete right bundle branch block or evidence of RVH are common. qR pattern in V_1 and very tall P waves with long PR segment due to prolonged intra-atrial conduction (P width/PR segment of < 1.0—Macruz index) in sinus rhythm are characteristic of huge RA.

Radiological Findings

Magnitude of the RA dilatation, SVC prominence, and distended azygos entry to SVC correlate with the severity of TR. Features of left heart lesion and of PH are seen in secondary TR. Right-sided pleural effusion is common. On fluoroscopy, systolic pulsation of RA may be seen.

Echocardiography

Echocardiography gives clear information regarding presence of TR, its severity and etiology, PA pressure, RV function, presence and severity of associated lesions, and indication for intervention. RA and RV are enlarged, the magnitude depends on the severity of TR. RV volume overload may produce paradoxical interventricular septal motion in early systole. Interatrial septum may be pushed to left side when the RA pressure exceeds the LA pressure. Continuous Doppler imaging measures TR jet velocity from which RV–RA pressure gradient and RV systolic pressure can be deducted. The features suggestive of severe TR are illustrated in **Box 5**.[1]

Pulmonary Valve Lesions

Pulmonary valve lesions are extremely rare (<4%) in RHD and is always associated with other valve lesions (refer topics on congenital heart disease for pulmonary valve lesions).

MULTIVALVULAR DISEASE

Involvement of multiple valves or combination of stenotic and regurgitant lesions in the same valve is commonly seen with rheumatic etiology; different combinations of valve lesions can occur. The clinical manifestations depend on relative severity of each of these lesions. The manifestations of the proximal valve lesion dominate as proximal lesion modifies the hemodynamics of the distal lesion. Recognition of multivalvular lesions is important because failure to correct all significant lesions may increase the mortality. Clinical examination alone may not be helpful in full assessment. Echo Doppler studies and other investigations are needed for complete evaluation. In some patients, hemodynamic studies by cardiac catheterization and angiography may be needed.

Mitral Stenosis plus Aortic Regurgitation

Nearly two-thirds of patients with MS have features of AR, with majority (90%) having mild AR which will not have much clinical significance. In about 10% of patients with MS, the AR is severe.[31] Severe MS with PH reduces the LV preload and thus can attenuate the clinical findings of AR except the low-diastolic blood pressure, but echo Doppler parameters of severe AR are not significantly affected. The effect of the AR jet striking the anterior mitral leaflet dampens the opening snap of MS. In the presence of severe AR, the LV diastolic pressure rises reducing the LA–LV gradient thereby under assessing the severity of MS by the usual echo parameters; planimetry and continuity equation are more reliable. How to assess the mid diastolic murmur over apex—MS versus Austin Flint—has been outlined earlier.

Mitral Stenosis plus Aortic Stenosis

Significant MS reduces the LV diastolic volume and the stroke volume;[31] hence, the symptoms of AS get exaggerated but the clinical findings become less impressive. The intensity and duration of mid-systolic murmur of AS get attenuated. In presence of severe AS, the LV diastolic pressure goes up, which modifies the hemodynamics of MS as in the case of associated AR. As the isovolumetric time is prolonged due to impaired relaxation, the A_2-OS interval and the mitral diastolic murmur get delayed. Echo Doppler studies help in diagnosing combined lesions.

Mitral Stenosis plus Regurgitation

The most common valvular lesion in RHD is mixed mitral valve lesion with dominance of either stenosis or regurgitation. Diagnosis of presence of MR is easy clinically by the presence of the murmur of MR; diastolic thrill, loud S_1, OS, and presystolic murmur favor associated MS. LV S_3 and decrescendo MDM without presystolic component suggest isolated severe MR. In mixed lesion LV type cardiomegaly, huge LA in X-ray and LV dominance in ECG favor dominant MR; absence of LV enlargement, severe PH, modest enlargement of LA, and right ward QRS axis suggest dominant MS. The issue to be sorted out is whether either or both lesions are hemodynamically significant and not which is dominant; this can be easily settled by a meticulous echo Doppler evaluation for planning the management protocol.

Aortic Stenosis plus Mitral Regurgitation

This combination is commonly seen with rheumatic etiology (however, mild-to-moderate secondary MR can occur in severe AS due to the high LV systolic pressure). The high LV systolic pressure of AS aggravates MR; hence, symptoms, signs, and radiological and echocardiographic findings of MR will be exaggerated. Severe MR reduces the forward stroke volume leading to aggravation of symptoms of AS, but the physical findings and echocardiographic parameters of AS will be attenuated. Mitral valve disease is one of the causes for paradoxical low-flow low-gradient AS.

Aortic Regurgitation plus Mitral Regurgitation

This combination is not infrequent in rheumatic etiology. There will be marked dilatation of LV. Usually, the clinical features of AR will dominate. The large LV volume with mitral annular dilatation and high LV systolic pressure of AR augment MR. As AR is a diastolic event, MR does not significantly modify the hemodynamics of AR except for the reduction in the stroke volume. Whether MR is secondary to LV dilatation or primary due to valve pathology needs to be assessed. Echo Doppler studies will help in the proper assessment.

Aortic Regurgitation plus Aortic Stenosis

The problem is same as in combination of MS and regurgitation. Diagnosis of mild AR in presence of severe AS is easy as findings of AS dominate with an audible EDM; the diastolic blood pressure and pulse pressure give us a clue whether the AR is mild or moderate. However, bedside diagnosis of AS in presence of severe AR may be difficult as the high-stroke volume of AR produces a prominent midsystolic murmur over aortic area; presence of slow upstroke of arterial pulse, sustained apex, systolic thrill, LV S_4, and long midsystolic murmur with late peaking favor associated significant stenosis. Echo evaluation of severity of AR is not that difficult, but assessment of severity of AS in presence of significant AR has limitations. Gradient is exaggerated by the high-stroke volume (high-flow high-gradient AS); hence, flow-independent parameters such as dimensionless index and planimetry have to be considered for assessing the severity of the obstruction.

Other Combined Lesions

Tricuspid valve lesions significantly modify the left heart lesions. In both TR and TS, the forward stroke volume to pulmonary circulation and thus to the left heart decreases thereby masking the symptoms and physical findings of MS, MR, and AR. Physical findings of AS get attenuated at the expense of worsening symptoms.

■ CONCLUSION

The cornerstone of clinical diagnosis is clinical history and physical examination. A proper detailed history and systematic clinical examination direct the clinician for appropriate investigations to make the correct diagnosis and plan the definite management protocol. The value of time taken to perform a physical examination in establishing and continuing the rapport of the physician–patient relationship should not be underestimated.

■ REFERENCES

1. Otto CM, Nishimura RA, Bonow RO, Carabello BA, Erwin JP, Gentile F, et al. 2020 ACC/AHA guideline for management of patients with valvular heart disease. Circulation. 2021;143:e1-156.

2. Vahanian A, Beyersdorf F, Praz F, Milojevic M, Bladus S, Bauersachs J, et al. 2021 ESC/EACTS Guidelines for the management of valvular heart disease. Eur Heart J. 2022;43:561-632.

3. Carmel MH, Brian PG. Physical Examination in Valvular Heart Disease. In: Joseph SA, James ED, Shahbudin HR (Eds). Valvular Heart Disease, 3rd edition. Philadelphia: Lippincott Williams & Wilkins; 2000. pp. 73-92.

4. Fang JC, O'Gara PT. History and Physical examination: An Evidence-Based Approach. In: Libby P, Bonow RO, Mann D, Tomaselli GF, Bhatt D, Solomon SD (Eds). Braunwald's Heart Disease: A Text Book of Cardiovascular Medicine, 12th edition. Amsterdam: Elsevier Inc; 2022. pp. 123-40.

5. Michael HG, Robert SB, Lloyd YT, Sable CA, Shulman ST, Carapetis J, et al. Revision of Jones Criteria for Diagnosis of Acute Rheumatic Fever in the Era of Doppler echocardiography—AHA Scientific Statement. Circulation. 2015;131:1806-18.

6. Krishnakumar R, Antunes MJ, Beaton A. Management of rheumatic heart disease: implications for closing the gap—AHA Scientific Statement. Circulation. 2020;142:e1-21.

7. Vasan RS, Srivastava S, Vijayakumar M, Narang R, Lister BC, Narula J. Echocardiographic evaluation of patients with acute rheumatic fever and rheumatic carditis. Circulation. 1996;94:73-82.

8. Wilson MJ, Neutze JM. Echocardiographic diagnosis of subclinical carditis in acute rheumatic fever. Int J Cardiol. 1995;50:1-6.

9. Soma Raju B, Zoltan GT. Rheumatic fever. In: Libby P, Bonow RO, Mann DL, Zipes DP (Eds). Braunwald's Heart Disease: A textbook of cardiovascular medicine. Philladelphia: Saunders; 2008. pp. 2079-86.

10. Chandrasekhar TS. Mitral Stenosis. In: Libby P, Bonow RO, Mann D, Tomaselli GF, Bhatt D, Solomon SD (Eds). Braunwald's Heart Disease: A text book of cardiovascular medicine, 12th edition. Amsterdam: Elsevier Inc; 2022. pp. 1441-54.

11. Kitchin A, Turner R. Diagnosis and treatment of tricuspid stenosis. Br Heart J. 1984;26:54-79.

12. Krishnan MN, Harikrishnan S, Gopalakrishnan A, Ahamed SZ, Deepti S, Naik N. Valvular Heart Disease. In: Prabhakaran D, Kumar RK, Naik N, Kaul U (Eds). Tandon's Text Book of Cardiology. New Delhi: Wolters Kluwer; 2019. pp. 1076-142.

13. Roy SB, Bhatia ML, Lazaro EJ, Ramalinga Swamy V. Juvenile mitral stenosis in India. Lancet. 1963;2:1193-5.

14. Otto CM. Mitral Stenosis. In: Otto CM (Ed). Valvular Heart Disease, 2nd edition. Philadelphia: Saunders; 2004. pp. 252-5.

15. Shaw TR, Sutaria N, Prendergast B. Clinical and hemodynamic profiles of young, middle aged and elderly patients with mitral stenosis undergoing mitral balloon valvotomy. Heart. 2003;89:1430-60.

16. Criley JM, Hermer AJ. The Crescendo presystolic murmur of mitral stenosis with atrial fibrillation. N Engl J Med. 1971;285:1284.

17. Iga K, Tomonaga G, Hori K. Continuous murmur in Lutembacher syndrome analysed by Doppler echocardiology. Chest. 1992;101:565-6.

18. Merendino KA, Hessel EA 2nd. The "murmur on top of the head" in acquired mitral insufficiency. Pathological and clinical significance. JAMA. 1967;199(12):892-6.

19. Enriquez–Sarano M, Schaff HV, Tajik AJ, et al. Chronic mitral regurgitation. In: Alpert JS, Dalen JE, Rahimtoola SH (Eds). Valvular Heart Disease, 3rd edition. Philadelphia: Lippincott Williams & Wilkins; 2000. pp. 113-42.

20. Enriquez–Sarano M, Avierinos JF, Messika–Zeitoun D, Detaint D, Capps M, Nkomo V, et al. Quantitative determinants of the outcome of asymptomatic mitral regurgitation. N Engl J Med. 2005;352:875-83.

21. Carabello BA. Progress in mitral and aortic regurgitation. Prog Cardiovasc Dis. 2001;43:457-75.

22. Bonow RO. Chronic aortic regurgitation. In: Alpert JS, Dalen JE, Rahimtoola SH, (Eds). Valvular Heart Disease, 3rd edition. Philadelphia: Lippincott Williams and Wilkins; 2000. pp. 245-68.

23. Otto CM. Aortic regurgitation. In: Otto CM (Ed). Valvular Heart Disease, 2nd edition. Philadelphia: Saunders; 2004. pp. 302-35.

24. Carabello BA. Evaluation and management of patients with aortic stenosis. Circulation. 2002;105:1746-50.

25. Gould KL, Carabello BA. Why angina in aortic stenosis with normal coronary arteriograms? Circulation. 2003;107:3121-3.

26. Bruns DL. A general theory of causes of murmur in the cardiovascular system. Am J Med. 1959;27:360-74.

27. Karliner JS, O' Rourke RA, Kearney J, Shabetai R. Hemodynamic explanation of why murmur of mitral regurgitation is independent of cycle length. Br Heart J. 1973;35:397-401.

28. Ewy GA. Tricuspid valve disease. In Alpert JS Dalen JE, Rahimtoola SH (Eds). Valvular Heart Disease, 3rd edition. Philadelphia: Lippincott Williams and Wilkins; 2000. pp. 377-92.

29. Mahapathra RK, Agarwal JB, Wasir HS. Rheumatic tricuspid stenosis. Indian Heart J. 1978;30:134-43.

30. Otto CM. Right sided valve disease. In: Otto CM (Ed). Valvular Heart Disease, 2nd edition. Philadelphia: Saunders; 2004. pp. 415-36.

31. Paraskos JA. Combined valve disease. In: Alpert JS, Dalen JE, Rahimtoola SH (Eds). Valvular Heart Disese, 3rd edition. Philadelphia: Lippincott Williams & Wilkins; 2000. pp. 291-337.

SUGGESTED READINGS

1. Chandrashekara Rao AS. Left parasternal heave. Karnataka J Med Science. 1998;1:75-6.

2. Craige E. Should auscultation be rehabilitated? N Engl J Med. 1998;318:1611-3.

3. Rao ASC. Auscultation in the new millennium. J Assoc Physicians India. 2001;49:731-3.

4. O'Brein KP, Cohen LS. Hemodynamic and phonocardiographic correlates of Austin Flint murmur. Am Heart J. 1969;77:603-9.

5. Fortuin NJ, Craige E. On the mechanism of Austin Flint murmur. Circulation. 1972;45:558-70.

6. Lochaya S, Igarashi M, Shaffer AB. Late diastolic mitral regurgitation secondary to aortic regurgitation: Its relationship to the Austin Flint murmur. Am Heart J. 1967;74:161-9.

7. Wooley CF, Fontana ME, Kilaman JW, Ryan JM. Tricuspid stenosis. Atrial systolic murmur, tricuspid opening snap and right atrial pressure pulse. Am J Med. 1995;78:375-84.

8. Gershlick AH, Leach G, Mills PG, Leatham A. The loud first sound in atrial myxoma. Br Heart J. 1984;52:403-7.

9. Green EW, Agruss NS, Adolph RJ. Right-sided Austin Flint murmur. Documentation by intracardiac phonocardiography, echocardiography and postmortem findings. Am J Cardiol. 1973;32:370-4.

10. Gold Farb B, Wang Y. Mitral stenosis and left to right shunt at the artial level. A broadened concept of Lutembacher syndrome. Am J Cardiol. 1966;17:319.

11. Gertsch M. ECG: A two-step approach to diagnosis, 1st edition. Berlin, Heidelberg: Springer-Verlag; 2004. p. 363.

12. Zoghbi WA, Enriquez-Sarano M, Foster E, Grayburn PA, Kraft CD, Levine RA, et al. Recommendations for the evaluation of the severity of native valvular regurgitation with two dimensional and Doppler echocardiography. J Am Soc Echocardiogr. 2003;37: 777-802.

13. Sagie A, Freitas N, Chen MH, Marshall JE, Weyman AE, Levine RA. Echocardiographic assessment of mitral stenosis and its associated valvular lesions in 205 patients and lack of association with mitral valve prolapse. J Am Soc Echocardiogr. 1997;10:141-8.

14. Wilkins GT, Wayeman AL, Abscal VM, Block PC, Palacios IF. Percutaneous balloon dilatation of mitral valve. An analysis of echocardiographic variables related to outcome and the mechanism of dilatation. Br Heart J. 1988;60:299-308.

15. Reimold SC, Rutherford JD. Valvular heart disease in pregnancy. N Engl J Med. 2003;349:52-9.

16. Hameed A, Karaalp IS, Tummala PP, Wani OR, Canetti M, Akhter MW, et al. The effect of valvular heart disease on the maternal and fetal out comes in pregnancy. J Am Coll Cardiol. 2001;37:893-9.

17. Kinsara AJ, Ismail O, Fawzi ME. Effect of balloon mitral valvuloplasty during preganancy on childhood development. Cardiol. 2002;97:155.

18. Kadem L, Dumesnil JG, Rieu R, Durand LG, Garcia D, Pibarot P. Impact of systemic hypertension on the assessment of patients with aortic stenosis. Heart. 2005;91:354-61.

19. Otto CM. Valvular aortic stenosis: Disease severity and timing of intervention. J Am Coll Cardiol. 2006;42:2141-51.

20. Hauck AJ, Freeman DP, Ackermann DM, Danielson GK, Edwards WD. Surgical pathology of tricuspid valve. A study of 363 cases spanning 25 years. Mayo Clin Proc. 1988;63:851-63.

21. Ha JW, Chung N, Jang Y, Rim SJ. Tricuspid stenosis and regurgitation. Doppler and color flow echocardiography and cardiac catheterization findings. Clin Cardiol. 2000;23:51-2.

22. El-Sherif N. Rheumatic tricuspid stenosis. A haemodynamic correlation. Br Heart J. 1971;33:16-31.

13

Role of Echocardiography in Rheumatic Heart Disease

IB Vijayalakshmi, Chitra Narasimhan

> *"The faculties developed by doing research are those most needed in diagnosis."*
>
> —**Francis Heed Adler** (1895–1975)
> US Ophthalmologist and Researcher, Philadelphia

INTRODUCTION

The long-term sequelae of acute rheumatic fever (ARF) is chronic rheumatic heart disease (RHD) continues to be a major health hazard in most developing countries like India.[1] The RHD is a neglected giant in children, adolescents, and young adults in India. It is estimated that globally >40 million people are affected by RHD and over 3 lakh die annually—by WHO Bulletin-2018. Nearly 60% of deaths are premature. Globally, India has the highest prevalence rate (27%), contributes nearly 25–50% of newly diagnosed cases, hospitalizations and deaths due to RHD—by WHO bulletin-2015. Unfortunately, India is in the phase of "epidemiological transition". On one hand there is a substantial burden due to RHD, on the other hand resources are scarce to treat the patients with RHD. The chronic RHD patients develop valve stenosis such as mitral stenosis, aortic stenosis, tricuspid stenosis with varying degrees of regurgitation of these valves. As a consequence to these valvular diseases they may develop atrial dilatation, atrial fibrillation, ventricular dilatation, ventricular dysfunction, and ultimately congestive heart failure (CHF). Echocardiography (ECHO) is the best noninvasive modality to assess the valvular lesions in RHD patients. Hence, it is very important to know echocardiographic features in RHD to diagnose and follow-up the cases for management at appropriate time.

BACKGROUND

Echocardiography with Doppler imaging is a noninvasive essential key tool for the diagnosis and evaluation of RHD. Assessment of the etiology, severity, hemodynamic consequences, and ventricular response to valvular abnormalities can be made out using appropriate echocardiographic techniques. ECHO also plays an important role in therapeutic decision making and provides prognostic information. In addition to two-dimensional (2D) ECHO, Doppler, transesophageal echocardiography (TEE) and three-dimensional (3D), and four-dimensional (4D) ECHO improve the precision in diagnosis and periprocedural or surgical management. It remains the principal modality for the diagnosis and follow-up of patients with multivalvular heart disease.

MITRAL STENOSIS

The most common cause of mitral stenosis (MS) worldwide is RHD. It is an important cause of cardiovascular morbidity and mortality especially in women. MS is an obstruction to left ventricular (LV) inflow at the level of the mitral valve (MV) as a result of a structural abnormality of the MV apparatus, which prevents proper opening during diastolic filling of the left ventricle (LV). In Wood's series, the latency period from

ARF until the onset of cardiac symptoms of MS was 19 years.[2] The youngest patient of RHD with MS with a mitral valve orifice area (MVOA) of 0.6 cm^2 and with combined tricuspid stenosis, was seen by us in a 2-year-3-month-old child. Isolated MS occurs in 40% of all patients presenting with RHD and a history of ARF can be elicited from approximately 60% of patients presenting with pure MS.[2,3] Isolated MS is twice as common in women as in men. Acquired causes of MV obstruction, other than RHD, are extremely rare. These include left atrial (LA) myxoma, ball valve thrombus, mucopolysaccharidosis, and severe annular calcification. All these conditions are easily distinguished from rheumatic MS by ECHO and Doppler.

Therapeutic decision making is based on ECHO assessment of the severity of valve stenosis. The pathological process in patients with MS due to RHD causes leaflet thickening, reduced mobility, commissural fusion, chordal fusion, and calcification or a combination of these processes. Instead of the normal fish mouth like mitral orifice, the orifice appears funnel shaped with a decrease in mitral valve area (MVA). Interchordal fusion obliterates the secondary orifices and commissural fusion narrows the principal orifice.[4,5] A normal MV area is 4.0–5.0 cm^2 in children, and 6.0 cm^2 in adults. Symptoms usually develop when the valve area decreases below 1.5 cm^2 and also below 2.5 cm^2, particularly when the heart rate is more, as during exercise.[6] Rheumatic mitral disease is often, but not always accompanied by rheumatic involvement of the aortic and tricuspid valves. For example, we had a case of RHD with critical MS with associated dextrocardia with bicuspid aortic valve with severe stenosis. RHD with MS associated with congenital atrial septal defect is called as "Lutembacher's syndrome".

Echocardiography is critical in the assessment of RHD with MS. 2D-ECHO will reveal the morphology of the MV, and allows determination of the parts of the MV apparatus that are involved. Doppler ECHO assesses the hemodynamic severity of MS, estimates pulmonary artery systolic pressure from the tricuspid regurgitation (TR) velocity signal, and assesses severity of concomitant mitral regurgitation (MR) or aortic regurgitation (AR). Hemodynamic exercise testing can be done using either a supine bicycle or an upright treadmill, with Doppler recordings of transmitral and tricuspid velocities. Recommendations for ECHO in MS are listed in **Table 1**.

Mitral valve is usually imaged by ECHO in the three primary planes:
1. The primary view to record the MV is the parasternal long-axis view **(Fig. 1A)**.
2. The MVOA is recorded in the parasternal short axis of the LV at the MV level **(Fig. 1B)**.
3. The third view is the apical four chamber view **(Fig. 1C)**.

Assessment of Mitral Valve

The ECHO is used to assess the morphology of the MV including mobility, thickness, and calcification of leaflets;

TABLE 1: Recommendations for echocardiography in mitral stenosis.[6]	
Class I	1. Echocardiography should be performed in patients for the diagnosis of MS, assessment of hemodynamic severity (mean gradient, MV area, and pulmonary artery pressure), assessment of concomitant valvular lesions, and assessment of valve morphology (to determine suitability for balloon mitral valvotomy) *(Level of Evidence: B)*
	2. Echocardiography should be performed for re-evaluation in patients with known MS and changing symptoms or signs *(Level of Evidence: B)*
	3. Echocardiography should be performed for assessment of the hemodynamic response of the mean gradient and pulmonary artery pressure by exercise Doppler echocardiography in patients with MS when there is a discrepancy between resting Doppler echocardiographic findings, clinical findings, symptoms, and signs *(Level of Evidence: C)*
	4. Transesophageal echocardiography in MS should be performed to assess the presence or absence of left atrial appendage thrombus and to further evaluate the severity of MR in patients considered for percutaneous mitral balloon valvotomy *(Level of Evidence: C)*
	5. Transesophageal echocardiography in MS should be performed to evaluate MV morphology and hemodynamics in patients when transthoracic echocardiography provides suboptimal data *(Level of Evidence: C)*
Class IIa	Echocardiography is reasonable in the re-evaluation of asymptomatic patients with MS and stable clinical findings to assess pulmonary artery pressure (for those with severe MS, every year; moderate MS, every 1–2 years and mild MS, every 3–5 years) *(Level of Evidence: C)*
Class III	Transesophageal echocardiography in the patient with MS is not indicated for routine evaluation of MV morphology and hemodynamics when complete transthoracic echocardiographic data are satisfactory *(Level of Evidence: C)*

(MR: mitral regurgitation; MS: mitral stenosis; MV: mitral valve)

subvalvular and commissural fusion. These features are important in considering the timing and type of intervention. The characteristic features of MS by 2D ECHO imaging are:[7-10]
- Thickened and deformed mitral leaflets with increased echogenicity **(Fig. 2A)**
- Fusion of the commissures
- Reduced diastolic excursion of the mitral leaflets especially posterior mitral leaflet (PML)
- Reduction in the MVOA
- Submitral fusion with stenosis **(Fig. 2B)**

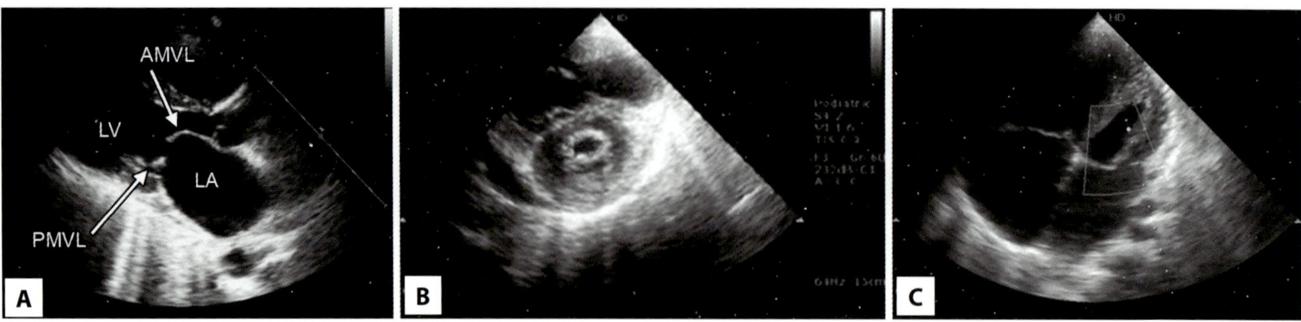

FIGS. 1A TO C: (A) Transthoracic echocardiography (TTE) in parasternal long-axis view shows thickened, deformed, and diastolic doming of anterior mitral leaflet (AML) with dilated left atrium (LA) in a case of mitral stenosis (MS) in a 15-year-old boy. (B) Parasternal short-axis view of the left ventricle at the mitral valve level shows fusion of both commissures with reduced mitral valve orifice area (MVOA) 0.7 cm². (C) Apical four-chamber view with dilated right atrium (RA) and right ventricle (RV) with dysfunction with small under filled left ventricle (LV) in a 12-year-old juvenile MS patient.

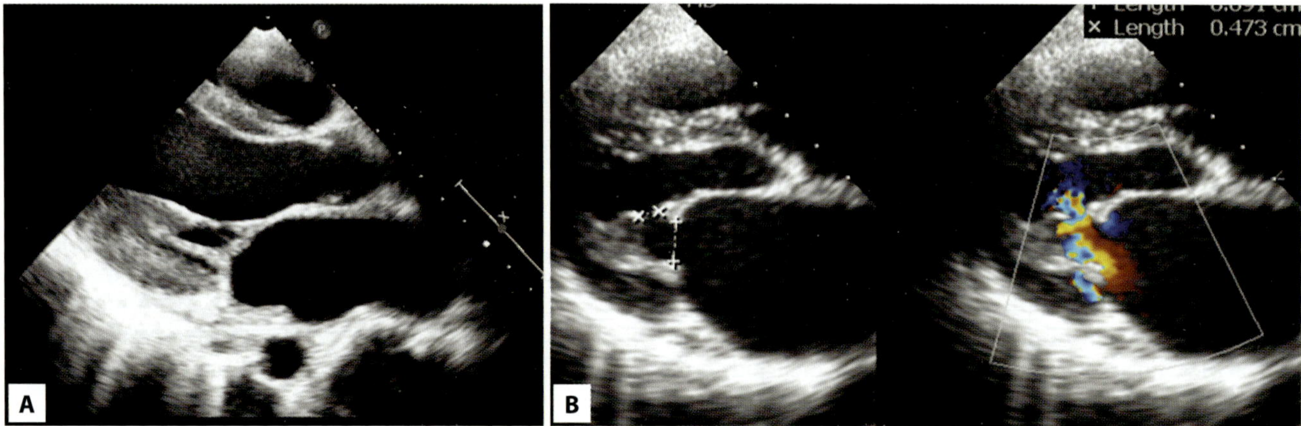

FIGS. 2A AND B: Parasternal long-axis (PLX) view shows thickened, deformed mitral leaflets with increased echogenicity of valve and submitral structures. (B) PLX view in diastole with color compare shows reduced diastolic excursion of the mitral leaflets especially PML with reduction in the mitral valve orifice area as well as very narrow submitral orifice.

With advances in 2D ECHO, the M mode is less routinely used in the evaluation of MS. Normal M mode of MV shows M pattern of anterior mitral leaflet (AML) and W pattern of PML as shown in **Figure 3A**. The characteristic M-mode findings of MS include increased echogenicity of the leaflets, a decreased E–F slope of MV **(Fig. 3B)**, anterior motion of the PML in early diastole, maintenance of fixed relationship of the two leaflets to each other throughout diastole, loss of M pattern of AML and W pattern of PML loss of A wave in the patients with normal sinus rhythm and in atrial fibrillation with irregular fast ventricular rate **(Fig. 3C)**, calcification of mitral valve and enlarged left atrium.[11] The decreased E–F slope, which is due to the decreased rate of diastolic closing of the AML, is nonspecific; however, it may also be present in the setting of impaired LV filling due to diastolic dysfunction.[12] The abnormal motion of the leaflets is apparent in early diastole. Fusion of commissures causes restriction in the motion of the tip of the anterior leaflet. However in the early phase of rheumatic process, the body of the anterior leaflet is pliable and continues to move anteriorly during diastole. This produces a dome-shaped leaflet, convex toward the interventricular septum **(Fig. 1A)**. With progressive fibrosis and calcification, the anterior leaflet becomes rigid and moves abruptly without appearing domed.[11]

Echocardiographically MS is characterized by diastolic doming of the AML **(Fig. 4A)**, with MV prolapse of only the tip producing "hockey stick" deformity **(Fig. 4B)**, fusion of the valve commissures and varying degrees of leaflet thickening, chordal involvement and with or without calcification.

Commissural fusion is assessed from the parasternal short-axis view. In short axis, the orifice of the MV appears funnel-shaped as opposed to a normal fish-mouth appearance **(Figs. 5A and B)** and the degree of commissural fusion can be best appreciated in this view and measure the MVOA **(Fig. 5C)**. In patients with severe valve deformity commissural anatomy may be difficult to assess and may be better visualized using real-time 3D ECHO.[13] Commissural fusion is an important feature to distinguish rheumatic MS from degenerative MS and to check the consistency of severity.

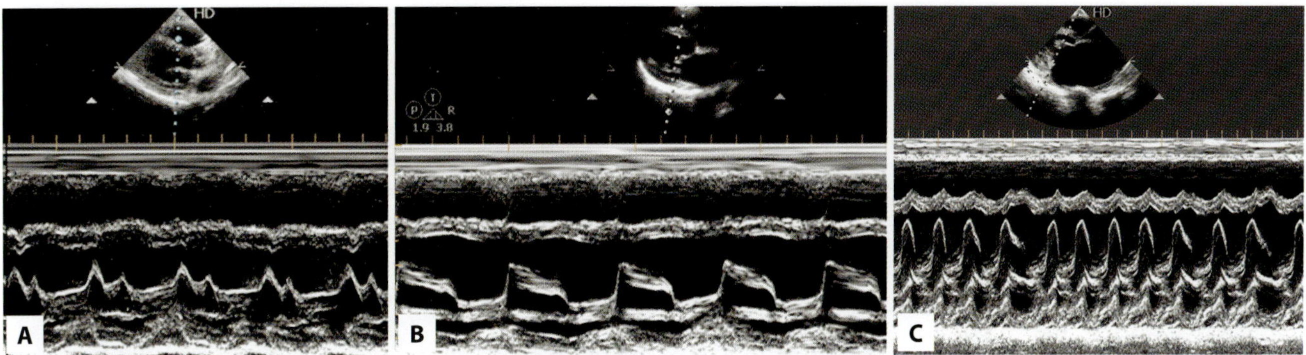

FIGS. 3A TO C: (A) M-mode of normal MV shows the M pattern of anterior mitral leaflet (AML) and W pattern of posterior mitral leaflet (PML); (B) increased echogenicity of AML and PML with decreased E-F slope of MV with loss of M pattern of AML and W pattern of PML in a case of MS; (C) M-mode of MV in a case of MS with atrial fibrillation with fast ventricular rate.

(MS: mitral stenosis; MV: mitral valve)

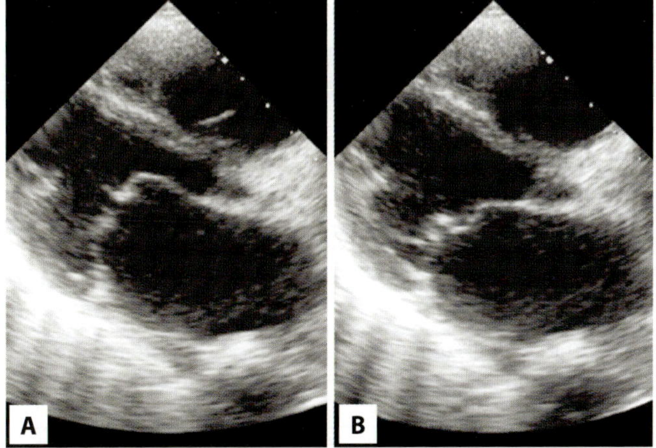

FIGS. 4A AND B: (A) Parasternal long-axis view shows diastolic doming of anterior mitral leaflet; (B) Shows "hockey stick" deformity.

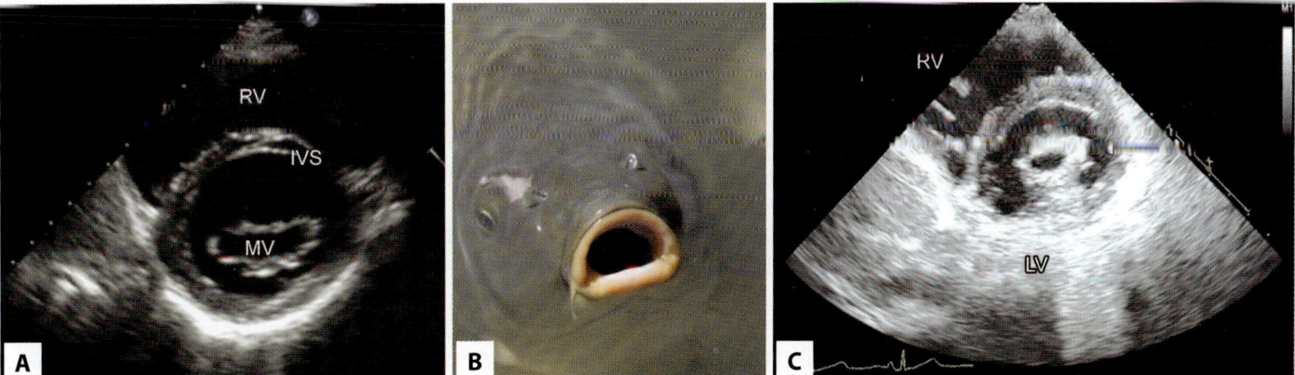

FIGS. 5A TO C: (A and B) Parasternal short-axis view shows normal MV with fish-mouth appearance; (C) Shows critical MS with commissural fusion and MVOA of 0.4 cm^2.

(MS: mitral stenosis; MV: mitral valve; MVOA: mitral valve orifice area)

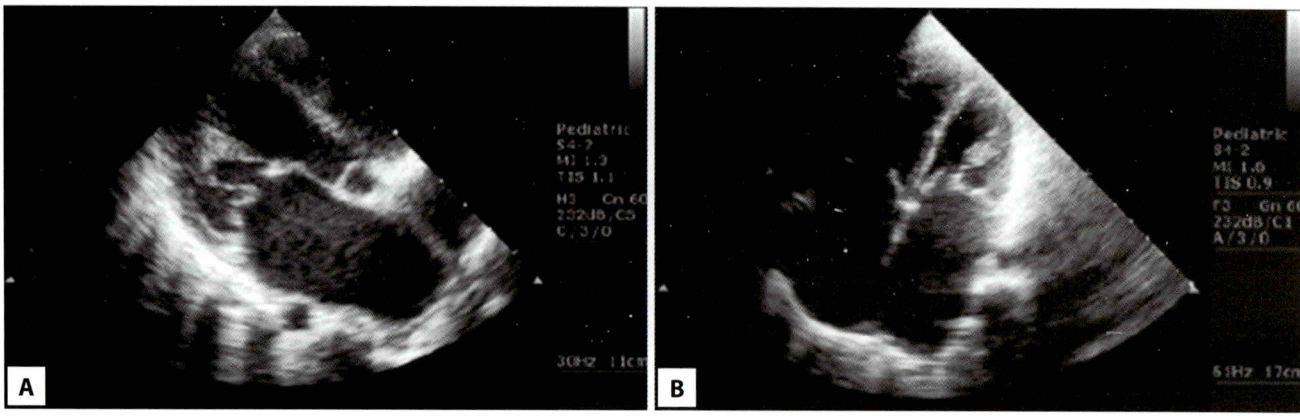

FIGS. 6A AND B: (A) Parasternal long-axis view shows hyperechogenic thick-fused chordae with dilated LA; (B). Apical four-chamber views chordal shortening and thickening with fusion of both papillary muscles almost looking like single papillary muscle with dilated LA, RA, and RV.

(LA: left atrium; RA: right atrium; RV: right ventricle)

TABLE 2: Assessment of mitral valve anatomy according to Wilkins score.[15]				
Grade	**Mobility**	**Thickening**	**Subvalvular thickening**	**Calcification**
1	Highly mobile valve with only leaflet tips restricted	Leaflets near normal in thickness (4–5 mm)	Minimal thickening just below the mitral leaflets	A single area of increased ECHO brightness
2	Leaflet mid and base portions have normal mobility	Mid-leaflets normal, considerable thickening of margins (5–8 mm)	Thickening of chordal structures extending up to one-third of the chordal length	Scattered areas of brightness confined to leaflet margins
3	Valve continues to move forward in diastole, mainly from the base	Thickening extending through the entire leaflet (5–8 mm)	Thickening extending to the distal third of the chords	Brightness extending into the mid-portion of the leaflets
4	No or minimal forward movement of the leaflets in diastole	Considerable thickening of all leaflet tissue (>8–10 mm)	Extensive thickening and shortening of all chordal structures extending down to the papillary muscles	Extensive brightness throughout much of the leaflet tissue

Total score is the sum of the four items and ranges between 4 and 16. Total score > 8 predicts unfavorable outcome after PTMC.

(PTMC: percutaneous transvenous mitral commissurotomy)

Complete fusion of both commissures generally indicates severe MS. On the other hand, the lack of commissural fusion does not exclude significant MS, as in degenerative etiologies or even rheumatic MS, where restenosis after previous commissurotomy may be related to valve rigidity with persistent commissural opening.[14] Chordal shortening and thickening are assessed using parasternal long axis and apical four-chamber views **(Figs. 6A and B)**.

Morphologic assessment of the MV with 2D imaging provides important information that guides therapy. Valves with significant calcification, chordal shortening and subvalvular stenosis are not good candidates for percutaneous or surgical commissurotomy. The Wilkins score[15] **(Table 2)** takes into account leaflet thickening, mobility, calcification, and the extent of subvalvular involvement, each graded on a scale of 1 (minimal involvement) to 4 (severe extensive involvement). The Wilkins score has been shown to be predictive of results with mitral commissurotomy.[16] Other scores have been developed **(Table 3)**, in particular taking into account the location of valve thickening or calcification in relation to commissures.[17] However, they have not been validated in large series. No score has been definitely proven to be superior to another and all have a limited predictive value of the results of balloon mitral commissurotomy, which depends on other clinical and echocardiographic findings.[15] Thus, the echocardiographic report should include a comprehensive description of valve anatomy and not summarize it using a score alone.

Associated Lesions

Echocardiography also provides information regarding the size of the left atrium (LA), right atrium (RA), and the size

TABLE 3: Assessment of mitral valve anatomy according to Cormier score.[17]

Echocardiographic group	Mitral valve anatomy
Group 1	Pliable noncalcified anterior mitral leaflet and mild subvalvular disease (i.e., thin chordae ≥ 10 mm long)
Group 2	Pliable noncalcified anterior mitral leaflet and severe subvalvular disease (i.e., thickened chordae < 10 mm long)
Group 3	Calcification of mitral valve of any extent, as assessed by fluoroscopy, whatever the state of subvalvular apparatus

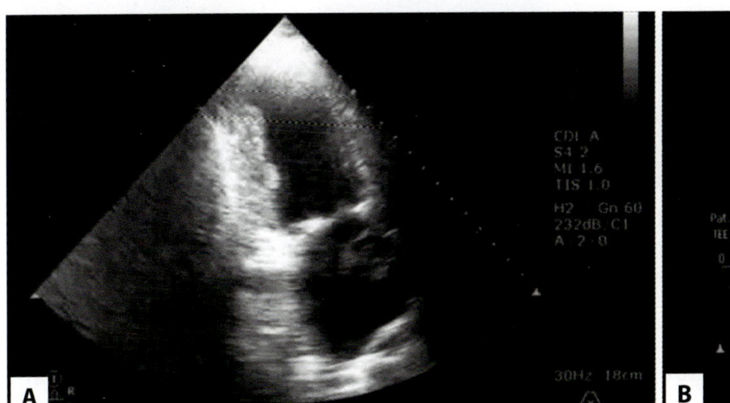
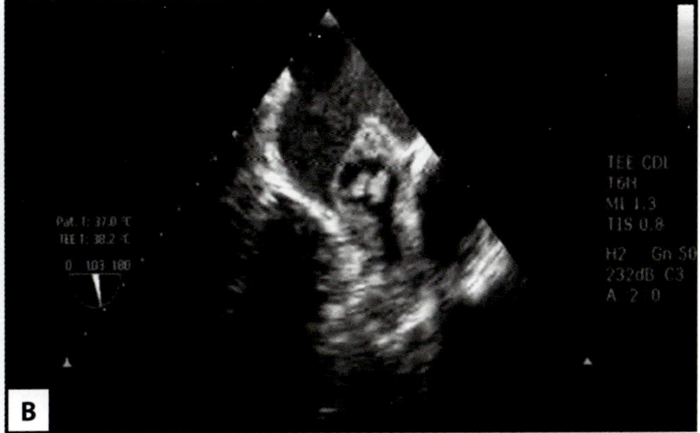

FIGS. 7A AND B: TTE in modified two chamber view shows doubtful thrombus in LAA; (B) TEE in this patient clearly shows partially organized mobile thrombus in LAA protruding into LA body with SEC in LA in a 35-year-old lady with RHD, MS, PAH, and atrial fibrillation.

(MS: mitral stenosis; PAH: pulmonary artery hypertension; RHD: rheumatic heart disease; TEE: transesophageal echocardiography; TTE: transthoracic echocardiography; LAA: left atrial appendage; SEC: spontaneous echo contrast)

and function of the LV and RV **(Fig. 6B)**. TEE assessment of left atrium is a better predictor of the thromboembolic risk than LA size.[18] TEE has a much higher sensitivity than the transthoracic approach to diagnose LA thrombus, in particular, when located in the LAA **(Figs. 7A and B)**. In presence of severe AR, the pressure half-time (T½) method for assessment of MS is not valid.[14] The analysis of the tricuspid valve should look for signs of involvement of the rheumatic process.

Associated MR has important implications for the choice of intervention. Quantification should combine semi-quantitative and quantitative measurements and be particularly careful for regurgitation of intermediate severity since more than mild regurgitation is a relative contraindication for balloon mitral commissurotomy.[19-21] The mechanism of rheumatic MR is due to restriction of leaflet motion, except after balloon mitral commissurotomy, where leaflet tearing rarely can cause severe MR. Hence, analysis of the mechanism of MR is important in patients presenting with moderate-to-severe MR after balloon mitral commissurotomy for MS **(Fig. 8)**. Other valve diseases are frequently associated with rheumatic MS. The severity of AS may be underestimated because of decreased stroke volume (SV) due to MS, as it reduces aortic gradient, thereby highlighting the need for the estimation of aortic valve area (AVA).

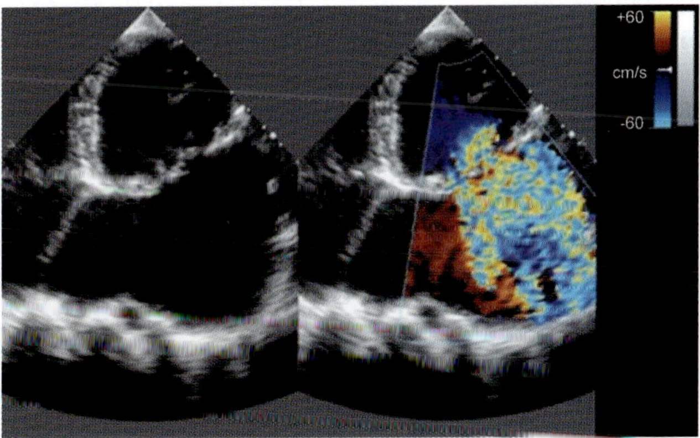

FIG. 8: Apical four-chamber view with color compare shows AML tear with severe MR with two jets one from the noncoapting valve and the other from AML tear or perforation in a 14-year-old boy with juvenile MS after BMV.

(AML: anterior mitral leaflet; BMV: balloon mitral valvotomy; MR: mitral regurgitation; MS: mitral stenosis)

More frequently, associated tricuspid disease is functional TR secondary to pulmonary artery hypertension (PAH). Methods for quantitating TR are not well established and highly sensitive to loading conditions. A diameter of the tricuspid annulus of 40 mm seems to be more reliable than

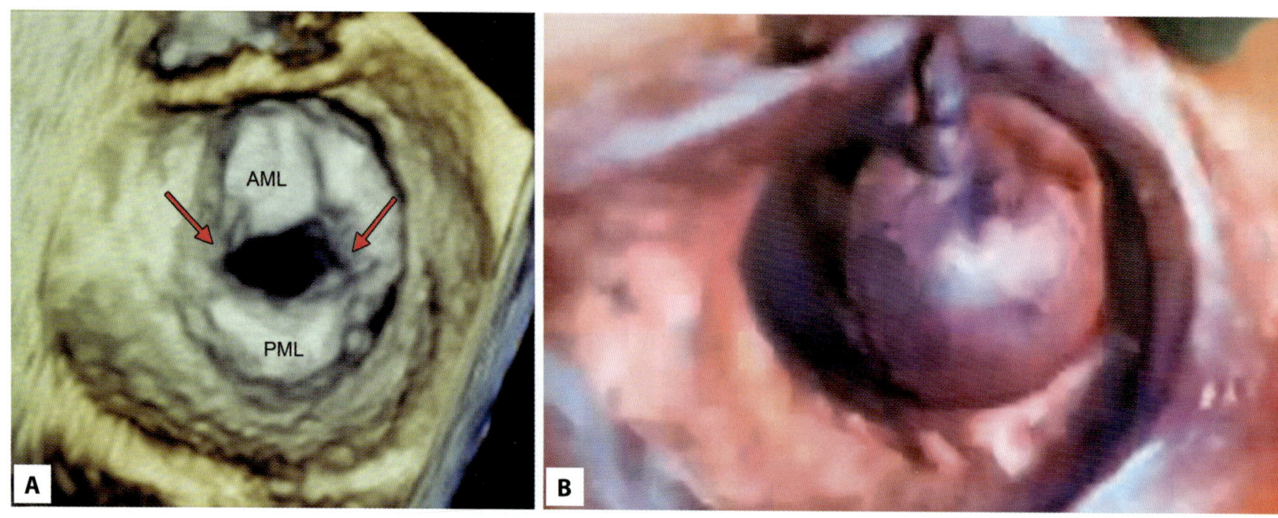

FIGS. 9A AND B: (A) Four-dimensional (4D) ECHO in short axis from LV side shows thickened AML and PML with fused commissures (Red arrows). (B) Inoue balloon across the MV from LV side shows balloon in appropriate position and not caught in chordae during BMV.

(AML: anterior mitral leaflet; BMV: balloon mitral valvotomy; LV: left ventricle; MV: mitral valve)

quantification of regurgitation to predict the risk of severe late TR after mitral surgery.[20,22]

Determination of Severity of Mitral Stenosis by ECHO

The severity of MS can be determined by 2D and 4D ECHO can visualize the valve from LA side or LV side and can illustrate quantifiable morphological features derived from even 4D-TEE analysis can effectively classify the etiology of MS and use it during successful BMV **(Figs. 9A and B)**. MVOA is frequently calculated to obtain a flow independent measure of the degree of narrowing. A number of methods have been proposed for this but none is entirely satisfactory. Moreover, it is questionable whether the complex hemodynamic disturbance to atrioventricular flow can be summed up in a simple statement of area.[23]

Mitral Valve Orifice Area by Planimetry

Mitral valve orifice area by planimetry is highly accurate when performed by an experienced echocardiographer. It has strong correlation with Gorlin formula and also has best correlation with anatomical valve area as validated with surgical and catheterization-determined valve areas. Parasternal short-axis view at mid-diastole, direct tracing of the mitral orifice including opened commissures has advantages: being a direct measurement of MVOA it is not affected by hemodynamics, associated valvular lesions, and unlike other methods, does not involve any hypothesis regarding flow conditions, cardiac chamber compliance, or associated valvular lesions.[14] In practice, 2D imaging of the diastolic orifice allows for planimetry of the valve area and has been shown to have the best correlation with anatomical valve area as validated with surgical and catheterization

determined valve areas.[24-26] Planimetry measurement involves direct tracing of the inner border of the MV opening in mid-diastole, including opened commissures, obtained from the parasternal short-axis view and can grade as mild, moderate, and severe/critical MS **(Figs. 10A to C)**. The classification of determination of severity of MS by ECHO by various methods is shown in **Table 4**.

Meticulous scanning from the apex to the base of the LV is required to ensure that the MV area is measured at the leaflet tips. The measurement plane should be perpendicular to the mitral orifice, which has an elliptical shape. Instrument factors such as gain and transmission power can affect the image. Gain setting should be just sufficient to visualize the whole contour of the mitral orifice.

Higher gain setting may cause overstating of the leaflet boundaries and hence underestimation of valve area, in particular when leaflet tips are dense or calcified. Image magnification, using the zoom mode, is useful to better delineate the contour of the mitral orifice. It is unclear whether the use of harmonic imaging improves planimetry measurement.[14] The normal MVOA is 4.0–6.0 cm^2. Planimetry has its limitations, particularly in the presence of significant leaflet tip calcification, poor border detection, highly deformed valve due to prior valvotomy **(Fig. 11)**, severe subvalvular obstruction, eccentric orifice, severe AR, and in atrial fibrillation. It is recommended to perform several different measurements, in particular in patients with atrial fibrillation and in those who have incomplete commissural fusion (moderate MS or after commissurotomy).[14]

Planimetry of MS may not be feasible in about 5%, even by experienced echocardiographers when there is a poor acoustic window or severe distortion of valve anatomy, in particular with severe valve calcifications of the leaflet tips.[17] Recent reports suggested that real-time 3D/4D

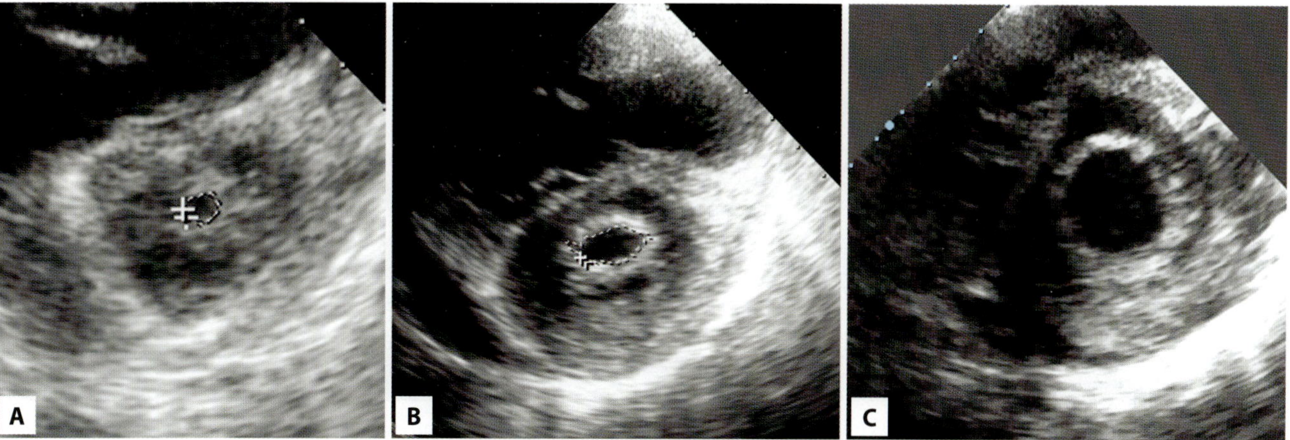

FIGS. 10A TO C: Two-dimensional (2D) ECHO in parasternal short axis planimetry of the mitral valve orifice in (A) shows critical stenosis—0.3 cm^2; (B) shows moderate stenosis—1.2 cm^2; and (C) mild stenosis with 1.8 cm^2.

TABLE 4: Classification of mitral stenosis (MS) severity.[14]

Grading of MS			
	Mild	**Moderate**	**Severe**
Specific findings valve area (cm^2)	>1.5	1.0–1.5	<1.0
Supportive findings: Mean gradient (mm Hg)	<5	5–10	>10
Pulmonary artery pressure (mm Hg)	<30	30-50	>50
Pressure half-time (ms)	100–150	150–220	>220
Exercise gradient mean >15 mm Hg			
Dobutamine stress gradient mean >18 mm Hg			

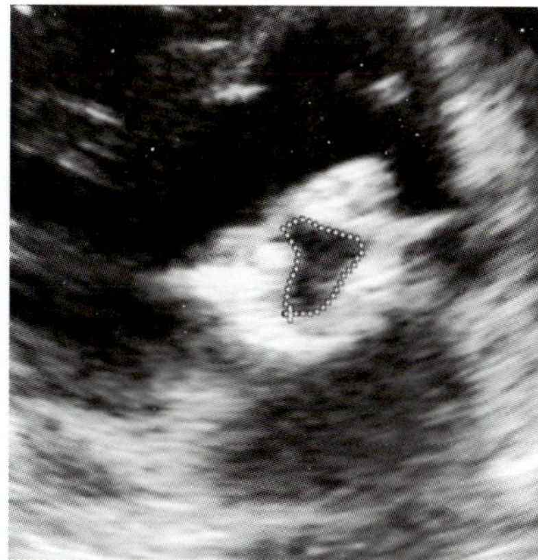

FIG. 11: mitral valve orifice area (MVOA) by planimetry shows 0.7cm^2 with highly deformed thick calcified valve in a 20-year-old lady with restenosis due to prior valvotomy 5 years ago.

ECHO-guided biplane imaging is useful in optimizing the positioning of the measurement plane and hence improving reproducibility especially when performed by less experienced echocardiographers.[13,27,28]

Pressure Gradient

The Doppler offers a noninvasive method for estimation of the diastolic pressure gradient across the MV **(Fig. 12A)**. The transmitral gradient can be determined by continuous wave (CW) Doppler of the mitral inflow during diastole and derived from the transmitral velocity flow curve using the simplified Bernoulli equation[29] where $P = 4V^2$. The magnitude of the pressure gradient depends not only on valve obstruction but also on volume flow rate. An increase in cardiac output, tachycardia, and coexistent MR can all increase the gradient across the MV. The use of CWD is preferred so as to ensure maximal velocities are recorded. When pulsed-wave Doppler is used, the sample volume should be placed at the level or just after leaflet tips.[14] Doppler gradient is assessed using the apical four-chamber view in most cases, as it allows for parallel alignment of the ultrasound beam and mitral inflow. The ultrasound Doppler beam should be oriented to minimize the intercept angle with mitral flow to avoid underestimation of velocities. The color Doppler flow in apical four-chamber view shows the classical "candle flame" appearance of the turbulent diastolic antegrade flow emerging from the LV through the stenotic MV **(Fig. 12B)**.

Color Doppler in apical four-chamber view is useful to identify eccentric diastolic mitral jets that may be seen in cases of severe deformity of valvular and subvalvular apparatus. In these cases, the Doppler beam is guided by the highest flow velocity zone identified by color Doppler. The gain settings, beam orientation, and good acoustic window should be optimized to obtain well-defined contours of the Doppler flow. Maximal and mean mitral gradients are calculated by integrated software using the trace of the Doppler diastolic mitral flow waveforms on the display screen **(Fig. 13)**. Mean gradient is the relevant hemodynamic finding. Maximal gradient is of little interest

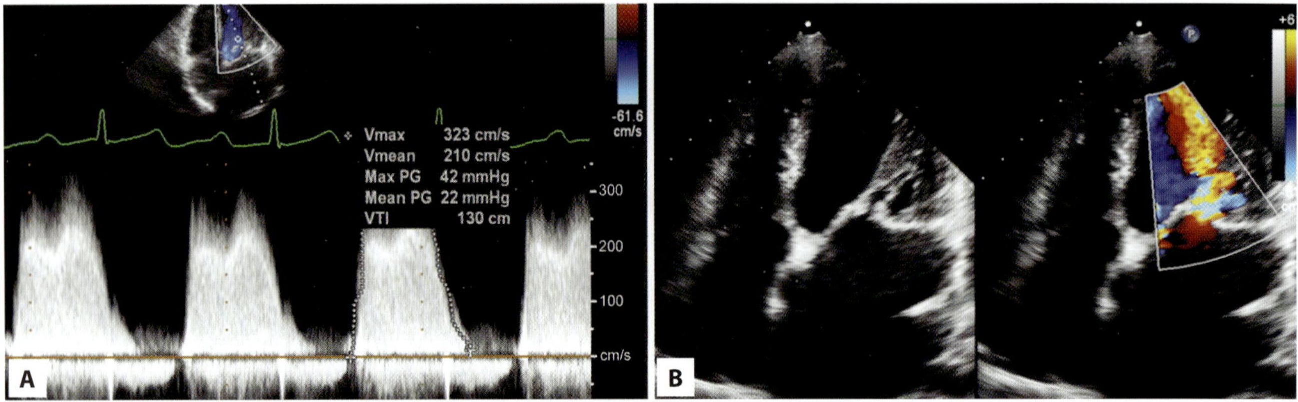

FIGS. 12A AND B: (A) The continuous wave (CW) Doppler of the mitral inflow during diastole shows maximum gradient of 42 mm Hg and mean gradient of 22 mm Hg in a 20-year-old lady with critical mitral stenosis (MS). (B) Apical four-chamber view shows severe deformity of valvular and subvalvular apparatus with "candle flame" appearance of the turbulent diastolic antegrade flow emerging through the stenotic mitral valve (MV).

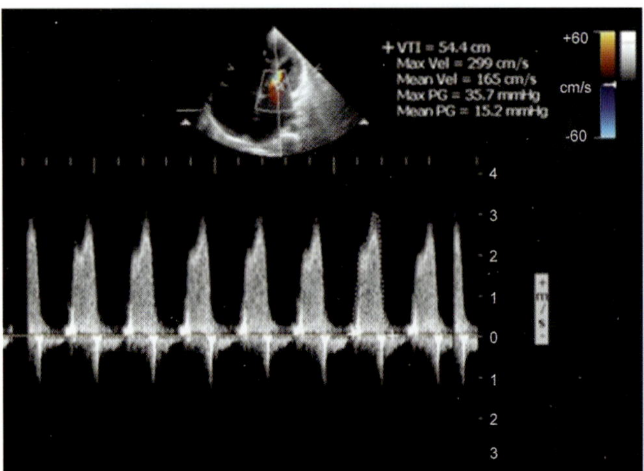

FIG. 13: Shows the Doppler diastolic mitral flow waveform to measure maximal 35 mm Hg and mean 15.2 mm Hg mitral gradients in a 16-year-old girl with critical mitral stenosis (MS) with sinus tachycardia.

as it derives from peak mitral velocity, which is influenced by the LA compliance and LV diastolic function.[30] Heart rate at which gradients are measured should always be reported. In patients with atrial fibrillation, mean gradient should be calculated as the average of five cycles with the least variation of R-R intervals and as close as possible to normal heart rate **(Figs. 14A and B)**.

The mean diastolic gradient obtained by Doppler has been shown to correlate well with hemodynamic measurement obtained during catheterization in patients with MS. But, mitral gradient assessed by Doppler is not the best marker of the severity of MS since it is dependent on the MVOA, as well as a number of other factors that influence transmitral flow rate, the most important being heart rate, cardiac output (determines the diastolic filling period), and associated MR.[31] The Doppler gradient does not correlate well the MV gradient measured using pulmonary capillary wedge pressure but there is good correlation with LA pressure obtained after transseptal perforation. The limitation of pressure gradient is that in patients with low cardiac output there may be an under estimation of the mean pressure gradient. It can also be underestimated if angle between the sample volume and the mitral flow is too large (>30°). Combined use of color flow and CW Doppler can overcome this problem. Gradients can be overestimated in patients with aortic regurgitation due to mixing of the mitral flow stream with the higher velocity aortic regurgitation flow. Color flow mapping can visualize the two streams and sampling can be done more accurately at the mitral orifice. However, the consistency between mean gradient and other echocardiographic findings should be checked, in particular in patients with poor quality of other variables (especially planimetry of valve area) or when such variables may be affected by additional conditions, point size, i.e., pressure half-time in the presence of LV diastolic dysfunction. In addition, mean mitral gradient has its own prognostic value, in particular following balloon mitral valvotomy (BMV).

Pressure Half-time

The Doppler determination of the mitral pressure half-time has gained widespread acceptance as a reliable estimate for MVA, despite little theoretical basis for its "independence" of other hemodynamic variables. A simple model of the left atrium and MV has been developed and a governing equation derived from fluid dynamics fundamentals. Solution of this equation indicates that the pressure half-time should vary inversely with MVA, but also proportionally to net LA and ventricular compliance and to the square root of the peak transmitral gradient.[32]

The rate of the pressure gradient decline also provides important information about the severity of stenosis. The pressure half-time, obtained from the CW Doppler inflow

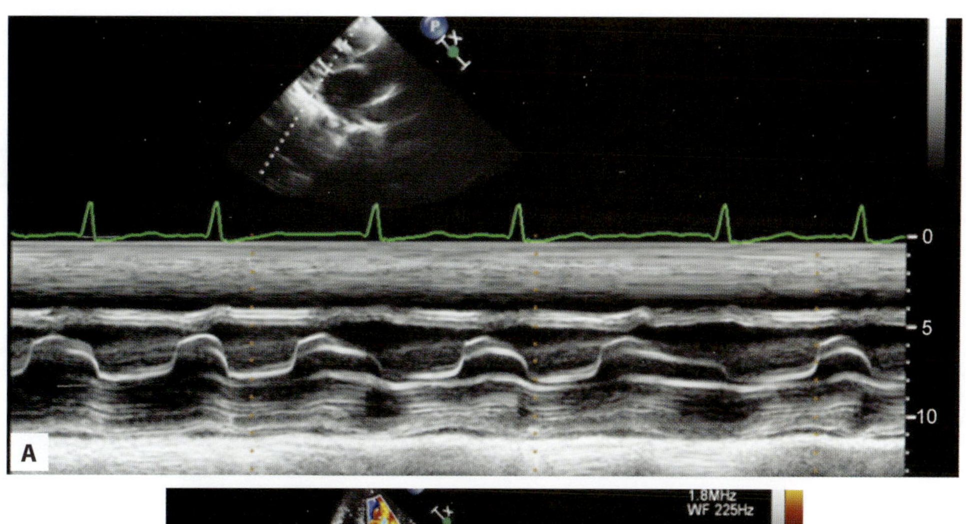

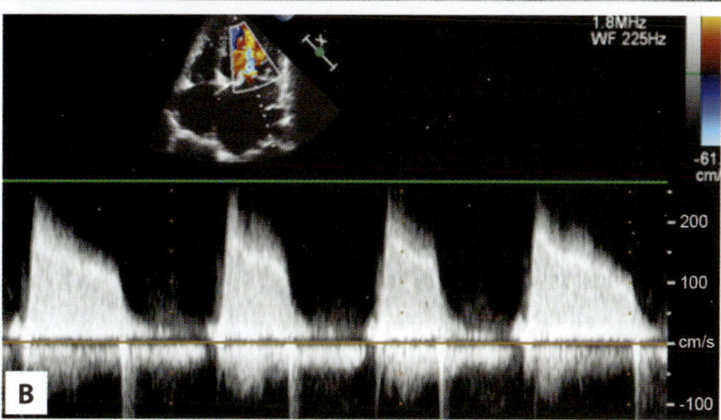

FIGS. 14A AND B: (A) M-mode of mitral valve in a patient with RHD, MS with atrial fibrillation with slow heart rate; (B) CW Doppler in case of RHD, MS with atrial fibrillation with slow ventricular rate.

(CW: continuous wave; MS: mitral stenosis; RHD: rheumatic heart disease)

signal is defined as the time (in milliseconds) that the initial pressure gradient decreases to half its maximum value.[33] Studies comparing Doppler half-time data with catheterization derived Gorlin valve areas found a linear relationship, with a half-time of 220 ms corresponding to a valve area of 1 cm^2 and have subsequently been shown to correlate well with invasive measurements of valve areas.[26,34,35] A pressure half-time of 220 ms represents a valve area of 1 cm^2. A pressure half-time of 440 ms represents a valve area of 0.5 cm^2. A pressure half-time of 110 ms represents a valve area of 2 cm^2. The decline of the velocity of diastolic transmitral blood flow is inversely proportional to valve area (cm^2) and MVOA is derived using the empirical formula:[32]

$$MVOA = 220/T\tfrac{1}{2}$$

The T½ is obtained by tracing the deceleration slope of the E wave on Doppler spectral display of transmitral flow and valve area is automatically calculated by the integrated software of currently used ECHO machines **(Figs. 15A and B)**. The Doppler signal used is the same as for the measurement of mitral gradient. As for gradient tracing, attention should be paid to the quality of the contour of the Doppler flow, in particular the deceleration slope. The deceleration slope is sometimes bimodal, the decline of mitral flow velocity being more rapid in early diastole than during the following part of the E-wave. In these cases, it is recommended that the deceleration slope in mid-diastole rather than the early deceleration slope be traced.[36] In the rare patients with a concave shape of the tracing, T½ measurement may not be feasible. In patients with atrial fibrillation, tracing should avoid mitral flow from short diastoles and average different cardiac cycles. The mitral pressure half-time is affected by anything that changes LV or atrial compliance or the driving pressure across the LA. Valve area calculation by pressure half-time is generally accurate in the setting of MR, although the early flow volume is dependent on cardiac output and MR.

The empirically determined constant of 220 is in fact proportional to the product of net compliance, i.e., the combined compliance of left atrium and LV and the square root of maximum transmitral gradient in a model that does not take into account active relaxation of LV.[37] The increase in mean gradient is frequently compensated by a decreased compliance and this may explain the rather good correlation between T½ and other measurements of MVOA in most series. In normal subjects, pressure half-time values range between 20 and 60 ms (mean 49 ms). In patients with MS,

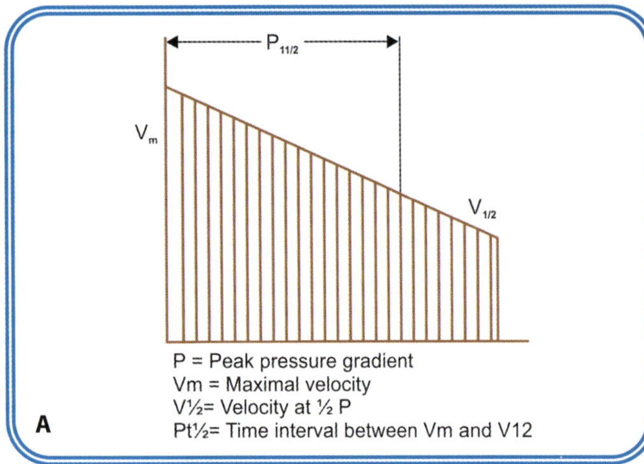

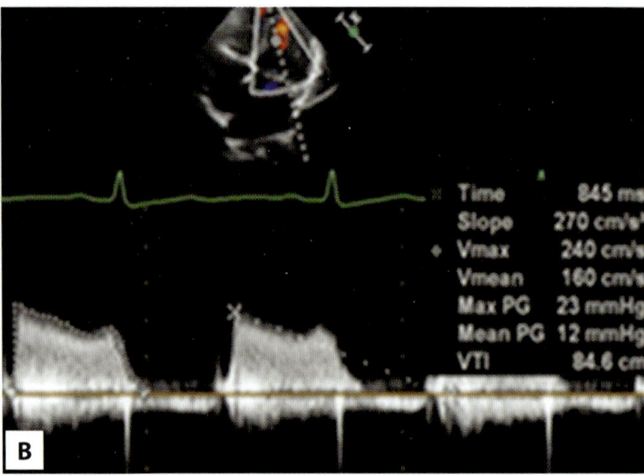

FIGS. 15A AND B: (A) Schematic diagram illustrating the method of calculating MVOA using pressure half-time. (B) PHT Doppler shows Hatle's method to calculate the functional orifice. It is useful because it gives information about both valvular and subvalvular obstructions.

(MVOA: mitral valve orifice area; PHT: pulmonary hypertension)

there is a marked delay and a strong correlation between the pressure half-time estimated from Doppler data and the MVA calculated from catheterization data using the Gorlin formula. Pressure half-time is relatively insensitive to the effects of exercise, atrial fibrillation or coexisting MR. Patients with MS had values from 90 to 383 ms, with the higher values seen in subjects with smaller valve areas. Pressure half-time >220 ms correlates well with a valve area <1.0 cm². Patients with isolated MR have values 35–80 ms.[33] Patients with abnormal myocardial relaxation have a prolonged pressure half-time but the peak E velocity is not increased and is usually <1 ms. Pressure half-time is not accurate immediately after percutaneous mitral commissurotomy due to opposing changes in LA and LV compliance immediately after the procedure.[37] After a period of 72 hours, the compliance of each chamber stabilizes and the pressure half-time can again be used for the calculation of MVA. Rapid decrease of mitral velocity flow, i.e., short T½ can be observed despite severe MS in patients who have a particularly low LA compliance.[38] The ability to calculate MVOA by pressure half-time is limited by significant coexistent AR **(Fig. 16)**. In this situation, if there is a more rapid rise in LV diastolic pressure, a shorter pressure half-time results. Conversely, if severe AR impairs mitral leaflet opening, functional MS may occur in conjunction with anatomical MS, resulting in a longer pressure half-time. However, mild-to-moderate AR does not significantly influence the pressure half-time measurement.[39] But, aortic insufficiency may preclude accurate measurement of pulmonary hypertension (PHT) as the regurgitant volume into the LV will lead to more rapid rate of rise of pressure in early diastole and lead to a shorter pressure half-time thereby underestimating severity. Alternatively, severe AR may lead to early closure of the MV and lengthen the PHT leading to overestimation of MS severity. The role of impaired LV diastolic function is more difficult to assess

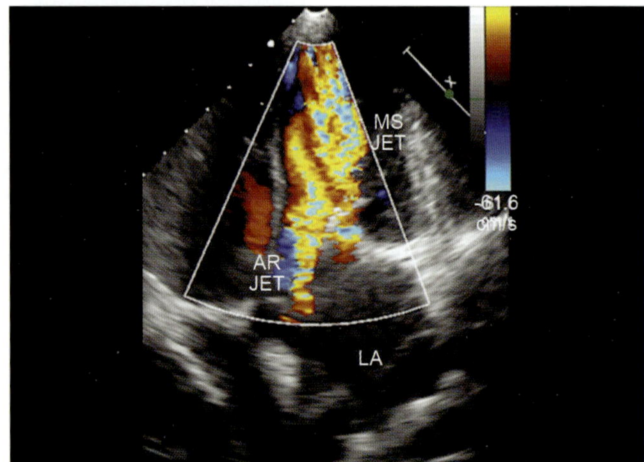

FIG. 16: Apical four-chamber view with color Doppler shows jet of mitral stenosis (MS) (candle flame appearance of MS jet) by the side of another jet of aortic regurgitation (AR jet).

because of complex and competing interactions between active relaxation and compliance as regard their impact on diastolic transmitral flow.[40] Early diastolic deceleration time is prolonged when LV relaxation is impaired, while it tends to be shortened in case of decreased LV compliance.[41] Impaired LV diastolic function is a likely explanation of the lower reliability of T½ to assess MVOA in the elderly.[42]

The continuity equation may also be used for the calculation of the MVA. It is based on the principle of mass and energy conservation. The flow at all points along a tube is constant and equals the product of mean velocity and cross-sectional area. MVA is calculated as the product of aortic or pulmonary annular cross-sectional area and the ratio of the respective valve velocity time integral to that of the mitral stenotic continuous wave velocity. Estimation of the stroke volume from the pulmonary artery is rarely performed in practice because of limited acoustic windows.[14,43]

$$MYA = \pi \left(\frac{D^2}{4} \right) \left(\frac{VTI_{aortic}}{VTI_{mitral}} \right)$$

Where D is the diameter of the LVOT (in cm) and VTI is in cm

Mitral valve area calculated by the continuity equation may be less reliable than planimetry, pressure half-time and proximal isovelocity surface area (PISA) methods.[24] The continuity equation cannot be used in cases of atrial fibrillation or associated significant MR or AR.

Proximal Isovelocity Surface Area Method

Proximal isovelocity surface area or flow convergence is used to calculate the transmitral volume flow rate. Blood flow through a narrowed orifice converges in a series of proximal isovelocity hemispheres (isovelocity surface area). In MS, it can be demonstrated by mosaic color Doppler on the atrial side in diastole. The narrowed orifice area can be calculated by dividing peak flow rate by maximal velocity through the orifice [obtained from the continuous wave Doppler (CWD)].

$$MVA = \pi\, r^2\, (V_{aliasing})/\text{Peak } V_{mitral} \text{ -}\alpha/180°$$

where r is the radius of the convergence hemisphere (in cm), Valiasing is the aliasing velocity (in cm/s), peak Vmitral the peak CWD velocity of mitral inflow (in cm/s) and α is the opening angle of mitral leaflets relative to flow direction.[44] MV area calculated by this method has been shown to correlate with that obtained by conventional catheterization. However, flow convergence method is subject to geometric complexities of the MVOA.[45] This method can be used in the presence of significant MR. But, it is technically demanding and requires multiple measurements. Its accuracy is impacted upon by uncertainties in the measurement of the radius of the convergence hemisphere and the opening angle. The use of color M mode improves its accuracy, enabling simultaneous measurement of flow and velocity.[44] The PISA method is rarely used in MS, in part because the single color image uses the volume flow rate at only one point in diastole rather than integrated over the entire diastolic filling period.

Other Indices of Severity

Mitral valve resistance is defined as the ratio of mean mitral gradient to transmitral diastolic flow rate, which is calculated by dividing SV by diastolic filling period. MV resistance is an alternative measurement of the severity of MS, which has been argued to be less dependent on flow conditions. This is, however, not the case. MV resistance correlates well with pulmonary artery pressure. However, it has not been shown to have an additional value for assessing the severity of MS as compared with valve area.[46] The estimation of pulmonary artery pressure, using Doppler estimation of the systolic gradient between right ventricle (RV) and right atrium,

reflects the consequences of MS rather than its severity itself. The degree of pulmonary artery pressure can be quantified from the velocity in the TR jet using the formula PASP = RAP + 4 (TR jet velocity)^2. 2D ECHO may show RV enlargement and hypertrophy, paradoxical septal motion, and TR. Although it is advised to check its consistency with mean gradient and valve area, there may be a wide range of pulmonary artery pressure for a given valve area. Nevertheless, pulmonary artery pressure is critical for clinical decision making and it is therefore very important to provide this measurement.

Exercise Echocardiography

It can be useful when symptoms of the patient are out of proportion to the severity of MS.[47] The restriction in LV diastolic filling in severe MS may result in low stroke volume and relatively low mean pressure gradients. With increases in volume flow rate during exercise, a significant increase in mean transmitral pressure over 15 mm Hg or an increase in pulmonary systolic pressure > 60 mm Hg suggests hemodynamically significant MS, regardless of the resting gradient.

The BMV is contraindicated in the presence of moderate to moderately severe MR and when a LA body thrombus is visualized **(Fig. 17)**. Complications of PTMC identified with ECHO include worsening of MR, a persistent atrial septal defect at the transseptal site and cardiac perforation and development of tamponade. The average reduction in MVA in the setting of rheumatic MS is 0.09 + 0.21 cm^2/year.[48] Predictors of more rapid progression include an ECHO score > 8 and a greater initial gradient. The average reduction in MVA after BMV is 0.08 cm^2/year by planimetry and 0.06 cm^2/year by pressure half-time. The ECHO morphology score is the strongest predictor of restenosis.[16]

Transesophageal echocardiography improves the visualization of the valvular structure and delineates the mechanism and severity of regurgitation. It is useful

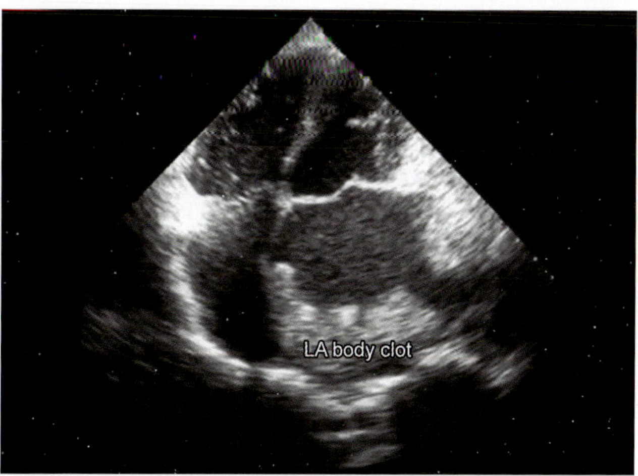

FIG. 17: Transthoracic echocardiography (TTE) in apical four-chamber view shows thrombus attached the roof of left atrium (LA).

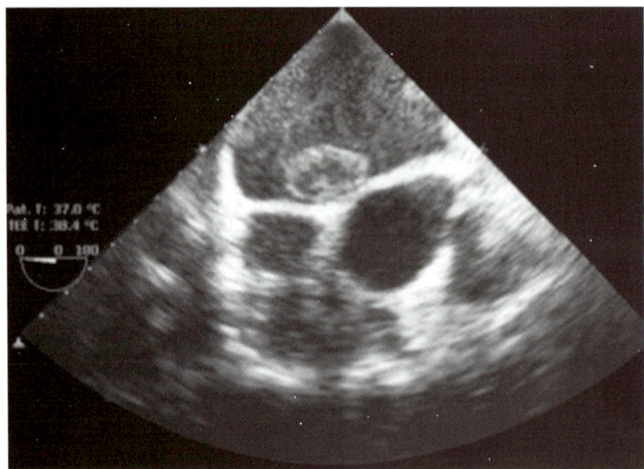

FIG. 18: Transesophageal echocardiography (TEE) shows thrombus in left atrial appendage (LAA) spontaneous echocardiography contrast (SEC) in the left atrium.

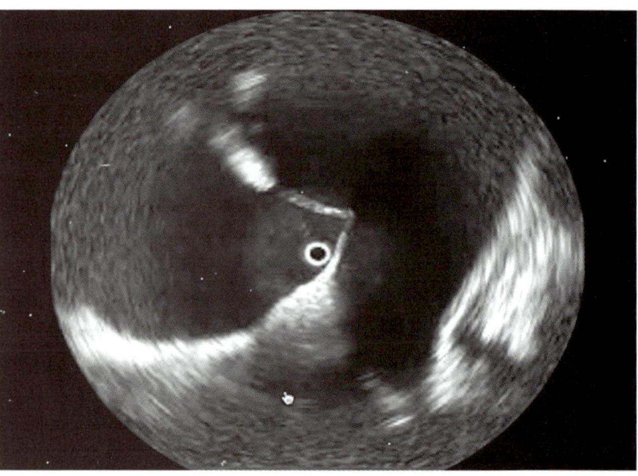

FIG. 19: Intracardiac echocardiography (ICE) illustrates transseptal puncture during balloon mitral valvotomy (BMV).

for the assessment of LA or left atrial appendage (LAA) thrombus **(Fig. 18)** particularly before percutaneous mitral commissurotomy. The specificity and sensitivity for detection of left atrial thrombus is both >99%.

Thrombus within the atrium is considered a contraindication to placement of a transseptal needle and a guidewire into the left atrium. TEE may detect spontaneous echocardiography contrast (SEC) in the left atrium or LAA. This is often described as "smoke" and appears as multiple tiny echoes with a swirling motion **(Fig. 18)**. This is probably due to low blood flow velocity with red blood cell Rouleaux formation. In patients with MS, SEC is commonly visualized by TEE as compared to transthoracic echocardiography (TTE). In the setting of MS, SEC is seen in most of the patients with atrial fibrillation and they are strongly associated with LA and LAA thrombus and they are more prone for embolic events. SEC can also been seen in other conditions like larger left atrium, depressed atrial appendage contractility, small MVOA and absence of moderate or severe MR.[49-52] SEC has been observed in patients with MS and in sinus rhythm. They have been associated with systemic embolization, independent from atrial or appendage thrombus.[51]

Transesophageal echocardiography can also be helpful for more definitive quantification of MR, particularly in the setting of heavy calcification when the degree of MR may be underestimated in transthoracic apical views because of acoustic shadowing. A limitation of TEE is underestimation of the degree of chordal involvement in the esophageal views because of masking by the stenotic MV. Transgastric views allow better visualization of the subvalvular apparatus. TEE or intracardiac echocardiography (ICE) can be used during BMV to guide proper position of the transseptal needle **(Fig. 19)** and placement of the balloon across the MV. Following inflation, Doppler can be used to assess the presence and severity of MR.[12]

Pitfalls of Using Echocardiography

When obtaining Doppler gradients and pressure half-time, care must be taken to have the ultrasound beam parallel to the jet of flow. If this is not done, the gradients and PHT will underestimate the severity of stenosis. Pressure half-time measurement cannot be used if there is concomitant MR or LV dysfunction. Both of these states alter the pressure gradient across the MV. The MR by virtue of raising LA pressure and LV dysfunction by raising LVEDP. Therefore, the pressure decay measured if one or both of these conditions are present will not reflect pure pressure decay across the MV.[53] Significant aortic insufficiency may preclude accurate measurement of PHT as the regurgitant volume into the LV will lead to more rapid rate of rise of pressure in early diastole and lead to a shorter pressure half-time thereby underestimating severity. Alternatively, severe AR may lead to early closure of the MV and lengthen the PHT leading to overestimation of MS severity. Finally, it is important to remember that pressure gradients vary with both valve area and flow rate (i.e., cardiac output). If the cardiac output is low due to restricted filling, one can underestimate the pressure gradient and the MVA, either by ECHO or by catheterization. Alternatively, if the diastolic filling period is diminished due to rapid heart rate, such as in atrial fibrillation, the gradient across the MV will be increased.

Three-dimensional and Four-dimensional Echocardiography

In clinical practice, 2D-ECHO with Doppler evaluation of MV gradient and pulmonary artery pressure has become the mainstay for evaluating MV disease and particularly MVOA. The MVOA is assessed directly by planimetry or indirectly by the PHT method. There are advantages and limitations to both methods. PHT derived MVOA can be obtained easily, but can be influenced by hemodynamic factors such as heart rate, cardiac index, cardiac rhythm, LV systolic and diastolic dysfunction, LV and atrial compliance, LV hypertrophy, and concomitant valvular disease.[33,54] MVOA by the planimetry method has the advantage of being relatively hemodynamically independent. The greatest limitation of this method is that measurements of MVOA are made in the short-axis view with no simultaneous independent imaging to verify that the imaging plane corresponds to the smallest and most perpendicular view of the mitral orifice. Hence, significant experience and operator skill is required to obtain the correct imaging plane that displays the true MVOA. This limitation is amplified in severely diseased valve and after PTMC. As valve orifice becomes more calcified and irregular with progression of the disease, making the tracing of the orifice becomes more challenging. After PTMC, if there is asymmetric commissural split, then tracing of the orifice is less reproducible between observers.[55] Many, but not all of these limitations, are overcome with the use of 3D/4D ECHO. In the last decade in the field of cardiac imaging, one of the most significant developments has been real-time three-dimensional echocardiography (RT3DE). Other methods of 3DE were used before to evaluate the MV, but the required reconstructive process made them much less practical. 3DE provides unique orientations of the cardiac structures not obtainable by standard 2DECHO. As 3DECHO can evaluate planimetry of the MVOA accurately in rheumatic MS, it has evolved from being only a research tool to having practical importance. It can provide not only adequate imaging of the anatomic structure of the MVOA (commissural splitting and leaflet tears),[56] but also information on the optimal plane of the smallest MVOA. Also, planimetry using 3DE can be done from the apical window and is not limited to the parasternal window as 2D ECHO.

Three-dimensional echocardiography performed with TEE and subsequent 3D reconstruction had shown promise for evaluating patients with MS before the advent of RT3DE. In one study, it showed good correlation between MVOA by this methodology and pressure half time.[57] In many studies, 3DE has shown that MVOA correlated closely with traditional methods, and visualization of the commissures was superior to what was seen by 2D ECHO.[58-62] Hence, RT3DE was the most accurate echocardiography parameter for measuring MVOA.[27] RT3DE allows a unique and superior evaluation of the MV apparatus, increasing the ability to obtain an accurate measurement of the MVOA, even after PMV.[28] RT3DE can accurately measure MVOA because of its ability to crop the volume data set in any position in space, and therefore, select the en face view that includes the smallest MVA. RT3DE is also useful to obtain accurate Wilkins score.[55]

Real-time 3D echocardiography or 4D and TEE is a major advance in cardiac imaging as it allows visualization of the entire MV apparatus and the optimal plane to measure the smallest MVOA. Currently, sufficient evidence has been compiled to prove that 3D imaging is superior to traditional 2D techniques and should be used routinely to quantify the MVOA in MS, particularly during BMV, postvalve replacement where other methods have been proven to be inaccurate.[28,63-65] RT3DE should be integrated into the routine echocardiographic examination and perhaps, in the near future, should replace Gorlin's method as the reference method to quantify the MVOA in rheumatic MS.

■ MITRAL REGURGITATION

Transthoracic echocardiography and Doppler are indispensable in the management of RHD patients with MR and should be used to assess the severity of MR, the LV response to volume overload, including LV size and systolic function, ejection fraction (EF) and end-systolic dimension, LA size, and pulmonary artery systolic pressure. ECHO may also identify the anatomic cause of MR, which is important for determining the feasibility of successful MV repair. ECHO allows an evaluation of the valvular structure as well as the impact of the volume overload on the cardiac chambers. Calcifications, tethering, flail motion or vegetations can be readily assessed, which can give indirect clues as to the severity of regurgitation.

Evaluation of the anatomy of the MV apparatus by 2D ECHO is critically important in the assessment of etiology and severity of MR. The MV apparatus includes the annulus, valve leaflets, chordae tendineae, papillary muscles and the LV myocardial wall. An abnormality in one or more of these structures may result in MR, although a mild amount of physiological regurgitation is present in 19–45% of normal MVs.[66,67] 2D ECHO evaluation is helpful in determining whether the MR is functional, related to dilatation of the LV or segmental wall motion abnormalities or due to primary structural abnormalities. In developing countries, the leading cause of MR is RHD. The other causes of organic MR include mitral valve prolapse (MVP) syndrome, infective endocarditis (IE), congenital anomalies such as cleft MVs, certain drugs and collagen vascular disease. MR may also occur secondary to a dilated annulus from dilatation of the LV (functional MR). In some cases, such as ruptured chordae tendineae **(Fig. 20)**, ruptured papillary muscle or infective endocarditis, MR may be acute and severe.

Indications for Transthoracic Echocardiography[6]

Class I

- Transthoracic echocardiography is indicated for baseline evaluation of LV size and function, RV and LA size, pulmonary artery pressure, and severity of MR in any patient suspected of having MR. *(Level of Evidence: C)*
- Transthoracic echocardiography is indicated for delineation of the mechanism of MR. *(Level of Evidence: B)*
- Transthoracic echocardiography is indicated for annual or semiannual surveillance of LV function (estimated by ejection fraction and end-systolic dimension) in asymptomatic patients with moderate to severe MR. *(Level of Evidence: C)*

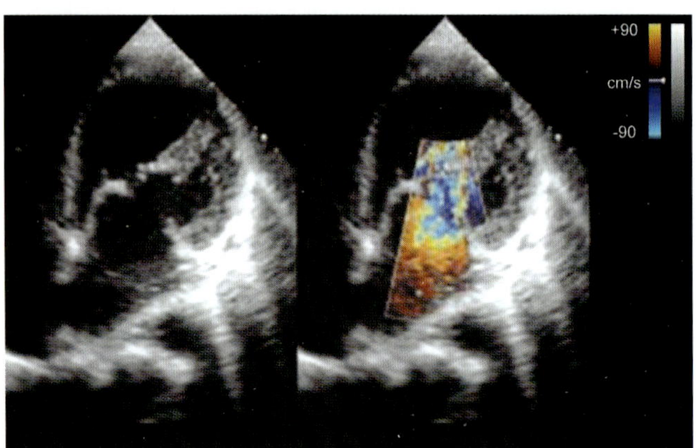

FIG. 20: Apical modified two-chamber view shows rolled uptorn chordae, anterior mitral leaflet (AML), and posterior mitral leaflet (PML) free from papillaries.

- Transthoracic echocardiography is indicated in patients with MR to evaluate the MV apparatus and LV function after a change in signs or symptoms. *(Level of Evidence: C)*
- Transthoracic echocardiography is indicated to evaluate LV size and function and MV hemodynamics in the initial evaluation after MV replacement or MV repair. *(Level of Evidence: C)*

Class IIa

Exercise Doppler echocardiography is reasonable in asymptomatic patients with severe MR to assess exercise tolerance and the effects of exercise on pulmonary artery pressure and MR severity. *(Level of Evidence: C)*

Class III

- Transthoracic echocardiography is not indicated for routine follow-up evaluation of asymptomatic patients with mild MR and normal LV size and systolic function. *(Level of Evidence: C)*

Two-dimensional echocardiography and Doppler echocardiogram are most useful in providing information on different aspects of MR. 2D ECHO helps in studying the etiology of MR and its effects on the rest of the cardiac chambers. Doppler/color Doppler helps in detection, quantification, and hemodynamic assessment of MR jet. Evaluation of MR can be approached by various ECHO techniques such as TTE, TEE, intraoperative TEE, and stress echocardiography.

Two-dimensional Echocardiography

The initial TTE should disclose the anatomic cause of the MR. Chronic rheumatic MV disease is characterized by varying degrees of thickening of the leaflets and chordae, fusion of the commissures, and calcification of valvular and subvalvular components. The posterior leaflet is retracted and tethered with limited mobility. The anterior leaflet may be doming in diastole from commissural fusion or be retracted limiting the

length of coaptation. Similar lesions of thickened, retracted, and immobile mitral leaflets may be observed with diet drugs or ergot toxicity. Similar leaflet thickening and retraction may result from "anticardiolipin antibody syndrome" with associated nonbacterial thrombotic endocarditis vegetations. MVP in chronic rheumatic MR may occur after chordal rupture, while acute rheumatic valvulitis causes MR by elongation of the chordae and dilatation of the annulus and associated AML prolapse.[68] Thus, thickened fibrotic valve with shortened scarred leaflets having some degree of MS or at least diastolic doming of AML would indicate a rheumatic pathology. However, in 10% of RHD there is no associated MS.[69] In contrast, diagnosis of MVP is diagnosed if the leaflets are thin or thick myxomatous, nonfibrotic, elongated and redundant with evidence of systolic sagging and noncoaptation in parasternal long-axis view.

In patients with MR in the setting of LV dilatation and/or systolic dysfunction, it is important to determine whether MR is functional due to LV dilatation or primary due to an abnormality of the valve apparatus. In functional MR, the leaflets are usually tethered by outward displacement of the LV walls and papillary muscles, with or without annular dilatation.[70,71] In patients with coronary artery, underlying wall motion abnormalities disease may also lead to functional MR.

In patients with organic MR, the echocardiogram should assess the presence of calcium in the annulus or leaflets, the redundancy of the valve leaflets and the MV leaflet involved (anterior leaflet, posterior leaflet, or bileaflet). These factors will help to determine the feasibility of valve repair if surgery is contemplated. The system proposed by Carpentier[72] allows the echocardiographer to focus on the anatomic and physiologic characteristics of the valve that aid the surgeon in planning the repair. The valve dysfunction is described on the basis of the motion of the free edge of the leaflet relative to the plane of the annulus: type I, normal; type II, increased, as in MVP; type IIIA, restricted during systole and diastole, and type IIIB, restricted during systole.[6]

The ECHO provides a baseline evaluation of the LA size and LV size and function which provides clues to the severity of MR, its acuteness or chronicity and which are important in determining the necessity and timing of surgery.[6,73] LV systolic function including ejection fraction, stroke volume can be assessed by 2D ECHO. Normal 2D ECHO derived values for LV size and function have been previously reported. Briefly, the end-diastolic minor axis dimension of the LV obtained from the parasternal window by 2D is normally ≤ 2.8 cm/m^2 while the normal end-diastolic LV volume is <82 mL/m^2.[74] For the LA, a normal anteroposterior diameter is ≤ 2 cm/m^2.[75] Increase in end-systolic dimensions on serial 2D ECHO may be considered as a sign of LV decompensation and even if the patient is asymptomatic, surgery is recommended.[76] Recent studies, however, have shown that determination of LA volumes with 2D ECHO from the apical views is generally more accurate in assessing LA size than the traditional anteroposterior dimension.[77] A normal maximal LA volume is ≤ 36 mL/m^2.[78]

Assessment of Severity of Mitral Regurgitation

The grading of MR by "eyeballing" the color flow jet area is not enough Doppler evaluation through multiple parameters should be used to diagnose severe MR,[21] including the color flow jet width and area **(Figs. 21A and B)**, the intensity of the CW Doppler signal **(Fig. 22)** the pulmonary venous flow contour, the peak early mitral inflow velocity and quantitative measures of effective orifice area and regurgitation volume.[79] Planimetry of the regurgitant jet should be abandoned, as this measurement is poorly reproducible and depends on numerous factors.

Color Flow Doppler

Color Doppler flow mapping is the most widely used technique to screen for the presence of MR. Small color flow jets are seen in roughly 40% of healthy normal volunteers and therefore are considered a normal variant.[66] Though color flow imaging jet detection is highly sensitive in diagnosing MR. It should be used with caution for MR severity assessment. The origin and direction of MR depends on the MR etiology and mechanism. For example, PML prolapse or flail is associated with an anteriorly directed jet whereas AML prolapse or flail causes a posteriorly directed jet of MR and functional MR has usually a central jet. Thus, clues regarding etiology of MR can be assessed by jet direction with flail or prolapsing leaflets resulting in regurgitation directed away from the leaflet pathology. Eccentric jets appear smaller than central jets of similar size as they do not entrain blood on both sides **(Fig. 23)**.[80,81] The extent of the jet into the LA is influenced by its momentum and thus by its regurgitant velocity and flow. Jet length into the LA, jet to jet area ratio, or jet area can be measured.[82] Small MR jets correspond consistently to mild MR. However, eccentric jets impinge on the LA wall and are constrained

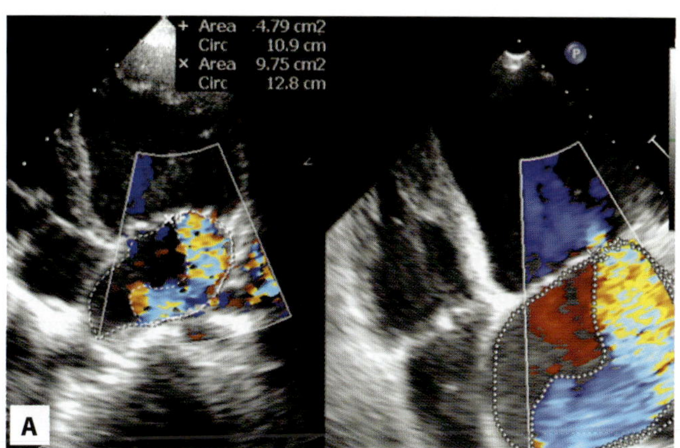
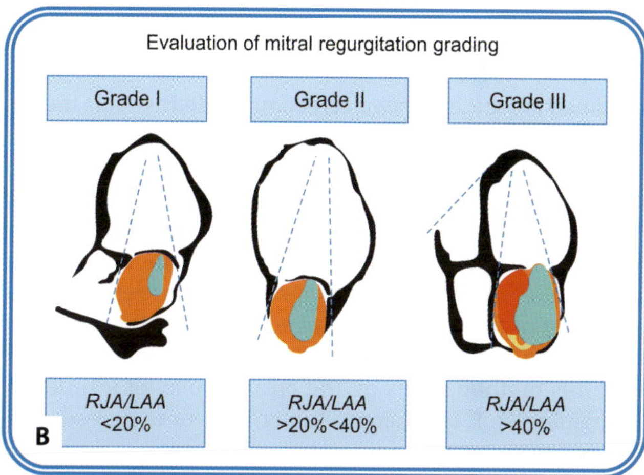

FIGS. 21A AND B: Apical four-chamber view with Color flow jet area measuring is shown; (B) Schematic diagram showing grading of MR with mitral RJA.

(LAA: left atrial appendage; MR: mitral regurgitant; RJA: regurgitant jet area)

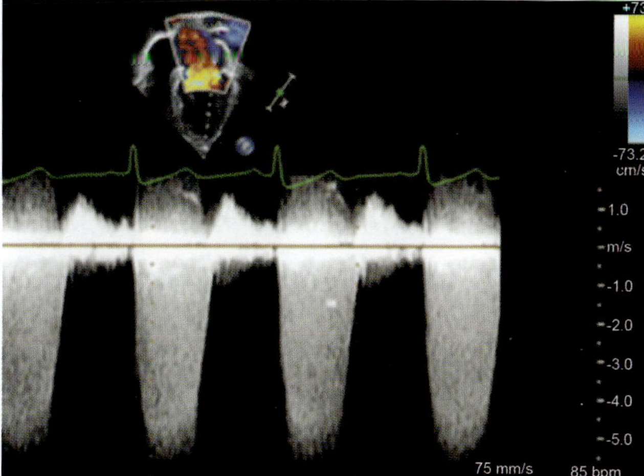

FIG. 22: The intensity of continuous wave (CW) Doppler signal shows severe mitral regurgitation (MR).

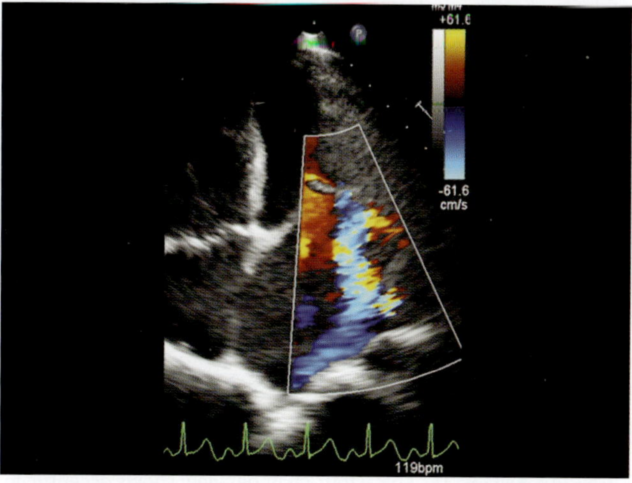

FIG. 23: Apical four-chamber view with color Doppler shows wall hugging eccentric jet with reflux into pulmonary veins indicating severe MR in a 14-year-old lady.

and MR may be underestimated, but reflux of MR jet in pulmonary veins indicates severe MR **(Fig. 23)**. Conversely, central jets are not constrained, expand more in large atria, and may overestimate regurgitant volume.[81] Therefore, for interpreting a jet as reflective of severe MR, it has to be large or reaching deep into LA and to be associated with wide vena contracta or large flow convergence. Because of the increased gradient between the LV and the LA during systole, the velocity of MR always exceeds the Nyquist limit, resulting in an aliasing pattern with a red–blue–green mosaic of color flow. Spurious signals can be mistaken for MR and include the normal posterior motion of blood in the LA from MV closure and the normal systolic inflow from the pulmonary veins. Jet direction provides clues about the etiology of MR.

There are three methods of quantifying MR severity by color flow Doppler mapping: regurgitant jet area, vena contracta **(Fig. 24)**, and flow convergence (PISA) method **(Fig. 19)**. Although jet area was the first method used for assessing MR severity, its sole use is less accurate than the latter two methods.

Regurgitant Jet Area Method

Planimetry of the jet area is not recommended as a sole means of quantification of MR. In general, large jets that extend deep into the LA correspond to more regurgitation than do smaller thin jets that appear just beyond the mitral leaflets. However, the correlation between jet area and MR severity is poor due to a variety of technical and hemodynamic limitations.[83] A regurgitant area of >8 cm^2 or relative area >40% that of the LA suggests severe regurgitation, whereas a jet area of <4 cm^2 or relative area <20% identifies mild MR. This method relies on the clear display of a uniform regurgitant jet. If used alone, it may over- or underestimate the regurgitation severity, particularly when the valve leaflets are flail and the jet uniformity is disrupted. Large jets that penetrate into the pulmonary veins are more likely to be hemodynamically significant, whereas eccentric, wall hugging jets should alert the observer to avoid the use of jet area as an index of severity and use other, more appropriate methods. Hence, determination of the severity of MR by "eyeballing" or planimetry of the MR color flow jet area only, is not recommended.[21] Jet areas studied by transesophageal technique also tend to overestimate valve regurgitation as LA is close to the transducer.

Mild, moderate, and severe MR corresponds to 3 cm^2, 3-6 cm^2, and >6 cm^2, respectively.[84] Also in patients with acute severe MR, with low systolic arterial blood and associated with elevated LA pressure, jet area may be small due to small eccentric color flow jet area, whereas patients with high systolic blood pressure with mild MR, jet area may be significant. Jet area can vary with echocardiography machine settings. Reducing the color scale and increasing the color gain can make even mild MR seem as moderate or at times severe.[85]

Vena Contracta Method

Vena contracta is measured as the narrowest cross-sectional area of the MR jet at the level of the regurgitant orifice **(Figs. 24A and B)**. The vena contracta method has been well validated for the assessment of MR.[86,87] It is superior to jet area in estimating MR severity via TTE or TEE.[88,89] The vena contracta should be imaged in high resolution, zoom views for the largest obtainable proximal jet size for measurements. As the MR jet is not usually circular and may be elongated along the zone of leaflet coaptation, vena contracta should not be measured in the apical two-chamber view as this

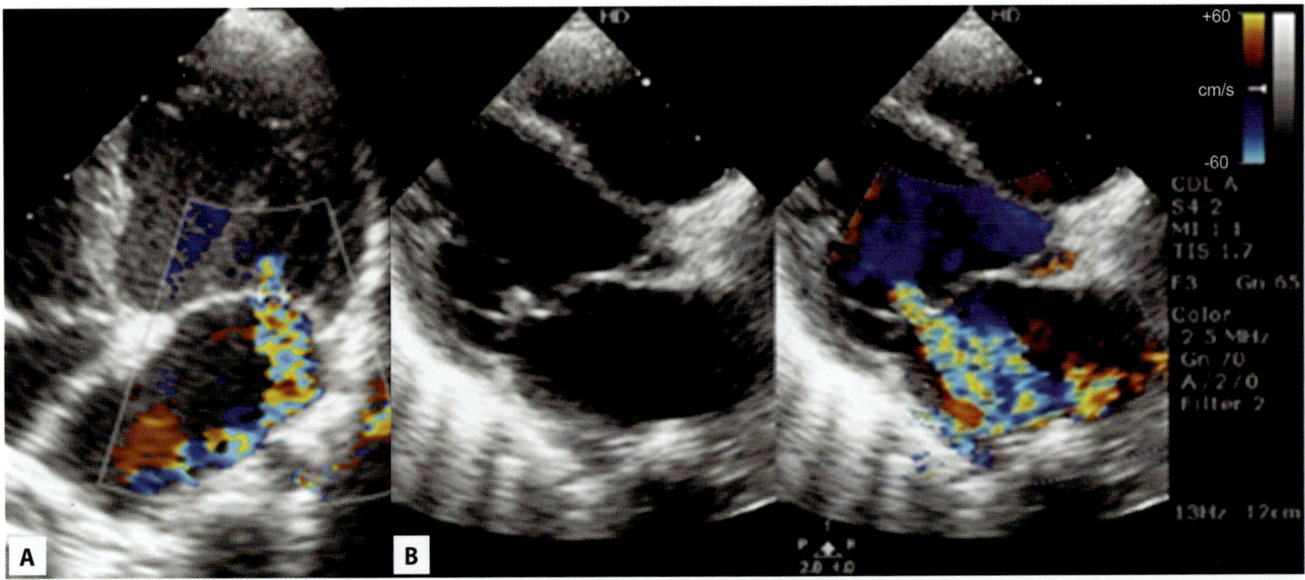

FIGS. 24A AND B: (A) Apical four-chamber view shows eccentric jet with 4 mm vena contracta; (B) Parasternal long-axis view shows vena contracta of 4 mm, illustrating moderate mitral regurgitation (MR) in a 14-year-old boy with rheumatic heart disease (RHD).

would show a wide vena contracta even in mild MR. Vena contracta is best measured in the parasternal long-axis view on TTE and examiner must search in multiple planes in this view.[12] Although the size of the vena contracta is independent of flow rate and driving pressure for a fixed orifice,[90] the regurgitant orifice in MR is often dynamic and therefore the vena contracta may change with hemodynamics or during systole.

The width of the vena contracta in long-axis views and its cross-sectional area in short-axis views can be standardized from the parasternal views.[91] A vena contracta <0.3 cm usually denotes mild MR whereas vena contracta ≥0.7 cm suggests severe MR **(Table 5)**. Vena contracta method works equally well for central and eccentric jets. Thus, in eccentric jets of severe MR, the width of the vena contracta along with flow convergence alerts one to the severity of regurgitation by color Doppler. In patients with multiple MR jets, the respective widths of the vena contracta are not additive, but their cross-sectional areas can be.[88] In the future, 3D imaging of the vena contracta should improve the accuracy of measuring effective regurgitant orifice area (EROA) by this technique.

Flow Convergence or Proximal Isovelocity Surface area Method

Most of the experience with the PISA method for quantitation of regurgitation is with MR. Qualitatively, the presence of proximal flow acceleration on the LV side of the MV at the usual Nyquist limit of 50–60 cm/s indicates significant MR. Several clinical studies have validated PISA measurements of regurgitant flow rate and EROA.[92-94] PISA is best measured from the apical views,[88,95] and in most cases, a single measurement in the apical four-chamber view is sufficient **(Figs. 25A and B)**. However, in the setting of a noncircular orifice, PISA can be measured in both apical four and two chambers for greater accuracy.[95] This methodology is more accurate for central regurgitant jets than eccentric jets and for a circular orifice than a noncircular orifice. The size of the PISA has meaning only in terms of the aliasing velocity that defines the color surface. Results vary widely for calculations at different aliasing velocities, and care must be taken to use the velocity at which the hemispheric formula applies best.[96,97] Furthermore, for determination of EROA, it is essential that the CW Doppler signal be well aligned with the regurgitant jet. Poor alignment with an eccentric jet will lead to an underestimation of velocity and an overestimation of the EROA. Using a radius during an earlier time in systole may help to correct for overestimation of MR in the setting of eccentric jets.[98] The PISA method is less reliable for measuring flow when there is calcification of the MV leaflets or annulus. In MVP or hypertrophic obstructive cardiomyopathy, MR may occur only during a portion of systole and the regurgitant volume obtained by

TABLE 5: Grading of mitral regurgitation (MR) by width of vena contracta.		
Mild	Moderate	Severe
<0.3	0.30–0.69	≥0.7
VC is 2.9mm mild MR	VC is 4mm moderate MR	VC is 8mm severe MR

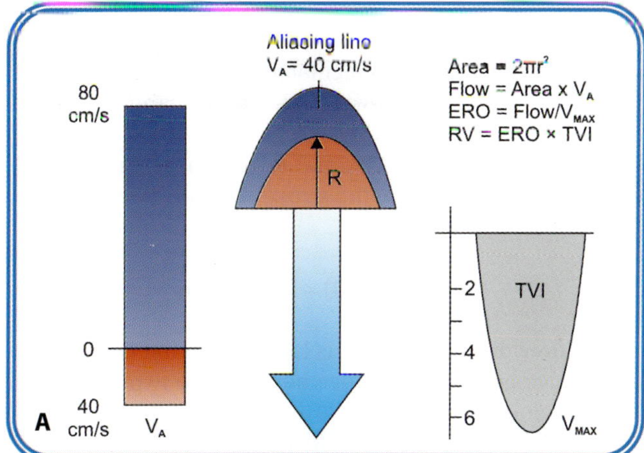

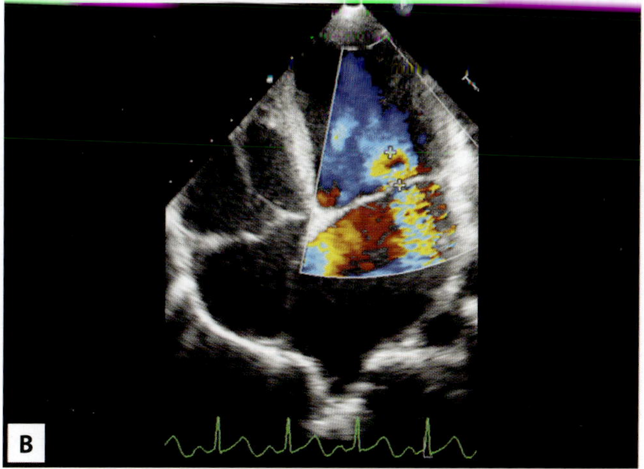

FIGS. 25A AND B: (A) Schematic diagram of proximal isovelocity surface area (PISA) or flow approaching a regurgitant orifice, increases velocity forming concentric hemispheric shells. (B) Apical four-chamber view with color Doppler with flow approaching a regurgitant orifice illustrates increased velocity forming concentric hemispheric shells.

(ERO: effective regurgitant orifice; RV: right ventricle; TVI: time-velocity integral)

PISA calculations will be overestimated unless adjusted by the fraction of systole during which regurgitation occurs.

$$\text{EROA is calculated by the formula} = \frac{\text{RV}}{\text{VTI MR}}$$

Generally, an EROA ≥ 0.4 cm^2 is consistent with severe MR, 0.20–0.39 cm^2 to moderate MR and <0.20 cm^2 to mild MR.[21]

Continuous Wave Doppler

In most patients, maximum MR velocity is 4–6 m/s due to the high systolic pressure gradient between the LV and LA. The velocity itself does not provide useful information about the severity of MR. The peak gradient between LV and LA can be calculated by using modified Bernoulli's equation. If this gradient is subtracted from the instantaneous systolic BP, one can calculate mean LA pressure. This is a sensitive test to measure LA pressure in the absence of aortic stenosis or left ventricular outflow tract (LVOT) obstruction. The contour of the velocity profile and its density are useful. The density of the CW Doppler signal is a qualitative index of MR severity. Denser is the signal more is the spectral broadening and indicates significant MR. Whereas a faint signal, with or without an incomplete envelope represents mild or trace MR, presuming the recording is made through the vena contracta. In eccentric significant MR, it may be difficult to record the full envelope of the jet because of its eccentricity, while the signal intensity shows dense features. Recently, the returning power of the regurgitant velocity signal, which is proportional to the area of the vena contracta, has been used to obtain instantaneous regurgitant orifice area and flow rate.[99] The shape of the classic MR jet trace is holosystolic. A truncated, triangular jet contour with early peaking of the maximal velocity indicates elevated LA pressure or a prominent regurgitant pressure wave in the LA. Using CW Doppler, an estimate of pulmonary artery pressure can be obtained from the TR peak velocity **(Fig. 26)**. The presence of PHT provides another indirect clue as to MR severity and compensation to the volume overload **(Table 6)**.

Pulsed Doppler

Pulsed Doppler tracings at the mitral leaflet tips are commonly used to evaluate LV diastolic function. Pulsed Doppler quantitative flow has been validated for the quantitation of MR in several studies.[100-102] Quantitative pulsed wave (PW) Doppler provides regurgitant volume, regurgitant fraction (RF), and orifice size. Determination of MR volume can be determined using a combination of 2D and PW Doppler. The mitral annulus is measured in its greatest dimension in diastole and the radius is used in the calculation of the mitral annular area. This is multiplied by the time-velocity integral of the mitral inflow obtained by PW Doppler at the level of the mitral annulus to determine the stroke volume across the mitral valve (TSV).

$$\text{TSV} = \text{VTI (MV)} \times \text{MV annulus area}$$

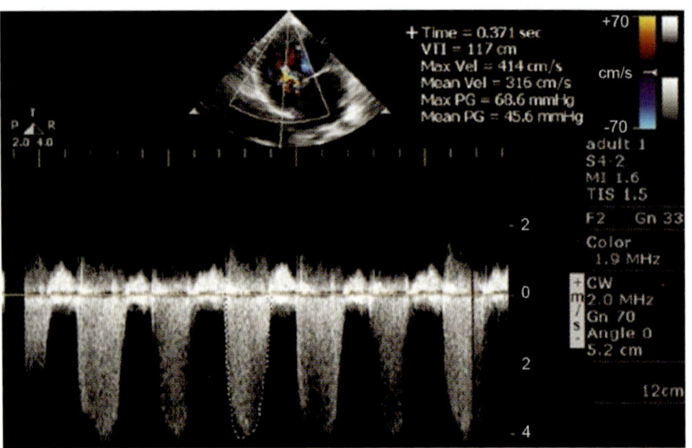

FIG. 26: Tricuspid regurgitation (TR) peak velocity is used to estimate pulmonary artery pressure.

TABLE 6: Grading mitral regurgitation by Doppler parameters.

	Doppler parameters		
	Mild	*Moderate*	*Severe*
Mitral inflow-PW	A wave dominant	Variable	E wave dominant
Jet density-CW	Incomplete or faint	Dense	Dense
Jet contour-CW	Parabolic	≈ Parabolic	Early peaking-triangular
Pulmonary vein flow	Systolic dominance	Systolic blunting	Systolic flow reversal
Regurgitant volume (mL)	<30	30–44	45–59
EROA (cm^2)	<0.20	0.20–0.29	0.30–0.39

(CW: continuous wave; EROA: effective regurgitant orifice area; PW: pulsed wave)

The LVOT area is then calculated by measuring the LVOT dimension in the parasternal long-axis view and multiplied by the LVOT time-velocity integral, obtained from PW Doppler sampled just proximal to the aortic valve in the apical view, to determine the stroke volume (SV) across the aortic valve.

$$\text{SV} = \text{VTI (AO)} \times \text{LVOT area}$$

The flow through the MV is larger than that through the aortic valve and the difference between the two represents the regurgitant volume.

Regurgitant volume (RV) in mL = TSV – SV
It is accurate for multiple jets and eccentric jets. RV < 30 mL is consistent with mild MR, 30–44 mL with moderate MR, 45–59 mL with moderately severe MR and ≥60 mL with severe MR.[21]

Regurgitant fraction is the regurgitant volume as a percentage of total stroke volume. It can be calculated by the formula:

$$RF = \frac{RV \times 100}{TSV} \text{ or } RF = \frac{(TSV - SV) \times 100}{TSV}$$

A RF of <30% is mild MR, 30–49% is moderate MR and ≥50% is severe MR.[21] Quantitative Doppler measurements may be more applicable to patients with a single regurgitant valve. The method is not valid with combined MR and AR unless pulmonary annular data are used. A regurgitant volume of 60 mL/beat and a RF of 50% suggest severe MR.[12] Quantitative PW Doppler method offers an advantage in the case of eccentric or multiple regurgitant MR jets as it evaluates MR during the entire duration of systole, whereas PISA is not as accurate and vena contracta is not applicable in the latter situation. PW Doppler also provides qualitative data regarding MR severity. A dominant early mitral inflow velocity is typical in severe MR due to increased diastolic flow across the MV.[103] In the setting of severe MR, the peak E velocity is usually >1.2 m/s and higher than the mitral A velocity. An increased peak mitral E wave velocity is not specific for MR, as E wave velocities are also influenced by LA pressure, LV compliance, MV stenosis, and heart rhythm abnormalities. However, a dominant A wave in the mitral filling pattern virtually excludes severe MR.[12]

Pulmonary Vein Flow

Pulsed Doppler evaluation of pulmonary venous flow is a useful adjunct to evaluating the hemodynamic consequences of MR. Normal pulmonary venous flow is characterized by a velocity during ventricular systole that is higher than during ventricular diastole. With increasing severity of MR, the velocity of forward systolic flow in the pulmonary vein decreases and eventually may be reversed in systole. Since the mitral regurgitant jet may selectively enter one or the other of the pulmonary veins, sampling through all pulmonary veins is recommended, especially during TEE. This sign is helpful in determining regurgitant severity only when the jet is not eccentric. It is not of great use in patients with severe LV disease in whom the systolic component of pulmonary venous flow is already poor and those with eccentric MR jet, e.g., posterior leaflet prolapse. Moreover, systolic flow in pulmonary veins is also affected by LA compliance, age and rhythm.[21,104] As a result, the use of pulmonary venous flow pattern should be used adjunctively with other parameters. Nevertheless, the finding of systolic flow reversal in more than one pulmonary vein is specific but not sensitive for severe MR **(Flowchart 1)**.

Supportive Signs

Echocardiography plays an important role in the management of MR and provides prognostic information. Organic MR tends to be progressive, and the LV responds to this volume load by developing eccentric hypertrophy and diastolic enlargement. Over time, LV contractile dysfunction occurs and is evident by increases in systolic dimensions. Survival following MV replacement is predicted by the preoperative LVEF[76,105,106] and postoperative LV systolic dysfunction is predicted by preoperative LVEF and LV end-systolic dimension.[76,107] A flail mitral leaflet is associated with adverse outcomes in nonsurgically treated patients, although the risk of death is lower in the segment of patients who were asymptomatic and had normal LVEF.[108] Indications for surgery include LVEF < 60%, LV end-systolic dimension > 45 mm, or symptoms.[19] It is estimated that end-systolic volume of >40 mL identifies patients with severe MR.[109] Asymptomatic patients not meeting these echocardiographic criteria should be followed with noninvasive studies. Exercise ECHO can be used in the setting of symptoms out of proportion to the MR severity and to assess functional status and hemodynamic changes in patients who are apparently asymptomatic.[110] In patients with PA systolic pressures > 60 mm Hg with exercise, MV surgery should be considered.[21] The feasibility of MV repair, which is preferred over replacement,[111] can be assessed echocardiographically. Repair is more likely when there is limited calcification of the leaflets or annulus, when prolapse of only one leaflet is present and when valve perforation or annular dilatation is the mechanism of MR.

Role of Transesophageal Echocardiography in Assessing Severity of Mitral Regurgitation[6]

Indications for transesophageal echocardiography

Class I

- Preoperative or intraoperative TEE is indicated to establish the anatomic basis for severe MR in patients in whom surgery is recommended to assess feasibility of repair and to guide repair. (*Level of Evidence: B*)

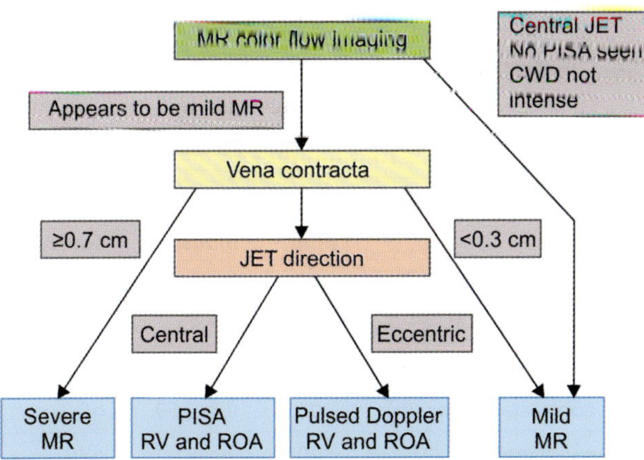

FLOWCHART 1: Mitral regurgitation by color flow.

(CWD: continuous wave Doppler; MR: mitral regurgitation; MV: mitral valve; PISA: proximal isovelocity surface area; ROA: regurgitant orifice area)

- Transesophageal echocardiography is indicated for evaluation of MR patients in whom TTE provides nondiagnostic information regarding severity of MR, mechanism of MR and/or status of LV function. *(Level of Evidence: B)*

Class IIa

Preoperative TEE is reasonable in asymptomatic patients with severe MR who are considered for surgery to assess feasibility of repair. *(Level of Evidence: C)*

Class III

- Transesophageal echocardiography is not indicated for routine follow-up or surveillance of asymptomatic patients with native valve MR. *(Level of Evidence: C)*

Transesophageal echocardiography is indicated to evaluate MR severity in patients in whom TTE is inconclusive or technically difficult. As the transducer is only a couple of mm away from LA, the cardiac structures especially the posterior ones like MV, MV apparatus are well visualized. Hence, TEE is superior to chest wall echocardiography in detailing the MV anatomy and in determining MR severity[112,113] and for planning MV surgery. All of the above methods of quantifying MR can also be used during TEE. In particular, the higher resolution of TEE, multiplane capabilities and proximity to the MV makes vena contracta imaging and PISA easier and probably more accurate. TEE does not overcome the limitations of jet expansion and may show larger jets, but can be useful in delineating extent of eccentric jets because of better resolution. Quantitative pulsed Doppler by TEE works well provided that a deep transgastric view is obtained to properly align the PW Doppler beam to the LV outflow tract. The latter, however, is more difficult than with the transthoracic approach. Interrogation of all pulmonary veins is generally feasible with TEE.[21]

Transesophageal echocardiography has played an important role in determining candidates for MV repair and guiding valve surgery. Hemodynamics are different in an anesthetized patient and can lead to the appearance of less severe regurgitation compared with an awake or mildly sedated patient. The goal of repair is a reduction of MR to mild or less, without creating significant valvular stenosis. A mean transmitral diastolic gradient of 2–4 mm Hg is generally acceptable following repair. It is a routine practice now to use intraoperative TEE that provides detailed perioperative assessment and detects early postoperative signs of valve dysfunction. Residual regurgitation can always be dealt with before closure of the chest and a second pump run can be established and the dysfunction corrected. A direct assessment of the mode of MV repair can be provided which includes: direct leaflet repair and chordal replacement with Gore-Tex suture or annuloplasty through insertion of a mitral ring. Intraoperative TEE also helps in assessing LV function before weaning off the bypass circulation. Finally, it identifies any entrapped air in the cardiac chambers.[114,115]

Integrative Approach to Assessment of Severity of Mitral Regurgitation

The approach to evaluation of MR severity should ideally integrate multiple parameters rather than depending on a single measurement. This helps to minimize the effects of technical or measurement errors that are inherent to each method previously discussed. It is also important to distinguish between the amount of MR and its hemodynamic consequences. For example, with acute MR, patient develops severe pulmonary congestion even with if a moderate regurgitant occurs acutely into a small, noncompliant LA. Conversely, some patients with chronic severe MR remain asymptomatic due to compensatory mechanisms and a dilated, compliant LA. Parameters that describe the amount of MR include vena contracta width, regurgitant volume and fraction, EROA calculated either by PISA or quantitative pulsed Doppler. Because regurgitant flows may be holosystolic or brief, as in valve prolapse,[92] color Doppler techniques should be adjusted for duration of MR. Thus, a wide vena contracta occurring briefly indicates only mild MR. On the other hand, the hemodynamic consequences of MR are reflected in several parameters including LA and LV volumes, the contour of the CW Doppler profile, and pulmonary venous flow pattern. The MR index has been devised that assigns different weights to six different indicators of MR,[116] using a score of 0–3 for jet penetration into the LA, PISA radius, CW jet intensity, pulmonary artery pressure, pulmonary venous flow pattern, and LA size. A score of 1.7 or less reliably separated mild MR from severe MR; a considerable overlap, however, was observed between moderate and severe MR. Although it may be impractical for routine clinical use, this scoring system emphasizes the need to evaluate multiple echocardiographic parameters. The Task Force[21] proposes a scheme of specific signs (>90% specificity), along with supportive signs and quantitative parameters to help grade the severity of MR **(Table 7)**. Specific signs have inherently a high positive predictive value for the severity of regurgitation. The supportive signs or clues may be helpful in consolidating the impression of the degree of MR,

TABLE 7: Quantitative parameters for evaluation of mitral regurgitation.

	Mild	*Moderate*	*Severe*
Regurgitant volume (mL/beat)	<30	30–59	≥60
Regurgitant fraction (%)	<30	30–49	≥50
EROA (cm^2)	<0.2	0.2–0.39	≥0.4
Vena contracta width (cm)	<0.3	0.3–0.69	≥0.7
Jet area/LA area (%)	<20	20–40	>40
Jet area (cm^2)	<4	4–9.9	>10

(EROA: effective regurgitant orifice area; LA: left atrium)
Source: Adapted from Tables 1 and 3 of Zoghbi WA et al.[21]

although their predictive value is more modest, since they are influenced by several factors. It is the consensus of the committee members that the process of grading MR should be comprehensive, using a combination of clues, signs, and measurements obtained by Doppler ECHO.

Follow-up

Asymptomatic patients with mild MR and no evidence of LV enlargement, LV dysfunction, or PHT can be followed on a yearly basis with instructions to alert the physician if symptoms develop in the interim.

In patients with moderate MR, clinical evaluation including ECHO should be performed annually and sooner if symptoms occur. Asymptomatic patients with severe MR should be followed up with history, physical examination, and ECHO every 6–12 months to assess symptoms or transition to asymptomatic LV dysfunction. Exercise stress testing may be used to add objective evidence regarding symptoms and changes in exercise tolerance especially if a good history of the patient's exercise capacity cannot be obtained. Measurement of pulmonary artery pressure and assessment of severity of MR during exercise may be helpful.[6]

Interpretation of LV ejection fraction in the patient with MR is made difficult because the loading conditions present in MR to facilitate ejection and increase ejection fraction, the standard guide to LV function. Ejection fraction in a patient with MR with normal LV function is usually ≥0.60. It has been observed that postoperative ventricular function is lower and survival is reduced in patients with a preoperative ejection fraction < 0.60 compared with patients with higher ejection fractions.[105,107]

Alternatively or in addition, echocardiographic LV end-systolic dimension (or volume) can be used in the timing of MV surgery. End-systolic dimension, which may be less load dependent than ejection fraction,[117] should be <40mm preoperatively to ensure normal postoperative LV function.[107,117-119] If patients become symptomatic, they should undergo MV surgery even if LV function is normal. Echocardiographic features in severe MR that determine timing of surgery are: (1) dilated LA, (2) dilated LV, EDV, ESV, EF, (3) jet area > 40% of LA, (4) E-wave dominant, (5) dense CW Doppler signal, (6) early peaking-triangular CW signal, (7) pulmonary vein flow reversal, (8) vena contracta ≥ 0.7 cm, (9) regurgitant volume ≥ 60 mL, (10) RF ≥ 50%, and (11) EROA ≥ 0.40 cm^2.

■ AORTIC STENOSIS

Two-dimensional and Doppler echocardiography is the imaging modality of choice for the diagnosis and quantification of aortic stenosis. Rheumatic disease of the aortic valve is less common than that of the MV and is almost invariably associated with rheumatic MV disease. The anatomic evaluation of the aortic valve is done with a combination of short- and long-axis images to identify the number of leaflets, for leaflet mobility, thickness, and

calcification. A normal aortic valve has three cusps and AVA is 3–4 cm^2. The normal cusp separation is 15–26 mm. Transthoracic imaging usually is adequate, although TEE may be helpful when image quality is suboptimal.

Rheumatic aortic leaflet involvement, like MV disease, is associated with commissural fusion which can clearly be seen from short-axis echocardiography of the aortic valve. As the disease progresses, the leaflets become fibrosed and calcified, resulting in valve stenosis. Thickening and calcification is most prominent along the edges of the aortic cusps. The presence of MS confirms the etiology of aortic stenosis as rheumatic. When associated with significant MS, the degree of aortic stenosis is usually clinically underestimated. Isolated rheumatic aortic stenosis is very rare.[120] Aortic stenosis causes chronic pressure load on the heart and which results in concentric LV hypertrophy and subsequent diastolic dysfunction. LA enlargement indicates concomitant diastolic dysfunction. Echocardiography can evaluate for presence of other valvular abnormalities of mitral, tricuspid, and pulmonary valve.

M-mode ECHO gives an idea about the severity of aortic stenosis by evaluating the average value of aortic leaflet cusp separation (normal aortic cusp separation is 19.4 ± 2.1 mm) with respect to the aortic root diameter, reduces with aortic stenosis **(Figs. 27A and B)**. The normal value is about 70% of the aortic root diameter. Mild stenosis is 50% and moderate to severe stenosis <30% of the aortic root diameter. This method has its limitations in overestimating the degree of valve stenosis in patients with severe leaflet calcification and those with significant LV disease and low cardiac output.[121-123] M mode can also measure the dimensions at LV. It also measures the degree of LV hypertrophy and mass from which mass index can be calculated.

Assessment of Severity of Aortic Stenosis

Although 2D can diagnose the presence of aortic stenosis, the severity of aortic stenosis cannot be determined by visualization of valve motion alone. Therefore, Doppler echocardiography must be used to further assess the severity of aortic stenosis **(Table 8)**. The primary hemodynamic parameters recommended for clinical evaluation of AS severity are: (1) AS jet velocity, (2) mean transaortic gradient, and (3) valve area by continuity equation.

Aortic Jet Velocity

Aortic jet velocity, which is the antegrade systolic velocity across the narrowed aortic valve, is measured using CW Doppler.[124-126] AS jet velocity is defined as the highest velocity signal obtained from any window. Multiple acoustic windows should be evaluated carefully in order to determine the highest velocity. Apical and suprasternal or right parasternal most frequently yield the highest velocity and rarely subcostal or supraclavicular windows may be required. Careful patient positioning and adjustment of transducer position and angle are crucial as velocity measurement assumes a parallel intercept angle between the ultrasound

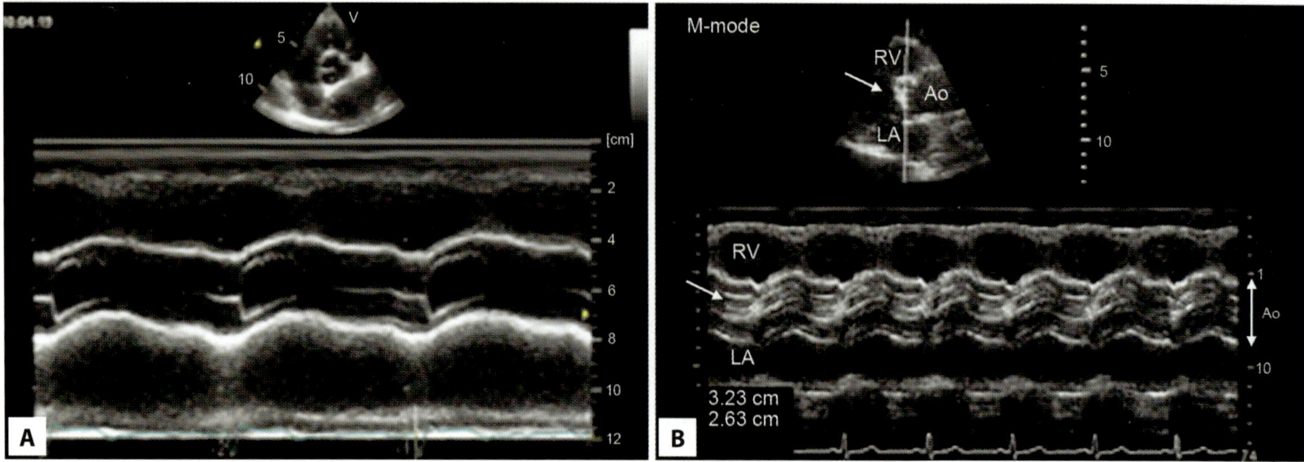

FIGS. 27A AND B: (A) M-mode of normal aortic valve opening; (B) thickened-aortic eccentric valve with reduced cusp separation in a 22-year-old man with rheumatic heart disease (RHD) and aortic stenosis (AS).

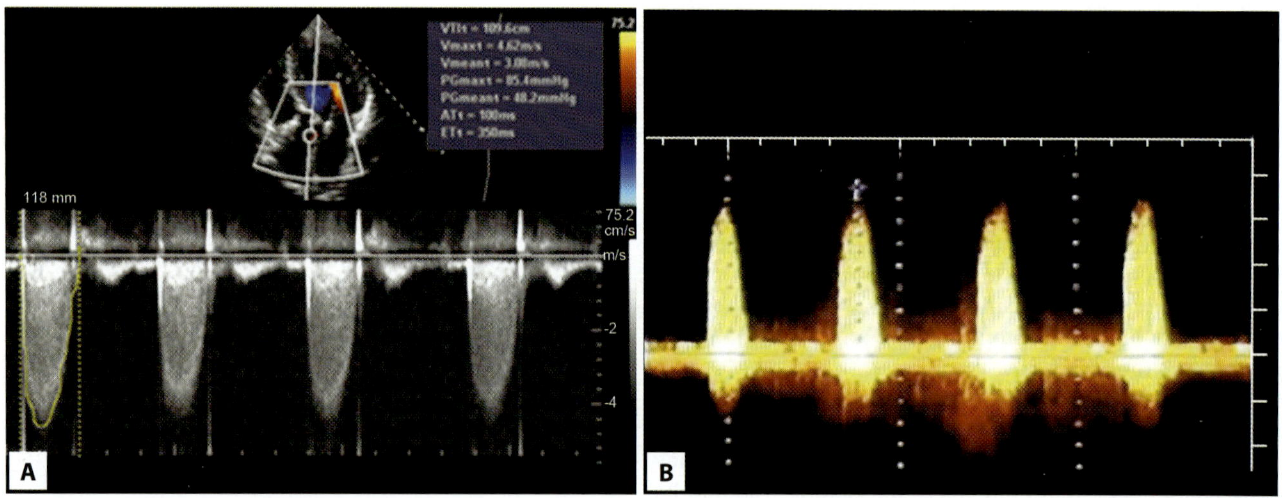

FIGS. 28A AND B: (A) Spectral Doppler signal shows a smooth velocity curve demonstrating maximum velocity in a case of AS critical aortic stenosis with cursor on aorta in apical five-chamber view. (B) Doppler signals obtained from transducer in suprasternal notch view.

TABLE 8: Assessment of severity of aortic stenosis.[6]			
Indicator	**Mild**	**Moderate**	**Severe**
Jet velocity (m/s)	<3.0	3.0–4.0	>4.0
Mean gradient (mm Hg)	<25	25–40	>40
Valve area (cm²)	>1.5	1.0–1.5	<1.0
Valve area index (cm²/m²)	>0.85	0.6–0.85	<0.6

fever, anemia, arteriovenous fistula, and aortic regurgitation will increase the peak aortic velocity but not the degree of stenosis. Conversely, when low cardiac output states exist, peak aortic velocity may be modestly elevated despite critical valve stenosis. The spectral Doppler signal should have a smooth velocity curve with a dense outer edge so that clear maximum velocity can be recorded **(Figs. 28A and B)**. The outer edge of the dark "envelope" of the velocity curve is traced to provide both the velocity time integral (VTI) for continuity equation and the mean gradient.

beam and direction of blood flow. Any deviation from a parallel intercept angle results in velocity underestimation. 3D direction of the aortic jet is unpredictable and usually cannot be visualized. Stenosis is only mild when velocity < 3 m/s and leaflet opening is well seen. Moderate AS when aortic jet velocity is 3.0–4.0 m/s and severe AS when aortic jet velocity is of >4 m/s.[6] High cardiac output states such as

Transesophageal Echocardiography: Planimetry Shows the Aortic Valve Orifice Area

The average of three or more beats in sinus rhythm and averaging of more beats is mandatory with irregular rhythms (at least five consecutive beats). Special care must be taken to select representative sequences of beats and to avoid postextrasystolic beats. The shape of the CW Doppler velocity curve is helpful in distinguishing the level and severity of obstruction. The time course of the velocity curve is similar at any level of obstruction but the maximum velocity occurs later in systole and the curve is more rounded in shape with more severe obstruction. While with mild obstruction, the peak is in early systole with a triangular shape of the velocity curve, compared with the rounded curve with the peak moving toward midsystole in severe stenosis, reflecting a high gradient throughout systole. Thus, in mild stenosis, velocities peak in early systole and in severe stenosis velocities peak in midsystole, in parallel with the rise in aortic pressure. The shape of the CWD velocity curve also can be helpful in determining whether the obstruction is fixed or dynamic. Dynamic subaortic obstruction shows a characteristic late peaking velocity curve, often with a concave upward curve in early systole.[14]

Another major technical issue in recording the aortic stenosis Doppler velocity profile is insuring measurement of the AS jet as opposed to an MR signal. The AS Doppler signal will start later than the MR signal due to isovolumic contraction and will have a shorter ejection time. The presence of AR in the spectral display diastolic flow signal may also be helpful in distinguishing AS from MR.

Mean Transaortic Pressure Gradient

The pressure gradient across a stenotic aortic valve is related to the velocity of blood flow across the stenotic orifice and is difference in pressure between the LV and aorta in systole. Both the maximal instantaneous gradient and the mean aortic valve gradient can be derived from CWD velocity. As mentioned above, a detailed meticulous study using multiple sites of interrogation should be done in order to ensure that the Doppler beam is parallel to the stenotic jet. One of the major pitfalls of Doppler ECHO is underestimation of the gradient when the Doppler beam is not parallel to the aortic velocity jet. The calculation of the mean gradient, which is the average gradient across the valve occurring during the entire systole, has potential advantages and should be reported. Though there is good correlation between peak gradient and mean gradient, the relationship between peak and mean gradient depends on the shape of the velocity curve, which varies with stenosis severity and flow rate. The Doppler derived maximum gradient is a peak instantaneous pressure gradient, which occurs at one point in time and is not the same as the "peak-to peak gradient" often reported in a cardiac catheterization report. The peak to peak catheter gradient refers to the pressure difference between peak LV pressure and peak aortic pressure, which are not simultaneous and not measured by continuous wave (CW) Doppler. Therefore, it should be no surprise that peak to peak catheter gradients are smaller and do not correlate well with peak Doppler instantaneous pressure gradients. Doppler mean gradients are more comparable to catheterization derived mean gradients. Many studies demonstrate a close correlation between simultaneous ECHO and catheterization derived mean gradients over a wide range of stenosis severity, from mild to critical aortic valve stenosis.[124,127-137]

The velocity obtained by CW Doppler across the aortic valve provides an accurate and reproducible measurement of valve gradient by application of the modified Bernoulli equation.

$$\text{Pressure grdient (mm Hg)} + 4V_2$$
$$\text{where } V \text{ is the peak Doppler velocity (m/s)}.$$

The maximum gradient is calculated from maximum velocity and the mean gradient is calculated by averaging the instantaneous gradients over the ejection period, a function included in most clinical instrument measurement packages using the traced velocity curve. The mean gradient requires averaging of instantaneous mean gradients and cannot be calculated from the mean velocity.

In addition, the simplified Bernoulli equation assumes that the proximal velocity can be ignored, a reasonable assumption when velocity is < 1 m/s because squaring a number < 1 makes it even smaller. When the proximal velocity is over 1.5 m/s or the aortic velocity is <3.0 m/s, the proximal velocity should be included in the Bernoulli equation so that when calculating maximum gradients. It is more problematic to include proximal velocity in mean gradient calculations as each point on the ejection curve for the proximal and jet velocities would need to be matched and this approach is not used clinically. In this situation, maximum velocity and gradient should be used to grade stenosis severity.

Aortic stenosis severity is graded on basis of mean gradient as mild < 25, moderate 25–40, and severe > 40 mm Hg.[6]

When stenosis is severe and cardiac output is normal, the mean transvalvular pressure gradient is generally >40 mm Hg. However, when cardiac output is low, severe stenosis may be present with a lower transvalvular gradient and velocity. Some patients with severe AS remain asymptomatic, whereas others with only moderate stenosis develop symptoms. Therapeutic decisions, particularly those related to corrective surgery, are based largely on the presence or absence of symptoms. Thus, the absolute valve area (or transvalvular pressure gradient) is not the primary determinant of the need for aortic valve replacement.[6] Depending on the flow across the aortic valve, the pressure gradient across the aortic valve increases or decreases. Increased flow increases the gradient and decreased flow decreases the gradient. Condition associated with decreased flow across the aortic valve and hence decreased gradient are: AS with MS, AS with MR, AS with subaortic stenosis, LV systolic dysfunction, atrial fibrillation, hypovolemia, and sedation. Conditions associated with increased flow across the aortic valve and hence increased gradient are exercise and dobutamine infusion.

Valve Area

Doppler velocity and pressure gradients are flow dependent for a given orifice area, velocity and gradient increase with an increase in transaortic flow rate and decrease with a decrease in flow rate. Calculation of the stenotic orifice area or AVA is helpful when flow rates are very low or very high, although even the degree of valve opening varies to some degree with flow rate. AVA is calculated based on the continuity equation concept that the stroke volume (SV) ejected through the LVOT all passes through the stenotic orifice (AVA) and thus SV is equal at both sites: Calculation of continuity equation valve area requires three measurements: AS jet velocity by CWD, LVOT diameter for calculation of a circular CSA, LVOT velocity recorded with pulsed Doppler. The LVOT diameter is measured from the parasternal long-axis view and converted to the LVOT area. From an apical approach with pulsed-wave Doppler, the LVOT velocity is obtained and traced to derive the time-velocity integral (TVI). The following formula is then used for calculation of AVA:

$$\text{Aortic valve area} = \frac{(\text{LVOT}_{\text{TVI}}) \times (\text{LVOT}_{\text{area}})}{(\text{AV}_{\text{TVI}})}$$

Calculation of AVA does require a skilled echocardiographer to ensure accurate measurement of the LVOT diameter and proper positioning of the same volume in the outflow tract. The largest source of variability in valve area calculation by the continuity equation lies in the measurement of the LVOT diameter, which is divided by two and then squared. Accurate measurement of the LVOT may not be possible in patients with poor acoustic windows and/or those with heavily calcified valves. Small errors in diameter measurement result in significant errors in the calculation of area. In each patient, there needs to be a correlation between the valve gradient, the valve area, and the stroke volume. Aortic valve stenosis is mild if valve area is >1.5 cm², moderate if it is 1.0–1.5 cm², and severe if it is <1.0 cm².[6] The mean coefficient of intraobserver and interobserver measurement variability has been reported at 5.1 and 7.9%, resulting in a valve area variability of 0.15 cm²

for a valve area of 1.0 cm².[138] For these reasons, the velocity ratio between the AS jet and the LVOT jet is also useful. The velocity ratio $VLVOT/VAS < 0.2$ suggests severe aortic stenosis. Coexistent AR results in increased transaortic flow and an increase in mean gradient. However, the valve area calculation by the continuity equation remains accurate. Clinical symptoms such as chest pain breathlessness predict prognosis not gradients or calculated valve areas. While the rate of hemodynamic progression is highly variable, studies reveal an increase in peak aortic jet velocity from 0.2 to 0.4 m/s per year, an increase in mean pressure gradient of 6–7 mm Hg/year and a decrease in AVA of 0–0.3.1 cm²/year.[139-146]

Transesophageal echocardiography can be utilized to measure AVA and for aortic valve morphology.[147] TEE is very useful in perioperative management of AS. It can display the stenotic aortic valve **(Fig. 29A)** and LV function, immediately before and after surgery. Especially TEE with 4D can detect paravalvular leaks and valve dysfunction. TEE allows monitoring of the LV function throughout surgery.[148]

If valve-sparing intervention like aortic balloon valvotomy (ABV) is considered, then TEE may be performed preoperatively to define the anatomy of the cusps and ascending aorta **(Fig. 29B)**.

Stress Echocardiography

Dobutamine stress ECHO (DSE) has been used to distinguish severe from nonsevere valvular aortic stenosis in patients with depressed LV function and low transvalvular gradients[149] (Class IIa indication). The investigation is also useful in patients with moderate aortic stenosis, based on pressure gradient, who are limited by symptoms. When there is increase in heart rate, the increased blood flow across the valve differentiates between severe valve narrowing and severe LV disease. When LV systolic dysfunction coexists with severe AS, the AS velocity and gradient may be low, despite a small valve area; a condition termed as "low-flow

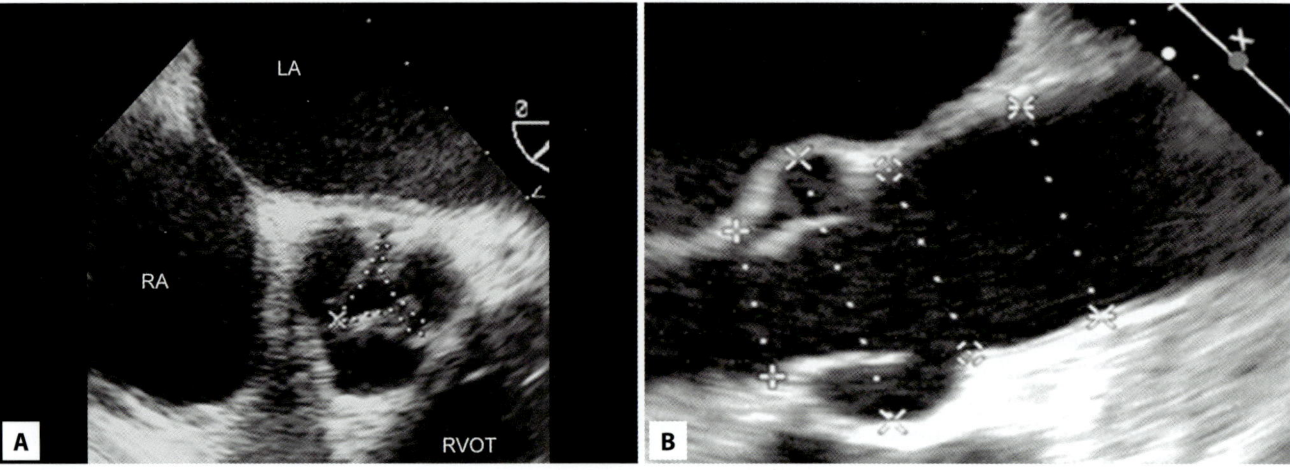

FIGS. 29A AND B: Transesophageal echocardiography (TEE)—planimetry shows the aortic valve orifice area.

TABLE 9: Dobutamine stress ECHO in low gradient and low-flow aortic stenosis.

	Severe aortic stenosis	Pseudostenosis	Indeterminate
Aortic valve area	No change	Increase > 0.3 cm^2	No change
Mean pressure gradient	Markedly increased	No change	No change
Stroke volume > 20%	Yes	Yes	No

low-gradient AS". A widely used definition of low-flow low-gradient AS includes the following conditions: Effective orifice area < 1.0 cm^2; LV ejection fraction < 40%; and mean pressure gradient < 30–40 mm Hg.[14] Dobutamine is infused in a graded fashion to a maximum dose of 20 µg/kg/min. At each stage, ventricular function is assessed by 2D imaging and Doppler data are obtained to reassess mean gradient and to calculate AV. The infusion should be stopped as soon as a positive result is obtained or when the heart rate begins to rise >10–20 bpm over baseline or exceeds 100 bpm. The three theoretical responses to dobutamine are as follows **(Table 9)**:

1. Transvalvular flow increases significantly, mean gradient increases to >40 mm Hg and valve area remains fixed at <1 cm^2.
2. Transvalvular flow increases, mean gradient increases modestly but remains <40 mm Hg, and valve area increases to >1 cm^2.
3. No significant change in transaortic flow, mean gradient, or valve area with dobutamine.

The patients demonstrating the second type of response have been termed as "pseudosevere AS". These patients are unable to augment stroke volume by 20% (as assessed by velocity–time integral in the LVOT) and hence prognosis is poor regardless of the severity of the aortic valve stenosis and suggests poor contractile reserve.[149-152] Recent studies suggest that those without LV contractile reserve by DSE have a high operative mortality, as high as 33%.[130,131] Thus, failure of aortic velocities to increase significantly with stress suggests impaired LV function as the cause of the low cardiac output and symptoms rather than aortic stenosis.[151] A valve area of <0.7 cm^2 that remains unchanged with stress is consistent with severe stenosis, particularly if there is evidence for adequate contractile reserve as evidenced by at least 50% increase in stroke volume.[153]

Associated Conditions

About 80% of adults with AS also have aortic regurgitation (AR). When AR is mild or moderate in severity and measures of AS severity are not significantly affected.

When severe AR accompanies AS, measures of AS severity remain accurate including maximum velocity, mean gradient, and valve area. However, because of the high transaortic volume flow rate, maximum velocity and mean gradient will be higher than expected for a given valve area. In this situation, reporting accurate quantitative data for the severity of both stenosis and regurgitation.[21] MS may result in low cardiac output and, therefore, low-flow low-gradient AS. MR severity does not affect evaluation of AS severity except for two possible situations. First, with severe MR, transaortic flow rate may be low resulting in a low gradient even when severe AS is present; valve area calculations remain accurate in this setting. Second, a high-velocity MR jet may be mistaken for the AS jet as both are systolic signals directed away from the apex. Timing of the signal is the most reliable way to distinguish the CWD velocity curve of MR from AS; MR is longer in duration, starting with MV closure and continuing until MV opening.[14] High cardiac output in patients on hemodialysis, with anemia, AV fistula, or other high-flow conditions may cause relatively high gradients in the presence of mild or moderate AS. In this situation, the shape of the CWD spectrum with a very early peak may help to quantify the severity correctly.

■ AORTIC REGURGITATION

Apart from aortic regurgitation caused by RHD, there are a number of other causes of AR. 2D ECHO is the principal diagnostic tool for detecting and assessing AR. The 2D ECHO, color-flow imaging, and pulsed and CW Doppler techniques are used for qualitative and quantitative measures that can be derived in a single examination to assess AR.

Indications for ECHO in AR6

Class I

- Echocardiography is indicated to confirm the presence and severity of acute or chronic AR *(Level of evidence: B)*.
- Echocardiography is indicated for diagnosis and assessment of the cause of chronic AR (including valve morphology and aortic root size and morphology) and for assessment of LV hypertrophy, dimension (or volume), and systolic function *(Level of evidence: B)*.
- Echocardiography is indicated in patients with an enlarged aortic root to assess regurgitation and the severity of aortic dilatation *(Level of evidence: B)*.
- Echocardiography is indicated for the periodic re-evaluation of LV size and function in asymptomatic patients with severe AR *(Level of evidence: B)*.
- Radionuclide angiography or magnetic resonance imaging is indicated for the initial and serial assessment of LV volume and function at rest in patients with AR and suboptimal echocardiograms *(Level of evidence: B)*.
- Echocardiography is indicated to re-evaluate mild, moderate, or severe AR in patients with new or changing symptoms *(Level of evidence: B)*.

Class IIa

- Exercise stress testing for chronic AR is reasonable for assessment of functional capacity and symptomatic response in patients with a history of equivocal symptoms *(Level of evidence: B)*.
- Exercise stress testing for patients with chronic AR is reasonable for the evaluation of symptoms and functional capacity before participation in athletic activities *(Level of evidence: C)*.
- Magnetic resonance imaging is reasonable for the estimation of AR severity in patients with unsatisfactory echocardiograms *(Level of evidence: B)*.

Class IIb

- Exercise stress testing in patients with radionuclide angiography may be considered for assessment of LV function in asymptomatic or symptomatic patients with chronic AR *(Level of evidence: B)*.

Rheumatic heart disease of the aortic valve results in thickening of the cusps and fusion of the commissures with retraction of the leaflets and hence noncooptation and regurgitation. The echocardiogram is able to demonstrate the size and function of the LV as well as the etiology of AR. Severe AR results in increase in LV filling pressure and as the LV is exposed to a significant volume overload, it adapts over time by increasing LV mass in an eccentric pattern, leading to progressive chamber dilatation. Ultimately, systolic dysfunction occurs and may be irreversible. An increase in LV end-diastolic volume and fall in end-systolic volume is compatible with a significant volume overload. The main difference between aortic and MR is that in the former ventricular loading occurs in early and mid-diastole whereas with MR it is predominantly early diastolic. An increase in LV minor axis end-systolic diameter > 5.0 cm or 2.5 cm/m² in the presence of any overload suggests independent ventricular disease even in the absence of significant symptoms.[154,155]

Coarse fluttering of anterior mitral leaflet: This is a common finding in aortic regurgitation. When the aortic regurgitant jet impinges on the AML in diastole, high-frequency fluttering of the leaflet can be appreciated on M-mode imaging, even in the setting of mild AR. This sign, however, is not sensitive in estimating regurgitation severity.[156] Diastolic noncoaptation of aortic valve leaflets, diastolic flutter of aortic valve, and LV volume overload can be recorded on M mode. Impaired AML opening can also occur, demonstrated by an increased distance between the "maximal anterior motion of the MV E-point and the most posterior motion of the ventricular septum" termed as "increased E-point septal separation" or EPSS. In the setting of severe and decompensated AR, there is a rapid increase in LV diastolic pressure and the MV closes before the onset of the QRS complex. This finding, termed as "systolic mitral preclosure", is best appreciated by M-mode imaging **(Figs. 30A and B)**.

Doppler Methods to Assess the Severity of Aortic Regurgitation

Color flow Doppler allows for both qualitative and quantitative assessment of AR. It directly shows the regurgitant flow through the aortic valve during diastole. Assessment of the regurgitant flow can be visualized through jet direction and size in the LV, the vena contracta through the regurgitant orifice and the flow convergence region in the aorta.

Regurgitant Jet Size

Imaging of the regurgitant jet is used in all patients with AR because of its simplicity and real-time availability.[157] The maximal length of the jet penetration is not accurate in determining AR severity.[158] Aortic regurgitation severity can roughly be assessed by measuring the distance of the regurgitant jet with respect to the valve level, either subvalvular (mild) or at midventricular cavity (moderate) or

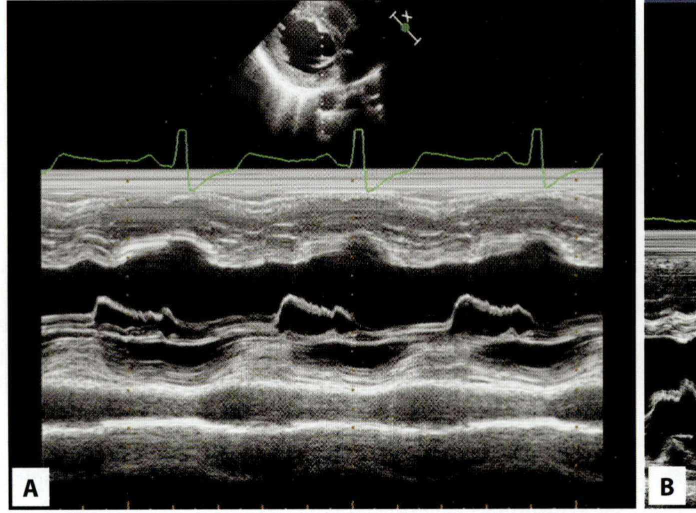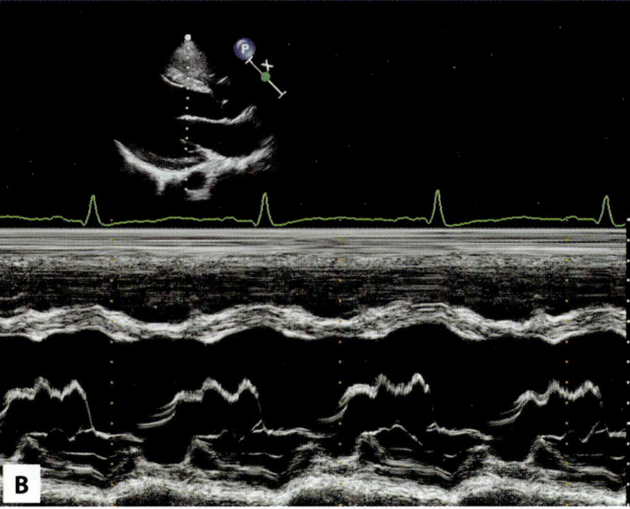

FIGS. 30A AND B: M-mode shows high-frequency fluttering of anterior mitral leaflet (AML) in a case of aortic regurgitation (AR).

approaching the apex (severe). A more accurate assessment of AR is based on the jet height or the cross-sectional area of the color jet proximal to the aortic valve within 1 cm of the valve. This is imaged in the parasternal long-axis view and compared to the LVOT width or area just below the valve.[158,159] Similarly, the cross-sectional area of the jet from the parasternal short-axis view and its ratio to the LV outflow tract area can also be used.[158] The criteria to define severe AR are ratios of >65% for jet width and >60% for jet area and mild AR is defined when the ratio is <25% **(Table 10)**.[21] The jet height is measured in the LVOT and must be distinguished from the vena contracta, which is measured immediately proximal to the flow convergence region **(Figs. 31A and B)**. Eccentric jets can be entrained along the LV wall, occupying a smaller portion of the outflow tract and may result in underestimation of severity. Diffuse jets arising from the entire coaptation line of the aortic valve can result in overestimation of regurgitation. Assessment of AR based on jet size in the LVOT is most often based on visual estimation rather than direct quantitative measurement and hence is used as a gross indicator of the degree of AR **(Fig. 32)**. This color-flow area of the regurgitant jet is not recommended to quantify the severity of AR. The color-flow imaging should only be used for a visual assessment of AR.

TABLE 10: Parameters for assessment of severity of aortic regurgitation.[21]

	Mild	Moderate	Severe
Jet width/LVOT width (%)	<25	25–64	≥65
Jet CSA/LVOT CSA (%)	<5	5–59	≥60
Vena contracta width (cm)	<0.3	0.3–0.6	>0.6
Regurgitant volume (mL/beat)	<30	30–59	≥60
Regurgitant fraction (%)	<30	30–49	≥50
EROA (cm^2)	<0.1	0.1–0.29	≥0.30

(CSA: cross-sectional area; EROA: effective regurgitant orifice area; LVOT: left ventricular outflow tract)

Vena Contracta

The vena contracta is defined as the smallest neck of the flow region at the level of the aortic valve, immediately below the flow convergence region. The measurement of vena contracta width is significantly smaller than that of jet width in the LVOT because the jet expands immediately after the vena contracta **(Fig. 33)**. Imaging of the vena contracta is obtained similarly from parasternal long-axis views.[160] Apical views should not be used due to as the splay of the color jet results in gross overestimation of the vena contracta. In the setting of eccentric jets, the vena contracta diameter should be measured perpendicular to the long axis of the jet rather than the long axis of the outflow tract. The vena contracta provides an estimate of the size of the EROA. To appropriately visualize the vena contracta, it is essential to see all three components of the regurgitant flow, i.e., the flow convergence, the vena contracta, and the jet. Measurement of vena contracta is simple and has a high feasibility both by transthoracic and TEE. The vena

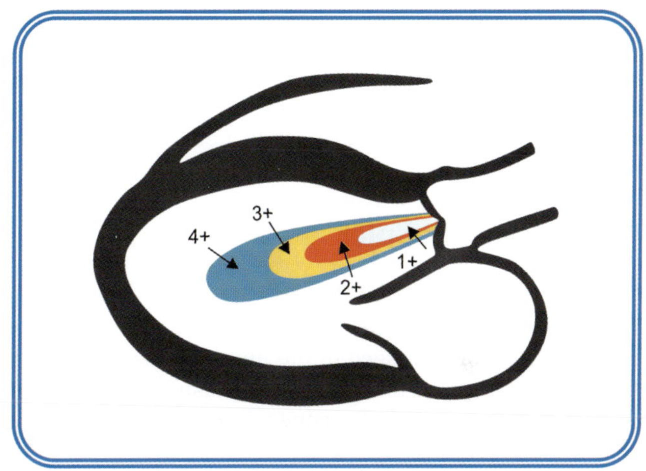

FIG. 32: Schematic jet width in LVOT/LVOT width (PLAX view). (LVOT: left ventricular outflow tract; PLAX: parasternal long axis)

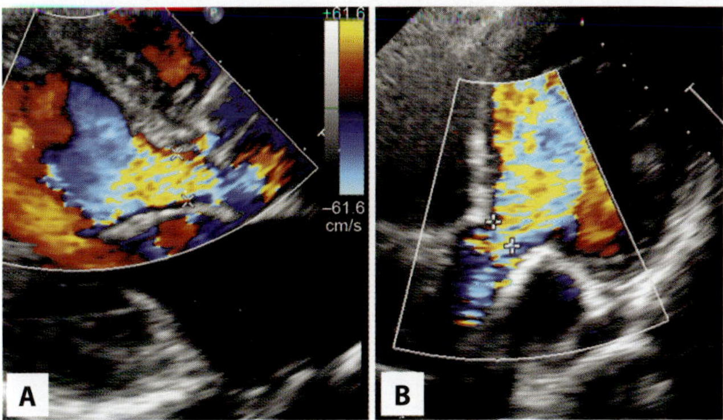

A   **B**

FIGS. 31A AND B: A parasternal long-axis view with color Doppler shows AR jet occupying LVOT indicating severe AR.

(AR: aortic regurgitation; LVOT: left ventricular outflow tract)

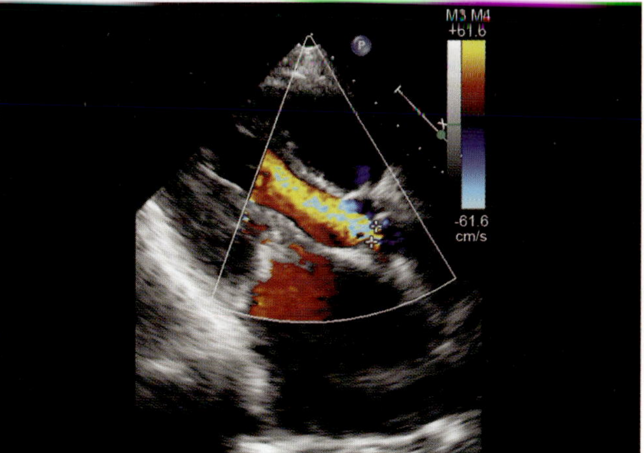

FIG. 33: Parasternal long-axis view with color Doppler illustrates measuring the narrowest portion of jet that occurs at or just downstream from orifice as vena contracta.

contracta has been shown to be a reliable measurement of the severity of aortic regurgitation when compared with other methods and is more robust than the jet height and area for AR severity.[159] Limitations of this parameter occur in the presence of multiple jets or jets with irregular shapes, where one diameter may not be reflective of the severity of the AR but, however, a short-axis view could provide a better appreciation of the regurgitation.[161] A vena contracta > 0.6 cm suggests severe aortic regurgitation.

Flow Convergence or Proximal Isovelocity Surface Area

There is limited experience using PISA for quantification of AR.[162]

Imaging of the proximal flow convergence region by TTE is done from apical, para-apical views, or the upper right sternal border, with images zoomed on the valvular and supravalvular region. The Nyquist limit is adjusted to obtain a rounded and measurable flow convergence zone and the aliasing radius is measured from the stop frame with the largest observable PISA. CW Doppler recording of the regurgitant peak velocity and velocity time integral allows calculation of the EROA and regurgitant volume. This method has been shown to provide accurate quantitation of AR.[162] Using the flow convergence method, severe AR is present when EROA $\geq$ 0.3 cm^2.

Pulsed Wave Doppler

Aortic Diastolic Flow Reversal

It is normal to observe a brief diastolic flow reversal in the aorta which is best imaged in the upper descending aorta at the aortic isthmus level using a suprasternal view or in the lower descending aorta using a longitudinal subcostal view as aortic regurgitation increases, the duration and the velocity of the reversal increases.[163] A holodiastolic reversal is usually a sign of at least moderate AR and appears to be more specific if recorded from the thoracoabdominal aorta. The velocity of flow reversal at end-diastole, the velocity time integral of the reversal and the ratio of reversal to forward velocity time integrals in the descending aorta have all been proposed as semi-quantitative indices of AR severity.[163,164] A prominent holodiastolic reversal with a diastolic time integral similar to the systolic time integral is a reliable qualitative sign of severe AR **(Figs. 34A and B)**.

Flow Calculations

Pulsed wave Doppler can be used in conjunction with 2D ECHO to calculate aortic regurgitant volume as the difference between transaortic and transmitral volume flow, provided there is only mild MR.[165,166] Total stroke volume (aortic stroke volume) can also be derived from quantitative 2D measurements of LV end-diastolic and end-systolic volumes (EDV and ESV). EROA can be calculated from the regurgitant stroke volume and the regurgitant jet velocity time integral by CW Doppler.[100,167] As with the PISA method, a regurgitant volume >60 mL is consistent with severe AR. PW Doppler can also be used at a single site in the proximal descending thoracic aorta to calculate forward and total stroke volume in AR.[163] The antegrade flow velocity integral is multiplied by the systolic cross-sectional aortic area. The flow-velocity integral of the flow reversal in diastole is then multiplied by diastolic cross-sectional area. Either 2D or M-mode imaging of the aortic arch can be used to determine both systolic and diastolic areas. A regurgitant volume $\geq$ 60 mL/beat and a RF $\geq$ 50% suggest severe AR.[21]

Continuous Wave Doppler

Signal Density

The density of the CW Doppler spectral display of the AR jet reflects the volume of regurgitation, especially in comparison to the antegrade spectral density. However, the AR jet density is also determined by the respective directions

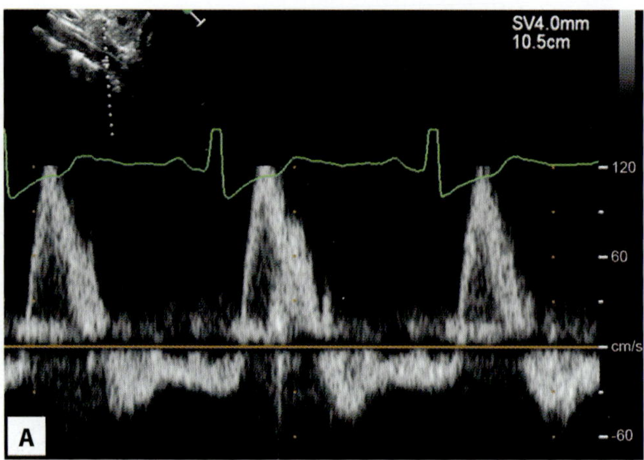

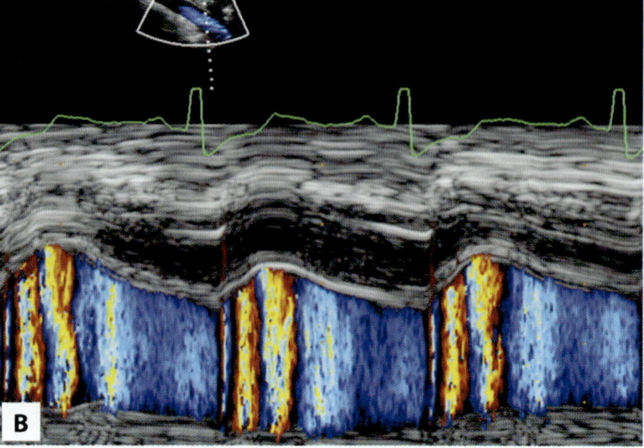

FIGS. 34A AND B: (A) Diastolic flow reversal in descending aorta; (B) color Doppler in descending aorta shows diastolic flow reversal in severe aortic regurgitation.

of initial and distal jet within the beam of ultrasound and also possibly by the ability of the jet to expand and mobilize adjoining red blood cells. While a faint spectral display is compatible with trace or mild AR, significant overlap between moderate and severe regurgitation exists in more dense jet recordings. Therefore, CW Doppler jet density is an imperfect indicator of severity of AR. The AR can be graded using spectral strength of the AR jet.[21]

Diastolic Jet Deceleration

The slope of deceleration of the CW Doppler signal provides a semi-quantitative assessment of AR.[168,169] The CW Doppler signal represents the pressure difference between the aorta and the LV during diastole. The pressure difference is highest at the beginning of diastole, with peak velocities of 4–6 m/s (corresponding to peak gradients of 64–144 mm Hg). In mild AR, there is a modest increase in LV pressure as diastole progresses and the slope of the CW signal is relatively flat. In severe and particularly acute AR, the aortic pressure is lower in diastole and the LVEDP increases sharply during diastole, resulting in a steeper deceleration slope **(Fig. 35)**. The rate of change of this index is defined as the pressure half-time, the time taken for the initial pressure gradient to decrease by half (or the velocity to decrease to 70% of its peak value). A flat slope (pressure half-time > 500 ms) is consistent with mild AR, while a steep slope (pressure half-time < 200 ms) is consistent with severe or acute, decompensated AR.[21] In extreme cases, the aortic and LV pressures equalize before the end of diastole, resulting in a deceleration signal that reaches the baseline. However, the diastolic AR velocity is also determined by LV diastolic compliance and pressure. For a given severity of AR, pressure half-time can be further shortened by an elevated LV diastolic pressure or by vasodilator therapy that reduces AR.[168,170] On the other hand, pressure half-time can be lengthened or normalized with chronic LV adaptation to severe AR.[171]

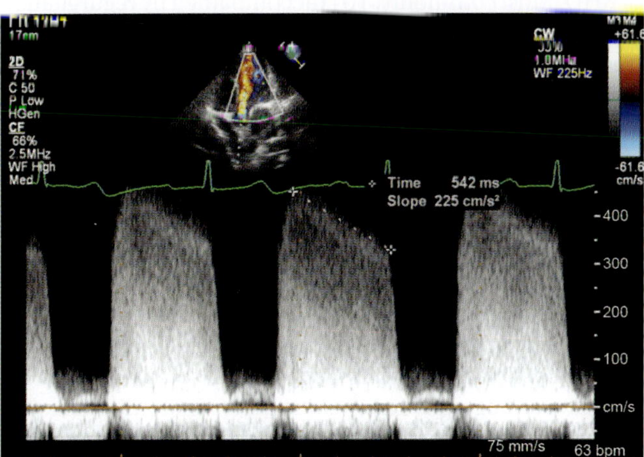

FIG. 35: Steeper slope (225 cm²) denotes severity of aortic regurgitation (AR).

Role of Transesophageal Echocardiography to Assess Aortic Regurgitation

Transesophageal echocardiography is seldom needed to evaluate severity of AR due to the proximity of the aortic valve to the chest from the parasternal window. However, in patients with poor acoustic windows. Color Doppler criteria on jet width and the size of the vena contracta apply equally to TEE. But, due to difficulty with TEE in obtaining views where the jet direction is parallel to the ultrasound beam, measurements of RF by PW Doppler and recording of the AR velocity with CW Doppler are more difficult to obtain reliably. Diastolic flow reversal can be recorded in the ascending aorta with PW Doppler from the upper esophageal views.[21]

Integrative Approach to Assess Severity of Aortic Regurgitation

The assessment of AR by Doppler ECHO is an integrative and comprehensive process based on all information collected during the examination. In all cases, one should perform routinely an evaluation of the aortic valve, LV size and function, **(Figs. 36A to C)** an assessment by color-flow imaging of the proximal jet width and, if possible, the vena-contracta. The LV outflow velocity and the velocity in the proximal descending aorta and/or abdominal aorta should be recorded by pulsed Doppler. CW Doppler of the AR jet should also be routinely recorded but only utilized if a complete signal is obtained. The Task Force[21] has proposed a scheme of specific signs with a specificity ≥ 90%, along with supportive signs whose predictive accuracy is more modest and quantitative parameters for AR severity. If the AR is definitely determined as mild or less using these signs, no further measurement is required. If there are parameters suggestive of more than mild AR and the quality of the primary data lends itself to quantitation, it is desirable for echocardiographers with experience in quantitative methods to measure quantitatively the degree of AR, including the regurgitant volume and fraction as descriptors of volume overload and the effective regurgitant orifice as a descriptor of the lesion severity. Invariably in RHD there will be combination of AS and AR with MV involvement also should be evaluated **(Fig. 37)**. Echocardiographic indications for surgical referral are LVEF < 50% or LV end-systolic dimension > 55 mm.[19] All patients with symptomatic severe AR should be considered for valve surgery.

■ TRICUSPID STENOSIS

Tricuspid valve stenosis (TS) is less prevalent than MS. But, rheumatic disease is the most common etiology of TS and is usually accompanied by MV involvement. ECHO can distinguish other rare causes of TS such as congenital causes, carcinoid, infective endocarditis, Whipple's disease or previous methysergide therapy from TS of RHD. A number of

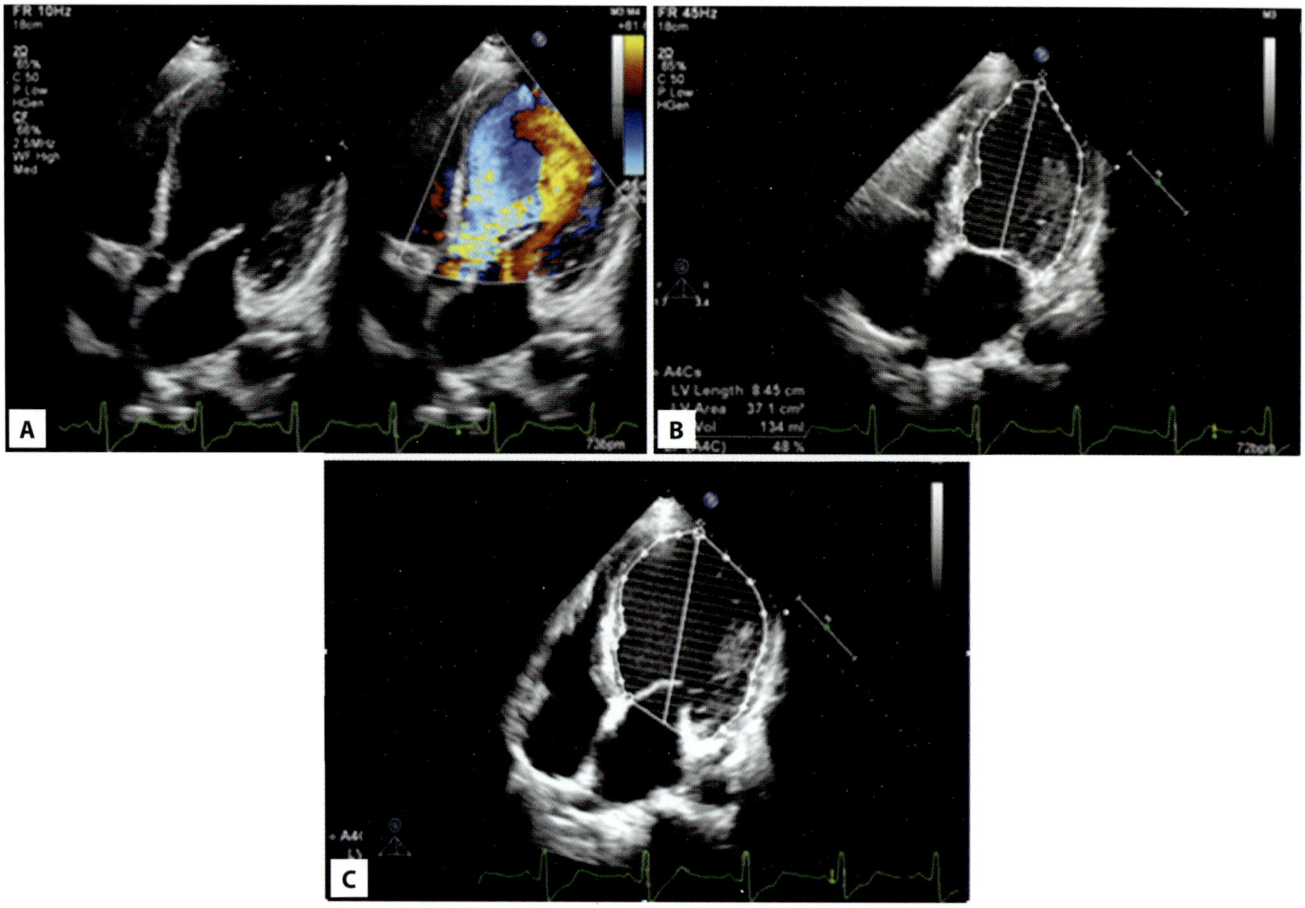

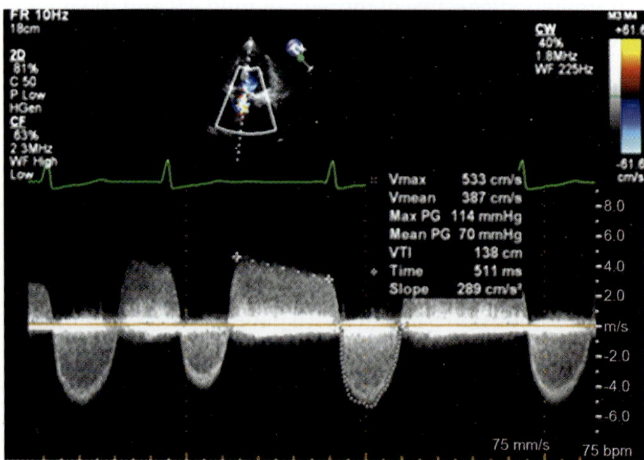

FIGS. 36A TO C: (A) Apical five-chamber with color Doppler shows severe aortic regurgitation (AR) with dilated left ventricle (LV), (B and C) show calculation of LV area in systole and diastole with ejection fraction (EF)—48%.

FIG. 37: Continuous wave (CW) Doppler shows aortic stenosis (AS) and aortic regurgitation (AR) in a case of rheumatic heart disease (RHD) with moderate mitral stenosis (MS) and mitral regurgitation (MR).

diseases that may contribute to the functional presentation of tricuspid stenosis such as a large atrial septal defect, localized pericardial effusion behind the right atrium and right atrial myxoma, and secondaries can also be differentiated from TS of RHD. Most commonly, TS is accompanied by regurgitation so that the higher flows through the valve further increase the transvalvular gradient and contribute to a greater elevation of right atrial pressures.[172] In rheumatic involvement, the cusps are thickened and the commissures fused so that the valve area becomes small. There is thickening of the leaflet tips and chordae. The valve leaflets, especially the anterior, domes toward the right ventricle in diastole, similar to rheumatic MV leaflets. The mid-portion of the leaflets typically has preserved mobility. In contrast to MV disease, the subvalvular apparatus is not usually involved[173-175] but the annulus may dilate. As the disease progresses, the right atrium dilates and becomes congested. This is always associated with some degree of TR. 3D echocardiography can provide better anatomical detail of the relation of the three leaflets to each other and assessment of the orifice area.[176]

Assessment of Severity of Tricuspid Stenosis

The evaluation of tricuspid stenosis severity is primarily done using the hemodynamic information provided by CW Doppler. The tricuspid inflow velocity is best recorded from either in apical four-chamber view or low-parasternal right ventricular inflow view. As the tricuspid inflow velocities are accentuated during inspiration, all measurements taken must be averaged throughout the respiratory cycle or recorded at end-expiratory apnea. In patients with atrial fibrillation, measurements from a minimum of five cardiac cycles should be averaged. It is ideal to assess the severity of TS at heart rates < 100 bpm, preferably between 70 and 80 bpm, because as with MS, faster heart rates make it impossible to appreciate the deceleration time (or pressure half-time). The hallmark of a stenotic tricuspid valve is an increase in transvalvular velocity recorded by CW Doppler. Peak inflow velocity through a normal tricuspid valve rarely exceeds 0.7 m/s. In patients with TS, it is common to record peak velocities >1.0 m/s that may approach 2 m/s during inspiration. The mean pressure gradient derived using the equation $4V_2$ is lower in tricuspid than in MS, because of the large tricuspid valve area. The usual range is between 2 and 10 mm Hg and averaging around 5 mm Hg. A mean diastolic gradient of 2 mm Hg obtained by CW Doppler can establish the diagnosis of TS and a mean gradients as low as 5 mm Hg can result in congestive symptoms. A mean gradient of ≥5 mm Hg is suggestive of severe TS. Supportive findings are dilated inferior vena cava and a dilated right atrium. Higher gradients may be seen with combined stenosis and regurgitation[177-179] **(Fig. 38)**.

The primary consequence of TS is elevation of right atrial pressure and development of right-sided congestion. Due to the frequent presence of TR, the transvalvular gradient is clinically more relevant for assessment of severity and decision making than the actual stenotic valve area. In addition, because anatomical valve orifice area is difficult to measure and TR is so frequently present, the typical CW Doppler methods for valve area determination are not very accurate. The pressure half-time method (T½) has been applied in a manner similar to MS. Some authors have used the same constant of 220, while others have proposed a constant of 190 with valve area determined as: 190/T½.[179]

Although validation studies with TS are less than those with MS, valve area by the T½ method may be less accurate than in MS. Probably, this is due to differences in atrioventricular compliance between the right and left side and the influence of right ventricular relaxation, respiration and TR on the pressure half-time. However, as a general rule, a longer T½ implies a greater TS severity with values > 190 frequently associated with significant (or critical) stenosis.

In theory, the continuity equation should provide a method for determining the effective valve area as SV divided by the tricuspid inflow VTI as recorded with CWD.[180] The main limitation of the method is obtaining an accurate measurement of the inflow volume passing through the tricuspid valve. In the absence of significant TR, one can use the SV obtained from either the left or right ventricular outflow and a valve area of 1 cm² is considered indicative of severe TS. The normal tricuspid valve area is 7 cm². However, as severity of TR increases, valve area is progressively underestimated by this method. Nevertheless, a value of 1 cm², although it is not accounting for the additional regurgitant volume, may still be indicative of a significant hemodynamic burden induced by the combined lesion. Spectral Doppler shows a prolonged deceleration slope of antegrade flow. Doppler quantification of TS compares well with cardiac catheterization.[181] The youngest child of MS in our experience was 2 years and 3 months old boy, presented with history of breathlessness. ECHO showed RHD with severe MS and TS **(Figs. 39A to D)**.

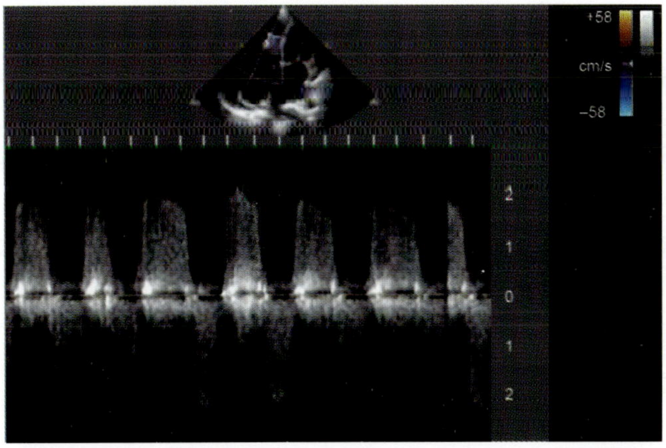

◼ TRICUSPID REGURGITATION

Tricuspid regurgitation is a common incidental echo-cardiographic finding and is readily detected using color-flow Doppler imaging **(Fig. 40)**.[67] Trivial degree of TR (physiological TR) is present in about 70% of normal individuals.[67,182,183] ECHO can differentiate rheumatic valvulitis cause of TR from, congenital, infective endocarditis, carcinoid, rheumatoid arthritis, radiation therapy, trauma (such as repeated endomyocardial biopsies), Marfan syndrome, tricuspid valve prolapse, tricuspid annular dilatation or congenital disorders such as Ebstein's anomaly[184] or a cleft tricuspid valve as part of atrioventricular canal malformations. TR is often a secondary phenomenon due to right ventricular (RV) and tricuspid annular dilatation secondary to PHT or RV dysfunction. It is then termed as "functional TR". Pressure or volume loading of the RV from pulmonary disease, left to right shunts, left heart disease or a combination of factors can cause functional or secondary TR.

FIG. 38: CW cursor on tricuspid valve to demonstrate TS, TR, in a patient of RHD with multivalvular disease with MS, MR, AS, AR, TS, and TR with atrial fibrillation with CHF.

(AR: aortic regurgitation; AS: aortic stenosis; CHF: congestive heart failure; MR: mitral regurgitation; MS: mitral stenosis; RHD: rheumatic heart disease; TR: tricuspid regurgitation; TS: tricuspid stenosis; CW: continuous wave)

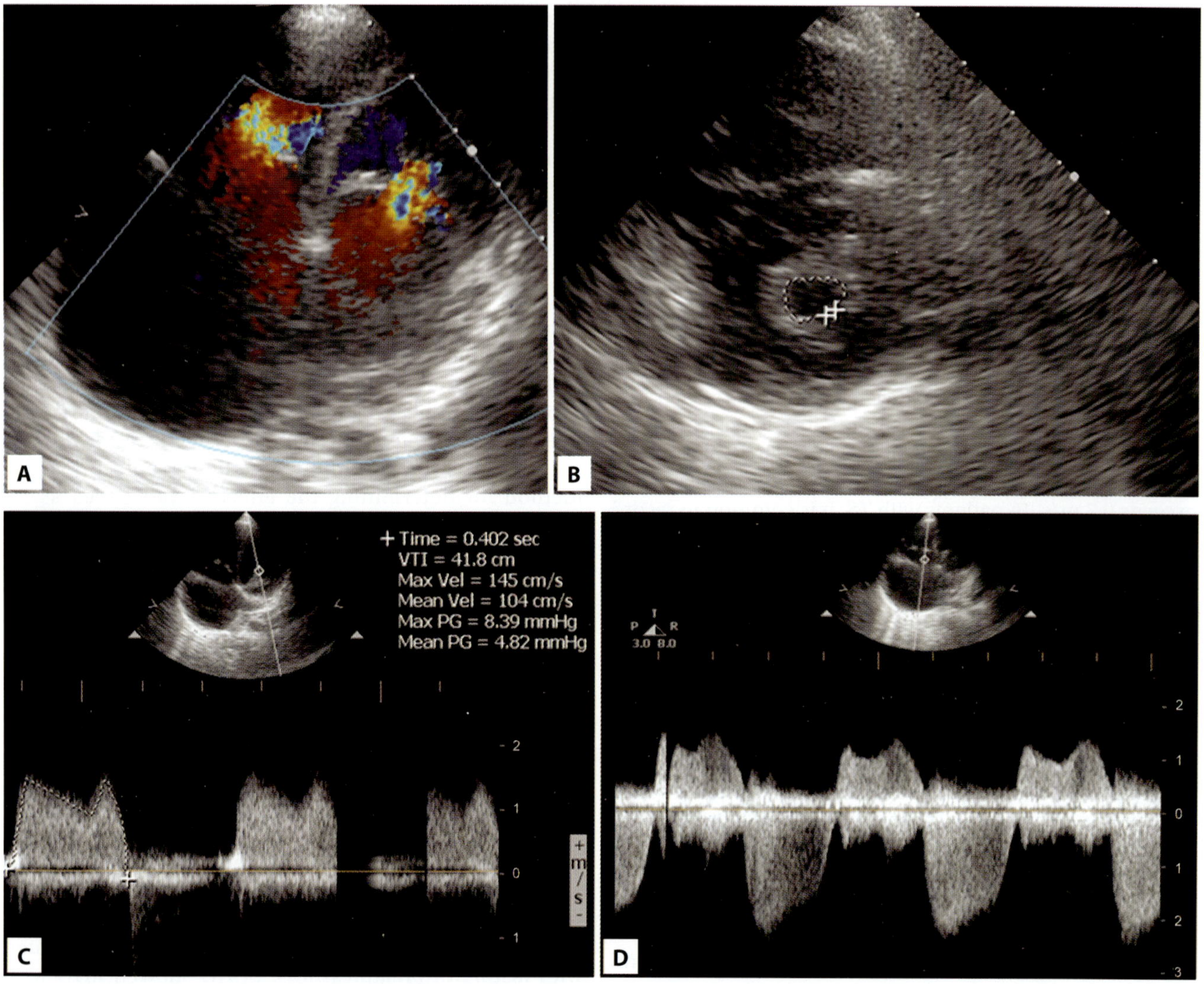

FIGS. 39A TO D: (A) Transthoracic echocardiography (TTE) in apical four-chamber view with color Doppler shows MS and TS in a 2 years and 3 months old boy. (B) TTE in parasternal short axis shows thickened MV with fused commissures with reduced MVOA of 0.4 cm². (C) The cursor is on MV and shows maximum gradient of 8.4 and mean of 4.8 mm Hg. (D) CW cursor on tricuspid valve to demonstrate TS, and TR in the same patient of extreme form of juvenile RHD.

(CW: continuous wave; MS: mitral stenosis; MV: mitral valve; MVOA: mitral valve orifice area; RHD: rheumatic heart disease; TR: tricuspid regurgitation; TS: tricuspid stenosis)

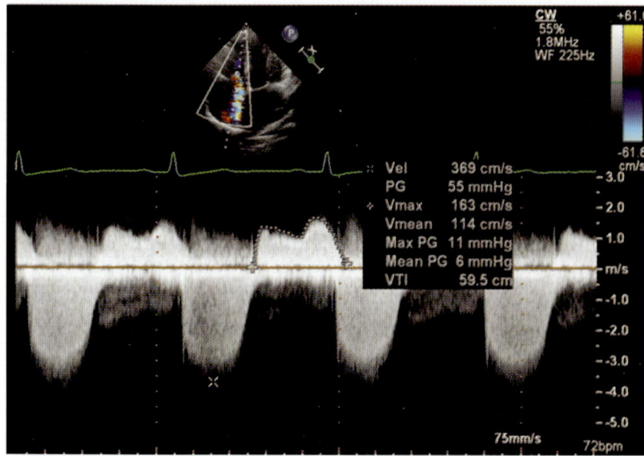

FIG. 40: Tricuspid stenosis and regurgitation.

Transthoracic echocardiography is the investigation of choice to confirm and document the presence of TR and define its severity and etiology. In 20–30% of cases with rheumatic valvular disease the tricuspid valve is involved, associated with MV and aortic valve disease, the most common findings in these cases being combined MS and TR. The standards for determining the severity of TR are hampered by the lack of a quantitative standard for severity. Hence, the assessment of the severity of TR is dependent on integration of multiple methods of evaluation. 2D ECHO helps to identify the etiology of the TR with a careful assessment of tricuspid leaflet morphology, leaflet mobility, tricuspid annular dimension, the subvalvular apparatus, and right ventricular size and function. The presence of pulmonary hypertension (PH) and coexisting left-sided valvular heart disease can be determined. Secondary findings like right atrial and RV enlargement are not specific for severe TR, but their absence suggests that TR is not severe. In severe TR, due to volume overload of RV, paradoxical ventricular septal motion may occur. But, this sign is not specific for TR, as it is affected by many factors.[185-187] Imaging of the inferior vena cava in the subcostal view for size and respiratory variation provides an evaluation of right-atrial pressure.[188-190]

Doppler Methods of Evaluation of Severity of Tricuspid Regurgitation

Color Flow Doppler

It detects the presence of TR **(Figs. 41A and B)**. Several views are evaluated to establish the characteristics, direction, and the size of the regurgitant jet. Transthoracic images usually are adequate and should include the parasternal RV inflow view, the parasternal short-axis view, the apical four-chamber view, and the subcostal four-chamber view. Jets that extend deep into the right atrium represent more TR than small central jets that appear just superior to the tricuspid leaflets. Color Doppler flow mapping of TR severity using jet area correlates well with angiographic evaluation[191] and clinical measures of regurgitant severity.[192,193] A dilated right atrium and a broad regurgitation jet that approaches the vena cava suggest significant TR. The TR jet area > 40% that of the right atrium is consistent with significant regurgitation.[194] Similar to MR, flow jets that are directed centrally into the right atrium generally appear larger by color Doppler than eccentric, wall impinging jets with similar or worse severity.

Color flow imaging also may be used to determine TR severity by the PISA method. Visualization of a measurable contour of the flow convergence zone is more challenging than with MR. The PISA method has been validated in small studies but is rarely used clinically.[191,195] The vena contracta can be used for assessment of TR severity[192] and correlates well with EROA, especially with greater degrees of TR.[196,197] Both PISA and vena contracta methods are less accurate in assessing TR severity in eccentric jets but in

central jets they appear to be more accurate than jet area. Underestimation of severe TR has been demonstrated in up to 20–30% of patients using PISA or jet area.[191] A jet width > 0.7 cm identifies severe TR with a sensitivity of 89% and a specificity of 93% and correlates well with EROA.[196,197] The systolic hepatic flow reversal is specific for severe TR. It represents the strongest additional parameter for evaluating TR. Assessment of myocardial function by TAPSE or systolic myocardial velocities is needed to know the RV dysfunction.

Continuous Wave Doppler

This records the pressure drop between the right ventricle and atrium in systole using the modified Bernoulli equation $4V_2$. In the absence of pulmonary valve or infundibular stenosis, recording of TR jet velocity provides a useful method for noninvasive measurement of RV or pulmonary artery systolic pressure. TR jet velocity is similar to velocity of other regurgitant lesions but is not related to the volume of regurgitant flow. In fact, massive TR is often associated with a low jet velocity (<2 m/s), as there is near equalization of RV and right atrial pressures. Whereas in patients with PHT, and mild regurgitation may have a very high jet velocity.[21] Estimation of the pulmonary artery systolic pressure is done by adding right atrial pressure to the transtricuspid pressure drop. The RA pressure can be estimated using the inferior vena cava (IVC) size and response to inspiration. With RA pressure < 10 mm Hg, the IVC diameter is <1.7 cm and demonstrates ≥50% collapse with inspiration. A dilated IVC that does not demonstrate >50% reduction in size with inspiration indicates RA pressure > 15 mm Hg.[12] Systolic pulmonary artery pressures > 55 mm Hg are likely to cause TR with anatomically normal tricuspid valves, whereas TR occurring with systolic pulmonary artery pressures < 40 mm Hg is likely to reflect a structural abnormality of the valve apparatus.[6]

The density and the contour of the CW Doppler signal provide qualitative data on the severity of TR. A characteristic dense systolic CWD signal is appreciated when TR is severe. Severe TR also results in a triangular or "dagger-shaped" early peaking TR jet profile due to early pressure equalization between the RA and RV. In severe TR and normal RV pressures, the antegrade and retrograde CW flow appear as near mirror images of each other, corresponding to the high velocity forward and low velocity retrograde flow across a severely incompetent TV.[198]

Pulsed Doppler

Pulsed wave Doppler cannot be used to accurately calculate TR volume because of complex structure of the annulus and significant respiratory variation in tricuspid inflow. Similar to MR, the severity of TR will affect the early diastolic tricuspid E velocity. In patients with severe TR, early diastolic TV velocity > 1.0 m/s is often recorded. Theoretically, TR volume can be calculated by subtracting the flow across a nonregurgitant valve from the antegrade flow across the tricuspid valve annulus. In contrast to MR

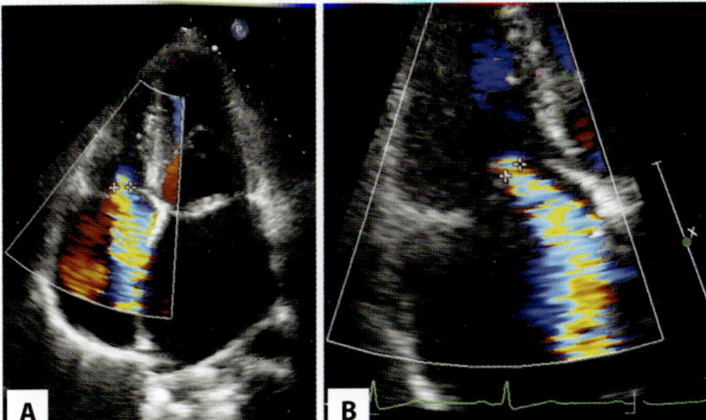

FIGS. 41A AND B: Apical four-chamber view with color Doppler shows tricuspid regurgitation (TR) with vena contracta (VC) of 5 mm; (B) Modified two-chamber view with color Doppler shows sever TR with VC of 7 mm.

and AR, because of errors in measuring the tricuspid valve annulus this approach is rarely utilized for TR. Similar to the use of pulmonary vein flow pattern in MR, PW Doppler examination of the hepatic veins helps to corroborate the assessment of TR severity. With increasing TR severity, normally dominant systolic wave of hepatic vein inflow is blunted in systole and there is development of systolic flow reversal in severe TR. The sensitivity of systolic flow reversal for identifying severe TR is as high as 80%.[193] Hepatic vein flow patterns can also be affected by abnormal RA and RV compliance, atrial fibrillation, phase of respiratory cycle, and preload.[199]

Role of Transesophageal Echocardiography

Transesophageal echocardiography complements TTE in the assessment of tricuspid valve regurgitation. Most often, TR can be adequately evaluated on transthoracic imaging and TEE may be helpful when transthoracic images are poor. Color-flow mapping can be done using the high esophageal four-chamber and short-axis views and the transgastric four-chamber and RV inflow views. Jet area may appear larger with TEE than with transthoracic imaging, similar to MR. CW Doppler signals can be recorded from high esophageal or transgastric views. Obtaining a parallel intercept angle can be problematic. Hepatic vein flow can be recorded by starting in a parasternal long-axis view of the RA and then following the inferior vena cava caudally until the hepatic veins are visualized.[21]

Intraoperative TEE can be used to assess tricuspid valve morphology prior to operation and should be used to evaluate the results of tricuspid repair immediately after cardiopulmonary bypass to detect residual TR or the development of tricuspid stenosis. Following tricuspid valve replacement, assessment of prosthetic valve function and prosthetic or periprosthetic regurgitation can be performed. There may be underestimation of TR severity due to the prevailing hemodynamic conditions related to general anesthesia in the operating room.

Integrative Approach to Assessment Severity of Tricuspid Regurgitation

An integrative approach is for evaluation of TR is recommended, similar to the assessment of other regurgitant lesions **(Table 9)**. This includes evaluation of the size of right-sided chambers, septal motion, and various Doppler parameters. Color Doppler flow mapping should be performed in at least two orthogonal planes, with particular attention to the vena contracta, flow convergence and the direction, and size of the jet. CW Doppler recording of the TR jet should be recorded to evaluate the signal intensity and contour of the jet, and to estimate pulmonary artery systolic pressure. Moreover, the size of the inferior vena cava and response to respiration as well as hepatic vein flow pattern help to evaluate right atrial pressure and adaptation to the

TABLE 11: Grading of tricuspid regurgitation.

	Mild	*Moderate*	*Severe*
Tricuspid valve morphology	Normal/abnormal	Normal/abnormal	Abnormal/flail, lack of coaptation
Color flow TR jet	Small and central	Intermediate	Very large central jet or eccenteric wall impinging jet
CW signal of TR jet	Faint/parabolic	Dense/parabolic	Dense/triangular with early peaking (peak < 2 m/s in massive TR)
Vena contracta width (mm)	Not defined	<7	≥7
PISA radius (mm)	≤5	6–9	>9
Hepatic vein flow	Systolic dominance	Systolic blurring	Systolic flow reversal
Tricuspid inflow	Normal	Normal	E wave dominant (≥1 cm/s)
EROA (mm^2)	Not defined	Not defined	≥40
R Vol (mL)	Not defined	Not defined	<45

(CW: continuous wave; EROA: effective regurgitant orifice area; PISA: proximal isovelocity surface area; TR: tricuspid regurgitation)

volume overload. The Task Force[21] recommends integration of information from all available parameters due to lack of extensive data on quantitation of TR. More attention needs to made toward the quality of the data obtained and to the physiologic conditions that can alter the accuracy of these parameters as indices of regurgitation severity **(Table 11)**. How to differentiate functional TR from pathological TR is given in **Table 12**.

The RHD is a neglected giant causing immense morbidity and untimely mortality in India.[200,201] The advent of echocardiographic screening for RHD has revealed a higher RHD burden than previously thought. In light of this global experience, the development of new International Echocardiographic Guidelines that address the full spectrum of the RHD process is opportune. Systematic differences in the reporting of and diagnostic approach to RHD exist, reflecting differences in local experience and disease patterns. The World Heart Federation Echocardiographic Criteria for RHD have, therefore, been developed and are formulated on the basis of the best available evidence.[202]

■ CONCLUSION

Echocardiography with Doppler imaging is an essential tool in the evaluation and management of RHD. Assessment of

TABLE 12: Differentiation of normal and pathological tricuspid regurgitation.

	Mild	*Moderate*	*Severe*
Tricuspid leaflets	Usually normal	Normal or abnormal	Abnormal/flail and lack of coaptation
RV, RA, and IVC size	Normal		Moderate or greater dilatation
Vena contracta width (cm)	Absent vena contracta		>0.7
Jet area (cm^2)	<5	5–10	>10
PISA radius (cm)	≤0.5	0.6–0.9	>0.9
Jet density–CW	Faint and parabolic	Dense	Dense and early peaking triangular
Hepatic vein	Systolic dominant flow	Blunting of systolic flow	Systolic flow reversal

(CW: continuous wave; IVC: inferior vena cava; PISA: proximal isovelocity surface area; RA: right atrium; RV: right ventricle)

Source: Adapted from Tables 8 and 9 of Zoghbi WA et al.21

the etiology, severity, hemodynamic consequences, and ventricular response to valvular abnormalities can be made with the use of appropriate echocardiographic techniques. While assessing the severity of RHD, it is necessary to check consistency between the different echocardiographic measurements, as well as the anatomy and mechanisms of RHD and clinical assessment. Echocardiographic evaluation should include a comprehensive evaluation of stenotic and regurgitant lesions of mitral, aortic, and tricuspid valves.

Echocardiography also plays an important role in therapeutic decision making and provides prognostic information. It remains the principal modality for the diagnosis and follow-up of patients with RHD. In addition TEE and 3D/4D ECHO help in decision making in difficult and complicated cases. Echocardiography is the key technique used to confirm, quantify, and monitor RHD valve analysis should integrate the assessment of etiology, lesion process, and type of dysfunction. A comprehensive evaluation of stenotic and regurgitant lesions of mitral, aortic tricuspid, and pulmonary valves is essential. All the four chambers, both appendages, pulmonary artery, aorta, and inferior vena cava must be interrogated thoroughly. Exercise and dobutamine echocardiography are sometimes needed for risk stratification and management strategy.

▪ REFERENCES

1. Sanyal SK, Berry AM, Duggal S, Hooja V, Ghosh S. Sequel of the initial attack of acute rheumatic fever in children from North India. A prospective 5-year follow-up study. Circulation. 1982;65:375 9.1.A.

2. Wood P. An appreciation of mitral stenosis. I: Clinical features. Br Med J. 1954;4870:1051-63.

3. Rowe JC, Bland EF, Sprague HB, White PD. The course of mitral stenosis without surgery: ten- and twenty-year perspectives. Ann Intern Med. 1960;52:741-9.

4. Roberts WC, Perloff JK. Mitral valvular disease: a clinicopathologic survey of the conditions causing the mitral valve to function abnormally. Ann Intern Med. 1972;77:939-75.

5. Rusted IE, Scheifley CH, Edwards JE. Studies of the mitral valve, II: certain anatomic features of the mitral valve and associated structures in mitral stenosis. Circulation. 1956;14:398-406.

6. Bonow RO, Carabello BA, Chatterjee K, Antonio CL Jr, David PF, Michael DF, et al. 2008 Focused update incorporated into the ACC/AHA 2006 guidelines for the management of patients with valvular heart disease: a report of the American College of Cardiology/American Heart Association Task Force on Practice Guidelines (Writing Committee to Develop Guidelines for the Management of Patients With Valvular Heart Disease). Circulation. 2008;118:e523-661.

7. Edler I, Gustafson A. Ultrasonic cardiogram in mitral stenosis: preliminary communication. Acta Med Scand. 1957;159(2): 85-90.

8. Nichol PM, Gilbert BW, Kisslo JA. Two-dimensional echocardiographic assessment of mitral stenosis. Circulation. 1977;55(1):120-8.

9. Wann LS, Weyman AE, Feigenbaum H, Dillon JC, Johnston KW, Eggleton RC. Determination of mitral valve area by cross-sectional echocardiography. Ann Intern Med. 1978;88(3): 337-41.

10. Martin RP, Rakowski H, Kleiman JH, Beaver W, London E, Popp RL. Reliability and reproducibility of two dimensional echocardiograph measurement of the stenotic mitral valve orifice area. Am J Cardiol. 1979;43(3):560-8.

11. James ED, Paul EF. Mitral stenosis. In: Joseph SA, James ED, Shahbudin HR (Eds). Valvular Heart Disease, 3rd Edition. Philadelphia: Lippincott Williams and Wilkins; 2000. pp. 92-3.

12. Gail EP, Lisa F. Echocardiographic Assessment of Native Valve Function. In: Andrew W, Thomas MB (Eds). Valvular Heart Disease. United States: Humana Press; 2009. pp. 123-64.

13. Messika-Zeitoun D, Brochet E, Holmin C, Rosenbaum D, Cormier B, Serfaty JM, et al. Three-dimensional evaluation of the mitral valve area and commissural opening before and after percutaneous mitral commissurotomy in patients with mitral stenosis. Eur Heart J. 2007;28:72-9.

14. Baumgartner H, Hung J, Bermejo J, Chambers JB, Evangelista A, Griffin BP, et al. Echocardiographic assessment of valve stenosis: EAE/ASE recommendations for clinical practice. J Am Soc Echocardiogr. 2009;22(1):1-23.

15. Wilkins GT, Weyman AE, Abascal VM, Block PC, Palacios IF. Percutaneous balloon dilatation of the mitral valve: an analysis of echocardiographic variables related to outcome and the mechanism of dilatation. Br Heart J. 1988;60:299-308.

16. Wang A, Krasuski RA, Warner JJ, Pieper K, Kisslo KB, Bashore TM, et al. Serial echocardiographic evaluation of restenosis after successful percutaneous mitral commissurotomy. J Am Coll Cardiol. 2002;39:328-34.

17. Iung B, Cormier B, Ducimetière P, Porte JM, Nallet O, Michel PL, et al. Immediate results of percutaneous mitral commissurotomy. A predictive model on a series of 1514 patients. Circulation. 1996;94:2124-30.

18. Black IW, Hopkins AP, Lee LC, Walsh WF. Left atrial spontaneous echo contrast: a clinical and echocardiographic analysis. J Am Coll Cardiol. 1991;18:398-404.

19. Bonow RO, Carabello BA, Chatterjee K, de Leon CC Jr, Faxon DP, Freed MD, et al. ACC/AHA 2006 guidelines for the management of patients with valvular heart disease: a report of the American College of Cardiology/ American Heart Association Task Force on Practice Guidelines (writing Committee to Revise the 1998 guidelines for the management of patients with valvular heart disease) developed in collaboration with the Society of Cardiovascular Anesthesiologists endorsed by the Society for Cardiovascular Angiography and Interventions and the Society of Thoracic Surgeons. J Am Coll Cardiol. 2006;48:e1-148.

20. Vahanian A, Baumgartner H, Bax J, Butchart E, Dion R, Filippatos G, et al. Guidelines on the management of valvular heart disease: The Task Force on the Management of Valvular Heart Disease of the European Society of Cardiology. Eur Heart J. 2007;28:230-68.

21. Zoghbi WA, Enriquez-Sarano M, Foster E, Grayburn PA, Kraft CD, Levine RA, et al. Recommendations for evaluation of the severity of native valvular regurgitation with two-dimensional and Doppler echocardiography. J Am Soc Echocardiogr. 2003;16:777-802.

22. Dreyfus GD, Corbi PJ, Chan KM, Bahrami T. Secondary tricuspid regurgitation or dilatation: which should be the criteria for surgical repair? Ann Thorac Surg. 2005;79:127-32.

23. Henein M, John P. The Mitral Valve Disease. In: Michael YH (Ed). Valvular Heart Disease in Clinical Practice. London: Springer-Verlag Limited; 2009. p. 16.

24. Faletra F, Pezzano A Jr, Fusco R, Mantero A, Corno R, Crivellaro W, et al. Measurement of mitral valve area in mitral stenosis: four echocardiographic methods compared with direct measurement of anatomic orifices. J Am Coll Cardiol. 1996;28:1190-7.

25. Henry WL, Griffith JM, Michaelis LL, McIntosh CL, Morrow AG, Epstein SE. Measurement of mitral orifice area in patients with mitral valve disease by real-time, two-dimensional echocardiography. Circulation. 1975;51:827-31.

26. Smith MD, Handshoe R, Handshoe S, Kwan OL, De Maria AN. Comparative accuracy of two-dimensional echocardiography and Doppler pressure half time methods in assessing severity of mitral stenosis in patients with and without prior commissurotomy. Circulation. 1986;73:100-7.

27. Zamorano J, Cordeiro P, Sugeng L, Perez de Isla L, Weinert L, Macaya C, et al. Real-time three-dimensional echocardiography for rheumatic mitral valve stenosis evaluation: an accurate and novel approach. J Am Coll Cardiol. 2004;43(11):2091-6.

28. Sebag IA, Morgan JG, Handschumacher MD, Marshall JE, Nesta F, Hung J, et al. Usefulness of three-dimensionally guided assessment of mitral stenosis using matrix-array ultrasound. Am J Cardiol. 2005;96(8):1151-6.

29. Holen J, Simonsen S. Determination of pressure gradient in mitral stenosis with Doppler echocardiography. Br Heart J. 1979;41:529-35.

30. Thomas JD, Newell JB, Choong CY, Weyman AE. Physical and physiological determinants of transmitral velocity: numerical analysis. Am J Physiol. 1991;260(5 Pt 2):H1718-31.

31. Rahimtoola SH, Durairaj A, Mehra A, Nuno I. Current evaluation and management of patients with mitral stenosis. Circulation. 2002;106:1183-8.

32. Thomas JD, Weyman AE. Doppler mitral pressure half time: a clinical tool in search of theoretical justification. J Am Coll Cardiol. 1987;10(4):923-9.

33. Hatle L, Angelsen B, Tromsdal A. Noninvasive assessment of atrioventricular pressure half time by Doppler ultrasound. Circulation. 1979;60:1096-104.

34. Come PC, Riley MF, Diver DJ, Morgan JP, Safian RD, McKay RG. Noninvasive assessment of mitral stenosis before and after percutaneous balloon mitral valvuloplasty. Am J Cardiol. 1988;61:817-25.

35. Chen CG, Wang YP, Guo BL, Lin YS. Reliability of the Doppler pressure half time method for assessing effects of percutaneous mitral balloon valvuloplasty. J Am Coll Cardiol. 1989;13:1309-13.

36. Gonzalez MA, Child JS, Krivokapich J. Comparison of two-dimensional and Doppler echocardiography and intracardiac hemodynamics for quantification of mitral stenosis. Am J Cardiol. 1987;60:327-32.

37. Thomas JD, Wilkins GT, Choong CY, Abascal VM, Palacios IF, Block PC, et al. Inaccuracy of mitral pressure half time immediately after percutaneous mitral valvotomy. Dependence on transmitral gradient and left atrial and ventricular compliance. Circulation. 1988;78:980-93.

38. Schwammenthal E, Vered Z, Agranat O, Kaplinsky E, Rabinowitz B, Feinberg MS. Impact of atrioventricular compliance on pulmonary artery pressure in mitral stenosis: an exercise echo-cardiographic study. Circulation. 2000;102:2378-84.

39. Robiolio PA, Rigolin VH, Harrison JK, Kisslo KB, Bashore TM. Doppler pressure half time method of assessing mitral valve area: aortic insufficiency does not adversely affect validity. Am Heart J. 1998;136:718-23.

40. Flachskampf FA, Weyman AE, Guerrero JL, Thomas JD. Calculation of atrioventricular compliance from the mitral flow profile: analytic and in vitro study. J Am Coll Cardiol. 1992;19:998-1004.

41. Karp K, Teien D, Bjerle P, Eriksson P. Reassessment of valve area determinations in mitral stenosis by the pressure half time method: impact of left ventricular stiffness and peak diastolic pressure difference. J Am Coll Cardiol. 1989;13:594-9.

42. Messika-Zeitoun D, Meizels A, Cachier A, Scheuble A, Fondard O, Brochet E, et al. Echocardiographic evaluation of the mitral valve

area before and after percutaneous mitral commissurotomy: the pressure half time method revisited. J Am Soc Echocardiogr. 2005;18:1409-14.

43. Nakatani S, Masuyama T, Kodama K, Kitabatake A, Fujii K, Kamada T. Value and limitations of Doppler echocardiography in the quantification of stenotic mitral valve area: comparison of the pressure half time and the continuity equation methods. Circulation. 1988;77:78-85.

44. Messika-Zeitoun Yiu D, Fung S, Cormier B, Iung B, Scott LC, Vahanian A, et al. Sequential assessment of mitral valve area during diastole using color M-mode flow convergence analysis: new insights into mitral stenosis physiology. Eur Heart J. 2003;24:1244-53.

45. Deng YB, Matsumoto M, Wang XF, Liu L, Takizawa S, Takekoshi N, et al. Estimation of mitral valve area in patients with mitral stenosis by the flow convergence region method: selection of aliasing velocity. J Am Coll Cardiol. 1994;24(3):683-9.

46. Izgi C, Ozdemir N, Cevik C, Ozveren O, Bakal RB, Kaymaz C, et al. Mitral valve resistance as a determinant of resting and stress pulmonary artery pressure in patients with mitral stenosis: a dobutamine stress study. J Am Soc Echocardiogr. 2007;20:1160-6.

47. Cheriex EC, Pieters FA, Janssen JH, de Swart H, Palmans-Meulemans A. Value of exercise Doppler-echocardiographyin patients with mitral stenosis. Int J Cardiol. 1994;45:219-26.

48. Gordon SP, Douglas PS, Come PC, Manning WJ. Two-dimensional and Doppler echocardiographic determinants of the natural history of mitral valve narrowing in patients with rheumatic mitral stenosis: implications for follow-up. J Am Coll Cardiol. 1992;19:968-73.

49. Beppu S, Nimura Y, Sakakibara H, Nagata S, Park YD, Izumi S. Smoke-like echo in the left atrial cavity in mitral valve disease: its features and significance. J Am Coll Cardiol. 1985;6(4):744-9.

50. Daniel WG, Nellessen U, Schröder E, Nonnast-Daniel B, Bednarski P, Nikutta P, et al. Left atrial spontaneous echo contrast in mitral valve disease: an indicator for an increased thromboembolic risk. J Am Coll Cardiol. 1988;11(6):1204-11.

51. Kasliwal RR, Mittal S, Kanojia A, Singh RP, Prakash O, Bhatia ML, et al. A study of spontaneous echo contrast in patients with rheumatic mitral stenosis and normal sinus rhythm: an Indian perspective. Br Heart J. 1995;74(3):296-9.

52. Li YH, Hwang JJ, Ko YL, Lin JL, Tseng YZ, Kuan P, Lien WP. Left atrial spontaneous echo contrast in patients with rheumatic mitral valve disease in sinus rhythm. Implication of an altered left atrial appendage function in its formation. Chest. 1995;108(1):99-103.

53. Selzer A, Cohn KE. Natural history of mitral stenosis: a review. Circulation. 1972;45:878-90.

54. Rodriguez L, Thomas J, Monterroso V, Weyman A, Harrigan P, Mueller L, et al. Validation of the proximal flow convergence method: calculation of orifice area in patients with mitral stenosis. Circulation. 1993;88:1157-65.

55. de Agustin JA, Nanda NC, Gill EA, de Isla LP, Zamorano JL. The use of three-dimensional echocardiography for the evaluation of and treatment of mitral stenosis. Cardiol Clin. 2007;25(2):311-8.

56. Applebaum RM, Kasliwal RR, Kanojia A, Seth A, Bhandari S, Trehan N, et al. Utility of three-dimensional echocardiography during balloon mitral valvuloplasty. J Am Coll Cardiol. 1998;32(5):1405-9.

57. Chen Q, Nosir YF, Vletter WB, Kint PP, Salustri A, Roelandt JR. Accurate assessment of MVA in patients with mitral stenosis by three-dimensional echocardiography. J Am Soc Echocardiogr. 1997;10:133-40.

58. Gill E, Bhola R, Carroll J, et al. Three-dimensional echocardiography predictors of percutaneous balloon mitral valvuloplasty success." Eur J Echocardiogr. 2000;1:S32.

59. Hozumi T, Yoshikawa J. Three-dimensional echocardiography using a multiplane TEE probe: the clinical applications. Echocardiography. 2000;17:757-64.

60. Singh V, Nanda NC, Agrawal G, Vengala S, Dod HS, Misra V, et al. Live three-dimensional echocardiographic assessment of mitral stenosis. Echocardiography. 2003;20:743-50.

61. Gill E, Bhola R, Carroll JD, et al. Live 3D echo and biplane evaluation of mitral stenosis for prediction of mitral valvuloplasty success. J Am Soc Echocardiogr. 2004;17:499.

62. Gorlin R, Gorlin SG. Hydraulic formula for calculation of the stenotic mitral valve, other cardiac valves and central circulatory shunts. Am Heart J. 1951;41:1-12.

63. Pérez de Isla L, Casanova C, Almería C, Rodrigo JL, Cordeiro P, Mataix L. Which method should be the reference method to evaluate the severity of rheumatic mitral stenosis? Gorlin's method versus 3D echo. Eur J Echocardiogr. 2007;8(6):470-3.

64. Herman Mannaerts FJ, Kamp O, Visser CA. Should mitral valve area assessment in patients with mitral stenosis be based on anatomical or on functional evaluation? A plea for 3D echocardiography as the new clinical standard. Eur Heart J. 2004;25:2073-4.

65. Sugeng L, Weinert L, Lammertin G, Thomas P, Spencer KT, Decara JM, et al. Accuracy of mitral valve area measurements using transthoracic rapid freehand 3-dimensional scanning: comparison with noninvasive and invasive methods. J Am Soc Echocardiogr. 2003;16:1292-300.

66. Yoshida K, Yoshikawa J, Shakudo M, Akasaka T, Jyo Y, Takao S, et al. Color Doppler evaluation of valvular regurgitation in normal subjects. Circulation. 1988;78:840-7.

67. Singh JP, Evans JC, Levy D, Larson MG, Freed LA, Fuller DL, et al. Prevalence and clinical determinants of mitral, tricuspid and aortic regurgitation (the Framingham Heart Study). Am J Cardiol. 1999;83:897-902.

68. Maurice ES, Vuyisile TN, Hector IM. Mitral Regurgitation. In: Andrew W, Thomas MB (Eds). Valvular Heart Disease. United States: Humana Press; 2009. pp. 221-46.

69. Selzer A, Katayama F. Mitral regurgitation: Clinical patterns, pathophysiology and natural history. Medicine. 1972;51:337-80.

70. Vijayalakshmi IB, Yavagal ST, Prabhudeva AN. Role of echocardiography in assessing the mechanism and effect of Ramipril on Functional Mitral Regurgitation in Dilated Cardiomyopathy. Echocardiography. 2005;22(4):289-95.

71. Otsuji Y, Handschumacher MD, Schwammenthal E, Jiang L, Song J, Guerrero JL, et al. Insights from three-dimensional echocardiography into the mechanism of functional mitral regurgitation: direct in vivo demonstration of altered leaflet tethering geometry. Circulation. 1997;96:1999-2008.

72. Carpentier A. Cardiac valve surgery—the "French correction. J Thorac Cardiovasc Surg. 1983;86:323-37.

73. Carabello BA, Crawford FA Jr. Valvular heart disease. N Engl J Med. 1997;337:32-41.

74. Schiller NB, Shah PM, Crawford M, De Maria A, Devereux R, Feigenbaum H, et al. Recommendations for quantitation of the left ventricle by two-dimensional echocardiography: American Society of Echocardiography Committee on Standards, Subcommittee on Quantitation of Two-Dimensional Echocardiograms. J Am Soc Echocardiogr. 1989;2:358-67.

75. Echocardiographic measurements and normal values. In: Feigenbaum H (Ed). Echocardiography. Philadelphia: Lea and Febiger; 1994. pp. 658-83.

76. Crawford MH, Souchek J, Oprian CA, Miller DC, Rahimtoola S, Giacomini JC, et al. Determinants of survival and left ventricular performance after mitral valve replacement. Department of Veterans Affairs Cooperative Study on Valvular Heart Disease. Circulation. 1990;81(4):1173-81.

77. Lester SJ, Ryan EW, Schiller NB, Foster E. Best method in clinical practice and in research studies to determine left atrial size. Am J Cardiol. 1999;84:829-32.

78. Wang Y, Gutman JM, Heilbron D, Wahr D, Schiller NB. Atrial volume in a normal adult population by two-dimensional echocardiography. Chest. 1984;86:595-601.

79. Cheitlin MD, Armstrong WF, Aurigemma GP, Beller GA, Bierman FZ, Davis JL, et al. ACC/AHA/ASE 2003 guideline update for the clinical application of echocardiography: summary article: a report of the American College of Cardiology/American Heart Association Task Force on Practice Guidelines (ACC/AHA/ASE Committee to Update the 1997 Guidelines for the Clinical Application of Echocardiography). J Am Coll Cardiol. 2003;42:954-70.

80. Chen CG, Thomas JD, Anconina J, Harrigan P, Mueller L, Picard MH, et al. Impact of impinging wall jet on color Doppler quantification of mitral regurgitation. Circulation. 1991;84:712-20.

81. Enriquez-Sarano M, Tajik AJ, Bailey KR, Seward JB. Color flow imaging compared with quantitative Doppler assessment of severity of mitral regurgitation: influence of eccentricity of jet and mechanism of regurgitation. J Am Coll Cardiol. 1993;21:1211-9.

82. Spain MG, Smith MD, Grayburn PA, Harlamert EA, De Maria AN. Quantitative assessment of mitral regurgitation by Doppler color flow imaging: angiographic and hemodynamic correlations. J Am Coll Cardiol. 1989;13:585-90.

83. Sahn DJ. Instrumentation and physical factors related to visualization of stenotic and regurgitant jets by Doppler color flow mapping. J Am Coll Cardiol. 1988;12:1354-65.

84. Sanjay M. Mitral regurgitation. In: Manoria PC (Ed). Echocardiography Update. Volume I–Valvular Heart Disease. Bhopal (India): Jainan Offset; 2002. pp. 32-48.

85. Smith MD, Grayburn PA, Spain MG, DeMaria AN. Observer variability in the quantification of color flow jet areas for mitral or aortic regurgitation. J Am Coll Cardiol. 1988;11:579-86.

86. Hall SA, Brickner ME, Willett DL, Irani WN, Afridi I, Grayburn PA. Assessment of mitral regurgitation severity by Doppler color flow mapping of the vena contracta. Circulation. 1997;95:636-42.

87. Heinle SK, Hall SA, Brickner ME, Willett DL, Grayburn PA. Comparison of vena contracta width by multiplane transesophageal echocardiography with quantitative Doppler assessment of mitral regurgitation. Am J Cardiol. 1998;81:175-9.

88. Tribouilloy C, Shen WF, Quéré JP, Rey JL, Choquet D, Dufossé H, et al. Assessment of severity of mitral regurgitation by measuring regurgitant jet width at its origin with transesophageal Doppler color flow imaging. Circulation. 1992;85:1248-53.

89. Mele D, Vandervoort P, Palacios I, Rivera JM, Dinsmore RE, Schwammenthal E, et al. Proximal jet size by Doppler color flow mapping predicts severity of mitral regurgitation. Clinical studies. Circulation. 1995;91:746-54.

90. Baumgartner H, Schima H, Kuhn P. Value and limitations of proximal jet dimensions for the quantitation of valvular regurgitation: an in vitro study using Doppler flow imaging. J Am Soc Echocardiogr. 1991;4:57-66.

91. Kizilbash AM, Willett DL, Brickner ME, Heinle SK, Grayburn PA. Effects of afterload reduction on vena contracta width in mitral regurgitation. J Am Coll Cardiol. 1998;32:427-31.

92. Schwammenthal E, Chen C, Benning F, Block M, Breithardt G, Levine RA. Dynamics of mitral regurgitant flow and orifice area: physiologic application of the proximal flow convergence method; clinical data and experimental testing. Circulation. 1994;90:307-22.

93. Enriquez-Sarano M, Miller FA Jr, Hayes SN, Bailey KR, Tajik AJ, Seward JB. Effective mitral regurgitant orifice area: clinical use and pitfalls of the proximal isovelocity surface area method. J Am Coll Cardiol. 1995;25:703-9.

94. Pu M, Prior DL, Fan X, Asher CR, Vasquez C, Griffin BP, et al. Calculation of mitral regurgitant orifice area with use of a simplified proximal convergence method: initial clinical application. J Am Soc Echocardiogr. 2001;14:180-5.

95. Utsunomiya T, Doshi R, Patel D, Mehta K, Nguyen D, Henry WL, et al. Calculation of volume flow rate by the proximal isovelocity surface area method: simplified approach using color Doppler zero baseline shift. J Am Coll Cardiol. 1993;22:277-82.

96. Schwammenthal E, Chen C, Giesler M, Sagie A, Guerrero JL, Vazquez de Prada JA, et al. New method for accurate calculation of regurgitant flow rate based on analysis of Doppler color flow maps of the proximal flow field: validation in a canine model of mitral regurgitation with initial application in patients. J Am Coll Cardiol. 1996;27:161-72.

97. Mele D, Schwammenthal E, Torp H, Nesta F, Pedini I, Vandervoort P, et al. A semiautomated objective technique for applying the proximal isovelocity surface area method to quantitate mitral regurgitation: clinical studies with the digital flow map. Am Heart J .2001;141:653-60.

98. Enriquez-Sarano M, Sinak LJ, Tajik AJ, Bailey KR, Seward JB. Changes in effective regurgitant orifice throughout systole in patients with mitral valve prolapse. A clinical study using the proximal isovelocity surface area method. Circulation. 1995;92:2951-8.

99. Buck T, Mucci RA, Guerrero JL, Holmvang G, Handschumacher MD, Levine RA. The power-velocity integral at the vena contracta: a new method for direct quantification of regurgitant volume flow. Circulation. 2000;102:1053-61.

100. Enriquez-Sarano M, Seward JB, Bailey KR, Tajik AJ. Effective regurgitant orifice area: a noninvasive Doppler development of an old hemodynamic concept. J Am Coll Cardiol. 1994;23:443-51.

101. Kizilbash AM, Hundley WG, Willett DL, Franco F, Peshock RM, Grayburn PA. Comparison of quantitative Doppler with magnetic resonance imaging for assessment of the severity of mitral regurgitation. Am J Cardiol. 1998;81:792-5.

102. Dujardin KS, Enriquez-Sarano M, Bailey KR, Nishimura RA, Seward JB, Tajik AJ. Grading of mitral regurgitation by quantitative Doppler echocardiography: calibration by left ventricular angiography in routine clinical practice. Circulation. 1997;96:3409-15.

103. Thomas L, Foster E, Schiller NB. Peak mitral inflow velocity predicts mitral regurgitation severity. J Am Coll Cardiol. 1998;31:174-9.

104. Klein AL, Obarski TP, Stewart WJ, Casale PN, Pearce GL, Husbands K, et al. Transesophageal Doppler echocardiography of pulmonary venous flow: a new marker of mitral regurgitation severity. J Am Coll Cardiol. 1991;18(2):518-26.

105. Enriquez-Sarano M, Tajik AJ, Schaff HV, Orszulak TA, Bailey KR, Frye RL. Echocardiographic prediction of survival after surgical correction of organic mitral regurgitation. Circulation. 1994;90:830-7.

106. Phillips HR, Levine FH, Carter JE, Boucher CA, Osbakken MD, Okada RD, et al. Mitral valve replacement for isolated mitral regurgitation: analysis of clinical course and late postoperative left ventricular ejection fraction. Am J Cardiol. 1981;48:647-54.

107. Enriquez-Sarano M, Tajik AJ, Schaff HV, Orszulak TA, McGoon MD, Bailey KR, et al. Echocardiographic prediction of left ventricular function after correction of mitral regurgitation: results and clinical implications. J Am Coll Cardiol. 1994;24:1536-43.

108. Ling LH, Enriquez-Sarano M, Seward JB, Tajik AJ, Schaff HV, Bailey KR, et al. Clinical outcome of mitral regurgitation due to flail leaflet. N Engl J Med. 1996;335:1417-23.

109. Ren JF, Kotler MN, De Pace NL, Mintz GS, Kimbiris D, Kalman P, et al. Two-dimensional echocardiographic determination of left atrial emptying volume: a non invasive index in quantifying the degree of nonrheumatic mitral regurgitation. J Am Coll Cardiol. 1983;2(4):729-36.

110. Armstrong GP, Griffin BP. Exercise echocardiographic assessment in severe mitral regurgitation. Coron Artery Dis. 2000;11:23-30.

111. Enriquez-Sarano M, Schaff HV, Orszulak TA, Tajik AJ, Bailey KR, Frye RL. Valve repair improves the outcome of surgery for mitral regurgitation. A multivariate analysis. Circulation. 1995;91:1022-8.

112. Lambert AS, Miller JP, Merrick SH, Schiller NB, Foster E, Muhiudeen-Russell I, et al. Improved evaluation of the location and mechanism of mitral valve regurgitation with a systematic transesophageal echocardiography examination. Anesth Analg. 1999;88:1205-12.

113. Enriquez-Sarano M, Freeman WK, Tribouilloy CM, Orszulak TA, Khandheria BK, Seward JB, et al. Functional anatomy of mitral regurgitation: accuracy and outcome implications of transesophageal echocardiography. J Am Coll Cardiol. 1999;34: 1129-36.

114. Czer LS, Maurer G, Bolger AF, De Robertis M, Resser KJ, Kass RM, et al. Intraoperative evaluation of mitral regurgitation by Doppler color flow mapping. Circulation. 1987;76(3 Pt 2):III108-16.

115. Reichert SL, Visser CA, Moulijn AC, Suttorp MJ, vd Brink RB, Koolen JJ, et al. Intraoperative transesophageal color-coded Doppler echocardiography for evaluation of residual regurgitationafter mitral valve repair. J Thorac Cardiovasc Surg. 1990;100(5):756-61.

116. Thomas L, Foster E, Hoffman JI, Schiller NB. The mitral regurgitation index: an echocardiographic guide to severity. J Am Coll Cardiol. 1999;33:2016-22.

117. Wisenbaugh T, Skudicky D, Sareli P. Prediction of outcome after valve replacement for rheumatic mitral regurgitation in the era of chordal preservation. Circulation. 1994;89:191-7.

118. Zile MR, Gaasch WH, Carroll JD, Levine HJ. Chronic mitral regurgitation: predictive value of preoperative echocardiographic indexes of left ventricular function and wall stress. J Am Coll Cardiol. 1984;3:235-42.

119. Flemming MA, Oral H, Rothman ED, Briesmiester K, Petrusha JA, Starling MR. Echocardiographic markers for mitral valve surgery to preserve left ventricular performance in mitral regurgitation. Am Heart J. 2000;140:476-82.

120. Henein M, Joseph M. Aortic Valve Disease. In: Michael YH (Ed). Valvular Heart Disease in Clinical Practice. London: Springer-Verlag Limited; 2009. p. 86.

121. Chang S, Clements S, Chang J. Aortic stenosis: echocardiographic cusp separation and surgical description of aortic valve in 22 patients. Am J Cardiol. 1977;39(4):499-504.

122. Lesbre JP, Scheuble C, Kalisa A, Lalau JD, Andrejak MT. Echocardiography in the diagnosis of severe aortic valve stenosis in adults. Arch Mal Coeur Vaiss. 1983;76(1):1-12.

123. Williams DE, Sahn DJ, Friedman WF. Cross-sectional echocardiographic localization of sites of left ventricular outflow tract obstruction. Am J Cardiol. 1976;37(2):250-5.

124. Currie PJ, Seward JB, Reeder GS, Vlietstra RE, Bresnahan DR, Bresnahan JF, et al. Continuous-wave Doppler echocardiographic assessment of severity of calcific aortic stenosis: a simultaneous Doppler-catheter correlative study in 100 adult patients. Circulation. 1985;71:1162-9.

125. Smith MD, Kwan OL, De Maria AN. Value and limitations of continuous-wave Doppler echocardiography in estimating severity of valvular stenosis. J Am Med Assoc. 1986;255:3145-51.

126. Burwash IG, Forbes AD, Sadahiro M, Verrier ED, Pearlman AS, Thomas R, et al. Echocardiographic volume flow and stenosis severity measures with changing flow rate in aortic stenosis. Am J Physiol. 1993;265(5 Pt 2):H1734-43.

127. Hegrenaes L, Hatle L. Aortic stenosis in adults. Non-invasive estimation of pressure differences by continuous wave Doppler echocardiography. Br Heart J. 1985;54:396-404.

128. Galan A, Zoghbi WA, Quinones MA. Determination of severity of valvular aortic stenosis by Doppler echocardiography and relation of findings to clinical outcome and agreement with hemodynamic measurements determined at cardiac catheterization. Am J Cardiol. 1991;67:1007-12.

129. Yeager M, Yock PG, Popp RL. Comparison of Doppler-derived pressure gradient to that determined at cardiac catheterization in adults with aortic valve stenosis: implications for management. Am J Cardiol. 1986;57:644-8.

130. Otto CM, Pearlman AS, Gardner CL, Enomoto DM, Togo T, Tsuboi H, et al. Experimental validation of Doppler echocardiographic measurement of volume flow through the stenotic aortic valve. Circulation. 1988;78:435-41.

131. Harrison MR, Gurley JC, Smith MD, Grayburn PA, De Maria AN. A practical application of Doppler echocardiography for the assessment of severity of aortic stenosis. Am Heart J. 1988;115:622-8.

132. Simpson IA, Houston AB, Sheldon CD, Hutton I, Lawrie TD. Clinical value of Doppler echocardiography in the assessment of adults with aortic stenosis. Br Heart J. 1985;53:636-9.

133. Stamm RB, Martin RP. Quantification of pressure gradients across stenotic valves by Doppler ultrasound. J Am Coll Cardiol. 1983;2:707-18.

134. Yoganathan AP, Valdes-Cruz LM, Schmidt-Dohna J, Jimoh A, Berry C, Tamura T, et al. Continuous-wave Doppler velocities and gradients across fixed tunnel obstructions: studies in vitro and in vivo. Circulation. 1987;76:657-66.

135. Hatle L, Angelsen BA, Tromsdal A. Non-invasive assessment of aortic stenosis by Doppler ultrasound. Br Heart J. 1980;43: 284-92.

136. Callahan MJ, Tajik AJ, Su-Fan Q, Bove AA. Validation of instantaneous pressure gradients measured by continuous wave Doppler in experimentally induced aortic stenosis. Am J Cardiol. 1985;56:989-93.

137. Smith MD, Dawson PL, Elion JL, Booth DC, Handshoe R, Kwan OL, et al. Correlation of continuous wave Doppler velocities with cardiac catheterization gradients: an experimental model of aortic stenosis. J Am Coll Cardiol. 1985;6:1306-14.

138. Otto CM. The Practice of Clinical Echocardiography, 2nd edition. Philadelphia: WB Saunders; 2002.

139. Lester SJ, McElhinney DB, Miller JP, Lutz JT, Otto CM, Redberg RF. Rate of change in aortic valve area duringa cardiac cycle can predict the rate of hemodynamic progression of aortic stenosis. Circulation. 2000;101:1947-52.

140. Bahler RC, Desser DR, Finkelhor RS, Brener SJ, Youssefi M. Factors leading to progression of valvular aortic stenosis. Am J Cardiol. 1999;84:1044-8.

141. Rosenhek R, Binder T, Porenta G, Lang I, Christ G, Schemper M, et al. Predictors of outcome in severe, asymptomatic aortic stenosis. N Engl J Med. 2000;343:611-7.

142. Otto CM, Pearlman AS, Gardner CL. Hemodynamic progression of aortic stenosis in adults assessed by Doppler echocardiography. J Am Coll Cardiol. 1989;13:545-50.

143. Roger VL, Tajik AJ, Bailey KR, Oh JK, Taylor CL, Seward JB. Progression of aortic stenosis in adults: new appraisalusing Doppler echocardiography. Am Heart J. 1990;119:331-8.

144. Faggiano P, Ghizzoni G, Sorgato A, Sabatini T, Simoncelli U, Gardini A, et al. Rate of progression of valvular aortic stenosis in adults. Am J Cardiol. 1992;70:229-33.

145. Peter M, Hoffmann A, Parker C, Luscher T, Burckhardt D. Progression of aortic stenosis. Role of age and concomitant coronary artery disease. Chest. 1993;103:1715-9.

146. Palta S, Pai AM, Gill KS, Pai RG. New insights into the progression of aortic stenosis: implications for secondary prevention. Circulation. 2000;101:2497-502.

147. Hoffmann R, Flachskampf FA, Hanrath P. Planimetry of orifice area in aortic stenosis using multiplane transesophageal echocardiography. J Am Coll Cardiol. 1993;22(2):529-34.

148. Otto CM, Burwash IG, Legget ME, Munt BI, Fujioka M, Healy NL, et al. Prospective study of asymptomatic valvular aortic stenosis. Clinical, echocardiographic, and exercise predictors of outcome. *Circulation.* 1997;95(9):2262-70.

149. deFilippi CR, Willett DL, Brickner ME, Appleton CP, Yancy CW, Eichhorn EJ, et al. Usefulness of dobutamine echocardiography in distinguishing severe from non severe valvular aortic stenosis in patients with depressed left ventricular function and low transvalvular gradients. Am J Cardiol. 1995;75:191-4.

150. Nishimura RA, Grantham JA, Connolly HM, Schaff HV, Higano ST, Holmes DR, Jr. Low-output, low-gradient aortic stenosis in patients with depressed left ventricular systolic function: the clinical utility of the dobutamine challenge in the catheterization laboratory. Circulation. 2002;106:809-13.

151. Monin JL, Monchi M, Gest V, Duval-Moulin AM, Dubois-Rande JL, Gueret P. Aortic stenosis with severe left ventricular dysfunction and low transvalvular pressure gradients: risk stratification by low-dose dobutamine echocardiography. J Am Coll Cardiol. 2001;37:2101-7.

152. Quere JP, Monin JL, Levy F, Petit H, Baleynaud S, Chauvel C, et al. Influence of preoperative left ventricular contractile reserve on postoperative ejectionfraction in low-gradient aortic stenosis. Circulation. 2006;113:1738-44.

153. Schwammenthal E, Vered Z, Moshkowitz Y, Rabinowitz B, Ziskind Z, Smolinski AK, et al. Dobutamine echocardiography in patients with aortic stenosis and left ventricular dysfunction: predicting outcome as a function of management strategy. Chest. 2001;119(6):1766-77.

154. Henry WL, Bonow RO, Rosing DR, Epstein SE. Observations on the optimum time for operative intervention for aortic regurgitation. II. Serial echocardiographic evaluation of asymptomatic patients. Circulation. 1980;61(3):484-92.

155. Chaliki HP, Mohty D, Avierinos JF, Scott CG, Schaff HV, Tajik AJ, et al. Outcomes after aortic valve replacement in patients with severe aortic regurgitation and markedly reduced left ventricular function. Circulation. 2002;106:2687-93.

156. Robertson WS, Stewart J, Armstrong WF, Dillon JC, Feigenbaum H. Reverse doming of the anterior mitral leaflet with severe aortic regurgitation. J Am Coll Cardiol. 1984;3(2 Pt 1):431-6.

157. Grayburn PA, Smith MD, Handshoe R, Friedman BJ, De-Maria AN. Detection of aortic insufficiency by standard echocardiography, pulsed Doppler echocardiography, and auscultation: a comparison of accuracies. Ann Intern Med. 1986;104:599-605.

158. Perry GJ, Helmcke F, Nanda NC, Byard C, Soto B. Evaluation of aortic insufficiency by Doppler color flow mapping. J Am Coll Cardiol. 1987;9:952-9.

159. Reynolds T, Abate J, Tenney A, Warner MG. The JH/LVOH method in the quantification of aortic regurgitation: How the cardiac sonographer may avoid an important potential pitfall. J Am Soc Echocardiogr. 1991;4:105-8.

160. Tribouilloy CM, Enriquez-Sarano M, Bailey KR, Seward JB, Tajik AJ. Assessment of severity of aortic regurgitation using the width of the vena contracta: a clinical color Doppler imaging study. Circulation. 2000;102:558-64.

161. Taylor AL, Eichhorn EJ, Brickner ME, Eberhart RC, Grayburn PA. Aortic valve morphology: an important in vitro determinant of proximal regurgitant jet width by Doppler color flow mapping. J Am Coll Cardiol. 1990;16:405-12.

162. Tribouilloy CM, Enriquez-Sarano M, Fett SL, Bailey KR, Seward JB, Tajik AJ. Application of the proximal flow convergence method to calculate the effective regurgitant orifice area in aortic regurgitation. J Am Coll Cardiol. 1998;32:1032-9.

163. Touche T, Prasquier R, Nitenberg A, de Zuttere D, Gourgon R. Assessment and follow up of patients with aortic regurgitation by an updated Doppler echocardiographic measurement of the regurgitant fraction in the aortic arch. Circulation. 1985;72: 819-24.

164. Tribouilloy C, Avinee P, Shen WF, Rey JL, Slama M, Lesbre JP. End diastolic flow velocity just beneath the aortic isthmus assessed by pulsed Doppler echocardiography: a new predictor of the aortic regurgitant fraction. Br Heart J. 1991;65:37-40.

165. Ciobanu M, Abbasi AS, Allen M, Hermer A, Spellberg R. Pulsed Doppler echocardiography in the diagnosis and estimation of severity of aortic insufficiency. Am J Cardiol. 1982;49:339-43.

166. Rokey R, Sterling LL, Zoghbi WA, Sartori MP, Limacher MC, Kuo LC, et al. Determination of regurgitant fraction in isolated mitral or aortic regurgitation by pulsed Doppler two-dimensional echocardiography. J Am Coll Cardiol 1986;7:1273-8.

167. Enriquez-Sarano M, Bailey KR, Seward JB, Tajik AJ, Krohn MJ, Mays JM. Quantitative Doppler assessment of valvular regurgitation. Circulation. 1993;87:841-8.

168. Teague SM, Heinsimer JA, Anderson JL, Sublett K, Olson EG, Voyles WF, et al. Quantification of aortic regurgitation utilizing continuous wave Doppler ultrasound. J Am Coll Cardiol. 1986;8:592-9.

169. Labovitz AJ, Ferrara RP, Kern MJ, Bryg RJ, Mrosek DG, Williams GA. Quantitative evaluation of aortic insufficiency by continuous wave Doppler echocardiography. J Am Coll Cardiol. 1986;8: 1341-7.

170. Padial LR, Oliver A, Vivaldi M, Sagie A, Freitas N, Weyman AE, et al. Doppler echocardiographic assessment of progression of aortic regurgitation. Am J Cardiol. 1997;80:306-14.

171. Griffin BP, Flachskampf FA, Siu S, Weyman AE, Thomas JD. The effects of regurgitant orifice size, chamber compliance, and systemic vascular resistance on aortic regurgitant velocity slope and pressure half time. Am Heart J. 1991;122:1049-56.

172. Yousof AM, Shafei MZ, Endrys G, Khan N, Simo M, Cherian G. Tricuspid stenosis and regurgitation in rheumatic heart disease: a prospective cardiac catheterization study in 525 patients. Am Heart J. 1985;110(1 Pt 1):60-4.

173. Daniels SJ, Mintz GS, Kotler MN. Rheumatic tricuspid valve disease: two-dimensional echocardiographic, hemodynamic, and angiographic correlations. Am J Cardiol. 1983;51(3):492-6.

174. Guyer DE, Gillam LD, Foale RA, Clark MC, Dinsmore R, Palacios I, et al. Comparison of the echocardiographic and hemodynamic diagnosis of rheumatic tricuspid stenosis. J Am Coll Cardiol. 1984;3(5):1135-44.

175. Shimada R, Takeshita A, Nakamura M, Tokunaga K, Hirata T. Diagnosis of tricuspid stenosis by M-mode and two-dimensional echocardiography. Am J Cardiol. 1984;53(1):164-8.

176. Pothineni KR, Duncan K, Yelamanchili P, Nanda NC, Patel V, Fan P, et al. Live/real time three-dimensional transthoracic echocardiographic assessment of tricuspid valve pathology: incremental value over the two-dimensional technique. Echocardiography. 2007;24:541-52.

177. Quinones MA, Otto CM, Stoddard M, Waggoner A, Zoghbi WA. Doppler Quantification Task Force of the Nomenclature and Standards Committee of the American Society of Echocardiography. Recommendations for quantification of Doppler echocardiography: a report from the Doppler Quantification Task Force of the Nomenclature and Standards Committee of the American Society of Echocardiography. J Am Soc Echocardiogr. 2002;15:167-84.

178. Hatle L. Noninvasive assessment of valve lesions with Doppler ultrasound. Herz. 1984;9:213-21.

179. Fawzy ME, Mercer EN, Dunn B, al-Amri M, Andaya W. Doppler echocardiography in the evaluation of tricuspid stenosis. Eur Heart J. 1989;10:985-90.

180. Karp K, Teien D, Eriksson P. Doppler echocardiographic assessment of the valve area in patients with atrioventricular valve stenosis by application of the continuity equation. J Intern Med. 1989;225:261-6.

181. Ha JW, Chung N, Jang Y, Rim SJ. Tricuspid stenosis and regurgitation: Doppler and color flow echocardiography and cardiac catheterization findings. Clin Cardiol. 2000;23:51-2.

182. Lavie CJ, Hebert K, Cassidy M. Prevalence and severity of Doppler-detected valvular regurgitation and estimation of right-sided cardiac pressures in patients with normal two dimensional echocardiograms. Chest. 1993;103:226-31.

183. Klein AL, Burstow DJ, Tajik AJ, Zachariah PK, Tallman CD, Taylor CL, et al. Age-related prevalence of valvular regurgitation in normal subjects: a comprehensive color flow examination of 118 volunteers. J Am Soc Echocardiogr. 1990;3:54-63.

184. Waller BF, Howard J, Fess S. Pathology of tricuspid valve stenosis and pure tricuspid regurgitation—part III. Clin Cardiol. 1995;18:225-30.

185. Veyrat C, Kalmanson D, Farjon M, Manin JP, Abitbol G. Noninvasive diagnosis and assessment of tricuspid regurgitation and stenosis using one and two dimensional echo-pulsed Doppler. Br Heart J. 1982;47:596-605.

186. Miyatake K, Okamoto M, Kinoshita N, Ohta M, Kozuka T, Sakakibara H, et al. Evaluation of tricuspid regurgitation by pulsed Doppler and two dimensional echocardiography. Circulation. 1982;66:777-84.

187. De Pace NL, Ross J, Iskandrian AS, Nestico PF, Kotler MN, Mintz GS, et al. Tricuspid regurgitation: noninvasive techniques for determining causes and severity. J Am Coll Cardiol. 1984;3: 1540-50.

188. Sakai K, Nakamura K, Satomi G, Kondo M, Hirosawa K. Hepatic vein blood flow pattern measured by Doppler echocardiography as an evaluation of tricuspid valve insufficiency. J Cardiogr. 1983;13:33-43.

189. Simonson JS, Schiller NB. Sonospirometry: a non-invasive method for estimation of mean right atrial pressure based on two dimensional echocardiographic measurements of the inferior vena cava during measured inspiration. J Am Coll Cardiol. 1988;11:557-64.

190. Abu-Yousef MM. Duplex Doppler sonography of the hepatic vein in tricuspid regurgitation. AJR Am J Roentgenol. 1991;156: 79-83.

191. Grossmann G, Stein M, Kochs M, Hoher M, Koenig W, Hombach V, et al. Comparison of the proximal flow convergence method and the jet area method for the assessment of the severity of tricuspid regurgitation. Eur Heart J. 1998;19:652-9.

192. Shapira Y, Porter A, Wurzel M, Vaturi M, Sagie A. Evaluation of tricuspid regurgitation severity: echocardiographic and clinical correlation. J Am Soc Echocardiogr. 1998;11:652-9.

193. Gonzalez-Vilchez F, Zarauza J, Vazquez de Prada JA, Martin DR, Ruano J, Delgado C, et al. Assessment of tricuspid regurgitation by Doppler color flow imaging: angiographic correlation. Int J Cardiol. 1994;44:275-83.

194. Suzuki Y, Kambara H, Kadota K, Tamaki S, Yamazato A, Nohara R, et al. Detection and evaluation of tricuspid regurgitation using a real-time, two-dimensional, color-coded, Doppler flow imaging system: comparison with contrast two-dimensional echocardiography and right ventriculography. Am J Cardiol. 1986;57(10):811-5.

195. Yamachika S, Reid CL, Savani D, Meckel C, Paynter J, Knoll M, et al. Usefulness of color Doppler proximal isovelocity surface area method in quantitating valvular regurgitation. J Am Soc Echocardiogr. 1997;10:159-68.

196. Rivera JM, Vandervoort P, Mele D, Weyman A, Thomas JD. Value of proximal regurgitant jet size in tricuspid regurgitation. Am Heart J. 1996;131:742-7.

197. Tribouilloy CM, Enriquez-Sarano M, Bailey KR, Tajik AJ, Seward JB. Quantification of tricuspid regurgitation by measuring the width of the vena contracta with Doppler color flow imaging: a clinical study. J Am Coll Cardiol. 2000;36:472-8.

198. Minagoe S, Rahimtoola SH, Chandraratna PA. Significance of laminar systolic regurgitant flow in patients with tricuspid regurgitation: a combined pulsed-wave, continuous-wave Doppler and two-dimensional echocardiographic study. Am Heart J. 1990;119:627-35.

199. Nagueh SF, Kopelen HA, Zoghbi WA. Relation of mean right atrial pressure to echocardiographic and Doppler parameters of right atrial and right ventricular function. Circulation. 1996;93: 1160-9.

200. Vijayalakshmi IB. Echocardiography in acute rheumatic fever and chronic rheumatic heart disease. In: Nanda NC (Ed). Comprehensive Textbook of Echocardiography. New Delhi: Jaypee Brothers Medical Publishers (P) Ltd; 2014. pp. 765-825. 5.

201. Vijayalakshmi IB. Rheumatic heart disease—A neglected giant. In: Deb PK (Ed). Cardiology update 2012. Kolkata: CSI; 2012. pp. 15-22.

202. Reményi B, Wilson N, Steer A, Ferreira B, Kado J, Kumar K, et al. World Heart Federation criteria for echocardiographic diagnosis of rheumatic heart disease an evidence-based guideline Nat Rev Cardiol. 2012;9(5):297-309.

14

Consensus and Controversies in the Management of Acute Rheumatic Fever: Introducing ARMOR to Prevent and Protect

Arati Dave Lalchandani, IB Vijayalakshmi

> *"… A good doctor is one who is shrewd in diagnosis and wise in treatment; but, more than that, he is a person who never spares himself in the interest of his patients."*
>
> **—Sir Hugh Cairns** (1896–1952)
> Australian-born British Neurosurgeon and
> Professor of Surgery, Oxford, UK

■ INTRODUCTION

Acute rheumatic fever (ARF) is a diffuse inflammatory disease of the joints, heart, blood vessels, brain, and subcutaneous tissue. Carditis is the most serious major manifestation of rheumatic fever (RF). The heart valves are the most commonly affected structures. The presence or absence of carditis is an important determinant of the course and prognosis of ARF. The prognosis worsens with increasing severity of the initial carditis and with recurrences.[1] Hence, the treatment of ARF is not just about relieving fever and joint pain but also to reduce the cardiac damage and prevent the recurrence. Although the prevention of ARF and the management of recurrences are well established, the optimal management of active rheumatic carditis is still unclear. Hence, there are both consensus and controversies in the management of various affections of ARF. The debate on optimal and safe management of RF and RHD can not be concluded without the mention of ARMOR Arati's Regime for Management of Rheumatic Fever. This regime is elaborated at the end of this chapter.

■ GENERAL MEASURES

All patients with suspected ARF (first episode or recurrence) with carditis should be hospitalized ideally. Hospitalization helps in ensuring that all investigations are done and for starting therapy. Also, the patient can be observed for a period prior to commencing treatment to confirm the diagnosis.

Bed rest to control rheumatic activity was first prescribed in the 1940s but not needed with application of ARMOR.[2] Common clinical practice is that physical activity should be restricted until the acute phase reactants have normalized and then ambulation is begun gradually. Bed rest contributes to the reduction of rheumatic activity.[3] Some experts advise that all patients with ARF should be placed on bed-chair-rest and monitored closely for the onset of carditis.[4]

In patients with carditis, a rest period of at least 4 weeks is recommended,[5] although physicians should make this decision on an individual basis. Ambulatory restrictions may be relaxed when there is no carditis and when arthritis has subsided.[6] Patients with chorea must be placed in a protective environment so that they do not injure themselves.

■ MAIN GOALS FOR SPECIFIC TREATMENT STRATEGY OF ARF

The main goals of management of ARF are:
- The management of the current infection with eradication of group A beta-hemolytic streptococcal (GABHS) infection.
- Anti-inflammatory treatment of the symptoms of ARF

- Treatment of carditis, cardiac failure, and chorea
- Prevention of recurring episodes of ARF with long-term secondary prophylaxis and infective endocarditis prophylaxis
- Surgery for severe regurgitations

Eradication of GABHS Infection

The primary prevention of ARF is accomplished by proper identification and adequate antibiotic treatment of GABHS tonsillopharyngitis. Diagnosis of GABHS pharyngitis is best accomplished by differentiating clinical presentation of streptococcal tonsillopharyngitis from other upper respiratory tract infections. The clinical judgment must be used with diagnostic test results, the criterion standard of which is the throat culture. Antimicrobials to be used for GABHS pharyngitis are penicillin (either oral penicillin V or injectable benzathine penicillin), which is the treatment of choice, because it is cost-effective, has a narrow spectrum of activity, and has long-standing proven efficacy and GABHS resistant to penicillin has not been documented.

For penicillin-allergic individuals, acceptable alternatives include a narrow-spectrum oral cephalosporin, oral clindamycin or various oral macrolides or azalides. The drugs used for eradication of GABHS pharyngitis are detailed in **Table 1**.[7] Tetracycline, sulfonamide, and chloramphenicol should not to be used to treat GABHS pharyngitis because of widespread prevalence of drug resistance.[8,9]

Although acute pharyngitis is one of the most frequent illnesses for which pediatricians and other primary care physicians are consulted, only a relatively small percentage of patients with this condition are infected by GABHS. Moreover, the signs and symptoms of group A streptococcal and nonstreptococcal pharyngitis overlap so broadly that accurate diagnosis on clinical grounds alone is usually impossible.[10] It is difficult to distinguish clinically between streptococcal pharyngitis and viral pharyngitis. However, an abrupt onset of tender cervical lymphadenopathy, tonsillopharyngeal exudate, headache, anorexia, abdominal pain, and vomiting suggests the possibility of streptococcal pharyngitis. Clinical presentation of streptococcal tonsillopharyngitis is as in **Table 2**.

TABLE 1: Treatment of streptococcal tonsillopharyngitis.

Agent	*Dose*	*Mode*	*Duration*
Penicillins			
Penicillin V (phenoxymethylpenicillin)	• *Children*: 250 mg two to three times daily for <27 kg (60 lb); children >27 kg (60 lb), adolescents, and adults • 500 mg two to three times daily	Oral	10 days
Or			
Amoxicillin	50 mg/kg once daily (maximum 1 g)	Oral	10 days
Or			
Benzathine penicillin G	600,000 U for patients <27 kg (60 lb); 1,200,000 U for patients >27 kg (60 lb)	Intramuscular	Once
For individuals allergic to penicillin:			
Narrow-spectrum cephalosporin[†] (cephalexin, cefadroxil)	Variable	Oral	10 days
Or			
Clindamycin	20 mg/kg/day divided in three doses (maximum 1.8 g/day)	Oral	10 days
Or			
Azithromycin	12 mg/kg once daily (maximum 500 mg)	Oral	5 days
Or			
Clarithromycin	15 mg/kg/day divided into BID (maximum 250 mg BID)	Oral	10 days

The following are not acceptable: Sulfonamides, trimethoprim, tetracyclines, and fluoroquinolones.

[†]To be avoided in those with immediate (type I) hypersensitivity to penicillin

TABLE 2: Clinical presentation of streptococcal tonsillopharyngitis.

Common findings	Findings not suggesting GABHS infection
Symptoms	
Sudden onset of sore throat	Coryza
Pain on swallowing	Hoarseness
Fever	Cough
Headache	Diarrhea
Abdominal pain	
Nausea and vomiting	
Signs	
Tonsillopharyngeal erythema	Conjunctivitis
Tonsillopharyngeal exudate	Anterior stomatitis
Soft palate petechiae ("doughnut" lesions)	Discrete ulcerative lesions
• Beefy red, swollen uvula • Anterior cervical adenitis • Scarlatiniform rash	
(GABHS: group A β-hemolytic *Streptococcus*)	

Recommendations

Patients with acute streptococcal pharyngitis should receive therapy with an antimicrobial agent at a dose and for a duration that is likely to eradicate the infecting organism from the pharynx. On the basis of its narrow spectrum of antimicrobial activity, the infrequency with which it produces adverse reactions and its modest cost, penicillin is the drug of choice for treatment of the patients who are not allergic to it.

There is a consensus in the treatment of acute streptococcal pharyngitis and primary prevention of ARF. But there is a paradigm shift over which drug to use and Azithromycin wins hands down.

Symptomatic persons with multiple, recurrent, episodes of pharyngitis, proven by culture or rapid antigen detection testing, are treated with the following oral antibiotics.

Treatment of Multiple, Recurrent Episodes of Group A Streptococcal Pharyngitis

- Oral clindamycin for 10 days in a dose of 20–30 mg/kg/day in three equally divided doses in children and in adults 600 mg/day in two to four equally divided doses.
- Amoxicillin–clavulanic acid for 10 days in a dose of 40 mg/kg/day in three equally divided doses in children and in adults 500 mg BID.
- Intramuscular benzathine penicillin G can be given as a single dose. 600,000 U for patients <27 kg; 1,200,000 U for patients >27 kg

- Combination of parenteral benzathine penicillin G with oral rifampin 20 mg/kg/day orally in two equally divided doses for 4 days[8]

Penicillin-resistant strains of GABHS have not been reported and follow-up cultures are not necessary.[11]

It is well established that appropriate treatment of streptococcal pharyngitis markedly decreases the risk of developing ARF if started within 9 days after the onset of symptoms.[12] But the problem is that as many as one-third to two-thirds of cases of ARF are preceded by a minimally symptomatic or asymptomatic GABHS pharyngitis, which makes effective primary prophylaxis impossible in many cases. Poor access to healthcare in developing countries, where the incidence of ARF is high, further decreases the likelihood of effective primary prophylaxis.

Difficulties in Eradication of GABHS Infection

- *GABHS* persists for up to 15 days on unrinsed toothbrushes and removable orthodontic appliances.[13] The pathogens are not isolated from rinsed toothbrushes after 3 days. Thus, instructing patients to rinse toothbrushes and removable orthodontic appliances thoroughly may help to prevent recurrent infections.[14]
- *Pets*: Transmission of GABHS occurs mainly through contact with respiratory secretions from an infected person. But, infection from family pets is rare and only a few cases have been reported.[15,16]
- *Close contacts*: During epidemics, 50% of the siblings and 20% of the parents of infected children develop streptococcal pharyngitis.[17] Asymptomatic contacts do not require cultures or prophylaxis. Symptomatic contacts may be treated with or without cultures.
- *Follow-up and carriers*: Routine throat cultures are not necessary after treatment. Nearly 5–12% of treated patients have a positive post-treatment culture, regardless of the therapy given.[18] A positive post-treatment culture represents the asymptomatic chronic carrier state. Carriers are not a significant source for the spread of GABHS. Also, they are not at risk of developing RF.[17] In general, asymptomatic carriers are not treated unless they are associated with treatment failure in a close contact index patient.
- *Contagion*: Patients with streptococcal pharyngitis are considered contagious until they have taken antibiotic for 24 hours.[19] Till the temperature subsides, children should not go back to their daycare center or school. The benefits of giving oral penicillin to eradicate group A streptococci from the pharynx of patients with ARF are largely based on anecdotal evidence. It has not been shown in controlled studies to change the outcome 1 year after the primary event. The recommended regimen for the treatment of streptococcal tonsillopharyngitis is as given in **Table 1**.

Treatment Features of ARF

The major issue on initial presentation in ARF is confirmation of the diagnosis. None of the treatments offered to patients with ARF has been proven to alter the outcome of the acute episode or the amount of damage to heart valves, except in the case of heart failure.[20,21] Hence, there is no urgency to begin definitive treatment.

Until the diagnosis is confirmed, it is recommended that joint pain be treated with paracetamol or codeine. It has been shown that paracetamol is more effective. The arthritis, arthralgia, and fever of ARF have been shown in controlled trials to respond dramatically to salicylate or other nonsteroidal anti-inflammatory drugs (NSAIDs).[22-24] The effect can be seen as early as a few hours and almost always within 3 days. If the symptoms and signs do not reduce substantially within 3 days of commencing anti-inflammatory medications, a diagnosis other than ARF should be considered.

Treatment of Arthritis

Thomas Maclagan discovered in 1876 that salicin quickly lowered fever, eased joint pain, and swelling, and lessened chest pain by decreasing pericardial fluid.[25] It had no effect on chorea. Shortly, many salicylates with slightly varying chemical constituents became available, including aspirin, which formed a mainstay of therapy for RF in the early 20th century. Relief from joint illness, prolonged fever, and chest pain brought excitement to doctors and patients alike and virtually overnight older therapies were cast aside. So effective was salicylate in alleviating distress that almost no physician critically analyzed its value to the injury that doctors feared most that is the cardiac involvement.

Salicylates remain the first-line drugs in the treatment of arthritis. The response is usually excellent.

Aspirin: It is the first line of therapy. It should be started in patients with arthritis or severe arthralgia as soon as the diagnosis of ARF has been confirmed. The dose is 100 mg/kg/day divided into four to five times. In children, the dose may be increased up to 125 mg/kg/day and to 6–8 g/day in adults.[11] After achieving the desired initial steady state concentration for 2 weeks, the dosage can be decreased to 60–70 mg/kg/day for an additional 3–6 weeks.[5,11,26] The initial doses of salicylate therapy should be continued until a satisfactory clinical response is obtained, i.e., there is complete relief of symptoms and signs of arthritis and the temperature has returned to normal. Thereafter, the dose may be reduced to two-thirds of the initial value and may be maintained till the laboratory investigations of inflammatory disease have returned to normal. For the remainder of the course of therapy, the dose may be reduced to half the initial daily dose. If relapse occurs when doses are reduced, it is advisable to return to the previous higher dosage that suppressed the process. Analgesia is optimally achieved with high doses of salicylates, often inducing dramatic clinical improvement. A lower dose may be required to avert symptoms of nausea and vomiting. The optimal aspirin dose should ensure an adequate response but avoid toxicity. The dose can be increased until serum salicylate levels of 20–30 mg/dL are reached. If symptoms of toxicity are present,

they may subside after a few days despite continuation of the medication, but blood levels could be monitored, if facilities are available.[11,26]

The duration of treatment is decided by the clinical response and improvement in the inflammatory markers such as erythrocyte sedimentation rate (ESR) and C-reactive protein (CRP). Most patients need aspirin for only 1–2 weeks, but some patients need it for up to 6 weeks. Most episodes of ARF subside within 6 weeks and 90% resolve within 12 weeks. Approximately, 5% of patients require salicylate therapy for 6 months or more.[27]

Some recommend low-dose aspirin of 30–60 mg/kg/day, given in four divided doses.[28] This dose is usually sufficient to affect dramatic relief of arthritis and fever and higher dosages carry a greater risk of side effects and there are no proven short- or long-term benefits of high doses that produce salicylate blood levels of 20–30 mg/dL.

There is also controversy over whether other nonsteroidal anti-inflammatory drugs or steroidal anti-inflammatory drugs are superior to aspirin. The various anti-inflammatory agents such as aspirin, corticosteroids, immunoglobulin, and pentoxifylline have been tried for preventing or reducing further heart valve damage in patients with ARF. It is advisable to avoid premature administration of salicylates or corticosteroids until the diagnosis of ARF is confirmed, as it may mask the development of migratory polyarthritis or the development of fever. No controlled trials comparing aspirin and other nonsteroidal anti-inflammatory agents have been conducted. However, in patients who are intolerant or allergic to aspirin, naproxen (10–20 mg/kg/day) has been used.[29] Naproxen has the advantage of twice daily dosing. One of the most common errors made by physicians is the early administration of anti-inflammatory therapy before the diagnosis has been finally established.

Treatment of Carditis and Heart Failure

Carditis

In the prepenicillin era, prolonged bed rest in patients with rheumatic carditis was associated with shorter duration of carditis, fewer relapses, and less cardiomegaly.[2] But now, strict bed rest is no longer recommended for most patients with rheumatic carditis. Ambulation should be gradual and as tolerated in patients with heart failure or severe acute valve disease, especially during the first 4 weeks, or until the serum CRP levels and the ESR have normalized or dramatically reduced. Patients with milder or no carditis should remain in bed only as long as necessary to manage other symptoms, such as joint pain.

Moderate-to-severe carditis is usually an indication for corticosteroids although efficacy in reducing sequelae has not been proven so far. In patient with severe carditis and congestive heart failure (CHF), corticosteroids may be lifesaving. Albert et al.[20] performed a meta-analysis of the literature on the treatment of rheumatic carditis, comparing corticosteroids and salicylates in preventing valvular damage. It seems clear that corticosteroids are superior to salicylates in rapidly resolving acute manifestations, but the advantage of the former in preventing a pathologic murmur at 1 year post-treatment was not statistically significant.[20] Prednisone, 1–2 mg/kg/day (maximum, 80 mg/day) is used for 2 weeks and after that, the dose is gradually tapered, reducing it by 20–25% of the previous dose every week.[5,26] Some advocate the concomitant use of salicylates to avoid rebound. In severe carditis, therapy may be initiated with intravenous (IV) methylprednisolone.[30,31] IV immunoglobulin seems not to alter the extent and severity of carditis or decrease chronic morbidity.[32] The treatment of acute carditis is given in **Box 1**.[33]

In rheumatic carditis, it should be emphasized that the primary hemodynamic abnormality is valvular incompetence rather than myocardial dysfunction. Diuretics, angiotensin-converting enzyme (ACE) inhibitors, and afterload reduction may be valuable as temporizing measures in patients with significant regurgitation and symptoms.

In disentangling the hormonal web connecting the pituitary and adrenal glands, endocrinologists had identified a pituitary hormone, adrenocorticotropic hormone (ACTH) that normally stimulated the adrenal glands to secrete cortisone. One property of cortisone was to reduce inflammation, the hallmark of symptoms in RF.

Physicians hoped to provide highly effective anti-inflammatory relief to patients either by administering ACTH, in doses that greatly exceeded the normal level of bodily hormone, or by giving large amounts of cortisone. The initial reception of these hormones was reminiscent of the introduction of salicylate 75 years earlier. First reports proclaimed dramatic deathbed rescues. Soon, concern over serious side effects and the reappearance of symptoms after stopping hormones or "rebound" dampened enthusiasm. Almost immediately, the American Heart Association (AHA) and the British Medical Research Council collaborated to study the comparative benefits of hormones and aspirin. Here, the epidemiological amelioration of RF, impeded determining whether hormones were superior to aspirin by limiting the number of critically ill children available for the study. When the multinational collaborators completed the first phase of their investigation in 1955, they announced a stalemate, which tempered some enthusiasm for cortisone but which paradoxically failed to convince many of those most closely involved in treating patients with RF. When the therapeutic dust settled in the mid-60s, there were so few children suffering from devastating carditis that most physicians selected therapy based on their experience rather than on rigorously vetted scientific proof. Many thought that the powerful drugs were no longer needed.[34]

Thus, corticosteroids should be reserved for the treatment of severe carditis. Corticosteroids are also recommended in patients who do not respond to salicylates and who continue to worsen and develop heart failure despite anti-inflammatory therapy.[6] Overlap with high-dose salicylate therapy is recommended as the dosage of the prednisone is tapered over a 2-week period. This is done to avoid poststeroid rebound.[6,35] In extreme cases, IV methylprednisolone may be used.

In a Cochrane review by Cilliers AM et al.,[21] eight randomized controlled trials involving 996 people were included. Several steroidal agents such as ACTH, cortisone, hydrocortisone, dexamethasone, prednisone, and IV immunoglobulin were compared to aspirin, placebo or no treatment in the various studies. Six of the trials were conducted between 1950 and 1965, while the remaining two were done in the last 10 years. The review showed no significant difference in the risk of cardiac disease at 1 year between the corticosteroid treated and aspirin treated groups (relative risk (RR) 0.87, 95% confidence interval (CI) 0.66–1.15). Similarly, use of prednisone (RR 1.78; 95% CI 0.98–3.34) or IV immunoglobulins (RR 0.87; 95% CI 0.55–1.39) when compared to placebo did not reduce the risk of developing heart valve lesions at 1 year.

Carditis is the most serious manifestation of the disease. It may culminate in chronic valvular disease and can lead to heart failure and ultimately death. Thus, there is no benefit in using corticosteroids or IV immunoglobulins to reduce the risk of heart valve lesions in patients with ARF. The antiquity of most of the trials restricted adequate statistical analysis of the data and acceptable assessment of clinical outcomes by current standards. New randomized controlled trials in patients with ARF to assess the effects of corticosteroids such

---

BOX 1 | **Treatment of acute carditis.**

- *General management*:
  - *Restricted activity*: Some recommend bed/chair rest for 4–6 weeks for carditis
  - Primary prophylaxis
  - Initiate secondary prophylaxis
  - Endocarditis prophylaxis
- *Carditis*:
  - Anti-inflammatory agents (see text for discussion of duration)
  - *Mild-to-moderate carditis*: Aspirin
  - 100–125 mg/kg/day in 4 divided doses for children
  - 6–8 g/day in adolescents and adults
  - Target salicylate levels 20–30 mg/dL
- *Severe carditis*:
  - Initial steroids (prednisone 1–2 mg/kg/day) for approximately 2 weeks then taper
  - Begin aspirin approximately 1 week prior to stopping steroids to prevent rebound
  - Follow acute phase reactants (ESR and CRP)
- *Cardiac treatment* depends on severity of involvement and symptoms:
  - *Moderate-to-severe*: Consider salt and fluid restriction, diuretics, afterload reduction as temporizing measures
  - *Intractable heart failure*: Surgery

as oral prednisone and IV methylprednisolone and other new anti-inflammatory agents are warranted.[21]

Heart Failure

Heart failure usually responds to steroids. Bed rest is always recommended and should be planned on an individual basis. Diuretics and vasodilators may be used in patients with more severe hemodynamic decompensation. Digoxin should be used with caution because of the risk of toxicity in the presence of active myocarditis.[11] Surgical treatment in the acute stage should be considered when clinical therapy is ineffective to control cardiac failure. Valve repair, although technically more difficult, is the first choice for younger patients.[36]

Carditis can cause heart failure and death. Various anti-inflammatory drugs have been used to treat carditis, including corticosteroids, aspirin, and immunoglobulins (immune therapy using antibodies). The review of trials found that there is no strong evidence to show that anti-inflammatory drugs can prevent heart damage that may occur following an episode of carditis.[21]

There is controversy about the value of steroids in patients with RF. Data available from several studies do not show an advantage of steroids over aspirin in the management of patients with mild or moderate carditis. It is recommended that aspirin should be used in patients with mild or moderate carditis and that steroids should be reserved for patients with severe carditis, particularly those with pancarditis and cardiac failure. The use of steroids in these patients is preferred because steroids produce a more prompt anti-inflammatory effect.[37] In view of the many controversies and uncertainties surrounding the use of anti-inflammatory agents in patients with acute RF, an up-to-date systematic review is indicated to clarify the most effective treatment strategy.

Heart Failure Management

Two meta-analyses have studied the use of glucocorticoids and other anti-inflammatory medications in rheumatic carditis.[20,21] All these studies of glucocorticoids were performed in the 1960s and did not use the commonly used drugs of today. These studies failed to suggest any benefit of glucocorticoids or intravenous immunoglobulin (IVIG) over placebo, or of glucocorticoids over salicylates, in reducing the risk of long-term heart disease. Studies also suggest that salicylates do not decrease the incidence of residual rheumatic heart disease (RHD) and hence salicylates are not recommended to treat carditis.[22-24]

The recommendation to use steroids in carditis is not supported by evidence, but is made because many clinicians believe that they may lead to more rapid resolution of cardiac compromise and even may be lifesaving in severe acute carditis.[21,38] The adverse effects of short courses of steroids include gastrointestinal bleeding and worsening of heart failure due to fluid retention.

Angiotensin-converting Enzyme Inhibitors[39]

Angiotensin-converting enzyme inhibitors are essential along with other medications including diuretics, digoxin, and beta-blockers. ACE inhibitors block the conversion of angiotensin I to angiotensin II which is an intrinsic (natural) substance that causes constriction of blood vessels and can lead to fluid retention. ACE inhibitors lower aortic pressure and systemic vascular resistance, do not affect pulmonary vascular resistance significantly, and lower left atrial and right atrial pressures in pediatric patients with heart failure. ACE inhibitors induce a small increase in left ventricular ejection fraction, left ventricular fractional shortening, and systemic blood flow in children with left ventricular dysfunction, mitral regurgitation, and aortic regurgitation. These beneficial effects usually persist long term without the development of tolerance.

Dose:
- Captopril is administered orally, usually every 8 hours. Daily doses range from 0.3 to 3 mg/kg/day in children.
- Enalapril is administered orally, once or twice a day and daily doses range from 0.1 to 0.5 mg/kg. Enalaprilat is administered intravenously, one to three times a day, in doses ranging from 0.01 to 0.05 mg/kg/dose.
- Ramipril is administered orally, once or twice a day, in the dose of 0.1–0.2 mg/kg/day, in children.

Side effects: The major side effect of ACE inhibitors is a dry nonproductive cough. Hypotension and renal failure usually occur within 5 days after starting ACE inhibition or on increasing the dose and in most cases, recovery is seen after reduction or cessation of the drug.

Heart failure usually responds to rest and corticosteroid therapy. In patients with severe symptoms, diuretics, ACE inhibitors and digoxin may be used.[11,26,40] Digoxin is usually used mainly for patients with atrial fibrillation. Some studies in children with valvular regurgitation have shown beneficial responses to ACE inhibitors, including decrease in left ventricular volume, mitral regurgitation, plasma atrial natriuretic peptide levels, and increases aortic stroke volume.[41] Long-term treatment with ACE inhibitors was effective in reducing not only left ventricular volume overload but also left ventricular hypertrophy.[42,43]

Surgery

However, in cases with intractable heart failure, surgical restoration of valvular competency (repair or replacement) may be lifesaving.[44,45] In particular, patients with a flail mitral valve after chordal rupture do not respond to medical management and require surgery.

Advances in echocardiography makes more objective and precise assessment of cardiac condition, e.g., 10 years old boy with ARF with severe MR in cardiac failure was put on high doses of corticosteroids by his pediatrician with no improvement in his condition. ECHO interrogation showed chordal tear of both anterior mitral leaflet and posterior mitral leaflet. He was successfully treated with surgical repair **(Figs. 1A to C)**.

Steroids are never a "lifesaving measure" in patients with a severe valvular lesion. It is argued that steroids are likely to make the tissues more friable and the task of the surgeon more difficult. Although steroids are frequently used, their use has not been shown to induce improvement in patients with fulminating rheumatic carditis.[3,45] The availability and use of echocardiography and other newer technologies will help greatly in providing more precise, valid and objective assessment of changes in the heart.[46]

Treatment Consensus and Controversies

- *Consensus*: Recommended therapies for ARF include bed rest, penicillin, and anti-inflammatory agents.
- *Controversies*:

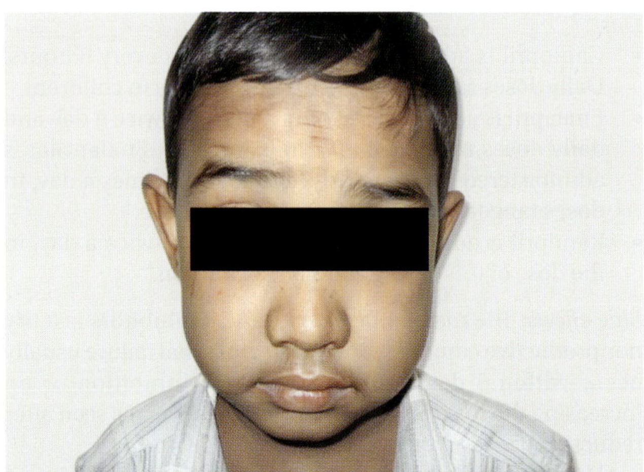

FIG. 1A: A 10-year-old boy with ARF and severe MR due to chordal tear, treated with steroids, shows features of steroid toxicity.

(ARF: acute rheumatic fever; MR: mitral regurgitation)

○ *Steroids*: At present, there is no clear consensus about the place of steroids in preventing RHD. Data available from several studies do not show an advantage of steroids over aspirin in the management of patients with mild or moderate carditis. Some authors recommend their use for patients with moderately severe carditis and heart failure.

○ *Aspirin (acetylsalicylic acid)*: There is controversy about the value of aspirin in patients with carditis in RF. It is recommended that aspirin should be used in patients with mild or moderate carditis and that steroids should be reserved for patients with severe carditis, particularly those with pancarditis and cardiac failure. The use of steroids in these patients is preferred because steroids produce a more prompt anti-inflammatory effect. Some books recommend low-dose aspirin for ARF.

In view of the many controversies and uncertainties surrounding the use of anti-inflammatory agents in patients with carditis in ARF, an up-to-date systematic review is indicated to clarify the most effective treatment strategy.

○ *Penicillin*: There is consensus that use of penicillin compared to other antibiotics is beneficial in the prevention of recurrent ARF and that intramuscular benzathine penicillin G (BPG) is superior to oral penicillin in the reduction of both recurrent ARF and streptococcal pharyngitis.[47] The dose for children is less clear. WHO recommends a dose of 600,000 U for children weighing <30 kg and 1,200,000 U for those weighing >30 kg.[4] AHA recommends 1,200,000 U for children >27 kg and 600,000 for children <27 kg.[7] Studies of BPG pharmacokinetics in children suggest that higher per kg doses are required to achieve sustained penicillin concentrations in serum

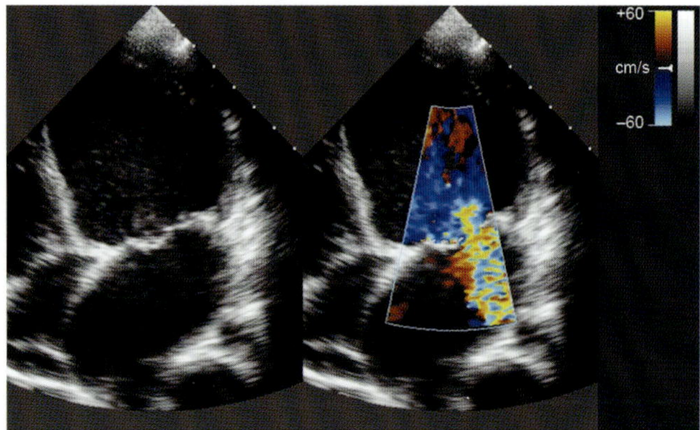

FIG. 1B: 2D ECHO shows dilated LV with free and prolapsing AML and PML due to chordal tear. Color Doppler shows severe mitral regurgitation.

(AML: anterior mitral leaflet; LV: left ventricle; PML: posterior mitral leaflet)

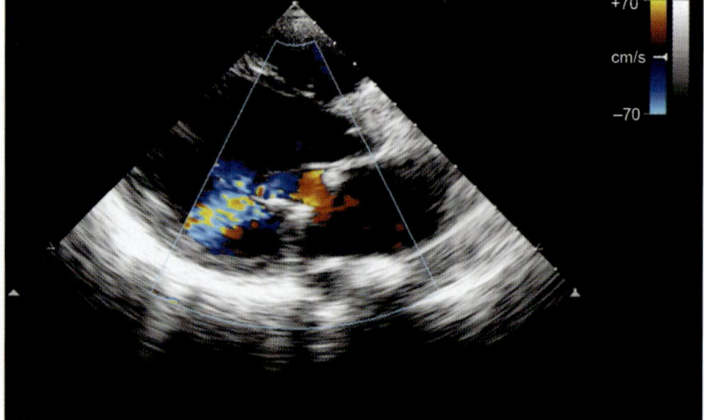

FIG. 1C: After mitral valve repair, 2D ECHO with Doppler shows mild MR.

(MR: mitral regurgitation)

and urine and that 600,000 U is insufficient for most children weighing <27 kg.[48,49] When BPG is usually administered in every 4 weeks, serum penicillin levels may be low or undetectable 28 days following a dose of 1,200,000 U.[50]

Fewer streptococcal infections and ARF recurrences occurred among patients receiving 3 weekly BPG.[47,51,52] In India, where ARF is endemic, it is preferable to administer penicillin prophylaxis once in 3 weeks. In some patients who are "fast excretors" of penicillin, prophylaxis may be needed once in 2 weeks.

Harmful Effects of Drugs

Massell[53] noted steroidal effects such as weight gain, moon face, buffalo hump, stria of the skin, and acne. Another group[54] found that both ACTH and cortisone groups had similar steroidal effects. Patients in the aspirin group experienced tinnitus, deafness, nausea, and hyperventilation. Dorfman[23] reported symptoms of nausea, emesis, and tinnitus in some of the patients receiving aspirin. Two patients receiving hydrocortisone and aspirin developed gastric ulceration. Bed rest may be an important cofactor in the success of corticosteroid therapy.

There is no evidence to support the benefit of using corticosteroids or IVIGs to prevent or reduce cardiac disease in patients presenting with ARF based on the findings of the reviewed studies. Although newer nonsteroidal anti-inflammatory agents such as naproxen[29] and high-dose methylprednisolone[55] have been used to treat patients with ARF in more recent studies, the outcomes have not been tested in a randomized and controlled manner.

Ultimately, there is no conclusive evidence to indicate that the use of corticosteroids in patients with ARF will prevent heart disease in the long term.

Chorea Management

Chorea is a self-limiting benign disease, requiring no therapy. Treatment is initiated only if the movements interfere with normal activities, place the person at risk of injury, or are extremely distressing to the patient, family, and friends.

Most cases will resolve within weeks and almost all cases within 6 months.[56] Rare cases may last as long as 2–3 years.[57,58] A prolonged course can lead to disability and/or social isolation.[59]

Anti-inflammatory agents do not have a significant effect on the signs and symptoms of chorea.[60] Neuroleptics, benzodiazepines, and antiepileptics are indicated, in combination with supportive measures such as rest in a quiet room. Manifestations of chorea may be exaggerated by emotional trauma. Sometimes, hospitalization may be helpful especially in reducing the stress that families

TABLE 3: Oral drug dosages for chorea.[64,65,67,69]	
Drug	**Dosage**
Haloperidol	• *Adults*: 0.5–2 mg PO BID/TID • *<3 years*: Not established for usage • *3–12 years*: Initial—0.05 mg/kg/day or 0.25–0.5 mg/day PO divided BID/TID may increase by 0.25–0.5 mg/day PO q 5–7 day • *Maintenance*: 0.05–0.15 mg/kg/day PO in two to three divided doses; not to exceed 0.15 mg/kg/day • *>12 years*: 0.5–30 mg/day (maximum 60 mg/day) in two divided doses
Valproic acid	15–20 mg/kg/day in three divided doses Can be increased up to 30 mg/kg/day
Carbamazepine	7–20 mg/kg/day in three divided doses
Phenobarbitone	3–5 mg/kg/day in two divided doses

face in dealing with abnormal movements and emotional liability.

Drugs

Haloperidol, diazepam, and carbamazepine have all been reported to be effective in the treatment of chorea.[61-63] Haloperidol was previously considered the first-line medical treatment for chorea. Carbamazepine and valproic acid are now preferred.[64,65] A small, prospective study of these three agents concluded that valproic acid was the most effective.[66] Oral drug dosages of medicine used in the treatment of chorea are given in **Table 3**.

Treatment with haloperidol[67] or valproic acid[64,65] is helpful in decreasing the severity of involuntary movements but may not improve the behavioral symptoms. Carbamazepine has also been suggested as a first-line treatment for Sydenham's chorea.[68]

Carbamazepine may be used initially for severe chorea requiring treatment and that valproic acid should be considered for refractory cases. This is because sometimes liver toxicity can occur with the usage of valproic acid. Alternatively, phenobarbital also may be used. Treatment is usually maintained for 8–12 weeks. IV immunoglobulin therapy has been suggested in some cases.[9]

Clinical response may take 1–2 weeks and initially may only reduce the symptoms. Medication should be continued for 2–4 weeks after chorea has subsided and then withdrawn. Recurrences of chorea are usually mild and can be managed conservatively but, in severe recurrences, the medication can be restarted if necessary.

PREVENTION OF RECURRING EPISODES AND ENDOCARDITIS PROPHYLAXIS

Secondary Prophylaxis

Secondary prevention of ARF is defined as the continuous administration of specific antibiotics to patients with previous attack of ARF or well-documented RHD. The purpose is to prevent colonization or infection of the upper respiratory tract with GABHS and the development of recurrent attacks of ARF. It is mandatory for all patients who have had an attack of ARF, whether or not they have rheumatic valvular heart disease **(Table 4)**.[7]

The prognosis is good for initial attacks of ARF, except for rare cases of death due to heart failure. Importance is stressed on compliance with the preventive antibiotic therapy, as correct prophylaxis prevents recurrences. Relapses are more frequent in the first 3–5 years following the first episode, further damaging the heart with each episode. Hence, duration of secondary prophylaxis is very important **(Table 5)**.[7]

TABLE 4: Antibiotics used in secondary prophylaxis of ARF.		
Agent	*Dose*	*Mode*
Benzathine penicillin G	600,000 U for children ? 27 kg (60 lb), 1,200,000 U for those >27 kg (60 lb) every 4 week*	Intramuscular
Penicillin V	250 mg twice daily	Oral
Sulfadiazine	0.5 g once daily for patients ? 27 kg (60 lb), 1.0 g once daily for patients >27 kg (60 lb)	Oral
For individuals allergic to penicillin and sulfadiazine macrolide or azalide	Variable	Oral

*In Indian subcontinent where ARF is endemic, penicillin prophylaxis once in 3 weeks is preferable.

TABLE 5: Duration of secondary rheumatic prophylaxis.	
Category	*Duration after last attack*
Rheumatic fever with carditis and residual heart disease (persistent valvular disease)	10 years or until 40 years of age (whichever is longer), sometimes lifelong prophylaxis
Rheumatic fever with carditis but no residual heart disease (no valvular disease)	10 years or until 21 years of age (whichever is longer)
Rheumatic fever without carditis	5 years or until 21 years of age (whichever is longer)

Endocarditis Prophylaxis

Endocarditis continues to be an important complication of RHD.[70,71] The AHA updated recommendations[72] regarding the use of prophylactic antibiotics to prevent infective endocarditis recommendation in certain conditions, such as patients with prosthetic valves, those with previous endocarditis, cardiac transplant recipients who develop cardiac valvulopathy, and specific forms of congenital heart disease as they are associated with the highest risk of adverse outcome from endocarditis.

Notably, the current AHA recommendations no longer suggest prophylaxis for patients with RHD, as in developed countries, the frequency of RHD has declined. However, the maintenance of optimal oral healthcare remains an important component of an overall healthcare program. But RHD is still endemic in developing countries, such as India and valvular lesions are common. Hence, even though the guidelines do not recommend, endocarditis prophylaxis is recommended for valvular heart disease **(Table 6)**. Since patients receiving chronic penicillin prophylaxis are likely to be colonized with amoxicillin-resistant organisms, clindamycin, clarithromycin, or azithromycin are recommended for indicated procedures.

SURGERY

Several current textbooks recommend the use of corticosteroids in patients with ARF and heart failure.[1,38,73] In contrast, other authors say that heart failure in patients with active rheumatic carditis occurs as a result of a hemodynamically severe valvular lesion that can be corrected only surgically and not by giving steroids.[44]

Surgery is usually postponed until active inflammation subsides. Surgery may be needed in cases of acute severe regurgitation due to valve leaflet or chordae tendineae rupture. Valve replacement is considered in patients with active carditis, especially in cases that are refractory to medical care or require high doses of vasodilators and diuretics. Valve repair is difficult because of the friable inflamed tissue and is done only by experienced surgeons. Regurgitant lesions respond to valve replacement, while pure stenotic lesions may benefit from more conservative balloon mitral commissurotomy.

Open-heart surgery may be needed to repair or replace heart valves in patients with severely damaged valves, the cost of which is exorbitant and a drain on the meager health resources of poor countries. Because of substantial evidence pointing to the inflammatory nature of the disease, anti-inflammatory agents such as corticosteroids and aspirin are used for its treatment. The treatment is, however, controversial.

Substantial contrary evidence points, however, against treating patients who have ARF with corticosteroid agents to prevent the complications of carditis. This evidence against corticosteroids is based largely on randomized-controlled

TABLE 6: Endocarditis prevention regimens for dental procedure.

Regimen: Single dose 30–60 min before procedure

Situation	Agent	Adults	Children
Oral	Amoxicillin	2 g	50 mg/kg
Unable to take oral medication	Ampicillin	2 g IM or IV	50 mg/kg IM or IV
	Or		
	Cefazolin or ceftriaxone	1 g IM or IV	50 mg/kg IM or IV
Allergic to penicillin or ampicillin: Oral	Cephalexin[*†]	2 g	50 mg/kg
	Or		
	Clindamycin	600 mg	20 mg/kg
	Or		
	Azithromycin or clarithromycin	500 mg	15 mg/kg
Allergic to penicillin or ampicillin and unable to take oral medication	Cefazolin or ceftriaxone[†]	1 g IM or IV	50 mg/kg IM or IV
	Or		
	Clindamycin	600 mg IM or IV	20 mg/kg IM or IV

(IM: intramuscular; IV: intravenous)

*Or other first- or second-generation oral cephalosporin in equivalent adult or pediatric dosage.

†Cephalosporins should not be used in an individual with a history of anaphylaxis, angioedema, or urticaria with penicillins or ampicillin.

studies performed 40–50 years ago and analyzed in a recent Cochrane review.[21]

ARMOR—ARATI'S REGIMEN FOR MANAGEMENT OF RHEUMATIC FEVER

Paradigm Shift in Diagnosis and Management of Rheumatic Fever and Rheumatic Heart Disease

From JONES to ARMOR

Diagnosis by ARMOR

For the past seven decades, we have been following the Jones Criteria for diagnosis and management of RF and RHD but today with modern diagnostic aids such as especially echocardiography Doppler, we can visualize the organic heart lesions of RHD directly and with 100% surety, consistency with ease in shortest time at an early stage of disease.

Vague-inconsistent unreliable and confusing features, which are major Jones criteria such as erythema marginatum subcutaneous nodules and most of the minor criteria which are not pathognomonic of RF have been removed from ARMOR.[74]

Since Chorea, which is considered a major diagnostic criterion of Jones, has most often no other features of RF in all literature scanned spanning several decades from Dr MMS Ahuja's Progress in Medicine to Dr BL Agarwal's monograph on RF; therefore, chorea of RF named Sydenham's chorea should be considered as Sydenham's chorea, a separate entity.

Considering all above facts, RF/RHD should be diagnosed in a patient who has arthralgia or arthritis:
- Carditis or evidence of cardiac involvement typically suggestive of RF/RHD
- Definitive evidence of cardiac involvement by 2D echocardiography Doppler study[75,76]

Management by ARMOR

Treatment of Arthritis by Aceclofenac

For decades, the only drug available and effective for arthritis in RF has been the good old aspirin but needless to say, aspirin is an extremely toxic drug with severe side effects such as peptic ulcer, rhinitis, gastric bleeding, tinnitus, headache, and can even be fatal as in Reye's syndrome in children.

Aspirin has to be given in high doses for prolonged periods and gradually tapered when the ESR comes to normal so as to avoid withdrawal symptoms.

As RF is a disease predominantly in children therefore, high doses of aspirin is indeed difficult to administer.

ARMOR—treatment of arthralgia and arthritis with aceclofenac or nimesulide instead of aspirin

ARMOR is a regimen where anti-inflammatory such as aceclofenac or nimesulide is given in doses of 200 mg twice a day for 5 days or more.

In over 14 years of usage of these NSAIDs, most patients recovered fully in 5 days or more without any side effects.[77]

Treatment, Primary Prevention, and Secondary Prevention of RF/RHD by Oral Azithromycin

The ARMOR consists of usage of azithromycin as antibiotic of choice for GABHS for primary prevention, treatment, and secondary prophylaxis of RF.

Azithromycin is given in a dose of 500 mg tablet or 12 mg/kg once daily for 5 days continuously followed by 1 tablet of azithromycin 500 mg once a week for 1 year only.[78]

Each time, the treatment and prophylaxis of RF/RHD must be started with 500 mg of azithromycin uninterrupted for 5 days followed by one tablet once a week. If the treatment is discontinued before 1 year, then again azithromycin should be given according to same regime. When shifting to ARMOR from other regimen, also this same pattern of administration of azithromycin must be followed.

Why benzathine penicillin G needs to be replaced with azithromycin?

- The best drug in terms of efficacy, reliability, and safety for GABHS till date is azithromycin.
- The availability of azithromycin is no issue whereas the manufacturing and supply of BPG greatly falls short of the demand.
- Whereas azithromycin has hardly any side effects, BPG causes fever, myalgia, joint pains, pain at injection site, and even abscess formation.
- Azithromycin oral tablet is as effective as BPG injection which is thick, oily, and difficult to inject in thin, cachectic children of RF.
- Azithromycin has immunosuppressant properties, cures valvulitis reverses ARF, whereas BPG causes transient valvulitis of mitral and aortic valves, therefore, perpetuates the destruction of valves.[79]
- Many drugs coprescribed in RF interact adversely with penicillin such as warfarin, diuretics, and lanoxin.
- Accidental IV BPG can cause cardiac arrest.
- Benzathine penicillin G may not be safe in pregnancy, whereas azithromycin has been proved to be safe in pregnancy and infants.
- Pseudomembranous enterocolitis and *Clostridium difficile* associated diarrhea (CDAD) is common with BPG.
- Many studies have shown that benzathine penicillin has no effect on recurrence of RF.[80]

Why azithromycin is the drug in ARMOR?

- Azithromycin 500 mg daily for five successive days results in persistence of the drugs in tissues for 6 days, therefore, if drug is given every 7th day then it results in total eradication of the bacteria from the tissues.
- Azithromycin has autoimmune suppressant properties.
- Azithromycin has anti-inflammatory effects; therefore, it cures ARF.
- Azithromycin is acid stable, therefore, has a prolonged action.
- Peak concentration is reached within 2–3.2 hours of administration of the drug. It is concentrated in the lungs tonsils and other upper respiratory tract tissues with minimum inhibitory concentration (MIC) >90 and concentration 50 times higher than in plasma.

- Its plasma clearance rate is 630 mL/min so its concentration declines in polyphasic pattern and a dose of 500 mg is eliminated in 68 hours due to large uptake and retarded release of the drug from tissue.
- Azithromycin is actively phagocytosed and reaches infection site in large quantities rapidly thus ensuring prompt scavenging of bacteria from the system.
- It is safe in hepatic disorders and pregnancy.
- As azithromycin is concentrated in tissues of tonsils, adenoid, and lungs, its efficacy which is 98% is not dependent on serum concentration of the drug.
- Overall, to summarize azithromycin is safe, cost-effective, easily available, and has high efficacy against GABHS.[81]

Azithromycin if started within 9 days of sore throat then all cases of RF/RHD can be prevented.

All patients with sore throat must be treated with azithromycin 500 mg once daily for 5 days or 12 mg/kg once daily for 5 days even if the sore throats of viral or bacterial etiology resolves before 5 days. This can result in total eradication of RF/RHD.[82]

■ CONCLUSION

For past several decades, we had been following the dictates of the Jones Committee with regard to diagnosis and management of RF and RHD although the disease has always been more prevalent in India than the west, and today more than ever before it has become imperative that we have our own guidelines for management of RF/RHD, as this disease has practically been eradicated in the developed countries of the world.

Valvular heart disease is more common in India than the rest of the world, the leading cause being RF.

So here what makes a grand entry is—

ARMOR: Arati's regimen for management of RF.

Diagnosis of RF/RHD is made by presence of:
- Arthralgia or arthritis typical of RF
- Carditis or evidence of cardiac involvement typically suggestive of RF/RHD
- Definitive evidence of cardiac involvement by 2D echocardiography Doppler study

Treatment of arthralgia and arthritis with aceclofenac or nimesulide instead of aspirin: In ARMOR, anti-inflammatory such as aceclofenac or nimesulide is given in doses of 200 mg twice a day for 5 days or more.

For primary prevention, treatment and secondary prophylaxis of RF: Azithromycin is given in a dose of 500 mg tablet or 12 mg/kg once daily for 5 days continuously followed by one tablet of azithromycin 500 mg once a week for 1 year only.

■ REFERENCES

1. El-Said GM, El-Rafaee MM, Sorour KA, El-Said HG. In: Garson A, Bricker JT, Fischer DJ, Neish SR (Eds). The Science and Practice of Pediatric Cardiology, 2nd edition. Baltimore: Williams and Wilkins; 1998. pp. 1691-724.

2. Taran LM. The treatment of acute rheumatic fever and acute rheumatic heart disease. Am J Med. 1947;2:285-95.

3. Barlow JB, Marcus RH, Pococketal WA. Mechanisms and management of heart failure in active rheumatic carditis. SAMJ. 1990;78:181-6.

4. WHO. Rheumatic fever and rheumatic heart disease: report of a WHO expert consultation, Geneva 29 October – 1 November 2001. Geneva: World Health Organisation; 2004.

5. Silva NA, Pereira BA. Acute rheumatic fever: still a challenge. Rheum Dis Clin North Am. 1997;23(3):545-68.

6. World Health Organization. Rheumatic fever and rheumatic heart disease. Report of a WHO Expert Committee. Geneva: World Health Organization; 1988 (WHO Technical Report Series, No. 764).

7. Gerber MA, Baltimore RS, Eaton CB, Gewitz M, Rowley AH, Shulman ST, et al. Prevention of rheumatic fever and diagnosis and treatment of acute Streptococcal pharyngitis: a scientific statement from the American Heart Association Rheumatic Fever, Endocarditis, and Kawasaki Disease Committee of the Council on Cardiovascular Disease in the Young, the Interdisciplinary Council on Functional Genomics and Translational Biology, and the Interdisciplinary Council on Quality of Care and Outcomes Research: endorsed by the American Academy of Pediatrics. Circulation. 2009;119:1541-51.

8. Bisno AL, Gerber MA, Gwaltney JM, Kaplan EL, Schwartz RH; Infectious Diseases Society of America. Practice guidelines for the diagnosis and management of group A streptococcal pharyngitis. Clin Infect Dis. 2002;35:113-25.

9. Danjani AS, Bisno AL, Chung KJ, Durack DT, Gerber MA, Kaplan EL, et al. Prevention of rheumatic fever. A statement for health professionals by the committee on rheumatic fever, endocarditis, and Kawasaki Disease of the Council on Cardiovascular Disease in the Young, the American Heart Association. Circulation. 1988;78(4):1082-6.

10. Wannamaker LW. Perplexity and precision in the diagnosis of streptococcal pharyngitis. Am J Dis Child. 1972;124:352-8.

11. Thatai D, Turi ZG. Current guidelines for the treatment of patients with rheumatic fever. Drugs. 1999;57:545-55.

12. Catanzaro FJ, Stetson CA, Morris AJ, Chamovitz R, Rammelkamp CH Jr, Stolzer BL, et al. The role of the Streptococcus in the pathogenesis of rheumatic fever. Am J Med. 1954;17:749-56.

13. Brook I, Gober AE. Persistence of group A beta-hemolytic streptococci in toothbrushes and removable orthodontic appliances following treatment of pharyngotonsillitis. Arch Otolaryngol Head Neck Surg. 1998;124:993-5.

14. Cynthia SH, Harold W. Management of Group A beta-Hemolytic Streptococcal Pharyngitis. Am Fam Phys. 2001;63(8):1557-64.

15. Mayer G, Van Ore S. Recurrent pharyngitis in family of four. Household pet as reservoir of group A streptococci. Postgrad Med. 1983;74(1):277-9.

16. Falck G. Group A streptococci in household pets' eyes—a source of infection in humans? Scand J Infect Dis. 1997;29:469-71.

17. Bass JW. Antibiotic management of group A streptococcal pharyngotonsillitis. Pediatr Infect Dis J. 1991;10(10 suppl):S43-9.

18. Pichichero ME, Marsocci SM, Murphy ML, Hoeger W, Green JL, Sorrento A. Incidence of streptococcal carriers in private pediatric practice. Arch Pediatr Adolesc Med. 1999;153:624-8.

19. Pichichero ME. Group A beta-hemolytic streptococcal infections. Pediatr Rev. 1998;19:291-302.

20. Albert DA, Harel L, Karrison T. The treatment of rheumatic carditis: a review and meta-analysis. Medicine (Baltimore). 1995;74:1-12.

21. Cilliers AM, Adler AJ, Saloojee H. Anti-inflammatory treatment for carditis in acute rheumatic fever. Cochrane Database Syst Rev. 2003;(2):CD003176.

22. Illingworth RS, Lorber J, Holt KS, Rendle-Short J. Acute rheumatic fever in children: a comparison of six forms of treatment in 200 cases. Lancet. 1957;2:653-9.

23. Dorfman A, Gross JI, Lorincz AE. The treatment of acute rheumatic fever. Pediatrics. 1961;27:692-706.

24. Bywaters EGL, Thomas GT. Bed rest, salicylates and steroid in rheumatic fever. BMJ. 1961;1:1628-34.

25. Maclagan T. The treatment of acute rheumatism by salicin. Lancet. 1876;1:342-3;2:601-4.

26. Dajani AS. Rheumatic fever. In: Braunwald E, Zipes DP, Libby P (Eds). Heart Disease, 6th edition. Philadelphia: Elsevier Saunders; 2001. pp. 2192-8.

27. Stollerman G. Rheumatic fever and Streptococcal infection. New York: Grune & Stra4on; 1975.

28. William WH, Myron JL, Judith MS, Robin RD. Cardiovascular Diseases. Current Diagnosis & Treatment Pediatrics, 19th edition. New York: The McGraw-Hill Companies, Inc.; 2009.

29. Uziel Y, Hashkes PJ, Kassem E, Padeh S, Goldman R, Wolach B. The use of naproxen in the treatment of children with rheumatic fever. J Pediatr. 2000;137:269-71.

30. Di Sciascio G, Taranta A. Rheumatic fever in children. Am Heart. 1980;99:635-58.

31. Herdy GV, Pinto CA, Olivaes MC, Carvalho EA, Tchou H, Cosendey R, et al. Rheumatic carditis treated with high doses of pulse therapy methylprednisolone. Results in 70 children over 12 years. Arq Bras Cardiol. 1999;72:601-6.

32. Voss LM, Wilson NJ, Neutze JM, Whitlock RM, Ameratunga RV, Cairns LM, et al. Intravenous immunoglobulin in acute rheumatic fever: a randomized controlled trial. Circulation. 2001;103:401-6.

33. Tani YL. Rheumatic Fever and Rheumatic Heart Disease. Moss and Adams Heart Disease in Infants, Children and Adolescents, 7th edition. Philadelphia: Wolters Kluwer; 2008. p. 1271.

34. English PC. Penicillin, Cortisone, and Heart Surgery. Rheumatic fever in America and Britain: a biological, epidemiological, and medical history. New Jersey, US: Rutgers University Press; 1999. p. 140.

35. Feinstein AR, Spagnuolo M, Gill FA. Rebound phenomenon in acute rheumatic fever. I. Incidence and significance. Yale J Biol Med. 1961;33:259-78.

36. Pomerantzeff PM, Brandao CM, Faberetal CM. Mitral valve repair in rheumatic patients. Heart Surg Forum. 2000;3:273-6.

37. Ayoub EM, Emmanouilides GC, Riemenschneider TA, Allen HD, Gutgesell HP (Eds). Moss and Adams' Heart Disease in Infants, Children, and Adolescents: Including the Fetus and the Young Adult, 5th edition. Baltimore: Williams and Wilkinson; 1995. pp. 1400-16.

38. Party RFW. The natural history of rheumatic fever and rheumatic heart disease: ten-year report of a cooperative clinical trial of ACTH, cortisone and aspirin. Circulation. 1965;32:457-76.

39. Momma K. ACE Inhibitors in Pediatric Patients with Heart Failure. Pediatr Drugs. 2006;8(1):55-69.

40. Bonow RO, Carabello B, de Leon AC Jr. ACC/AHA guidelines for the management of patients with valvular heart disease. J Am Coll Cardiol. 1998;32:1486-588.

41. Kura S, Tunaoglu FS, Olgunturk R, Gokcora N. Atrial natriuretic peptide levels in rheumatic mitral regurgitation and response to angiotensin-converting enzyme inhibitors. Canad J Cardiol. 2003;19(4):405-8.

42. Mori Y, Nakazawa M, Tomimatsu H, Momma K. Long-term effect of angiotensin converting enzyme inhibitor in volume overloaded heart failure during growth: a controlled pilot study. J Am Coll Cardiol. 2000;36(1):270-5.

43. Alehan D, Ozkutlu S. Beneficial effects of 1-year captopril therapy in children with chronic aortic regurgitation who have no symptoms. Am Heart J. 1988;135(4):598-603.

44. Kalangos A, Beghetti M, Baldovinos A, Vala D, Bichel T, Mermillod B, et al. Aortic valve repair by cusp extension with the use of fresh autologous pericardium in children with rheumatic aortic insufficiency. J Thorac Cardiovasc Surg. 1999;118:225-36.

45. Kingsley RH, Pocock WA. Perspectives on the Mitral Valve. In: Barlow JB (Ed). Philadelphia: F. A. Davis Company; 1987. pp. 227-45.

46. Vijayalakshmi IB, Mithravinda J, Deva AN. The role of echocardiography in diagnosing carditis in the setting of acute rheumatic fever. Cardiol Young. 2005;15:583-8.

47. Manyemba J, Mayosi BM. Penicillin for secondary prevention of rheumatic fever. Cochrane Database Syst Rev. 2002;(3):CD002227.

48. Ginsburg C, McCracken GH Jr, Zweighaft TC. Serum penicillin concentrations after intramuscular administration of benzathine penicillin G in children. Pediatrics. 1982;69:452-4.

49. Meria Z, Mota Cde C, Tonelli E, Nunan EA, Mitre AM, Moreira NS. Evaluation of secondary prophylactic schemes, based on benzathine penicillin G, for rheumatic fever in children. J Pediatr. 1993;123:156-8.

50. Kaplan E, Berrios X, Speth J, Siefferman T, Guzman B, Quesny F. Pharmacokinetics of benzathine penicillin G: serum levels during the 28 days after intramuscular injection of 1,200,000 units. J Pediatr. 1989;115:146-50.

51. Lue HC, Wu MH, Hsieh KH, Lin GJ, Hsieh RP, Chiou JF. Rheumatic fever recurrences: controlled study of 3 week versus 4 week benzathine penicillin prevention programs. J Pediatr. 1986;108:299-304.

52. Padmavati S, Gupta V, Prakash K, Sharma KB. Penicillin for rheumatic fever prophylaxis 3 weekly or 4 weekly schedule. J Assoc Physicians India. 1987;35:753-5.

53. Massell BF, Jhaveri S, Czoniczer G, Barnet R. Treatment of rheumatic fever and rheumatic carditis. Observations providing a basis for the selection of aspirin or adrenocortical steroids. Med Clin N Am. 1961;45:1349-68.

54. A joint report by the Rheumatic Fever Working Party of the Medical Research Council of Great Britain and the Subcommittee of Principal Investigators of the American Council on Rheumatic Fever and Congenital Heart Disease, American Heart Association. The Treatment of Acute Rheumatic Fever in Children. A Cooperative Clinical Trial of ACTH, Cortisone and Aspirin. Circulation. 1955;2:343-71.

55. Herdy GVH, Pinto CA, Olivaes MC, Carvalho EA, Tchou H, Cosendey R, et al. Rheumatic carditis treated with high doses of pulse therapy methylprednisolone. Arq Bras Cardiol. 1999;72:604-6.

56. Lessof MH, Bywaters EG. The duration of chorea. BMJ. 1956;1:1520-3.

57. Carapetis JR, Currie BJ. Rheumatic chorea in northern Australia: A clinical and epidemiological study. Arch Dis Child. 1999;80:353-8.

58. al-Eissa A. Sydenham's chorea: a new look at an old disease. Brit J Clin Pract. 1993;47:14-6.

59. Swedo SE, Leonard HL, Schapiro MB, Casey BJ, Mannheim GB, Lenane MC, et al. Sydenham's chorea: Physical and psychological symptoms of St Vitus dance. Pediatrics. 1993;91:706-13.

60. Markowitz M, Gordis L. Rheumatic Fever, 2nd edition. Philadelphia: WB Saunders; 1972.

61. Mivakava M, Ohkubo O, Fuchigami T, Fujita Y, Moriuchi R, Hiyoshi K, et al. Effectiveness of haloperidol in the treatment of chorea minor. No To Hattatsu. 1995;27:191-6.

62. Zecharia HL, Zecharia A, Straussberg R, Volovitz B, Amir J. Successful treatment of rheumatic chorea with carbamazepine. Pediatr Neurol. 2000;23(2):147-51.

63. Ronchezel MV, Hilario MO, Forleo LH, Len CA, Terreri MT, Vilanova LC, et al. The use of haloperidol and valproate in children with Sydenham chorea. Indian Pediatr. 1998;35(12):1215-8.

64. Daoud AD, Zaki M, Shakir R, al Saleh Q. Effectiveness of sodium valproate in the treatment of Sydenham's chorea. Neurology. 1990;40:1140-1.

65. Genel F, Arslanoglu S, Uran N, Saylan B. Sydenham's chorea: clinical findings and comparison of the efficacies of sodium valproate and carbamazepine regimens. Brain Dev. 2002;24:73-6.

66. Pena J, Mora E, Cardozo J, Molina O, Montiel C. Comparison of the efficacy of carbamazepine, haloperidol and valproic acid in the treatment of children with Sydenham's Chorea. Arq Neuropsiquiatr. 2002;60:374-7.

67. Marques-Dias MJ, Mercadante MT, Tucker D, Lombroso P. Sydenham's chorea. Psychiatr Clin North Am. 1997;20:809-20.

68. Harel L, Zecharia A, Straussberg R, Volovitz B, Amir J. Successful treatment of rheumatic chorea with carbamazepine. Pediatr Neurol. 2000;23:147-51.

69. Lennon D. Acute rheumatic fever in children: recognition and treatment. Pediatr Drugs. 2004;6:363-73.

70. Carapetis JR, Steer AC, Mulholland EK, Weber M. The global burden of group A streptococcal diseases. Lancet Infect Dis. 2005;5:685-94.

71. Deshpande J, Vaideeswar P, Amonkar G, et al. Rheumatic heart disease in the past decade: An autopsy analysis. Indian Heart J. 2002;54:676-80.

72. Wilson W, Taubert KA, Gewitz M, Lockhart PB, Baddour LM, Levison M, et al. Prevention of infective endocarditis: guidelines from the American Heart Association: a guideline from the American Heart Association Rheumatic Fever, Endocarditis, and Kawasaki Disease Committee, Council on Cardiovascular Disease in the Young, and the Council on Clinical Cardiology, Council on Cardiovascular Surgery and Anesthesia, and the Quality of Care and Outcomes Research Interdisciplinary Working Group. Circulation. 2007;116:1736-54.

73. Abraham MT, Cherian G. In: Chatterjee K, Cheitlin MD, Karliner J, Parmley WM, Rapaport E, Scheinman M (Eds). Cardiology: An Illustrated Text/Reference. London; Gower Medical.

■ REFERENCES FOR ARMOR

74. Lalchandani A, Shameem M, Sondhi P, Agarwal A, Agarwal V, Neelam P, et al. A paradigm shift in diagnosis of RF: A Review of 200 patients of RF with a view to scrap Jones Criteria. Indian Heart J. 2005;57:463.

75. Saxena A, Zuhike L, Wilson N. Echocardiographic Screening for Rheumatic Heart Disease. Global Heart. 2013;8(3):197-202.

76. Vijayalakshmi IB. Efficacy of echocardiographic criteria for diagnosis of carditis in acute rheumatic fever. Medica Innovatica. 2012;1(1).

77. Lalchandani A, Rana M, Mehrotra N, et al. Use of aceclofenac instead of aspirin in arthritis of rheumatic fever. Circulation. 2010;122:715. (e115; originally published online, June 14, 2010).

78. Donde S, Mishra A, Kochhar P. Azithromycin in Acute Bacterial URTI: An Indian Noninterventional Study. Indian J Otolaryngol Head Neck Surg. 2014;66(Suppl 1):225-30.

79. Thomson WO. Sudden Death Following injection Penicillin. Brit Med J. 1952;2(4775):70-2.

80. Seckeler, Hoke TR, Gurka MJ, Barton LL. No demonstrable effect of benzathine penicillin on recurrence of RF in pacific island population. Pediatr Cardiol. 2010;31(6):849-52.

81. Lalchandani A, Rana M, Mehrotra M, Prabhu K, Lalchandani T. Benzathine Penicillin must be substituted with Azithromycin for treatment and prophylaxis of RF. Circulation. 2010;122: e115-712. Downloaded from http://circ.ahajournals.org/ December 16, 2011.

82. Schaad UB. Acute Streptococcal tonsillopharyngitis: A review of clinical efficacy and bacteriological eradication. J Int Med. 2004;32:1-13.

15

Medical Management of Rheumatic Heart Disease and Management during Pregnancy, Noncardiac Surgery, and Infective Endocarditis

Chandrakant B Patil, IB Vijayalakshmi

> *"The principles of medical management are essentially the same for individuals of all ages, albeit the same problem is handled differently in different patients."*
>
> —**Dana W Atchley**, (1892–1982),
> US Physician

INTRODUCTION

Rheumatic heart disease (RHD) is more prevalent in underdeveloped and developing countries than in developed countries and among the population with multiple social issues such as poverty, low socioeconomic status, overcrowded dwellings, undernutrition, poor sanitation, cultural constraints, and suboptimal medical care.[1] As per the global burden of cardiovascular (CV) diseases, 40.5 million people were affected in 2019, which reflect increased global awareness, availability of echocardiograms for case definition, improved survival in some places, and chronic nature of RHD. Its burden has heterogeneity and burden is highest among world's most disadvantaged, most marginalized poorest populations regionally, nationally, and at subnational levels not showing signs of improvement and continue to die early from RHD.[2] In most endemic regions, affected patients present with heart failure (HF). Echo screening helps to detect patients earlier when prophylaxis is more likely to be effective. Hence, Registries help to give optimal care and secondary penicillin prophylaxis within their resources.[3] WHO recommends registries as vital adjunct for prevention and control of RHD. Global registries such as REMEDY (Global Rheumatic Heart Disease Registry), regional or subregional registry, e.g., VALVAFRIC as in western and central Africa covering small fraction of the affected population are helpful in studying disease burden and have improved management within available resources, close follow-up and counseling for timely interventions in needy people including surgery and catheter-based interventions and helped to improve the necessary care and research activities also. There are challenges of a good primary healthcare network and to train personnel involved, comprehensive service delivery, and their integration in to mainstream health system, and to keep pace with rapid technology remains a big task with limited resources.[3]

Rheumatic valvular heart disease (VHD) is common and often requires intervention. Continuous decline of acute rheumatic fever (ARF) owing to better prophylaxis of streptococcal infections has decreased the incidence of rheumatic valve diseases, whereas incidence of endocarditis remains stable. Diagnosis is now dominated by echocardiography and treatment is not only developed through the continuing progress in prosthetic valve technology, but has also been reoriented by the development of conservative surgical approaches and the introduction of percutaneous interventional techniques. When compared to other heart diseases, there are few trials in the field of RHDs and randomized clinical trials are particularly scarce. The same is true with guidelines and there is a real gap between the existing guidelines and their effective application.[4]

Medical management has a limited role to play in RHD and their complications and hence, it is an attempt to describe the medical management of various valvular lesions caused by RHD and their complications.

BACKGROUND

Streptococcal infections are to be diagnosed and treated fully, and those who have carditis with or without valve disease should receive antibiotic prophylaxis against recurrent streptococcal infections and it is continued even after interventions. The prophylaxis against infective endocarditis is a lifelong requirement. **Figure 1** describes the gradual progression of RHD from its detection to the symptoms and if not treated at a proper stage leading to death in that individual.

Heart failure develops after a chronic asymptomatic period of progressive valve disease when severe or moderate when associated with multivalvular disease or with associated comorbidities. There is no RHD-specific evidence of optimal drug therapy for HF, but is derived from existing HF guidelines and principles of management are more complex, expensive, and need multidisciplinary teams (MDTs) involving cardiologists, cardiothoracic-surgeons, physician, pediatrician, dentistry, obstetrics, anesthesia and infectious disease specialist. Long-term management to be done by a specialist trained in RHD management by proper history, clinical evaluation, periodic structural assessment by ECHO including right ventricle (RV)/left ventricle (LV) function, timely referral for interventions, monitoring of anticoagulation in atrial fibrillation (AF) and prosthetic valves, annual influenza vaccination, and secondary prevention with penicillin prophylaxis to avoid complications of underlying VHD.[5]

Heart failure results from underlying moderate-to-severe valvular lesions causing breathlessness, fatigue, decreased exercise tolerance, and congestion. Functional class is New York Heart Association (NYHA) based and staging is as per American College of Cardiology/American Heart Association (ACC/AHA) guidelines, which stress on the progressive nature of VHD and its timely treatment **(Table 1 and Fig. 2)**.

GENERAL MANAGEMENT OF HEART FAILURE

Aim is to improve functional class and quality of life.

Lifestyle modification by control of body weight, stopping smoking and alcohol, salt (<6 g/day) and water restriction in needy cases. If hypertension >140/90 mm Hg needs any of angiotensin-converting enzyme inhibitor (ACEI), angiotensin receptor blockers (ARBs), or angiotensin receptor-neprilysin inhibitor (ARNI), a beta-blocker, diuretics, mineralocorticoid receptor antagonists (MRAs), or calcium channel blockers (CCBs)-like amlodipine or felodipine to control to a goal BP of 130/80 mm Hg. Anemia if Hb% <12 g% needs evaluation of the type of anemia and its underlying etiology and correction accordingly.

Pharmacological Therapy

For heart failure with reduced ejection fraction (HFrEF) guideline-based medical therapy (GDMT) including loop diuretics for edema/congestion, ACEI/ARBs or ARNI in their place, beta-blockers, MRAs is useful. If ACEI is intolerant then hydralazine/isosorbide dinitrate and digoxin may also help. Randomized controlled trials (RCTs) have shown

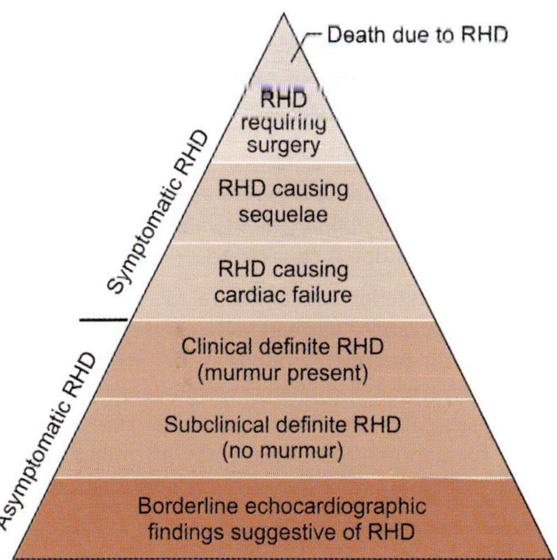

FIG. 1: Progression of rheumatic heart disease (RHD).

TABLE 1: Stages of valvular heart diseases.

Stage	Definition	Description
A	At risk	Patients with risk factors for development of VHD
B	Progressive	Patients with progressive VHD (mild-to-moderate severity and asymptomatic)
C	Asymptomatic severe	Asymptomatic patients who have the criteria for severe VHD: • C1: Asymptomatic patients with severe VHD in whom the LV or RV remains compensated • C2: Asymptomatic patients with severe VHD with decompensation of the LV or RV
D	Symptomatic severe	Patients who have developed symptoms as a result of VHD

(VHD: valvular heart disease; LV: left ventricle; RV: right ventricle)

Source: Otto CM, Nishimura RA, Bonow RO, Carabello BA, Erwin JP 3rd, Gentile F, et al. 2020 ACC/AHA Guideline for the Management of Patients With Valvular Heart Disease: Executive Summary: A Report of the American College of Cardiology/American Heart Association Joint Committee on Clinical Practice Guidelines. Circulation. 2021;143;e35-71.

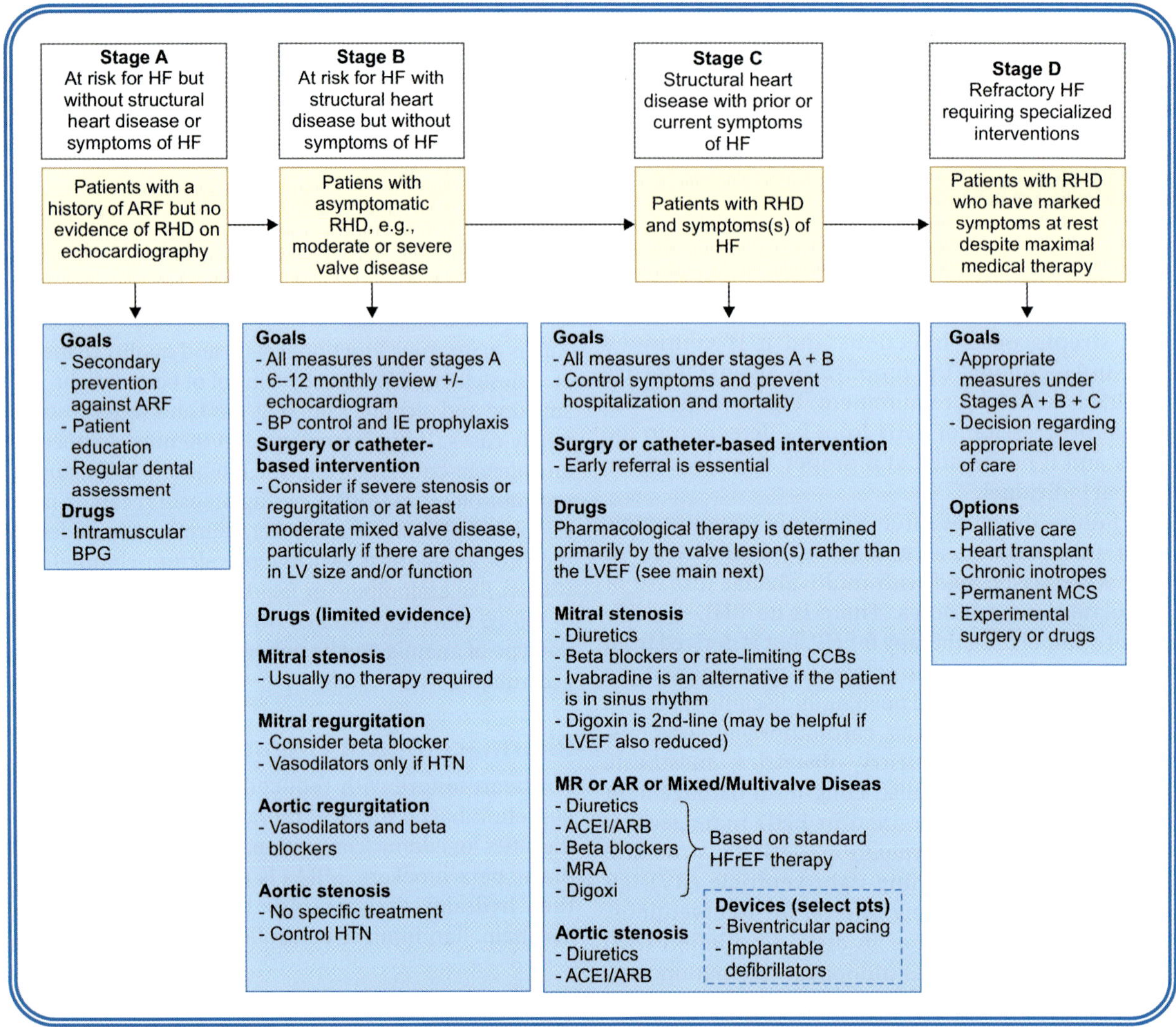

FIG. 2: General principles of medical management.[6]

(ACEI: angiotensin-converting enzyme inhibitor; ARB: angiotensin receptor blocker; BPG: benzathine penicillin G; CCBs: calcium channel blockers; HF: heart failure; HFrEF: heart failure with reduced ejection fraction; HTN: hypertension; IE: infective Endocarditis; LV: left ventricle; LVEF: left ventricular ejection fraction; MCS: mechanical circulatory support; MRA: mineralocorticoid receptor antagonist; RHD: rheumatic heart disease;

improved survival with above drugs except diuretics and digoxin. Recent additions are ARNI and selective sinus node inhibitor such as ivabradine, which decrease HF hospitalizations and mortality probably in RHD patients with HFrEF also, but do not alter the natural history of RHD or their need for timely interventions. Digitalis is used only for heart rate (HR) control in AF with rapid ventricular rate and associated HFrEF. It decreases HF hospitalizations and improves symptoms. Decision regarding timely interventions has to be taken by a multidisciplinary heart team approach depending on the severity **(Table 2)**.

MITRAL STENOSIS

In RHD, mitral stenosis (MS) commissural fusion is characteristic, often seen in females (80% in REMEDY study), symptoms occur when mitral valve (MV) area is

TABLE 2: Recommendations for the multidisciplinary heart valve team and heart valve centers.

COR	LOE	Recommendations
1	CEO	Patients with severe VHD should be evaluated by a multidisciplinary heart valve team (MDT) when intervention is considered
2a	CLD	Consultation with or referral to a primary or comprehensive heart valve center is reasonable when treatment options are being discussed for: (1) asymptomatic patients with severe VHD, (2) patients who may benefit from valve repair versus valve replacement, or (3) patients with multiple comorbidities for whom valve intervention is considered[1,4,7-23]

(COR: class of recommendation; LOE: level of evidence; VHD: valvular heart disease)

Source: Otto CM, Nishimura RA, Bonow RO, Carabello BA, Erwin JP 3rd, Gentile F, et al. ACC/AHA VHD Guidelines, 2020. Circulation. 2021;143:e35-71.

<2.0 cm^2. Latent period can be short in endemic regions, prognosis depends on functional class, valve anatomy whether suitable for balloon mitral commissurotomy or for open mitral valvotomy. Rarely, LV dysfunction occurs due to hypertension, mixed MV disease with mitral regurgitation (MR) or aortic regurgitation (AR). MV gradient increases as HR increases following exercise, new onset AF, sepsis increased cardiac output (CO) as in pregnancy or anemia can worsen moderate or severe MS acutely causing pulmonary edema and hypotension. Chronic increase in left atrial (LA) pressure leads to LA enlargement, LA thrombosis, increased pulmonary venous hypertension (PVH), and pulmonary arterial hypertension (PAH) leading to right HF. 60% of deaths in MS occur due to progressive HF and remaining deaths due to thromboembolism (TE).

Medical Management: Prevention of Symptoms and Complications and to Evaluate for Timely Intervention[5]

Overall management depends on symptomatic status, degree of stenosis, and suitability of the valve for percutaneous transluminal mitral commissurotomy (PTMC). Mild MS patients are managed medically. They do not require endocarditis prophylaxis, but secondary prophylaxis for rheumatic fever is mandatory. Annual re-evaluation is required, but echocardiogram is not needed until there is a change in clinical status. Patients with mild MS and symptoms of exertional dyspnea are treated with salt restriction, diuretics to lower LA pressure and PVH. In symptomatic patients with MS in sinus rhythm (SR) if tachycardia HR control with beta-blockers may blunt the chronotropic response to exercise and may improve exercise capacity by improving diastolic filling period, decreases LA pressure of the heart, but should not be used with normal HR. Greater efficacy of beta-blockers versus HR regulating nondihydropyridine CCBs such as verapamil or diltiazem is reported. But, their effect on exercise tolerance is uncertain. One should avoid arterial vasodilators. Some MS patients have increased bronchial reactivity, which responds to inhaled corticosteroids. Ivabradine as an add-on or alternative to beta-blockers improves hemodynamics, exercise performance, and dyspnea in symptomatic MS with SR. AF exacerbates symptoms. Embolism is a much-feared complication of MS and occurs in up to 20% of patients and the risk increases with advancing age and AF. Cerebral embolism is a devastating complication. It accounts for 60–70% of episodes of systemic embolism. Episodes of systemic embolism can occur with any degree of MS and risk increases markedly when AF develops. In the series of patients with MS followed by Rowe et al. 19% of the deaths were attributed to arterial embolism. Increasing age and LA size increase the risk of systemic embolism.[5,7]

If AF is present, digitalis plays a critical role in controlling ventricular rate. In selected patients, beta-adrenergic blocking drugs, diltiazem or amiodarone may be added, if digoxin alone is not satisfactory in controlling ventricular rate to increase diastolic filling time at rest or exercise. Loop diuretics, furosemide, metolazone, and torsemide decrease preload and reduce pulmonary congestion and right HF and peripheral edema. Cardioversion of AF and maintenance of SR using antiarrhythmic therapy with either digitalis and quinidine or digitalis and amiodarone should be offered to these patients. In patients who need interventional therapy, cardioversion is performed after interventional procedure. Antiarrhythmic drug therapy may be used in an attempt to restore SR, but long-term efficacy may depend on correction of the MS.

It is controversial whether long-term anticoagulation therapy to be given on the basis of LA enlargement or spontaneous echo contrast (SEC) on transesophageal echocardiography (TEE). But, very large LA, dense SEC, and decreased LA appendage velocity have higher TE events. Rheumatic disease affects atrial muscle thus increased risk of blood flow stasis and thrombosis in LA appendage and body of LA also. They are prone for atrial arrhythmias especially AF causing acute hemodynamic changes, decreased diastolic filling, and increased LA pressure. They need immediate cardioversion and anticoagulation. In the stable patient, rate versus rhythm control depends on duration of AF, hemodynamic response to AF, LA size, prior episodes of AF, and history of embolic events. Rhythm control is difficult because of progressive fibrosis, enlargement of atria, fibrosis of internodal and interatrial tracts, and damage to SA node. Use of negative dromotropic agents such as beta-blockers is controversial even though HR is decreased, prolongation of diastolic filling period decreases transmitral gradient, but may decrease exercise tolerance because of limitation of CO because of limited stroke volume (SV) and chronotropic incompetence. But RCTs have shown improvement of symptoms and exercise duration on beta blockers/Ivabradine or both in younger patients with higher resting exercise-induced HR.[24]

Anticoagulation with warfarin is imperative for patients with paroxysmal, persistent, or chronic AF and MS, because they are at high risk for TE and it is also indicated in those with a history of prior embolism even in SR or known LA thrombus (ACC/AHA Class I). Newer, less emphatic recommendation (ACC/AHA Class IIb) has been made for MS with large atrial diameter (55 mm) or those with severe MS and enlarged LA size and evidence of spontaneous contrast on echocardiogram.[5,8]

Anticoagulation with warfarin is usually begun about 3 weeks in advance of cardioversion and continued for 4 weeks after the procedure. Alternately, if LA thrombus is excluded by TEE, 2 or 3 days of IV heparin should be instituted, the patient should be cardioverted to SR, and warfarin therapy should be continued for at least 4 weeks. Patients with chronic AF and those with a previous history of embolism should receive anticoagulation with warfarin to maintain INR of 2-3. Systemic embolization necessitates permanent anticoagulation. A single systemic embolic episode is not an absolute indication for MV surgery as embolism can and does occur in patients with mild MS.[4]

Role of PTMC in patients with new onset of AF and moderate-to-severe MS who are otherwise asymptomatic is controversial. Indications for percutaneous mitral balloon commissurotomy (PMBC) are severe symptoms, MV area ≤1.5 cm², and a favorable morphology for intervention in absence of contraindications. If symptoms are >NYHA Class II, it implies patient has significant MS, then the patient should be referred for percutaneous therapy or surgery. MV surgery is indicated in severely symptomatic patients with severe MS, MVA < 1.5 cm², stage D who are not at high risk for surgery and who are not candidates for balloon mitral valvuloplasty (BMV) or failed previous BMV. An asymptomatic patient with moderate-to-severe MS and evidence of pulmonary hypertension at rest or with exercise should also be referred for percutaneous therapy, if valve is suitable. Mortality increases as the symptoms progress. Natural history studies, before valvotomy procedures were developed, suggest that young symptomatic patients have about 40% mortality at 10 years and almost 80% mortality at 20 years. Elderly patients have 60–70% mortality at 10 years. Marked pulmonary hypertension (PA systolic pressure > 60 mm Hg) is an indication for mechanical treatment even in the absence of symptoms in moderate-to-severe MS.[5,9]

◼ MEDICAL THERAPY OF ATRIAL FIBRILLATION

Atrial fibrillation is a critical factor diagnosing RHD. AF hinders the prognosis. Its prevalence with MV disease increases with age. It is present in 29% of patients with MS, 6% with MR, 1% with aortic valve (AV) disease, 52% with mixed MV disease, 70% in combined MS, MR and TR, and patients with MV disease with AF have higher NYHA class, larger LV, LA size versus without AF. AF significantly impacts event-free survival both prior to and following an intervention on MV.

Patients with MS are prone for atrial arrhythmias, particularly AF and atrial flutter. 30–40% of patients with symptomatic MS develop AF. Incidence of AF is 3% when LA size <40 mm versus 54% ≥40 mm. Structural changes from the pressure and volume overload of LA alter electrophysiological properties of left atrium and the rheumatic process may lead to fibrosis of the internodal and interatrial tracts and damage to the sinoatrial (SA) node. Slowing velocities of conduction, increased dispersion of refractoriness, and automaticity initiate and perpetuate AF. AF tends to be persistent in MS and is less dependent on pulmonary veins foci. Electrical remodeling is partially influenced by atrial stretch secondary to LA overload. Significant hemodynamic changes occur due to rapid ventricular rate and this shortens diastolic filling period and causes elevation of LA pressure.[25]

Thromboembolism and Oral Anticoagulation

Systemic embolization occurs in 10–20% of MS patients. It depends on age and presence of AF. One-third of embolic events occur within 1 month of onset of AF and two-thirds occur within 1 year. The frequency of embolic events does not seem to be related to severity of MS, CO, size of LA or even presence or absence of HF symptoms. In patients who have embolic events, the frequency of recurrence is as high as 15–40 events/100 patient months. Retrospective studies have shown 4–15-fold decrease in incidence of embolic events with anticoagulation in these patients. Embolic events are thought to originate from LA thrombi; the presence or absence of LA thrombus does not appear to correlate with embolic events. It has been suggested that timely commissurotomy reduces the incidence of future embolic events. One prospective study has reported decreased risk of arterial embolism after mitral commissurotomy.[8]

Atrial fibrillation is responsible for one-third of all strokes ≥65 years of age. Nonvalvular AF increases risk of strokes five times. AF with MV disease stroke risk increases 17 times. Lifetime recurrence rate of stroke is as high as 30–75%. MR has lower risk of SEC in TEE versus MS and hence lower risk of TE. Clots are seen in 20% of MS patients but none in MR and clots are found in LA body and its appendage in MV disease versus 90% in LA appendage only in nonvalvular AF. Hence, in absence of contraindications, anticoagulation with vitamin K antagonists to keep the INR in a therapeutic range of 2.5–3 is very essential in all cases of MS and AF and risk decreases after successful commissurotomy. Role of direct oral anticoagulants (DOACS) is not known in moderate-to-severe MS as they were excluded from NOAC RCTs. The INVICTUS-VKA (investigation of rheumatic atrial fibrillation treatment using vitamin K antagonists, rivaroxaban versus VKA in RHD with AF/AF. The role of LAA occlusion in young patients with RHD and AF is unknown.[3,25]

Management

Atrial fibrillation starts as paroxysmal later turns in to persistent AF. Symptoms depend on duration of AF and because of rapid irregular HR, HF, and systemic TE. Control ventricular rate maintains SR by aggressive therapy and continues anticoagulation. Whenever feasible, correct underlying VHD, balloon commissurotomy in MS, valve repair or replacement in MR. If any reversible factors are there, they need corrections. Complications of AF are HF, stroke, and peripheral TE and premature death. Small RCTs have favored electrical or pharmacological cardioversion or catheter ablation in addition to valve interventions. This may not be possible in low- and middle-income countries (LMICs). Control of ventricular rate when SR is not feasible is done by beta-blockers such as propranolol, metoprolol, CCBs such as verapamil/diltiazem in absence of LV dysfunction. Digitalis increases vagal tone and acts on AV node but ineffective during exercise but can be combined with above drugs to control HR during peak exercise. In drug refractory cases, catheter ablation of AV junction and implantation of rate-responsive PPI may be considered. It is still not clear which strategy is best in VHD and AF patients.[25]

Rhythm Control

The results of BMV or surgery are inferior versus when SR is present or restored before intervention as shown by a study of Vaturi et al. following MVR and Nair et al. following BMV. Restoration of SR is effective following correction of underlying VHD. Drugs are ineffective in long-standing AF. Antiarrhythmic drugs of Class IA, IC, or III are effective. Reported success rates of flecainide, propafenone, and amiodarone are around 60%. Class III agents such as IV ibutilide, IV/oral dofetilide are not effective in recent onset atrial flutter/atrial fibrillation (AF). Short-term treatment with amiodarone with or without electrical cardioversion is effective in rhythm control in chronic AF after MV surgery. Prophylactic use of oral amiodarone and sotalol is shown to prevent AF immediately after cardiac surgery. There is no conclusive data regarding best management of rhythm control in RHD AF. Nonpharmacological methods include both surgical and radiofrequency catheter ablation after valve interventions maintain SR. In those who are hemodynamically stable and not requiring valve intervention again, their role is vague. Pharmacological rhythm control has its own limitations. Still, there is no consensus on the optimal approach of achieving SR.[25] AF occurs commonly in elderly and has poor prognosis with a 10-year survival rate of 25% versus 46% with SR. The risk of arterial embolism especially stroke is significantly increased in patients with AF. Treatment of an acute episode of AF with rapid HR consists of anticoagulation with heparin and control of HR response. IV digoxin, rate-limiting CCBs, or beta-blockers should be used to control ventricular response by slowing conduction through the AV node. IV or oral amiodarone can also be used when beta-blockers or CCBs cannot be used. If there is hemodynamic instability, electrical cardioversion should be undertaken urgently with IV heparin before, during, and after the procedure. In selected patients, chemical cardioversion may also be attempted. Patients who have been longer than 24–48 hours without anticoagulation are at an increased risk for embolic events after cardioversion, but embolization may also occur with <24 hours of AF also. Decision for cardioversion depends on multiple factors including duration of AF, hemodynamic response to the onset of AF, prior episodes of AF, and history of prior embolic events. If it lasts for >48 hours, then patient needs either TEE for LA thrombus or anticoagulation with warfarin for more than 3 weeks followed by elective cardioversion. Recurrent AF is treated with class IC or Class III antiarrhythmic drugs; however, beta-blockers and CCBs are effective in controlling exercise-induced increase in HR.

In them, long-term anticoagulation with warfarin is required to prevent embolism.[25]

■ MITRAL REGURGITATION

In a compensated state, most patients are asymptomatic, which lasts several years till left ventricular end-diastolic diameter (LVEDD) < 60-mm size and left ventricle end-systolic dimension (LVESD) < 40 mm and left ventricular ejection fraction (LVEF) ≥ 60%. It is better to intervene before LV decompensation, PA systolic pressure > 50 mm Hg with or without appearance of symptoms. Because chronic MR with LV dysfunction will have higher postoperative mortality and persistent LV dysfunction later also.[25]

Medical Treatment

In chronic asymptomatic MR, there is some evidence of beta-blockers benefit. In an Indian study of RHD, chronic MR, metoprolol decreased NYHA class, left ventricular end-diastolic volume (LVEDV), left ventricular end-systolic volume (LVESV), and brain natriuretic peptide (BNP) over 3 months versus controls and over 6 months MR decreased from severe-to-moderate in 11% versus none in control group. In symptomatic moderate or severe MR and LVEF, ≤60% needs standard GDMT of HFrEF. Vasodilators are not useful in asymptomatic MR with normal LVEF. There is no consistent improvement in LV volumes and severity of MR in small studies that have examined the effect of ACEI in MR. Beneficial effect seen in some studies may be more related to blockade of tissue angiotensin rather than its vasodilatory effect. They are indicated in systemic hypertension with MR with preserved LV function. However, in patients with functional or ischemic MR, preload reduction may be beneficial. If LV dysfunction is present then ACEI, beta-blockers (carvedilol), spironolactone, and biventricular pacing have all been shown to reduce the severity of functional MR. Best data exists for beta-blockers with better surgical outcomes and delayed onset of LV dysfunction versus not on beta-blockers. In patients with symptomatic MR with preserved LV function, surgery is the most appropriate therapy.[5,24]

Indications for Cardiac Surgery in Mitral Regurgitation

Usually, MV repair is preferred over replacement to avoid risks of mechanical valve complications such as TE, bleeding, adherence to anticoagulation, and its problems in women of childbearing age and use of bioprosthetic valve in children and its early degeneration. Higher the LVESV Z-score, higher is the risk of late postoperative LV dysfunction. ACC/AHA guidelines apply to high- and mid-income countries with good resources and good healthcare facilities. As per these guidelines, indications are: (1) MV surgery is indicated for symptomatic chronic severe primary MR and LVEF ≥ 30%.

and valve rupture cause abrupt and severe symptoms. Mechanical valve dysfunction may present with HF, shock, TE, hemolysis, or change in auscultatory findings. Acute or subacute presentation because of thrombus formation, impairment of leaflet opening and closure can occur and patient prosthetic mismatch and functional stenosis of a repaired native valve to be considered and to be evaluated with TTE and its comparison with postoperative TTE transvalvular velocity, gradient, area, LV volumes, LVEF, PA pressure, and RV function. TEE is better for valve thrombus, pannus, vegetation, and abscess. Fluoroscopy and CT imaging are required for mechanical valve obstruction and reduced motion. In AVR, 30% valve dysfunction occurs over 10 years of follow-up. Increase in mean gradient of >10 mm Hg or worsening of transprosthetic regurgitation ≥ I grade when compared with previous TTE/TEE. If accelerated degeneration <5 years, then young age <60 years at implantation, AF, smoking, diabetes mellitus (DM), chronic kidney disease CKD, initial gradient of ≥ 15 mm Hg gradient and on valve type have to be considered as risk factors. 13% of AVR patients develop hemodynamic valve dysfunction at a median of 6.7–9.9 years after implantation. Data for TAVI is not robust and TTE in hospital, at 30 days and at 1 year, is reasonable. Choice of prosthetic valve type depends on age, durability, need for and timing of reintervention, long-term VKA after mechanical valves and its complications and monitoring.[24]

Antithrombotic Therapy for Prosthetic Valves

Antithrombotics are needed for those with mechanical valve replacement, those with AF, and those in SR with other specific risk factors for TE. Annual rate of mechanical valve thrombosis is 0.1–5.7% depending on valve types more often in the first 3 months. Aim is to prevent valve/leaflet thrombosis and TE and to be balanced against risk of bleeding. Lifelong VKAs are needed for mechanical valve prosthesis. An addition of antiplatelets for acute coronary syndromes (ACSs) or percutaneous coronary interventions (PCIs) is done with caution. A target INR with a range of 0.5 and depending on comorbidities to be fixed. For a bileaflet mechanical AVR prosthesis on VKA, TE events of 0.53 per patient year occur between INR range of 2 and 4.5. INR of 2.5 is appropriate for current generation of mechanical prosthetic AV. If risk of AF, previous TE, hypercoagulable state and older generation prosthesis, severe LV dysfunction then INR to be maintained at around 3 (range 2.5–3.5). Incidence of TE is highest with MV prosthesis. In a German GELIA study, a lower INR range had lower survival versus higher INR range (2.5–4.5). Patient's compliance is challenging with higher INR. Target of INR is 3 (range 2.5–3.5) which is reasonable in mechanical MV prosthesis).[24]

Risk of TE is 0.7%/year in biological valves with SR. MV bioprosthesis has higher rates of TE versus aortic bioprosthesis (2.4% vs. 1.9% per patient year).

In bioprosthetic AV in SR without another indication for VKA, incidence of TE bleeding and death was similar with antiplatelets versus VKA, which may apply to MV bioprosthesis in SR also. Because following bioprosthetic valve surgery of MVR or AVR, there is a need for decreasing ischemic stroke risk between 90 and 180 days. No studies on long-term effects of antiplatelets in MV repair. Surgical implantation of bioprosthetic MV or AV will not require lifelong anticoagulation in absence of independent indication such as AF. But in the initial 90–180 days, there is an increased risk of ischemic stroke; hence, there is a need of anticoagulation till valve gets endothelialization and risk of bleeding needs to be assessed by HASBLED score and drugs and other associated risk factors for higher bleeding. Additional antiplatelet for a mechanical prosthetic valve on anticoagulation to be decided on risk of bleeding and presence of other risk factors. In mechanical Aortic On X valve, INR to be targeted at lower values between 1.5 and 2 with aspirin 81 mg for long-term management. Following surgery, INR is kept around 2.5 for the first 3 months. Novel oral anticoagulants and antithrombotics have no role as on today.[24]

■ MANAGEMENT OF VALVULAR HEART DISEASE IN PREGNANCY

Rheumatic valve diseases may increase the maternal and fetal risks associated with pregnancy. Adverse outcomes are related to the type and severity of maternal valvular disease and the resulting abnormalities of functional capacity, LV function, and pulmonary pressure. Evaluation and management require an understanding of the normal physiological changes associated with gestation, labor, delivery and the early postpartum period. On an average, there is 50% increase in circulating blood volume during pregnancy along with CO peaking before the mid-portion of the second-and third-trimester. There is smaller increase in HR averaging 10–20 bpm. Because of effects of uterine circulation and endogenous hormones, SVR decreases with disproportionate decrease in diastolic blood pressure leading to wide pulse pressure. IVC obstruction from a gravid uterus results in abrupt decrease in cardiac preload, which leads to hypotension with weakness and lightheadedness. These symptoms resolve quickly with a change in position.

There is further abrupt increase in CO during labor and delivery related in part to the associated anxiety and pain. Uterine contractions can lead to marked increases in both systolic and diastolic blood pressure. After delivery, there is an initial surge in preload related to the autotransfusion of uterine blood into the systemic circulation and to caval decompression. Cardiac filling pressures may increase. Cardiovascular adaptations associated with pregnancy regress by approximately 6 weeks after delivery.

Pregnancy is also associated with a hypercoagulable state due to relative decreases in protein S activity, stasis, and venous hypertension. Estrogens can interfere with collagen deposition within the media of the large muscular arteries. Circulating elastase can break up the elastic lamellae and weaken aortic media predisposing to dissection.[8]

Murmurs develop in nearly all women during pregnancy. They are usually soft midsystolic and heard along left sternal border. Their intensity may increase during pregnancy. Echocardiography is warranted when diastolic or continuous or loud systolic murmurs (more than grade 2/6) during pregnancy are detected or when murmurs are associated with symptoms or an abnormal ECG.[11]

Consequences of Valvular Heart Disease during Pregnancy

Prevalence of clinically significant maternal heart disease is low during pregnancy (<1%). Its presence increases the risk of adverse maternal, fetal, and neonatal outcomes. AHA/ACC has classified maternal and fetal risk during pregnancy on the basis of the type of valvular abnormality and NYHA functional class.

The absolute risk conferred on a given women by pregnancy also depends on additional clinical features. Recent analysis of the outcomes of pregnancy in Canada identified predictors of adverse maternal and fetal outcomes in a heterogeneous group of women with congenital or acquired heart diseases (546 women and 579 pregnancies). Approximately, 40% of the women had a primary valve disorder. Adverse maternal cardiac events such as pulmonary edema, arrhythmia requiring therapy, stroke, cardiac arrest, or death occurred in 13% of completed pregnancies and were significantly more likely among women with reduced LV systolic function (EF < 40%), left heart obstruction such as AS with valve area <1. 5 cm^2 or MS with a valve area <2 cm^2, previous CV events such as HF, transient ischemic attacks or stroke or disease of NYHA Class II or higher.[12]

Abnormal functional capacity (NYHA Class II or higher) and left heart obstruction were also predictors of neonatal complications including premature birth, intrauterine growth retardation (IUGR), respiratory distress syndrome, intraventricular hemorrhage, and death. Other predictors of adverse fetal outcomes included the use of anticoagulant drugs, smoking during pregnancy and multiple gestations. Fetal mortality was 4% among pregnancies in women with one or more of these risk factors as compared with 2% among those with none of these risk factors. Maternal age <20 years and >35 years also mattered for such complications with similar risk factors.

Secondary pulmonary hypertension due to valvular disease is associated with an increased rate of adverse maternal events, but the absolute risk of such events is unclear. A systolic pulmonary artery pressure (PAP) >75% of systemic pressure places the woman at high risk.

Valvular heart disease is an important contributor for maternal cardiac disease causing 50–90% of maternal complications in LMICs. MS being single most cause for

mortality up to 34% when diagnosed during pregnancy. Physiological changes such as 30% increase in SV, 10–20% increase in HR, 30–50% increase in CO early in pregnancy, which plateaus between second and third trimester. Decreased SVR up to second trimester by 35–40%, which accommodates increased CO. Plasma volume increases by 6th week of pregnancy and reaches 50% above baseline value by second trimester. Red cell mass does not rises correspondingly; hence, there is physiological anemia and a hyperdynamic circulation, which leads to worsening of symptoms of left-sided valvular stenosis but regurgitant lesions are well tolerated. Pregnancy is an arrhythmogenic and a thrombogenic state because of increased concentration of clotting factors, which decrease PT by 20%, activated partial thromboplastin time (APTT), increased platelet adhesiveness, and decreased fibrinolysis. Risk of thrombosis is more during puerperium during first 6 weeks than during pregnancy which is dangerous to underlying mechanical heart valves, MS, and AF patients.

There is 30% increase in CO in first stage of labor. 60–80% immediately postdelivery because of increase in HR (pain and anxiety) and SV as 300–500 mL of blood is autotransfused to systemic circulation with each uterine contraction, and increase in preload after delivery as IVC compression is relieved. Shifts in maternal hemodynamics peak between first 24 and 72 hours postpartum and are more rapid after cesarean section. Hence, in women having heart disease, HF chances are more during this period. HF risk, thrombotic events, and bleeding risk last up to 1 year postpartum leading to late maternal deaths also.[26]

Preconception Evaluation

Many women are unaware of underlying VHD and present after 20 weeks when hemodynamic decompensation occurs due to pregnancy. Delayed diagnosis of VHD is a risk factor for maternal death. Unplanned pregnancies lead to poor outcomes for mother and fetus. During counseling, risk of death, embryopathy, whether to stop and to take new medicines, risk of thrombosis, and postpartum bleeding to be discussed. Some may require interventions/surgery before planned pregnancy. If at higher risk, better advice is to avoid pregnancy.[26]

Risk Stratification

Apart from clinical examination and routine blood tests, ECG, ECHO, X-ray chest if need be CT chest, exercise test for functional class, maternal cardiac and obstetrical risk, fetal, neonatal risk, long-term effect of pregnancy on the heart, maternal life expectancy and any modification of cardiac drugs have to be assessed.

General and Lesion-specific Risk Factors

General risk factors for adverse maternal cardiac events are NYHA functional class cyanosis, previous cardiac events (pulmonary edema, TIA, and stroke), arrhythmias, LVEF, left heart obstruction such as MS with valve area <2 cm^2, AV area <1.5 cm^2, peak LVOT gradient >30 mm Hg, prosthetic mechanical heart valves, and significant MR/TR. Most frequent complications during pregnancy are HF, arrhythmias, and TE. CARPREG (cardiac disease in pregnancy) is an established general risk index derived from observational prospective cohort study of pregnant women with underlying congenital and acquired heart disease which establishes the severity of the risk depending on the number of risk factors present in that particular individual. Another established risk index is the modified WHO classification which incorporates both general and lesion-specific diagnosis and is the most accurate risk assessment currently in use even though better suited to high-income countries rather than LMICs (moderate prediction) and risks are additive, e.g., mixed valve disease, LV dysfunction, noncardiac risk factors such as hypertension, obesity or CKD will add to the risk score **(Box 1)**.[26]

Women at low risk as per modified World Health Organization (mWHO) can be managed by a local cardiologist and obstetrical team. Those at moderate-to-high-risk mWHO Class II-IV has to be referred to a tertiary care center before pregnancy itself where they can be counseled and managed appropriately **(Table 3)**.

In LMICs, 88.9% antenatal heart disease is RHD. In South Africa RHD MS/MR, prior MV repair accounted for 71.84%. 8.28% of heart diseases were unmasked by pregnancy.

BOX 1	The cardiac disease in pregnancy (CARPREG) risk score.

Risk factor:
- Prior cardiac *event* or arrhythmia
- NYHA Class III or IV or cyanosis
- Left heart obstruction
- Systemic ventricular dysfunction (EF < 40%)

Score and risk of cardiac complications:
- *Score 0:* 5% risk
- *Score 1:* 27% risk
- *Score > 1:* 62% risk

(EF: ejection fraction; NYHA: New York Heart Association)

TABLE 3: Modified World Health Organization (mWHO) classification of maternal cardiovascular risk.

	mWHO I	mWHO II	mWHO II-III	mWHO III	mWHO IV
Diagnosis (if otherwise well and uncomplicated)	• Trivial MR • Uncomplicated mitral valve prolapse • Trivial AR • Mild TR • Mild PS PR • Isolated atrial or ventricular ectopic beats	• Mild MS, MR • Mild AS, AR • Mild TS • Moderate TR • Moderate PS, PR • Most arrhythmias (supraventricular arrhythmias)	• Moderate MR • Moderate AS • Moderate AR • Severe PR • Mild LVSD (EF 45–54%)	• Mechanical valve • Moderate MS • Severe MR • Severe, asymptomatic AS • Severe AR • Severe TS, TR • Severe PS • Ventricular tachycardia • Moderate LVSD (EF 30–44%)	• Severe MS • Severe symptomatic AS • Critical AS • Pulmonary hypertension • Severe systemic ventricular dysfunction (EF < 30% or NYHA Class III or IV)
Risk	No detectable increased risk of maternal mortality and no/mild increased risk in morbidity	Small increased risk of maternal mortality or moderate increase in morbidity	Intermediate increased risk of maternal mortality or moderate-to-severe increase in maternal morbidity	Significantly increased risk of maternal mortality or severe morbidity	Extremely high risk of maternal mortality or severe morbidity
Maternal cardiac event rate	2.5–5%	5.7–10.5%	10–19%	19–27%	40–100%
Counseling	Yes	Yes	Yes	Expert counseling required	Pregnancy is contraindicated. If pregnancy occurs, termination should be discussed
Care during pregnancy and delivery	Local hospital	Local hospital	Referral hospital	Expert center for pregnancy and cardiac disease	Expert center for pregnancy and cardiac disease
Minimal follow-up visits during pregnancy	Once or twice	Once per trimester	Bimonthly	Monthly or bimonthly	Monthly

(AS: aortic stenosis; AR: aortic regurgitation; MS: mitral stenosis; MR: mitral regurgitation; NYHA: New York Heart Association; PS: pulmonary stenosis; PR: pulmonary regurgitation)

Hemodynamic stresses of pregnancy such as increased SV, HR, CO are poorly tolerated by severe valve stenosis causing adverse events in mother and neonatal prematurity, low-birth weight and death.[27]

Rheumatic Heart Disease and Pregnancy Outcomes

Findings from ROPAC (Registry of Pregnancy and Cardiac disease) registry are a large prospective cohort of pregnant women (n-390) with RHD to date. Key features of the study are: (1) women with mild/asymptomatic MV disease tolerate pregnancy well with few complications; (2) MS is less well tolerated than MR resulting in high rates of HF and need for hospitalizations. Rates of hospitalizations were highest in severe MS (49.1%) and moderate MS (MVA: 1–1.5 cm^2)—31.8%. Symptomatic MS is an independent predictor of maternal adverse cardiac events. (3) mixed moderate-to-severe MS/MR had similar adverse pregnancy outcomes similar to that of severe MS. (4) severe MS is an independent risk factor for adverse fetal outcomes including preterm birth and low-birth weight. ROPAC showed increased complications with greater severity of stenosis and higher functional class. Increase in mortality and HF in moderate-to-severe MR is notable as this lesion is well tolerated in pregnancy, if LV function and NYHA class are normal. Even REMEDY study reported that 25% of adults with RHD had decreased LV function and 20% had antenatal HF. Hence, pregnancy with MR and increased functional class and decreased LV function comes under WHO III category with increased risk of adverse events. In mixed MV, disease there is paucity of data. 56 patients with mixed moderate-to-severe MR with MS whose baseline characteristics and pregnancy outcomes were similar to those of severe MS including antenatal AF in 9%, elevated PH in 48%, HF in 28%, peripartum AF in 10%, HF in 34%. Options for pure MR and mixed MV disease, which are more common in younger patients of childbearing age, are exclusively surgical which option is limited in poor countries and difficult choice of mechanical versus bioprosthetic valves has to be entertained in these women. Burden of RHD on maternal and fetal health is underestimated in this study for three reasons: (1) discrepancy on healthcare facilities and data available from different countries, which will not give a correct picture of this disease and its complications; (2) MVR cases were excluded from this study, which are at high risk for morbidity and mortality; (3) only 56% of ROPAC study had follow-up after 1 week, hence, postpartum and rate of maternal deaths would have been underestimated because of insufficient follow-up.[27] Hence, there are number of opportunities to improve by counseling during pregnancy as in this study, 75% of RHDs were diagnosed preconception, 34% antenatal HF which stress importance of counseling for optimization of treatment and preconception interventions. 20% moderate and 34% severe MS patients had HF. As per GDMT, PBMC is needed for symptomatic patients and preconception PBMC in asymptomatic patients. Even beta-blockers decrease HR, MV gradients, LA pressure, and reduce symptoms in >90% of patients. In ROPAC registry, hardly 40% of MS patients were treated with beta-blockade and, hence, education of physicians and optimization of medications should be the goals. It is an ongoing registry, which includes the burden of RHD in LMICs and developing world and endemic population with poor public health systems. Prevention is cheap, readily available, and cost-effective and helps political and financial commitments at global and local levels with the goal of eradicating RHD.[27]

Medical Therapy

Women with severe VHD are at risk for HF, arrhythmias, and effect of cardiac drugs to be assessed. Even though beta-blockers control HR and treat arrhythmias but can cause fetal growth retardation but less with metoprolol. Diuretics decrease volume overload but can decrease placental blood flow also. In ROPAC registry, diuretics use was associated with low-birth weight and fetal mortality. ACEI and ARBs are contraindicated because of fetal malformations.[24] Medical management of women before, during, and after pregnancy with unoperated or operated RHD is a challenge and requires an MDT of physician, cardiologist, obstetrician, anesthesiologists, and CT surgeons. Unoperated RHD is often diagnosed because of increased CO and decreased peripheral vascular resistance (PVR), which unmask moderate or severe lesions and contribute to maternal mortality within 42 days after delivery and late maternal death up to 1 year postpartum. Hence, all women with RHD have increased risk of poor maternal and fetal outcomes, which increase further if there is RV/LV dysfunction or PAH, AF, and any signs of HF. Stenotic lesions are less well tolerated than regurgitant lesions and may require interventions including BMV, CT surgery, or termination of pregnancy, if maternal risk is very high. Suitable preconception counseling including advice of contraception. The REMEDY study showed that only 5% of women with prosthetic heart valves and 2% of those with severe MS were on contraception. In a recent study of 3,506 pregnant women having Echo scoring in second and third trimester in Uganda, 1.7% had cardiac disease, 88% were RHD, and <5% were aware of their diagnosis. 50% required intervention or change in delivery planning and attributed risk of heart disease on maternal mortality was 11% and increased fetal mortality also. Women with mechanical prosthetic valves require OAC including warfarin and heparin. If warfarin dose is <5 mg, medication can be continued till the end of pregnancy; in others, more complex treatment algorithm needs to be followed (Circulation. 2020;e357-72).

■ EVALUATION

Assessment of a woman with clinically significant VHD should ideally occur before conception including echocardiography. History of patients' exercise capacity, current or past evidence of HF and associated arrhythmias,

TABLE 4: Signs and symptoms of normal pregnancy and pregnancy with cardiac compromise.

Signs and symptoms that may occur in normal pregnancy	Signs and symptoms suggesting cardiac decompensation during pregnancy
Breathlessness on exertion	Marked breathlessness, e.g., minor exertion, talking, and eating
Difficulty sleeping due to discomfort	Orthopnea and paroxysmal nocturnal dyspnea
Increased heart rate <100 bpm (10–20 bpm higher than prepregnancy)	Sinus tachycardia persistently >100 bpm
Chest discomfort due to reflux	Exertional, tearing, or pleuritic chest pain
Vasovagal syncope, postural hypotension	Exertional or palpation-related syncope
Palpation due to atrial and ventricular ectopics	Sustained tachyarrhythmias
Jugular venous pulse visible—2 cm	Jugular venous pulse raised >2 cm
3rd heat sound	4th heart sound
Mild peripheral edema	Marked peripheral edema

cardiac hemodynamics including PA pressure, and the severity of valve dysfunction should be assessed by echocardiography. During pregnancy, they should be evaluated each trimester for any change in symptoms in order to evaluate any deterioration in maternal cardiac status **(Table 4)**.[11]

In VHD, hemodynamic changes associated with pregnancy may cause significant burden. Hence, pregnancy evaluation of VHD is needed with TTE and its anatomic and hemodynamic assessment of VHD and risks to mother and fetus, functional class, severity of lesion status, LV/RV function, PH, medication review, and any interventions required before pregnancy itself. If asymptomatic severe VHD exercise testing for risk assessment and if symptoms occur on exercise, they should be treated like symptomatic VHD (stage D).[24]

◼ GENERAL MANAGEMENT

In VHDs with high maternal mortality, pregnancy should be discouraged. Individual counseling usually requires a multidisciplinary approach and should include information regarding contraception, maternal and fetal risks of pregnancy, and expected long-term outcomes. However, many patients with VHD can be successfully managed throughout pregnancy and during labor and delivery with conservative medical measures designed to optimize intravascular volume and systemic loading conditions.

Simple interventions such as bed rest and avoidance of supine position should be advised. Whenever possible symptomatic and severe valve lesions should be corrected before conception and pregnancy.[8]

Medical therapy for VHDs in the nonpregnant patients includes vasodilators, diuretics, anticoagulants, and antiarrhythmics.

During pregnancy, many of these drugs are associated with an increased risk to the fetus but if the benefits to the mother are more than the risks, then they are used **(Table 5)**.

Bacteremia after uncomplicated vaginal delivery occurs in approximately 2% of patients. Antibiotic prophylaxis at the time of delivery is recommended in women with VHDs. Patients at high risk for endocarditis may receive higher antibiotics at the discretion of the physician.[11]

Prepregnancy Interventions in Valvular Heart Disease

In severe VHD with symptoms, asymptomatic severe MS, if suitable for PBMV, severe AS, severe MR, choice of valve, its risk of thrombosis and need for OAC and its effects on pregnancy, on fetus, if bioprosthetic valve, its early degeneration in young women to be counseled. Mild-to-moderate AS may tolerate pregnancy well. In severe AS, 10–44% may have HF and arrhythmias in 25%. Sudden deterioration can occur and fetal complications are frequent. Interventions are palliative aortic balloon dilatation followed by AVR later or MVR surgery for severe MR. Asymptomatic severe MR tolerates well with normal LV function, whereas if LV dysfunction or PAH > 50 mm Hg needs MV repair or replacement before conception itself or if pregnant should be referred to comprehensive valve center for further management **(Flowchart 1)**.[24]

During Pregnancy Interventions

In pregnant women with severe VHD, intractable symptoms (NYHA III-IV) despite medical therapy surgical or percutaneous interventions are necessary. Severe MS with HF or symptoms or sudden deterioration needs PBMV with suitable morphology, which is a high-risk procedure to both mother and the fetus and to be performed in a comprehensive valve center under the guidance of an MDT. In regurgitant valve lesions only if severe symptoms, NYHA IV HF refractory to maximal medical therapy needs valve repair or replacement surgery as it carries up to 9% maternal mortality and 30–40% fetal mortality. Severe AS, if symptomatic, needs temporary balloon dilatation to relieve immediate symptoms later to be followed by AVR surgery or immediate high-risk AVR surgery which carries both maternal and fetal mortality.[24]

Prosthetic Valves in Pregnant Women

Pregnancy in women with mechanical heart valves is classified as WHO category III and carries risk to mother and

TABLE 5: Fetal effects maternal indications and risks associated with drugs used in treatment of maternal valvular heart disease.

Drug	Fetal effects	Indications in pregnant patients with valve disease	Risk category
Diuretics			
Furosemide	Increased urinary sodium and potassium level	To decrease congestion associated with valvular heart disease	C_m
Antihypertensive			
Beta-blockers	Possible decreased heart rate, possible lower birth weight	Hypertension, supraventricular arrhythmias, to control heart rate in women with clinically significant mitral stenosis	D_m
Methyldopa	No major adverse effects	Hypertension	C
Vasodilator agents			
Angiotensin-converting enzyme inhibitors	Urogenital defects, death, intrauterine growth retardation	Not indicated during pregnancy and should be discontinued	D_m
Hydralazine	No major adverse effects	For vasodilatation is case of aortic regurgitation and ventricular dysfunction	
Nitrates	Possible bradycardia	Rarely used to decrease venous congestion	$B\text{-}C_m$
Anticoagulant and antithrombotic agents			
Warfarin	Hemorrhage, development abnormalities when used between week 6–12 of gestation	For anticoagulation of mechanical heart valves, valvular heart disease with associated atrial fibrillation during week 12–36 of pregnancy	D_m
Unfractionated heparin	Hemorrhage, no congenital defects	For anticoagulation of mechanical heart valves, valvular heart disease with associated atrial fibrillation during week 6–12 and after week 36 of pregnancy	C_m
Low-molecular weight heparin	Hemorrhage	Not currently indicated during pregnancy	D_m
Aspirin	Hemorrhage, prolongation of labor, low-birth-weight when taken in high doses	Low-dose aspirin (81 mg/day) occasionally used as an adjunct in patients with previous embolic events or prosthetic–valve thrombosis	C
Antiarrhythmic agents			
Digoxin	No major adverse effects	For suppression of supraventricular arrhythmias	C
Adenosine	No major adverse effects	For immediate conversion of supraventricular arrhythmias	C_m
Quinidine	High doses may be oxytocic	Occasionally used for suppression of ventricular arrhythmias	C_m
Procainamide	No major adverse effects	Occasionally used for suppression of ventricular arrhythmias	C_m
Amiodarone	Hypothyroidism, intrauterine growth retardation, premature birth	Rarely used during pregnancy because of side effects; may be used to suppress atrial or ventricular arrhythmias in high risk patients	C_m

fetus also. Maternal mortality is up to 1%, chance of valve thrombosis is 5%, and high risk to fetus also. Preconception TTE for valve function, ventricular function, PA pressure, and their risk can be explained. There is higher risk of prosthetic valve thrombosis as pregnancy is a hypercoagulable state and needs a good INR control keeping its risks on mother and fetal outcomes also. Hence, MDT approach, high suspicion of valve thrombosis with embolic event, clinical deterioration, HF, increase in valve gradients, or regurgitation is important in its detection. TEE is more useful for leaflet motion and thrombus burden. Fluoroscopy and gated cardiac CT are useful in suspected valve thrombosis.[24]

Anticoagulation for Mechanical Prosthetic Heart Valves

There is increased risk of maternal complications such as valve thrombosis, valve failure, TE, stroke, hemorrhage, and death. Risk of poor fetal outcomes is high with increased risk of spontaneous abortions, fetal death, fetal hemorrhage, and teratogenicity. When warfarin dose is >5 mg/day, more than 3rd of women have serious maternal or fetal complications. They need uninterrupted therapeutic anticoagulation, which is safe to mother and fetus also. Warfarin is most effective anticoagulation to prevent TE complications but

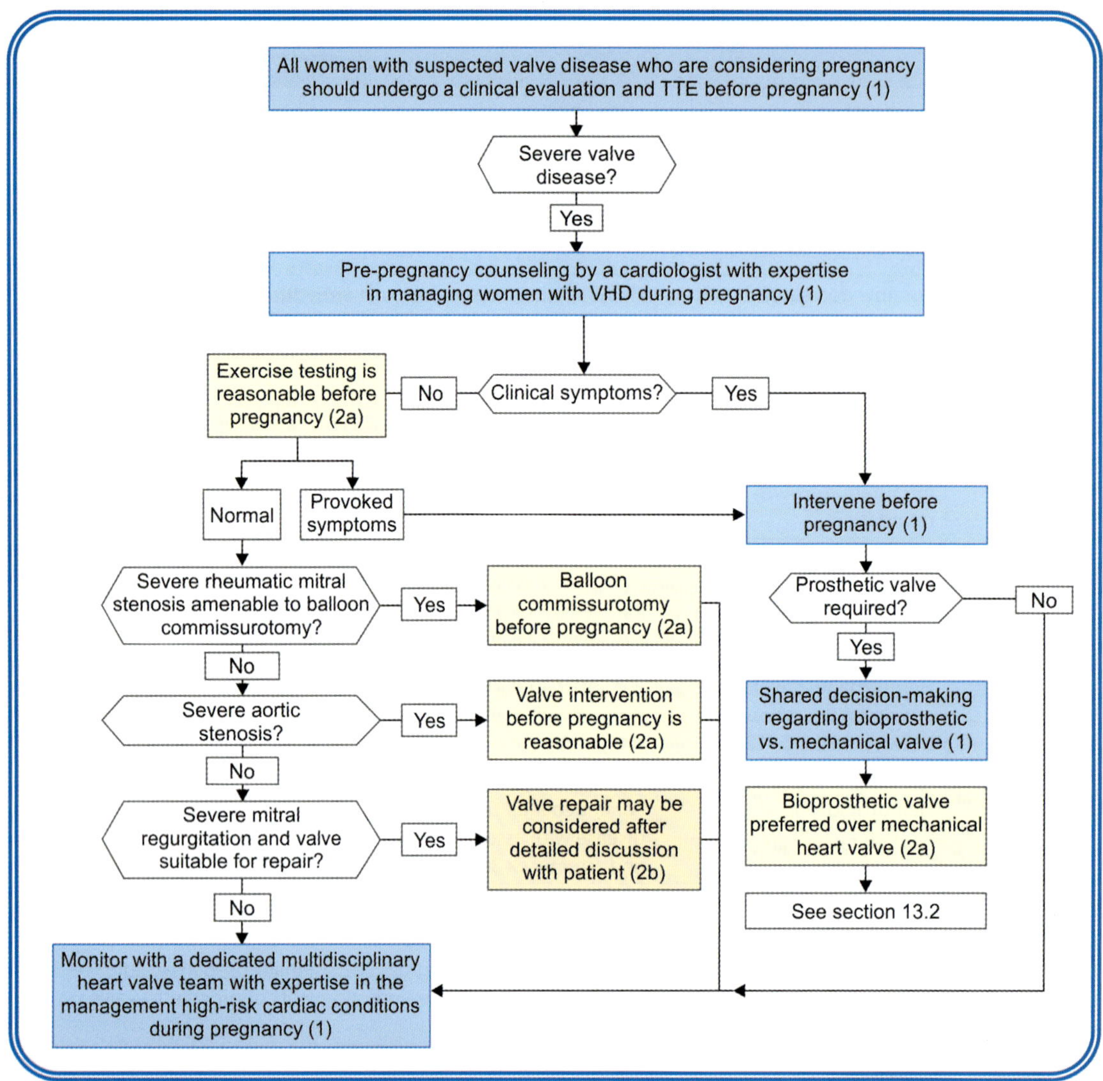

FLOWCHART 1: Preconception management of women with native valve disease.

(TTE: transthoracic echocardiogram; VHD: valvular heart disease)

Source: Otto CM, Nishimura RA, Bonow RO, Carabello BA, Erwin JP 3rd, Gentile F, et al. ACC/AHA VHD Guidelines, 2020. Circulation. 2021;143:e35-71.

crosses placenta and can cause miscarriage, spontaneous abortion warfarin embryopathy when the dose is >5 mg/day in the first trimester, and fetal intracranial hemorrhage. Although low-molecular weight heparin (LMWH) is not teratogenic but when not monitored properly, it can lead to thrombotic events. Hence, there are three strategies: (1) continue Warfarin throughout pregnancy; (2) use heparin throughout pregnancy as it does not cross placenta; (3) sequential therapy of heparin during first trimester and warfarin during second and third trimester. Hence, proper counseling regarding proper choice of anticoagulation and its monitoring is very important for both mother and fetus. If on warfarin, switch to heparin 1 week prior to delivery, but maternal hemorrhage risk is high on heparin. Hence, before delivery, switch to unfractionated heparin (UFH) infusion to keep APTT more than two times control levels and stop UFH

6 hours before delivery to decrease maternal hemorrhage. If on warfarin in therapeutic range, risk of fetal intracranial hemorrhage is more on vaginal delivery. Hence, reverse anticoagulation and planned cesarean section decreases intracranial hemorrhage. Teratogenicity is dose dependant. Warfarin embryopathy <3%, if dose <5 mg, has a lowest risk to both mother and fetus also throughout pregnancy. If warfarin dose >5 mg in first trimester for INR in a therapeutic range, there is >30% risk of fetal loss or embryopathy. Replacing to LMWH in first trimester with XA levels monitoring every week decreases fetal loss. Fixed dosing is not appropriate and has more maternal morbidity and mortality. After first trimester, switching to warfarin is safer for mother and fetus also. If monitoring is not possible and warfarin dose >5 mg, it is better to give UFH in first trimester to maintain APTT two times the control, but line infections, osteoporosis,

heparin-induced thrombocytopenia (HIT) are problems. Subcutaneous UFH is associated with valve thrombosis, stroke, and death in pregnant women with mechanical heart valves during second and third trimester. If mechanical valve thrombosis occurs during pregnancy, low-dose slow infusion of tPa is an alternative to surgical valve replacement in women who are stable hemodynamically or with TE complications in nonobstructive valve thrombosis with thrombus >10 mm as cardiac surgery carries high rates of fetal loss. Even in second and third trimester on warfarin, there is chance of pregnancy loss and fetal hemorrhage. Hence, dose-adjusted LMWH is a better alternative but has a higher thrombotic complication than warfarin. Low-dose aspirin is safe during pregnancy and can be continued with mechanical heart valves, if needed for other indications including prevention of preeclampsia. Anti-XA agents are not safe during pregnancy.[24]

■ VALVE-SPECIFIC RISK STRATIFICATION AND MANAGEMENT

Mitral Stenosis

Mitral stenosis is the most common clinically significant valvular abnormality and may be associated with pulmonary congestion, edema, and atrial arrhythmias during pregnancy or soon after delivery. Increased volume load and increased CO associated with pregnancy lead to an increase in LA volume and pressure, elevated pulmonary venous filling pressures, dyspnea and decreased exercise tolerance, increased maternal HR, decreased diastolic filling period, further increasing LA pressure. Mortality among pregnant women with minimal symptoms is <1%. Predictors of adverse maternal outcomes are MV area <1.5 cm^2 and abnormal functional class before pregnancy. 35–74% deteriorate during pregnancy. Asymptomatic mild MS is low-risk mWHO II although events can still occur. As per ROPAC registry, MS during pregnancy mortality is 1.9% where half with severe MS (<1 cm^2) and one-third with moderate MS (1–1.5 cm^2) developed HF during second trimester of pregnancy when CO is at its peak. Other predictors of maternal complications are functional class NYHA III-IV, systolic PA pressure > 30 mm Hg, history of pulmonary edema, TIA/stroke, decreased LVEF, and older age. Death is 0.3% in LMICs. Persistent AF is in <10% of pregnancies which precipitates HF. PAH secondary to PVH due to left-sided VHD increases maternal mortality to 16–30%. Rapid fluid shifts and tachycardia associated with labor and postpartum up to 72 hours can cause pulmonary edema and low-output state. Mixed MV disease also had adverse clinical outcomes. Fetal mortality increases with deteriorating maternal functional capacity. Fetal risks include prematurity (20–30%), IUGR (5–20%), and fetal death (1–5%). Risks are higher if mother's functional class was NYHA III-IV during pregnancy.[26] Fetal mortality is 30% when there is NYHA class IV symptoms in the mother. Penicillin prophylaxis is indicated as in nonpregnant state.

Avoidance of excess salt, reduction of physical activity, and diuretics are recommended in mild-to-moderate MS. Beta-blockers (metoprolol or atenolol) attenuate the increase in HR and prolong diastolic filling period, which provides symptomatic benefit. Development of AF requires prompt treatment including cardioversion, beta-blockers, and digoxin for rate control. If suppressive antiarrhythmic therapy is needed, procainamide and quinidine are used and to prevent TE, anticoagulant therapy is indicated.

Patients with Class III or IV NYHA or tight MS with valve area <1 cm^2 need BMV, if valve is suitable or valve surgery before conception. Those who present with severe symptoms during pregnancy, successful PTMC can be performed in second trimester and has been associated with normal subsequent deliveries and excellent fetal outcomes. Risk to the fetus associated with exposure to radiation may be reduced by proper shielding of the pelvis and abdomen of the mother with lead apron while doing the procedure and avoiding the procedure in first half of pregnancy **(Fig. 3)**. PTMC is also done using echocardiography, 23-year-old full-term pregnant lady presented with pulmonary apoplexy, losing almost half liter blood in hemoptysis for the past 4 days. On ECHO interrogation, MV orifice area was just 0.4 cm^2. Emergency PTMC was done in the morning and in the evening; she developed labor pains and had a normal vaginal delivery at night. Emergency PTMC literally saved both the mother and the child **(Fig. 4)**. Open cardiac surgery has been performed which has maternal outcomes similar as nonpregnant women but fetal loss occurs in 10–30% of cases. Vaginal delivery is the usual approach with the use of epidural anesthesia for effective pain relief and use of assist devices such as forceps during second stage of delivery, eliminating the need for pushing. Cesarean section should be performed for obstetrical indications

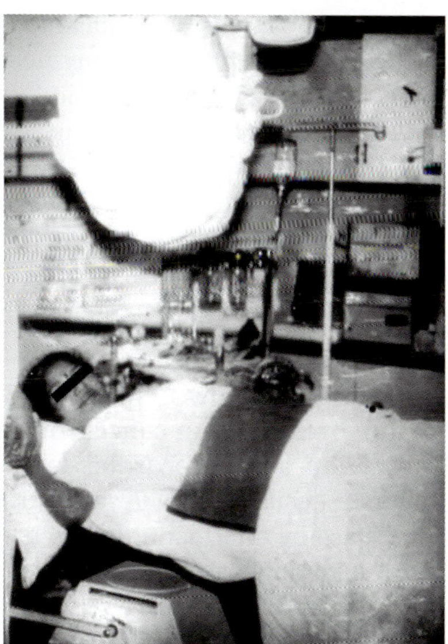

FIG. 3: The abdomen is covered with lead shield in a 25-year-old, 7 months pregnant lady undergoing PTMC for severe MS.

(MS: mitral stenosis; PTMC: percutaneous transvenous mitral commissurotomy)

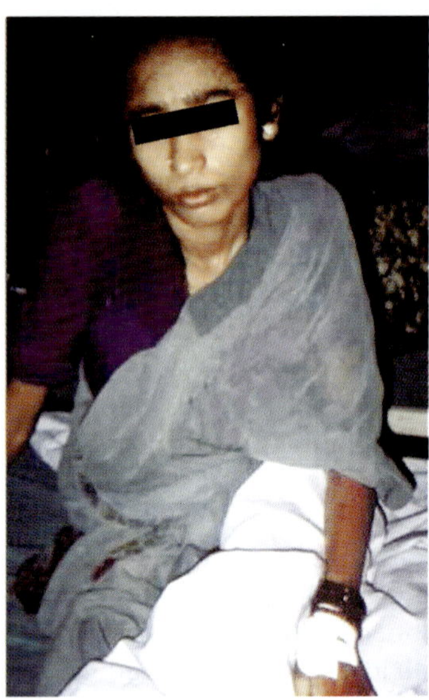

FIG. 4: A 23-year-old lady with RHD, critical MS with MVOA 0.4 cm^2, who presented with pulmonary apoplexy, delivered 12 hours after emergency PTMC.

(MS: mitral stenosis; MVOA: mitral valve orifice area; PTMC: percutaneous transvenous mitral commissurotomy; RHD: rheumatic heart disease)

only. Labor is associated with an increase of 8–10 mm Hg in LA pressure and pulmonary capillary wedge pressure (PCWP). Some may need hemodynamic monitoring with advanced disease.[11]

Mitral Regurgitation/Aortic Regurgitation

Mild lesions are well tolerated. If severe with symptoms, decreased EF, LV dilatation, or PAH can develop HF in 20–25%. If LVEF < 30% or any pulmonary hypertension should avoid pregnancy. Obstetrical risk does not increase with these lesions. IUGR in 5–10%.[26] It is usually well tolerated because of decreased SVR. If symptomatic, it may need diuretics. Vasodilators are used only for hypertension. Hydralazine is safe. Avoid ACEI because of their multiple adverse effects on fetal development. Women with symptomatic MR benefit by valve surgery especially repair before pregnancy, whereas if LV dysfunction does not improve even after surgery then it increases maternal risk during pregnancy.

Aortic Stenosis

The obstruction to LV outflow imposed by valvular AS results in pressure overload with concentric hypertrophy. Diastolic dysfunction and myocardial oxygen supply–demand imbalance ensue, followed later in the natural history of the disease by afterload mismatch and systolic pump dysfunction. Pathophysiologic deterioration may be accelerated by the superimposition of systemic hypertension that can occur during pregnancy and/or AF. Severe AS is poorly tolerated. If mild or moderate asymptomatic severe AS with normal exercise tolerance usually tolerate pregnancy well with low risk of HF (<10%). One-fourths of symptomatic AS will develop HF, miscarriage, and fetal death risk <5%. Other fetal risks are prematurity, IUGR, low-birth weight in 20–25% in moderate AS and more in severe AS.[26] If moderate or severe stenosis with peak gradient >50 mm Hg, they are advised to delay the pregnancy until the surgical correction. If symptomatic before the end of first trimester, it is better to advise termination of pregnancy. AV surgery or balloon aortic valvuloplasty (BAV) is done during pregnancy with some maternal and fetal risks. Women with severe AS, if asymptomatic or have mild symptoms, are managed conservatively with bed rest, oxygen, and beta-blockers. If they develop symptoms, percutaneous aortic balloon valvuloplasty or surgery before labor and delivery can be undertaken but they are associated with maternal and fetal risks.[8]

Tricuspid Valve Disease

Maternal risk is determined by left-sided valve lesions or pulmonary hypertension. Mild or moderate TR is tolerated well. Severe TR is at risk for right-sided HF and arrhythmias. Prognosis depends on associated valve diseases. TR with HF may require diuretics, which should be used with caution to avoid hypoperfusion.

■ MIXED VALVE LESIONS

There is lack of data on this subset. Risk depends on most hemodynamically significant lesion and risk of the lesions is additive as per mWHO risk index.

Prosthetic Heart Valves

Bioprosthetic valves are not as durable as mechanical prosthesis but if normally functioning with normal LV function, pregnancy is well tolerated. Risk increases if there is bioprosthetic dysfunction; chances of event-free pregnancy and live birth are 79%. Pregnancy in a woman with mechanical valve, risk is very high mWHO III and chances of event-free pregnancy with live birth are 58% versus 78% with LV disease without a prosthetic valve.[26] This added risk is because of hemorrhage due to anticoagulation and associated with an estimated maternal mortality of 1–4% with death usually resulting from complications of prosthetic valve thrombosis.[11] Hence, the patients with mechanical valves with pregnancy are put on daily heparin injection to avoid valve thrombosis, instead of anticoagulants due to the fear of teratogenicity. Rest of the management aspects are already discussed above under prosthetic valves section.

Following strategies help to decrease the risk during labor and delivery:

- Use of epidural anesthesia decreases pain and sympathetic induced tachycardia
- Hemodynamic monitoring from 24 to 72 hours
- Assisted vaginal delivery
- Avoid bolus dose of oxytocin
- Avoid ergometrine
- Planned elective cesarean section with postpartum ICU care.

■ MANAGEMENT OF VALVULAR HEART DISEASES DURING NONCARDIAC SURGERY

Management depends on type and severity of VHD depending on: (1) presence or absence of symptoms, (2) severity of VHD, (3) risk of noncardiac surgery, (4) response of LV and/or RV to the overload caused by VHD, and (5) PA systolic pressure. If patient meets standard criteria for valve intervention, defer elective noncardiac procedures and patient should undergo the valve intervention prior to surgery. In emergencies, heart team consisting of cardiologist, cardiac anesthetist, cardiac surgeon, and concerned surgeon have to decide its management. If severe VHD undergoing low-risk procedure or in mild-to-moderate VHD, noninvasive monitoring under cardiac anesthesiologist and in severe VHD and high-risk noncardiac surgery whether to do under invasive hemodynamic monitoring and TEE monitoring required intra- and postoperatively in ICU has to be decided by heart team. After clinical evaluation, ECG, TTE for severity of VHD and for LV/RV size and function, and PA pressure to be assessed.[24]

Risk of noncardiac surgery increases especially with severe AS. AS is present in 1–2% in patients >65 years and 3–8% in >75 years of age. Clinical predictors of perioperative CV risks depend on symptomatic status, presence of arrhythmias, severity of valve lesions, LV function, level of PAP, and comorbidities including ischemic heart disease. Cardiovascular risk can also be stratified according to the different noncardiac surgical procedures. And their risks also. Left-sided regurgitant lesions are better tolerated but still have a high risk **(Flowchart 2)**.

Preoperative Clinical Evaluation

Symptoms such as dyspnea, angina, syncope or HF, and arrhythmias such as AF should be recorded. Physical examination, ECG, echocardiogram for severity of valve disease, LV function, PAP, etc. to be evaluated.

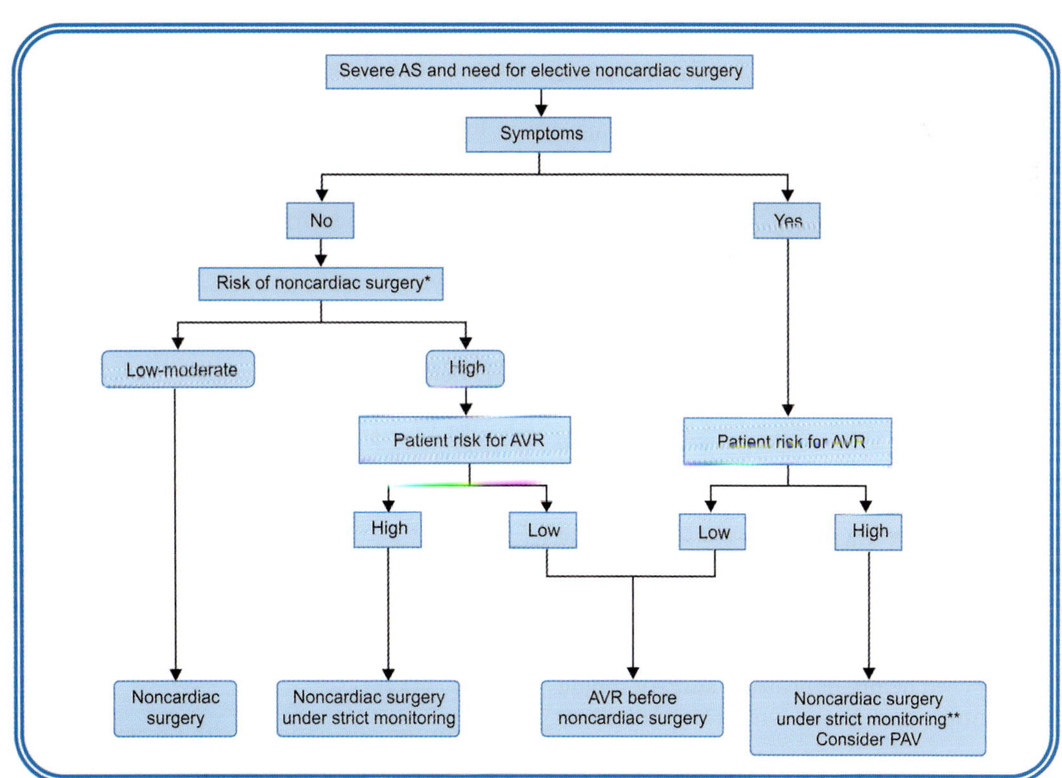

* See legend.

** Noncardiac surgery performed only if strictly needed.

FLOWCHART 2: Algorithm for noncardiac surgery in severe aortic stenosis patients.

(AS: aortic stenosis; AVR: aortic valve replacement; PAV: percutaneous aortic valvuloplasty)

Factors	Criteria for diagnosis or threshold
Coronary artery disease	Distant myocardial infarct, positive exercise test, current angina, use of nitrates, and Q waves
Heart failure	History of heart failure, S3 and rales, chest X-ray evidence
Cerebrovascular disease	History of stroke or transient ischemic attack
Diabetes	On insulin
Renal failure	Creatinine >l.60 µmol/L
Age	>70

Note: The presence of two or more factors is taken as high risk.

Management of symptomatic patients with VHD undergoing noncardiac surgery: They benefit from valve interventions before the surgery. They have to be assessed further as per revised cardiac index risk score and out of the following factors, if two or more factors are present then the risk is high and to be counseled accordingly **(Table 6)**.

SPECIFIC VALVE LESIONS

Mitral Stenosis

Rheumatic heart disease MS may be poorly tolerated because of altered hemodynamics of anesthesia and noncardiac surgery. In nonsignificant MS (Mv area >1.5 cm^2), noncardiac surgery can be performed at low risk. In asymptomatic patients with significant MS and PA systolic pressure <50 mm Hg, noncardiac surgery can be performed at low risk except if AF develops, then there can be a sharp deterioration. Still, severe MS patients undergoing surgery need invasive hemodynamic monitoring to optimize loading conditions. Maintenance of LV preload and SR is required in perioperative phase to avoid pulmonary edema and to maintain CO and PCWP. Tachycardia has to be avoided.

In asymptomatic severe MS with PA pressure > 50 mm Hg and symptomatic severe MS patients with PA systolic pressure >50 mm Hg, correction of MS by means of PTMC, whenever possible depending on the suitability of the valve, should be attempted before noncardiac surgery. This recommendation is stronger before high-risk noncardiac procedures.

If surgery, in particular valve replacement, is needed, then decision to proceed before noncardiac surgery should be taken with caution and based on strict individual considerations.

Aortic Stenosis

Several studies have shown that severe AS with AV area (<1 cm^2) increases the risk of noncardiac surgery. Risk is 10–30%. Recommendations for the management are in significant AS with normal LV function who need urgent noncardiac surgery where surgery has to be performed under careful hemodynamic monitoring both intra- and postoperatively, better to optimize periprocedural loading conditions and avoiding hypotension and tachycardia which can increase ischemia, arrhythmias, myocardial injury, cardiac failure, and death. Hence, right heart catheter and intraoperative TEE help and continue monitoring 24–48 hours after noncardiac surgery. General anesthesia is safe. Anesthetic agents are chosen to maintain SR and normotension. Phenylephrine, noradrenaline to increase BP if no significant CAD. For hypertension, CCBs are useful. Epidural and spinal anesthetic interventions to be modified to avoid rapid changes in systemic pressures using only high dilution neuraxial local anesthetic agents in combination with opioids. When elective surgery is required, the risk of cardiac complications during surgery should be balanced with the risk and benefit of having the valve replaced (Surgical AVR/TAVI) before noncardiac surgery.

If moderate or severe AS, hemodynamic effects of anesthesia and surgery are poorly tolerated. Predictors of adverse outcomes are severity of AS, coexisting MR, PAH, and CAD. They need hemodynamic monitoring and optimization of loading conditions in AS.

In asymptomatic patients with severe AS, a noncardiac procedure of low- or moderate-risk can be performed safely. If high-risk noncardiac surgery is needed, then patient should be carefully evaluated for AVR before noncardiac surgery including coronary angiogram (CAG) to rule out associated coronary artery disease (CAD).

In asymptomatic patients who are poor candidates for AVR because of comorbidities or poor life expectancy, noncardiac surgery to be carefully discussed and, if really needed, to be performed under strict intraoperative and perioperative hemodynamic monitoring.

In symptomatic patients with severe AS undergoing noncardiac surgery, valve replacement (SAVR/TAVI) should always be considered depending on age and associated CAD before noncardiac surgery at low-to-moderate risk. If valve replacement is contraindicated, noncardiac surgery should be performed only, if absolutely necessary. In hemodynamically unstable patients with high risk for AVR, percutaneous BAV as a bridging strategy may be an option to create a time window of reduced cardiac risk during which the noncardiac surgery can be considered and may have a role depending on local expertise.[24]

Aortic Regurgitation and Mitral Regurgitation

In asymptomatic patients with preserved LV function and severe MR/AR, with PA pressure <50 mm Hg, noncardiac surgery can be performed at low risk. But, avoid increase afterload bradycardia. General anesthesia decreases SVR. Hence, invasive hemodynamic monitoring and intraoperative TEE monitoring to optimize LV-filling pressures during operation and postoperatively up to 72 hours in ICU also, monitoring is required. In severe AR, increased volume load can lead to increased myocardial wall stress because of noncardiac surgery, hypotension, arrhythmias, HF, postoperative MI, stroke, pulmonary edema can occur versus patients without AR. Decreased LV function, serum creatinine >2 mg/dL, and intermediate-to-high-risk noncardiac surgery were predictors of cardiopulmonary complications and death. Hence, they need intra- and postoperative monitoring strictly. In symptomatic patients with standard indications, valve repair/replacement to be performed before noncardiac surgery. In patients with depressed LV function (EF < 30%), noncardiac surgery should be performed only if strictly needed. The medical therapy of HF should be optimized before surgery with drugs for HFrEF as per GDMT which are particularly useful in such patients.[24]

Prosthetic Valves

If there are no symptoms or signs of prosthetic valve dysfunction by clinical examination and echocardiogram, noncardiac surgery can be safely performed. However, there is a high risk mostly related to the changes in anticoagulation regimen in patients with mechanical valves. Thus, management of anticoagulation is of utmost importance in these circumstances. Although prophylactic antibiotic therapy is aimed primarily at reducing staphylococcal infection and is now routinely used at the time of prosthetic valve implantation, few studies have evaluated prophylactic measures against the development of PVE. Because the presence of a prosthetic heart valve is a predisposition to the development of endocarditis, antibiotic therapy, or prophylaxis, at the time of healthcare-related procedures, has been a mainstay of care of the patient with a prosthetic valve. However, prophylaxis is recommended only for patients with prosthetic heart valves prior to dental procedures, but not before gastrointestinal or genitourinary procedures.[13]

Endocarditis Prophylaxis

In valve disease patients, all surgical procedures even minor require scrupulous asepsis and avoidance of wound hematoma formation. Antibiotic prophylaxis should be prescribed for those patients undergoing noncardiac procedures at high bacteremic risks.[9]

Perioperative Monitoring

Patients requiring moderate- or high-risk noncardiac surgical procedures need hemodynamic monitoring and perioperative care to avoid volume overload or volume depletion and hypotension, especially in patients with AS. In patients with moderate-to-severe AS or MS, MR, AR, it is better to electively admit such patients to intensive care postoperatively even if they appear to be doing well.[4]

Summary

Management depends on the type and urgency/emergency of noncardiac surgery, the revised cardiac index risk score, stage of valve disease, presence of symptoms, functional class, urgency or necessity of noncardiac surgery, and presence of comorbidities. Adverse events of noncardiac surgery often occur with presence of coronary artery disease and hemodynamic aspects of valve disease and if VHD is severe and symptomatic, it needs surgery or interventions before a noncardiac surgery.[29]

■ INFECTIVE ENDOCARDITIS

Burden of Infective Endocarditis

Total number of DALYs due to endocarditis has risen steadily since 1990 reaching 1.72 million DALYs and 66.300 deaths in 2019. Global burden of CV diseases estimated 1.09 million incident cases of endocarditis in 2019. Age-standardized rates show an increase in incidence from 9.9/100,000 as well as deaths from 0.7/100,000 to 0.9/100,000. This may be explained by an increasing proportion of endocarditis caused by virulent organisms such as *Staphylococcus* or complex infection patients who are not fit for surgery. At global level, more DALYs were lost by men than women till a peak 55–59 years for men and 65–69 years for women, where women >75 years had more DALYs versus men. Lowest DALYs for endocarditis were seen in central and east Asia. Epidemiology of endocarditis including predisposing conditions is heterogeneous. *Staphylococcus* endocarditis is the predominant pathogen in most parts of the world and is extremely virulent and a marker of worst outcomes. Hence, efforts to be focused on management and prevention of this life threatening condition.[2]

The incidence of IE has not decreased over the past 30 years. It is recognized as a disease associated with poor dentition and RHD. The development of IE involves a complex interaction between the host and the invading microorganisms, which includes the vascular endothelium, hemostatic mechanisms, cardiac anatomical and hemodynamic characteristics, the surface properties, and the enzyme and toxin production by the microorganisms and the host immune system.[14] The endothelial lining of the heart and valves is generally resistant to bacterial or fungal infection. A few highly virulent organisms such as *Staphylococcus aureus* are capable of infecting apparently normal heart valves but this is uncommon. The majority of patients who develop IE have preexisting structural abnormalities, mostly due to RHD. A detailed description of the clinical microbiology is beyond the scope of this chapter. The diagnosis of IE is based upon clinical suspicion derived from signs and symptoms and, most importantly, the demonstration of associated bacteremia. The modified Duke criteria are used for making the diagnosis of IE as given in **Table 7**.[15]

It is relatively uncommon and a severe disease carrying high mortality of 30% at 1 year. Epidemiology and management have drastically changed in past two decades in western countries where infective endocarditis (IE) is a healthcare-related disease in elderly patients early after heart valve surgery. True burden is unknown because of scarcity of data from low-income countries (LIC). In few studies, RHD was found to be the underlying valve disease in 5.4–77% of cases. It differs between countries in which RHD is eradicated versus endemic countries. Guidelines have reduced role of antibiotic prophylaxis before dental procedures because of lack of scientific evidence of reduction of IE burden while using prophylaxis. Uncertain to be the same in LMICs where dental hygiene is much poorer. Higher incidence of IE caused by *Streptococcus* species in endemic RHD population raises questions regarding indication for prophylaxis before dental procedures. Dental health policies to be promoted as a general recommendation for all RHD patients in LMICs.[3]

Infective endocarditis is fatal unless treated appropriately. All are symptomatic. In-hospital mortality is 15–20% with 1-year mortality nearing 40%. For diagnosis and management of patients' heart valve MDT including infectious disease experts. Cardiac imaging, TTE, TEE, CT, and CT/PET imaging are critical for diagnosis of IE and transfer to comprehensive valve center for management. Blood cultures are positive in 90% provided ≥2 blood culture samples obtained at different times with all aseptic techniques ideally >6 hours apart at peripheral sites before

TABLE 7: Modified Duke criteria and case definitions of infective endocarditis (IE).

Modified Duke criteria	*Case definitions*
Major criteria *Blood culture positive for IE*: • Typical microorganisms consistent with IE from two separate blood cultures: Viridans streptococci, *Streptococcus bovis*, HACEK group, *Staphylococcus aureus* or community acquired enterococci in the absence of a primary focus • Microorganisms consistent with IE from persistently positive blood cultures defined as follows: at least two positive cultures of blood samples drawn >12 hours apart or all of three or a majority of ≥4 separate cultures of blood (with first and last sample drawn at least 1 h apart) • Single positive blood culture for *Coxiella burnetii* or anti-phase 1 IgG antibody titer > 1:800 *Evidence of endocardial involvement*: Echocardiogram positive for IE [TEE recommended for patients with prosthetic valves, rated at least "possible IE" by clinical criteria or complicated IE (paravalvular abscess); TTE as first test in other patients] defined as follows: • Oscillating intracardiac mass on valve or supporting structures, in the path of regurgitant jets or on implanted material in the absence of an alternative anatomic explanation • Abscess • New partial dehiscence of prosthetic valve • New valvular regurgitation (worsening or changing or preexisting murmur not sufficient) **Minor criteria:** • *Predisposition*: Predisposing heart condition or injection drug use • Fever, temperature > 38°C • Vascular phenomena, major arterial emboli, septic pulmonary infarcts, mycotic aneurysm, intracranial hemorrhage, conjunctival hemorrhages, and Janeway's lesions • *Immunologic phenomena*: Glomerulonephritis, Osler's nodes, Roth's spots, and rheumatoid factor • *Microbiological evidence*: Positive blood culture but does not meet a major criterion as noted above or serological evidence of active infection with organism consistent with IE	**Definite infective endocarditis** *Pathological criteria*: • Microorganisms demonstrated by culture or histological examination of a vegetation, a vegetation that has embolized or an intracardiac abscess specimen • *Pathological lesions*: Vegetation or intracardiac abscess confirmed by histological examination showing active endocarditis *Clinical criteria*: • two major criteria • one major criterion and three minor criteria • five minor criteria *Possible IE*: • one major criterion and one minor criterion or • three minor criteria *Rejected*: • Firm alternative diagnosis explaining evidence of IE • Resolution of IE syndrome with antibiotic therapy for <4 days • No pathological evidence of IE at surgery or autopsy, with antibiotic therapy for <4 days • Does not meet criteria for possible IE as above

antimicrobial therapy. In 10% culture negative patients, serological testing including polymerase chain reaction (PCR) helps to identify etiological agent. Modified Dukes criteria are well validated. Three-fourths of IE patients are diagnosed within 30 days of onset of IE even though peripheral signs and embolic/immunological phenomenon are rare. Stroke (16.9%), peripheral embolism other than stroke (22.6%), HF (32.3%), intracardiac abscess (14.4%), and need for surgery (48.2%) remain common. TTE sensitity 50–90%, specificity >90% for vegetation in native valve endocarditis but sensitivity of 36.69% in prosthetic valve endocarditis (PVE) but quantifies valve dysfunction, paravalvular leaks, ventricular size, systolic function and PA pressures and for AV assessment, but TEE is better for vegetations and abscesses, pericardial effusion. TEE sensitivity 90–100% in native valve endocarditis (NVE), slightly less in PVE, to detect complications, valve regurgitation, fistulae, intracardiac thrombi, intraoperative assessment and management. HF, paravalvular extension, and embolic events are three most severe complications and main indications for early surgery, which are performed in 50% of patients. Hence, repeat examination and imaging should be indicated to detect these complications. Paravalvular fistula and pseudoaneurysms occur over time and repeat TEE required to detect them because of long active phase and fluctuating course of the disease. Intraoperative TEE for assessment of anatomic, hemodynamic, and as a monitoring tool during surgery and quality of intended surgical result.[24]

In recently published randomized POET trial (Partial Oral Treatment of Endocarditis), 4,000 patients of stable left-sided IE caused by *Streptococcus, Enterococcus faecalis, Staphylococcus aureus*, or coagulase-negative *Staphylococcus* on IV antibiotics for initial 10 days randomized to usual care or discharged to ambulatory treatment with oral antibiotics and reassessed by TEE within 1–3 days of completion of therapy to confirm sufficient response to therapy. Primary outcome was composite of all-cause mortality, unplanned cardiac surgery, embolic events, or relapse of bacteremia with primary pathogen. At 6 months after antibiotic treatment completion, the switch to early oral antibiotic therapy was noninferior to traditional long-term IV therapy. IE with *S. aureus* bacteremia involves normal cardiac valves, and clinical examination may not be sufficient and TEE helps to diagnose IV catheter-associated *S. aureus* bacteremia. Intracardiac electronic devices or high-risk IE such as PVE or their associated complications. It has disabling, life-threatening sequelae, and has mortality of 19–65%, HF (20–50%), paravalvular cardiac abscess (30–40%), and systemic embolization (40%). In contrast, PVE has lower incidence of vegetation in mechanical prosthesis and high incidence of annular abscess and other paravalvular complications. Even clinical examination has limited help, TEE is helpful in these high-risk patients with serial evaluations. ECG synchronized MDCT to detect complications of IE and in right-sided IE to detect septic pulmonary infarcts and abscesses and paravalvular complications, but less effective in valve vegetation or perforations. Preoperative

evaluation for AV infective endocarditis and coronary arteries and aortic involvement. CT evaluates mechanical valve occluders motion with fluoroscopy as an adjunct for obstructive valve disease. Abnormal 18-FDG PET/CT uptake at initial presentation of PVE enabled to diagnose definite IE by experienced in technology as false positives can occur because of sterile inflammation can occur in implanted prosthetic valves. It can be complimentary also in native valve IE (NVIE). TEE helps in the setting of *Staphylococcus* bacteremia in 30% of cases.[24]

"Culture-negative" Endocarditis

Blood cultures are negative in only approximately 5–10% of patients with IE confirmed by strict diagnostic criteria.[16,17] This may be due to several factors: (1) the prior administration of antibiotics, (2) cultures taken toward the end of a chronic course (longer than 3 months), (3) uremia supervening in a chronic course, (4) mural endocarditis as in ventricular septal defects, postmyocardial infarction thrombi, or infection related to pacemaker wires, (5) slow growth of fastidious organisms such as anaerobes, (6) subacute right-sided endocarditis, (7) fungal endocarditis, and (8) endocarditis caused by obligate intracellular parasites, such as *Rickettsiae, Chlamydiae, Tropheryma whipplei*, and perhaps viruses or noninfective endocarditis or an incorrect diagnosis.[18]

Echocardiography is standard clinical practice in evaluating patients with suspected IE. Echocardiographic findings that provide specific evidence of IE include vegetations, evidence of periannular tissue destruction (abscess), aneurysm, fistula, leaflet perforation, and valvular dehiscence. **Table 8** outlines specific definitions of these characteristics.[19] Both transthoracic and transesophageal echocardiography have an important role in the diagnosis and management of patients with suspected IE **(Figs. 5 and 6)**.

General Management including Antibiotic Therapy in Infective Endocarditis

Infective endocarditis has evolved over the last few decades with the improvements in diagnostic capabilities and therapy.[20,21] Rapid diagnosis, early risk stratification, and institution of appropriate antibiotic therapy have improved survival in IE by 70–80% and have been shown to reduce the incidence of complications of IE. Detailed descriptions of antibiotic regimens for specific causative IE organisms are found in recent, comprehensive guidelines by the AHA and the European Society of Cardiology.[15,22] Although the choice of antimicrobial therapy is mainly guided by the infecting organism and its antibiotic susceptibilities, there are basic tenets of antibiotic treatment for the eradication of native valve infection. First, a prolonged course of antibiotic treatment (4–6 weeks) is necessary to eradicate infection because bacterial concentration within vegetations is as high as 10^9-10^{11} CFUs/g of tissue and organisms deep

TABLE 8: Echocardiographic findings in infective endocarditis.

Echocardiographic finding	Description
Vegetation	• Highly mobile, irregular, fuzzy echogenic mass • Adherent to leaflets or prosthetic valve • Oscillation of mass (supportive, not mandatory)
Abscess	• Thickened area or mass within the myocardium or valve annulus • Evidence of flow into region (supportive, not mandatory)
Aneurysm	ECHO lucent space with thin surrounding tissue
Fistula	Blood flow between two distinct cardiac blood spaces or chambers through abnormal path/channel
Leaflet perforation	Defect in body of valve leaflet with flow through defect
Valve dehiscence	Prosthetic valve with abnormal rocking motion/excursion >15° in at least one direction

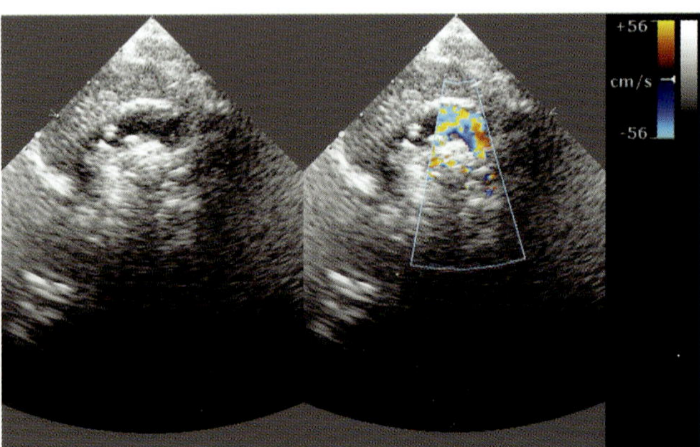

FIG. 5: A 6-year-old sick looking boy with rheumatic heart disease, who came for fitness for surgery, had multiple vegetations in the aortic arch.

within vegetations are inaccessible to phagocytic cells.[23,30] If surgery is performed for IE, completion of the 4–6 weeks course of antibiotic therapy is generally favored to reduce the risk of recurrent IE. Second, parenteral administration of antibiotic therapy is necessary to achieve adequate drug levels required to eradicate infection. Parenteral therapy is typically initiated in the hospital setting and the patient may receive outpatient, parenteral treatment for the remaining duration after an initial period of observation to assess for clinical response to therapy (e.g., clearance of bacteremia and absence of complications).

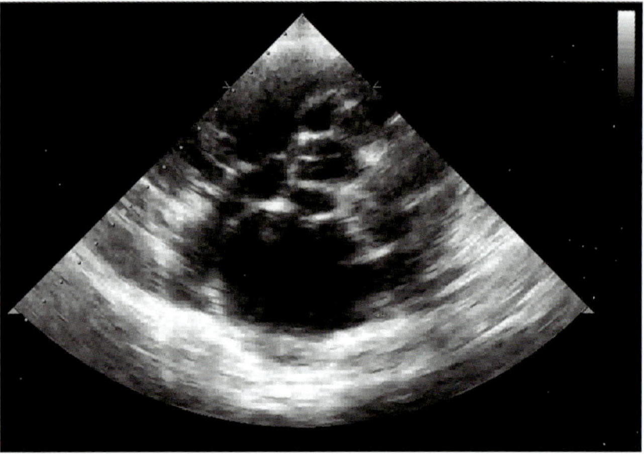

FIG. 6: A 28-year-old pregnant lady with rheumatic heart disease with multiple aortic annular abscesses.

Antimicrobial Therapy

Optimal management requires multidisciplinary approach involving IE team on the levels of heart team for quick inter-faculty consultation and rapid initiation of definitive therapy. In observation studies, mortality has decreased by 50% versus controls over 1–3 years of observational studies by MDT. Drawbacks of antimicrobial therapy, antibiotic resistance, longer duration of therapy, prolonged hospital stay, and antecedent mortality. Resistance (1) biofilm by bacteria especially coagulase negative *Staphylococcus* hindering the bacterial penetration. New treatment of combination of monoclonal antibody-TRLI 1068 and daptomycin appears promising. IV antibiotics for 4–6 weeks as per culture sensitivity reports and dose advocated as per guidelines are the standard. For infections with selected species of *Streptococcus* or methicillin-sensitive *Staphylococcus* with MIC of antibiotics as per c/s reports have shown a cure over 2 weeks especially those who have undergone surgery. Oral antibiotic therapy with a combination of rifampicin and ciprofloxacin in the right-sided IE caused by methicillin-sensitive *Staphylococcus* of native valve has good results in IV drug abusers. As told before in POET trial, partial oral treatment of endocarditis, which enrolled patients with gram positive (*Streptococcus, Staphylococcus,* and *Enterococcus*) IE to receive initial IV antibiotics therapy for 10 days followed by TEE and by oral therapy versus continued IV therapy with a composite endpoint of death, embolism, and recurrence of IE. Switchover to oral therapy was noninferior to continued IV therapy. OPAT outpatient parenteral antibiotic therapy—initial in-hospital IV followed by outpatient or home-based IV therapy under strict vigil may be offered to selected stable patients who have shown excellent clinical response and have shown rapid culture negativity and not having HF, large vegetation, annular abscess, conduction abnormality, or renal derangement.[31]

Specific Recommendations

Apart from guideline-based antibiotic regimen, rifampicin should be used in foreign body infection, such as PVE after 3–5 days of IV antibiotics use (once the bacteremia has cleared) as rifampicin has antagonistic effect with other antibiotics for replicating bacteria and synergistic effect on dormant bacteria in biofilms, which are prevalent in PVE. Aminoglycoside use is now not recommended for Staphylococcal NVE as its benefit is less and has renal toxicity. Daptomycin > 10 mg/kg/day and fosfomycin are recommended for staphylococcal infections and netilmycin for streptococcal IE but have limited availability. Empirical treatment for both native as well as late PVE should cover Staphylococci, Streptococci, and Enterococci. Early PVE should cover methicillin-resistant *Staphylococcus aureus* (MRSA), *Enterococcus*, and non-HACEK organisms.

Surgery in Infective Endocarditis

Surgical intervention may be performed either in the acute/active phase of IE or after the eradication. A major controversy regarding cardiac surgery in IE is the potential risk of neurologic deterioration caused by cardiopulmonary bypass in patients who have experienced a cerebrovascular complication from embolization of vegetation on the valve **(Fig. 7)**. Surgery during the active phase is generally considered for: (1) those patients in whom the likelihood of cure of infection with antibiotic therapy alone is low or (2) those in whom severe complications of IE have or are likely to occur.[32] Surgery after eradication of infection is predominantly performed for adverse hemodynamic effects of valvular regurgitation that results from valve damage.

Indications for Surgery in Infective Endocarditis

In uncontrolled HF, uncontrolled infection, and complications of IE such as abscess, heart blocks, and recurrent emboli and women who had higher in-hospital and 1-year mortality than men despite similar comorbidities as per ACC/AHA 2020 guidelines, ESC has indicated timings for interventions as emergent within 24 hours, urgent within 7 days, or elective after 1–2 weeks of antibiotic therapy. Up to 50% of patients require surgery for IE. The principal indications are: (1) HF: (A) cardiogenic shock as a result of progressive native or prosthetic valve obstruction/regurgitation or fistula formation—emergency surgery (<24 hours), (B) severe valve disease and symptoms of HF and a poor hemodynamic response—urgent surgery (<7 days); (2) Failure to control infection—urgent surgery: (A) local ongoing infection—aortic root abscess, Aneurysm or fistula formation, expanding vegetation size, (B) infection with a difficult to treat organism

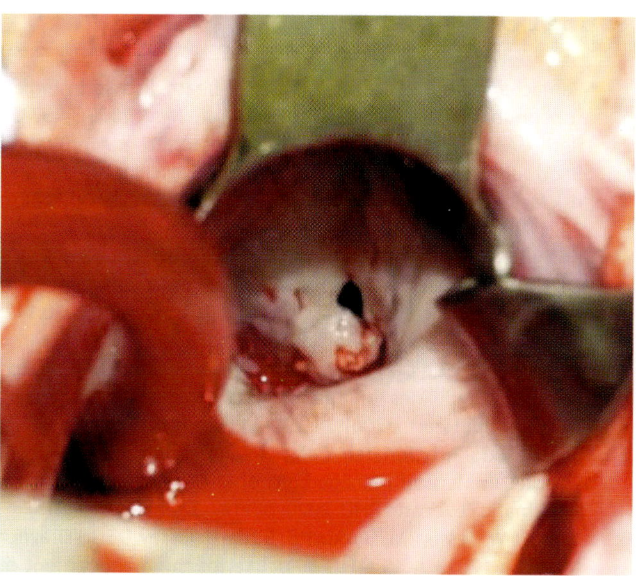

FIG. 7: Vegetation on the mitral valve, as seen on the operating table.

(fungi or multiresistant organism, staphylococci or non-HACEK gram-negative bacilli on a prosthetic valve), (C) persistance of positive blood cultures despite appropriate antibiotics or inadequate control of metastatic septic foci. (3) prevention of septic emboli—urgent surgery: (A) vegetation >10 mm with an embolic event while on appropriate antibiotic therapy, (B) vegetation > 30 mm, (C) vegetation >10 mm and severe native or prosthetic valve disease and patient is at a low-operative risk.[33]

■ CONCLUSION

The medical management of patients with RHD requires an integrated understanding of pathophysiology and natural history and prevention of IE. While surgical intervention is often required, medical treatment may, in some circumstances, retard the progression of valvular and ventricular dysfunction and reduce associated complications. Patients with RHD commonly require treatment for other associated conditions especially during pregnancy and during noncardiac surgery, as severe hemodynamic changes causing acute burden on the heart can occur. The medical treatment of patients with RHD is closely linked to an established schedule of clinical and echocardiographic follow-up, as dictated by the specific valve lesion and its anticipated natural history. There are, at present, no specific medical therapies available to arrest the progression of native valve disease. Prevention of IE is very important as management after IE has occurred is very tedious and difficult.

◼ REFERENCES

1. Ramachandran M, Ponniah T. Valvular heart disease in Indian subcontinent: Social issues. Indian J Comm Med. 2009;34:57-8.

2. Roth GA, Mensah GA, Johnson CO, Addolorato G, Ammirati E, Baddour LM, et al. Global burden of cardiovascular disease and risk factors, 1990-2019: Update From the GBD 2019 Study. JACC. 2020;76(25):2982-3021.

3. Krishna Kumar R, Antunes MJ, Beaton A, Mirabel M, Nkomo VT, Okello E, et al. Contemporary diagnosis and management of RHD: A Scientific statement from AHA. Circulation. 2020;142; e337-57.

4. Vahanian A, Baumgartner H, Bax J, Butchart E, Dion R, Filippatos G, et al. Guidelines on the management of valvular heart diseases. Eur Heart J. 2007;28: 230-68.

5. Scott Dougherty,Jonatan Carapetis,Liesl zuhlke,Ngel Wilson. Chapter 6: Medical management of RHD. Textbook on Acute Rheumatic Fever and RHD. 2020. pp. 107-32.

6. Yancy CW, Jessup M, Bozkurt B, Butler J, Casey DE Jr, Drazner MH, et al. 2013 ACCF/AHA guideline for the management of heart failure. Circulation. 2013;128(16);1810-52.

7. Topol EJ. Textbook of Cardiovascular Medicine, 3rd edition. Philadelphia: Lippincott Williams & Wilkins; 2007.

8. Bonow RO, Carabello BA, Kanu C, de Leon AC Jr, Faxon DP, Freed MD, et el. ACC/AHA 2006 Guidelines for the management of patients with Valvular Heart Disease. Circulation. 2006;114:e84-231.

9. Halley CM, Thamilarasan M, Griffin BP. Mitral valve disease. In: Griffin BP, Topol EJ (Eds). Manual of Cardiovascular Medicine. Philadelphia: Lippincott Williams & Wilkins; 2009. pp. 234-5.

10. Libby P, Bonow RO, Mann DL, Zipes DP. Braunwald`s Heart Disease: A Textbook of Cardiovascular Medicine, 8th edition. Philadelphia: Saunders; 2008.

11. Reimold SC, Rutherford JD. Valvular Heart Disease in Pregnancy. N Engl J Med. 2003;349:52-9.

12. Nishimura RA, Carabello BA, Faxon DP, Freed MD, Lytle BW, O'Gara PT, et al. ACC/AHA 2008 Guideline Update on Valvular Heart Disease. J Am Coll Cardiol. 2008;52;676-85.

13. Wilson W, Taubert KA, Gewitz M, Lockhart PB, Baddour LM, Levison M, et al. Prevention of infective endocarditis. Guidelines from the American Heart Association. A Guideline From the American Heart Association Rheumatic Fever, Endocarditis, and Kawasaki Disease Committee, Council on Cardiovascular Disease in the Young, and the Council on Clinical Cardiology, Council on Cardiovascular Surgery and Anesthesia, and the Quality of Care and Outcomes Research Interdisciplinary Working Group. Circulation. 2007;116:1736-1754.

14. Moreillon P, Que YA. Infective endocarditis. Lancet. 2004;363(9403):139-49.

15. Baddour LM, Wilson WR, Bayer AS, Fowler VG Jr, Bolger AF, Levison ME, et al. Infective endocarditis: diagnosis, antimicrobial therapy, and management of complications: a statement for healthcare professionals from the Committee on Rheumatic Fever, Endocarditis, and Kawasaki Disease, Council on Cardiovascular Disease in the Young, and the Councils on Clinical Cardiology, Stroke, and Cardiovascular Surgery and Anesthesia, American Heart Association: endorsed by the Infectious Diseases Society of America. Circulation. 2005;111(23):e394-434.

16. Hoen B, Selton-Suty C, Lacassin F, Etienne J, Briançon S, Leport C, et al. Infective endocarditis in patients with negative blood cultures: analysis of 88 cases from a one year nationwide survey in France. Clin Infect Dis. 1995;20(3):501-6.

17. Tunkel AR, Kaye D. Endocarditis with negative blood cultures. N Engl J Med. 1992;326(18):1215-7.

18. Bashore TM, Cabell C, Fowler V Jr. Update on infective endocarditis. Curr Probl Cardiol. 2006;31:274-352.

19. Sachdev M, Peterson GE, Jollis JG. Imaging techniques for diagnosis of infective endocarditis. Cardiol Clin. 2003;21:185-95.

20. Durack DT, Lukes AS, Bright DK. New criteria for diagnosis of infective endocarditis: utilization of specific echocardiographic findings. Duke Endocarditis Service. Am J Med. 1994;96(3):200-9.

21. Daniel WG, Mugge A, Martin RP, Lindert O, Hausmann D, Nonnast-Daniel B, et al. Improvement in the diagnosis of abscesses associated with endocarditis by transesophageal echocardiography. N Engl J Med. 1991;324(12):795-800.

22. Horstkotte D, Follath F, Gutschik E, Lengyel M, Oto A, Pavie A, et al. Guidelines on prevention, diagnosis and treatment of infective endocarditis executive summary; the task force on infective endocarditis of the European society of cardiology. Eur Heart J. 2004;25(3):267-76.

23. Durack DT, Beeson PB. Experimental bacterial endocarditis. II. Survival of a bacteria in endocardial vegetations. Br J Exp Pathol. 1972;53(1):50-3.

24. Otto CM, Nishimura RA, Bonow RO, Carabello BA, Erwin JP 3rd, Gentile F, et al. 2020 ACC/AHA clinical practice guidelines on the management of patients with Valvular heart disease. Circulation 2021;143;e35-e71.

25. Krishnakumar S, Hari Krishnan S. Chapter 16: Atrial fibrillation in RHD. Essentials of PG Cardiology. 2019. pp. 115-7.

26. Mocumbi A, et al. Chapter 9: RHD in pregnancy. Book on ARF and RHD. 2020. pp. 171-93.

27. Katherine A, Poppas A. Rheumatic Heart Disease in Pregnancy: Global Challenges and Clear Opportunities. Circulation. 2018;137;817-9.

28. Boersma E, Kertai MD, Schouten O, Bax JJ, Noordzij P, Steyerberg EW, et al. Perioperative cardiovascular mortality in noncardiac surgery: validation of the Lee cardiac risk index. Am J Med. 2005;118:1134-41.

29. Chambers JB. Valve disease and Noncardiac surgery. Heart. 2018;0:1-10.

30. Hamburger M, Stein L. *Streptococcus viridans* subacute bacterial endocarditis; two week treatment schedule with penicillin. J Am Med Assoc. 1952;149(6):542-5.

31. Dwiwedi SK, Saran M. Chapter 24: Infective endocarditis: What is new. Essentials of Postgraduate Cardiology. 2019pp. 204-8.

32. Andrew W, Christopher HC. Infective Endocarditis. In: Andrew W, Thomas MB (Eds). Valvular Heart Disease. Totowa, New Jersey: Humana Press; 2009. pp. 123-64.

33. Rajani R, Klein JL. Infective Endocarditis: A contemporary update. Clin Med (Lond). 2020;20(1);31-5.

16

Echocardiographic Screening for Rheumatic Heart Disease

Nicola Culliford-Semmens, Bo Remenyi,
Nigel Wilson

INTRODUCTION

Acute rheumatic fever (ARF) and its long-term sequelae chronic rheumatic heart disease (RHD) are still major health problems in children, adolescents, and young adults in many developing countries. The World Health Organization (WHO) has reported in its bulletin that nearly 50% of patients with ARF carditis and RHD detected in surveys and health checkup camps are unaware of their disease.[1] More than 70% do not receive secondary prophylaxis regularly.

BACKGROUND

There are many clinical scenarios where established RHD is found in children and in adults without any prior history of ARF. Up to 50% of adults with symptomatic RHD never recall an episode of ARF and others present with bacterial endocarditis, embolic strokes, atrial arrhythmias and sudden or unexpected death.[2] Echocardiography now reveals that over half the patients with Sydenham's chorea have evidence of carditis[3,4] and 58% will progress to established RHD.[3] Indolent carditis has been recognized as a presentation of ARF[5] and these cases have usually come to attention due to symptoms and are due to continued recurrence of ARF. These multiple presentations support the notion that rheumatic carditis frequently occurs at a subclinical level with minimal or no joint symptoms.

WHY SCREEN FOR RHEUMATIC HEART DISEASE?

Bland et al.[6] followed 1,000 ARF patients meticulously from 1928 for 20 years. They found that 44% (154/347) of cases with ARF and no murmur developed mitral stenosis, most without a recognized recurrence of ARF. It seems very likely that those patients had subclinical carditis with mitral regurgitation (MR) that evolved to mitral stenosis over time. This was in the era before penicillin prophylaxis and provides evidence that subclinical cardiac involvement can progress without the intervention of secondary penicillin prophylaxis.

EVOLUTION OF SCREENING FOR RHEUMATIC HEART DISEASE

Traditional screening for RHD has been by auscultation in high prevalence regions: Pakistan,[7,8] South Africa,[9] Republic of Congo,[10] Tonga,[11] India,[12,13] and Samoa.[14] In the Waikato region in New Zealand, screening was undertaken in the 1970s but it was considered that detection rates of 6/1,000 (0.6%) would not justify screening.[15] The advent of echocardiography showed that auscultation is unreliable for RHD screening. It is neither sensitive nor specific and had significantly underestimated the burden of RHD.[16-21] Echocardiographic screening has solved the paradox of low RHD detection rates by auscultation in the face of high ARF/RHD[16-21] and is now considered to be the gold standard. Since 2004, the WHO has recommended echocardiographic screening for RHD in high prevalence regions.[22]

Studies from Cambodia,[19] Mozambique,[19] and New Zealand[21] demonstrate a 9–11% sensitivity by highly trained auscultators to detect RHD compared to echocardiography. This would imply that potentially up to 90% of the children with RHD would miss out on penicillin prophylaxis if echocardiography is not used as a first-line screening tool. Although in the New Zealand study[21] the specificity of normal examination for exclusion of pathological regurgitation was 97%, a good screening test requires high sensitivity not specificity.

Resource-limited countries tend to preselect patients with pathological murmurs for echocardiography. This allows a much larger population to be screened for the same dollar value.[23-25] Sadiq et al.[24] were able to screen an impressive 24,980 Pakistani children using this model. However, it is important to note that this model will invariably underestimate the burden of disease. An excellent summary of the optimal active and passive surveillance appears in the National Institute of Health (NIH)/WHO document.[26]

In 2008, Carapetis et al.[17] tested three different models of screening. A total of 980 Tongan children underwent auscultation by a medical student, then by a trained physician followed by a focused echocardiogram. The results showed that detection of a murmur by a medical student (simulating a primary healthcare worker) neither increased nor decreased the likelihood of RHD. This was due to the high prevalence of innocent murmurs among Tongan children. Even the pediatrician failed to detect pathological regurgitation and stenosis and incorrectly labeled innocent murmurs as regurgitant. In this study, the sensitivity and the specificity of a highly trained auscultator was 46% and 65%, respectively, for RHD. Their data showed that the most sensitive and specific model of screening was echocardiography, independent of clinical examination findings.

■ REQUIREMENTS FOR A POPULATION SCREENING TEST

At first sight, echocardiographic screening for RHD meets the three main requirements for disease screening listed in **Box 1**. Firstly, there is a suitable condition (RHD), secondly the condition is detectable (by echocardiography), and thirdly, it is treatable (by long-acting benzathine penicillin). A more detailed list of requirements for screening suggested by New Zealand National Health Committee[27] and the Council of Europe[28] are found on their respective websites.

BOX 1	Ideal requirements for population screening.

- Suitable condition in a latent or preclinical phase
- Suitable test
- Effective and accessible intervention
- Potential benefit of screening outweighs harm
- Health system can support all steps in screening pathway
- Consideration of social and ethical issues
- Consideration of cost-benefit issues
- High-quality evidence, ideally from randomized controlled trials, that screening reduces mortality and morbidity

Source: Screening to improve Health in New Zealand: Criteria to assess screening programs by National Health Committees.[27]

The first requirement is met par excellence as most subjects positive for RHD by echocardiography have subclinical disease which is latent and mild. They have most to gain from such a program by prevention of progressive RHD. Is the test suitable? The lack of specificity and sensitivity has previously been the "Achilles heel" of screening. The lower limit of what constitutes RHD by echocardiography is discussed later. The treatment or intervention is by long-acting penicillin which prevents recurrences of ARF[29] and progression of RHD.[30] It follows that it is unethical to begin a screening program if secondary penicillin delivery is not available in the region being screened. It is important to be aware that in short term, RHD screening will increase the prevalence of RHD within the region and additional resources will need to be allocated to effectively deliver secondary prophylaxis.

Disease Progression of Echocardiography-detected Rheumatic Heart Disease

The hypothesis that screening will reduce mortality and morbidity of RHD for the individual and subsets of the population is based on first principles of the pathogenesis of rheumatic fever, and this underpins the rationale of screening. Obtaining high-level evidence that screening reduces the incidence of severe RHD in a high-prevalence ARF and RHD region, using a large program with good follow-up over 5–10 years is achievable.

There have been at least 10 longitudinal follow-up studies of children with latent RHD reported, with median follow-up between 2 and 7 years.[31] Follow-up data show variable outcomes in terms of disease progression; however, studies are difficult to compare due to use of differing definitions of progression and inclusion criteria. Some studies which have shown benzathine penicillin to be ineffective in preventing progression of latent RHD have been underpowered to show a difference in progression between groups or have included children with moderate-to-severe RHD.

By 2021, Beaton et al. completed the GOAL trial,[32] a randomized controlled trial of secondary antibiotic prophylaxis in Uganda for 800 children with mild RHD using 4-weekly injections of benzathine benzyl penicillin G or no prophylaxis. The study excluded those with moderate or severe RHD, assigning them as missed clinical cases. Thus, only mild RHD cases were randomized. After only 2 years follow-up, there was a statistically significant difference in rates of progression of RHD. Fewer than 1% of the prophylaxis group progressed, compared with an 8% progression in the control group.[33] This landmark study, with its large cohort, is the missing data required to confirm all requirements for population screening: there is an effective treatment for mild echocardiographically-detected RHD. Logistical issues will remain for roll out of programs in most regions with high prevalence RHD.

ECHOCARDIOGRAPHIC CRITERIA

When the first echocardiographic screening studies were performed, there was not a standardized guideline for echocardiographic diagnosis of RHD, and thus different criteria were adopted. In 2005, a consensus case definition of RHD was established by a WHO expert panel consultation at the 16th Lancefield Symposium in Cairns, Australia.[26]

In 2012, the World Heart Federation (WHF) criteria for echocardiographic diagnosis of RHD were published. These criteria were based on the best echocardiographic, surgical, and pathologic evidence available.[34] The WHF criteria classify echocardiograms as *Definite RHD, Borderline RHD* or *Normal*. These criteria have been widely adopted by screening programs and used by clinicians as the current gold standard for definitions of mild RHD. The criteria have been found to enable reproducible categorization for RHD in a study of 200 cases read by 15 echocardiographic readers.[35]

Echocardiographic criteria for definite RHD require both morphological and color-Doppler abnormality of either the aortic or mitral valves, pathological mitral stenosis, or borderline disease of both the mitral and aortic valves. Borderline RHD, a category used for individuals under the age of 20 years, is defined as either regurgitation on color-Doppler (usually) or morphological changes (less frequently) but not both **(Table 1)**.

For left heart valve regurgitation to be regarded as pathological, the regurgitation jet must meet the four color-Doppler criteria listed in **Table 2**. These four color-Doppler features require further explanation:

1. *Mitral regurgitation and aortic regurgitation (AR) must be seen in a minimum of two views:* Any two of the parasternal long axis (PSLA), parasternal short axis (PSSA), apical four-chamber (A4C) or apical two-chamber (A2C) views. Eccentric jets of color Doppler can be missed from any window unless the operator uses sweeps as utilized in pediatric or congenital echocardiographic imaging.

2. *Mitral regurgitation jet length*: The spatial determinants of the regurgitant jet depend on orifice size, pressure difference, and whether the jet travels freely into the left atrium (LA) or hits a wall of the LA before its energy dissipates.[36-39] In assessment of severe lesions, cardiology practice places more importance on the proximal jet width than length.[40] RHD screening more often involves mild MR and length is more useful as a discriminator. There is a tendency for a recorded freeze frame image of a color jet to appear more impressive than the same color jet reviewed on a cine-loop.

   Aortic regurgitation jet length: Physiological AR occurs in about 1% of children with a normal trileaflet aortic valve.[41-43] To avoid false positive diagnosis of RHD, a minimum jet length of 1 cm is required.

3. *High velocity > 3 m/s*: Confirm that the jet is high velocity using imaging windows that are parallel to the blood flow (A4C or A2C for MR and A5C for AR). Due to the principles of Doppler physics, this feature needs confirmation in one view only.

4. *Holosystolic (MR) or holodiastolic (AR)*: This needs confirmation in one view only. The best imaging window to confirm whether an MR jet is holosystolic (or AR is

TABLE 2: World Heart Federation (WHF) criteria for pathological regurgitation.[34]

Pathological mitral regurgitation (all four Doppler criteria must be met)	Pathological aortic regurgitation (all four Doppler criteria must be met)
Seen in two views	Seen in two views
In at least one view, jet length ≥ 2 cm	In at least one view, jet length ≥ 1 cm
Velocity ≥ 3 m/s for one complete envelope	Velocity ≥ 3 m/s for one complete envelope
Pansystolic jet in at least one envelope	Pandiastolic jet in at least one envelope

TABLE 1: World Heart Federation (WHF) criteria for diagnosis of borderline and definite rheumatic heart disease (RHD).[34]

Individuals aged ≤20 years		Individuals aged >20 years
Definite RHD	**Borderline RHD**	**Definite RHD**
A. Pathological MR and at least two morphological features of RHD of the MV	A. At least two morphological features of RHD of the MV without pathological MR or MS	A. Pathological MR and at least two morphological features of RHD of the MV
B. MS mean gradient ≥4 mm Hg	B. Pathological MR	B. MS mean gradient ≥4 mm Hg
C. Pathological AR and at least two morphological features of RHD of the AV	C. Pathological AR	C. Pathological AR and at least two morphological features of RHD of the AV (only in individuals <35 years)
D. Borderline disease of both the AV and MV		D. Pathological AR and at least two morphological features of the MV

(AR: aortic regurgitation; AV: aortic valve; MR: mitral regurgitation; MS: mitral stenosis; MV: mitral valve)

TABLE 3: World Heart Federation (WHF) morphological criteria for rheumatic heart disease.[34]

Mitral valve morphologic features	Aortic valve morphologic features
AMVL thickening ≥ 3 mm (age specific)[34]	Irregular or focal thickening
Chordal thickening	Coaptation defect
Restricted leaflet motion	Restricted leaflet motion
Excessive leaflet tip motion during systole	Prolapse
(AMVL: anterior mitral valve leaflet)	

BOX 2 — Differential diagnosis of rheumatic heart disease in school aged children.

- Upper limit of physiological mitral valve regurgitation
- Congenital heart disease with mitral regurgitation, e.g., primum or secundum atrial septal defect
- Congenital mitral valve prolapse or floppy mitral valve syndrome*
- Infective endocarditis
- Congenital malformation of the mitral valve, e.g., double orifice MV, parachute MV, Hammock MV, funnel-shaped MV or cleft MV

*May be associated with abnormal body habitus, Marfan syndrome or other connective tissue disorders.

(MV: mitral valve)

holodiastolic) is the A4C (A5C for AR) view as the jet is well aligned to the Doppler beam.

In the authors' experience, reviewing many individual echocardiograms from screening programs undertaken prior to the development of the WHF criteria, requirements 3 and 4 are frequently omitted which place undue reliance on color in borderline lesions. If the regurgitant jet is not high velocity and holosystolic, then by definition the jet should be classified as physiological.

The morphological features of RHD as described in the WHF criteria are listed in **Table 3**.

It is of great importance that physicians who are part of RHD screening programs are familiar with the differential diagnoses of RHD; these are listed in **Box 2**. Unskilled or overzealous echocardiography interpretation, without understanding the range of differential diagnosis, can lead to false positive diagnosis of RHD.

In summary, echocardiography is more accurate than auscultation for RHD screening but as outlined above, there are some limitations. The WHF criteria provide the gold standard for echocardiographic identification of RHD and have allowed standardization between screening programs.

MODELS OF SCREENING

Most echocardiographic screening programs have been school-based, primarily for logistical reasons. The optimal age for screening for RHD is still debated. Screening new school entrants at the age of 5 or 6 will be ineffective as the prevalence of RHD is low. The peak incidence of ARF is 10–12 years and this is a practical age to perform echocardiography as body habitus is not large, which means few children have difficult echocardiographic images. Screening of older adolescents may reveal a higher prevalence of RHD, but in many countries the proportion attending school will have fallen significantly by the age of 15 years. Targeted screening for high-risk groups such as family members of RHD cases[44,45] and pregnant women[46] have been proposed and could have the most impact in terms of numbers screened.

EQUIPMENT: EVOLUTION OF ECHOCARDIOGRAPHY MACHINES

Hospital-based large echocardiography machines are not usually available for RHD screening programs as they are in use in busy cardiology departments. The cost of a modern echocardiogram machine can be several hundred thousand dollars, and this, with the cost of fully trained echocardiography technicians, makes their use for RHD screening nonviable on an economic basis. The advent of lower cost portable echocardiography equipment has meant that population-based RHD screening in the "field" has become a reality. RHD screening is usually school based, but epidemiologically sound community-based programs such as that in Leon, Nicaragua are achievable in the hospital or clinic setting.[20] There is now a choice of second and third generation portable machines weighing between 5 and 12 kg, the size of a laptop computer. The next evolution was to use handheld machines.[47-49] This makes RHD screening feasible even in remote areas without electricity, using machines with long-battery duration or with the aid of small portable generators. Beaton et al. in Uganda using handheld machines showed high accuracy when compared to standard portable echocardiography.[47] Of note, the handheld ultrasound machines currently available do not have the Doppler capabilities required to diagnose RHD as per the WHF criteria so a confirmatory full echocardiogram may be required.

LOGISTIC AND PRACTICAL ISSUES OF RHEUMATIC HEART DISEASE ECHOCARDIOGRAPHY SCREENING

It is important to note that the echocardiographic modalities required for RHD echocardiography screening are basic two dimensional and color-Doppler imaging. Several studies have shown that noncardiac expert healthworkers, such as nurses, can be trained to perform simplified echocardiograms to detect RHD.[50-54] This has been termed as "task-shifting". Online courses are available for RHD echocardiographic training.[55-57]

The majority of RHD echocardiograms are taken "in the field" usually in school rooms. It is essential to ensure that the rooms are darkened to standards used in hospital settings, as acquiring images in a lit room impairs image quality and compromises interpretation. Interpretation of RHD echocardiograms frequently involves mild disease, which can be subtle. Final interpretation of echocardiograms should be by those experienced in RHD, congenital heart disease, and the variations of physiological regurgitation. The interpretation of abnormality is usually straightforward when hemodynamically significant mitral or AR is found but experience and care are needed in assessment of abnormality at the minor end of the RHD spectrum. Remote reporting by experts has been utilized.[58] Those performing the full echocardiogram need to understand the principle of two-dimensional and color sweeps in all views, with careful Doppler interrogation of regurgitant jets, both important diagnostically even though the hemodynamic lesion is mild.

CONSIDERATIONS FOR ESTABLISHING NEW ECHOCARDIOGRAPHIC SCREENING PROGRAMS

There is no place for individuals starting screening programs without buy in from their local Ministry of Health and clinical teams. Logistics must be carefully established in advance with consideration of prescreening information for schools and families, practical considerations of scan location and infrastructure required including areas for changing. Echocardiogram logistics with portable versus handheld technology, sonographer/technician workforce and appropriately experienced reporting clinicians must all be considered. Screening protocols (very abbreviated versus more detailed scans) may differ between programs, but there should be a clear pathway for more detailed imaging and follow-up of abnormal scans. Information sharing with families regarding results must be timely and appropriate counseling regarding abnormal scans provided. The threshold for benzathine penicillin prophylaxis must be considered in advance, with appropriate surveillance and sore throat management for those with borderline RHD not commenced on secondary prophylaxis. Consideration must be given to nonrheumatic abnormalities (e.g., congenital or other acquired cardiac disease) which may be detected by screening and to treatment pathways for any participants with severe RHD.[31]

Children who have participated in screening along with their parents and teachers have been supportive of RHD screening in their feedback.[59,60] For some families, however, a positive screening result increases anxiety[61] and decreases quality of life for children[62,63] and parents.[63] A New Zealand study reported 20% of participants with positive results had long-term changes in physical activity.[61] It is important that counseling emphasizes there should not be any exercise restriction for those with mild or moderate RHD disease.

CURRENT LIMITATIONS OF RHEUMATIC HEART DISEASE ECHOCARDIOGRAPHIC SCREENING

There is no laboratory test that is specific for ARF. Similarly, there is no well-defined cut-off for what constitutes the lower limit of echocardiographic changes that are categorically rheumatic in origin. Long-term follow-up of the various subclinical valvular morphological and Doppler echocardiographic patterns is required to calculate both the risk of recurrence of ARF and the risk of progression to more severe RHD.

CONCLUSION

Portable echocardiography is a relatively new screening tool for RHD with evolving strategies over the past 15 years. It has been helpful for better understanding the epidemiology of RHD. It has increased awareness and advocacy for better RHD control.

If echocardiographic screening is widely applied, with effective delivery of secondary prophylaxis via a registry-based program, it should decrease the prevalence of severe RHD in high RF regions. The requirements of a screening test are met with the evidence-based WHF diagnostic criteria enabling standardization between screening programs. The model for future RHD screening program is likely to involve initial school-based portable echocardiography with handheld devices with remote specialist reporting and local counseling, for positive cases.

REFERENCES

1. Strasser T, Dondog N, El Kholy A, Gharagozloo R, Kalbian VV, Ogunbi O, et al. The community control of rheumatic fever and rheumatic heart disease: report of a WHO international cooperative project. Bull World Health Organ. 1981;59(2):285-94.
2. Zuhlke L, Engel ME, Karthikeyan G, Rangarajan S, Mackie P, Cupido B, et al. Characteristics, complications, and gaps in evidence-based interventions in rheumatic heart disease: the Global Rheumatic Heart Disease Registry (the REMEDY study). Eur Heart J. 2015;36(18):1115-22a.
3. Carapetis JR, Currie BJ. Rheumatic chorea in northern Australia: a clinical and epidemiological study. Arch Dis Child. 1999;80(4):353-8.

4. Kiliç A, Unüvar E, Tatli B, Gökçe M, Omeroğlu RE, Oğuz F, et al. Neurologic and cardiac findings in children with Sydenham chorea. Pediatr Neurol. 2007;36(3):159-64.

5. Dajani A, Ayoub E, Bierman F, Bisno A, Denny F, Durack D, et al. Guidelines for the diagnosis of rheumatic fever. Jones Criteria, 1992 update. Special Writing Group of the Committee on Rheumatic Fever, Endocarditis, and Kawasaki Disease of the Council on Cardiovascular Disease in the Young of the American Heart Association. JAMA. 1992;268:2069-73.

6. Bland EF, Duckett Jones T. Rheumatic fever and rheumatic heart disease; a twenty year report on 1000 patients followed since childhood. Circulation. 1951;4(6):836-43.

7. Abbasi AS, Hashmi JA, Robinson RD Jr, Suraya S, Syed SA. Prevalence of heart disease in school children of Karachi. Am J Cardiol. 1966;18(4):544-7.

8. Ilyas M, Peracha MA, Ahmad R, Khan N, Ali N, Janjua M. Prevalence and pattern of rheumatic heart disease in the frontier province of Pakistan. J Pak Med Assoc. 1979;29(8):165-8.

9. Maharaj B, Dyer RB, Leary WP, Arbuckle DD, Armstrong TG, Pudifin DJ. Screening for rheumatic heart disease amongst black schoolchildren in Inanda, South Africa. J Trop Pediatr. 1987;33(1):60-1.

10. Kimbally-Kaky G, Gombet T, Voumbo Y, Ikama-Méo S, Elenga-Mbola B, Mbika-Cardorelle A, et al. Rheumatic heart disease in schoolchildren in Brazzaville. Med Trop (Mars). 2008;68(6):603-5.

11. Finau SA, Taylor L. Rheumatic heart disease and school screening: initiatives at an isolated hospital in Tonga. Med J Aust. 1988;148(11):563-7.

12. Kumar P, Garhwal S, Chaudhary V. Rheumatic heart disease: a school survey in a rural area of Rajasthan. Indian Heart J. 1992;44(4):245-6.

13. Thakur JS, Negi PC, Ahluwalia SK, Sharma R. Integrated community-based screening for cardiovascular diseases of childhood. World Health Forum. 1997;18(1):24-7.

14. Steer AC, Adams J, Carlin J, Nolan T, Shann F. Rheumatic heart disease in school children in Samoa. Arch Dis Child. 1999;81(4):372.

15. Talbot RG. Rheumatic fever and rheumatic heart disease in the Hamilton health district: II. Long term follow-up and secondary prophylaxis. N Z Med J. 1984;97(764):634-7.

16. Bhaya M, Panwar S, Beniwal R, Panwar RB. High prevalence of rheumatic heart disease detected by echocardiography in school children. Echocardiography (Mount Kisco, NY). 2010;27(4):448-53.

17. Carapetis JR, Hardy M, Fakakovikaetau T, Taib R, Wilkinson L, Penny DJ, et al. Evaluation of a screening protocol using auscultation and portable echocardiography to detect asymptomatic rheumatic heart disease in Tongan schoolchildren. Nat Clin Pract Cardiovasc Med. 2008;5(7):411-7.

18. Marijon E, Celermajer DS, Tafflet M, El-Haou S, Jani DN, Ferreira B, et al. Rheumatic heart disease screening by echocardiography: the inadequacy of World Health Organization criteria for optimizing the diagnosis of subclinical disease. Circulation. 2009;120(8):663-8.

19. Marijon E, Ou P, Celermajer DS, Ferreira B, Mocumbi AO, Jani D, et al. Prevalence of rheumatic heart disease detected by echocardiographic screening. N Engl J Med. 2007;357(5):470-6.

20. Paar JA, Berrios NM, Rose JD, Caceres M, Pena R, Perez W, et al. Prevalence of rheumatic heart disease in children and young adults in Nicaragua. Am J Cardiol. 2010;105(12):1809-14.

21. Webb RH, Wilson NJ, Lennon DR, Wilson EM, Nicholson RW, Gentles TL, et al. Optimising echocardiographic screening for rheumatic heart disease in New Zealand: not all valve disease is rheumatic. Cardiol Young. 2011;21(4):436-43.

22. World Health Organization. Rheumatic fever and rheumatic heart disease: Report of a WHO expert consultation. Geneva, Switzerland: World Health Organization; 2004. Contract No.: World Health Organisation Technical Report Series 923.

23. Longo-Mbenza B, Bayekula M, Ngiyulu R, Kintoki VE, Bikangi NF, Seghers KV, et al. Survey of rheumatic heart disease in school children of Kinshasa town. Int J Cardiol. 1998;63(3):287-94.

24. Sadiq M, Islam K, Abid R, Latif F, Rehman AU, Waheed A, et al. Prevalence of rheumatic heart disease in school children of urban Lahore. Heart. 2009;95(5):353-7.

25. Steer AC, Kado J, Wilson N, Tuiketei T, Batzloff M, Waqatakirewa L, et al. High prevalence of rheumatic heart disease by clinical and echocardiographic screening among children in Fiji. J Heart Valve Dis. 2009;18(3):327-35; discussion 36.

26. Carapetis JR, Paar JA, Cherian T. Standardization of epidemiologic protocols for surveillance of post-streptococcal sequelae: acute rheumatic fever, rheumatic heart disease and acute post-streptococcal glomerulonephritis. NIH: National Institute of Allergy and Infectious Diseases; 2006. pp. 1-32.

27. National Advisory Committee on Health and Disability. (2003). Screening to Improve Health in New Zealand: Criteria to assess screening programmes 2003:(1-49). [online] Available from http://nhc.health.govt.nz/ [Last accessed August, 2022].

28. Council of Europe CoM. (1994). Recommendation No. R (94) 11 on Screening as a Tool of Preventive Medicine (Oct. 10, 1994): University of Minnesota Human Rights Center and Library. [online] Available from http://hrlibrary.umn.edu/instree/coerecr94-11.html [Last accessed August, 2022].

29. Frankish JD. Rheumatic fever prophylaxis:Gisborne experience. N Z Med J. 1984;97:674-5.

30. Feinstein AR, Spagnuolo M, Wood HF, Taranta A, Tursky E, Kleinberg E. Rheumatic fever in children and adolescents. A long-term epidemiologic study of subsequent prophylaxis, streptococcal infections, and clinical sequelae. VI. Clinical features of streptococcal infections and rheumatic recurrences. Ann Intern Med. 1964;60(Suppl 5):68-86.

31. Beaton A, Engelman D, Mirabel M. Chapter 13—Echocardiographic Screening for Rheumatic Heart Disease. In: Dougherty S, Carapetis J, Zühlke L, Wilson N (Eds). Acute Rheumatic Fever and Rheumatic Heart Disease. San Diego (CA): Elsevier; 2021. pp. 261-74.

32. Beaton A, Okello E, Engelman D, Grobler A, Scheel A, DeWyer A, et al. Determining the impact of Benzathine penicillin G prophylaxis in children with latent rheumatic heart disease (GOAL trial): Study protocol for a randomized controlled trial. Am Heart J. 2019;215:95-105.

33. Beaton A, Okello E, Rwebembera J, Grobler A, Engelman D, Alepere J, et al. Secondary antibiotic prophylaxis for latent rheumatic heart disease. N Engl J Med. 2022;386(3):230-40.

34. Remenyi B, Wilson N, Steer A, Ferreira B, Kado J, Kumar K, et al. World Heart Federation criteria for echocardiographic diagnosis of rheumatic heart disease--an evidence-based guideline. Nat Rev Cardiol. 2012;9(5):297-309.

35. Remenyi B, Carapetis J, Stirling JW, Ferreira B, Kumar K, Lawrenson J, et al. Inter-rater and intra-rater reliability and agreement of echocardiographic diagnosis of rheumatic heart disease using the World Heart Federation evidence-based criteria. Heart Asia. 2019;11(2):e011233.

36. Chao K, Moises VA, Shandas R, Elkadi T, Sahn DJ, Weintraub R. Influence of the Coanda effect on color Doppler jet area and color encoding. In vitro studies using color Doppler flow mapping. Circulation. 1992;85(1):333-41.

37. Zhang J, Jones M, Shandas R, Valdes-Cruz LM, Murillo A, Yamada I, et al. Accuracy of flow convergence estimates of mitral regurgitant flow rates obtained by use of multiple color flow Doppler M-mode aliasing boundaries: an experimental animal study. Am Heart J. 1993;125(2 Pt 1):449-58.

38. Zhang J, Shiota T, Shandas R, Deng YB, Weintraub R, Paik J, et al. Effects of adjacent surfaces of different shapes on regurgitant jet sizes: an in vitro study using color Doppler imaging and laser-illuminated dye visualization. J Am Coll Cardiol. 1993;22(5):1522-9.

39. Ginghină C. The Coandă effect in cardiology. J Cardiovasc Med (Hagerstown). 2007;8(6):411-3.

40. Flachskampf FA, Frieske R, Engelhard B, Grenner H, Frielingsdorf J, Beck F, et al. Comparison of transesophageal doppler methods with angiography for evaluation of the severity of mitral regurgitation. J Am Soc Echocardiogr. 1998;11(9): 882-92.

41. Ayabakan C, Ozkutlu S, Kilic A. The Doppler echocardiographic assessment of valvular regurgitation in normal children. Turk J Pediatr. 2003;45(2):102-7.

42. Berger M, Hecht SR, Van Tosh A, Lingam U. Pulsed and continuous wave doppler echocardiographic assessment of valvular regurgitation in normal subjects. J Am Coll Cardiol. 1989;13(7):1540-5.

43. Choong CY, Abascal VM, Weyman J, Levine RA, Gentile F, Thomas JD, et al. Prevalence of valvular regurgitation by Doppler echocardiography in patients with structurally normal hearts by two-dimensional echocardiography. Am Heart. 1989;117(3): 636-42.

44. Aliku T, Sable C, Scheel A, Tompsett A, Lwabi P, Okello E, et al. Targeted echocardiographic screening for latent rheumatic heart disease in Northern Uganda: Evaluating familial risk following identification of an index case. PLoS Negl Trop Dis. 2016;10(6):e0004727.

45. Culliford-Semmens N, Tilton E, Wilson N, Stirling J, Doughty R, Gentles T, et al. Echocardiography for latent rheumatic heart disease in first degree relatives of children with acute rheumatic fever: Implications for active case finding in family members. E Clinical Medicine. 2021;37:100935.

46. Otto H, Saether SG, Banteyrga L, Haugen BO, Skjaerpe T. High prevalence of subclinical rheumatic heart disease in pregnant women in a developing country: an echocardiographic study. E chocardiography. 2011;28(10):1049-53.

47. Beaton A, Aliku T, Okello E, Lubega S, McCarter R, Lwabi P, et al. The utility of handheld echocardiography for early diagnosis of rheumatic heart disease. J Am Soc Echocardiogr. 2014;27(1):42-9.

48. Ploutz M, Lu JC, Scheel J, Webb C, Ensing GJ, Aliku T, et al. Handheld echocardiographic screening for rheumatic heart disease by non-experts. Heart. 2016;102(1):35-9.

49. Zuhlke LJ, Engel ME, Nkepu S, Mayosi BM. Evaluation of a focussed protocol for hand-held echocardiography and computer-assisted auscultation in detecting latent rheumatic heart disease in scholars. Cardiol Young. 2016;26(6): 1097-106.

50. Beaton A, Nascimento BR, Diamantino AC, Pereira GT, Lopes EL, Miri CO, et al. Efficacy of a standardized computer-based training curriculum to teach echocardiographic identification of rheumatic heart disease to nonexpert users. Am J Cardiol. 2016;117(11):1783-9.

51. Colquhoun SM, Carapetis JR, Kado JH, Reeves BM, Remenyi B, May W, et al. Pilot study of nurse-led rheumatic heart disease echocardiography screening in Fiji: a novel approach in a resource-poor setting. Cardiol Young. 2013;23(4):546-52.

52. Engelman D, Kado JH, Remenyi B, Colquhoun SM, Carapetis JR, Donath S, et al. Focused cardiac ultrasound screening for rheumatic heart disease by briefly trained health workers: a study of diagnostic accuracy. Lancet Glob Health. 2016;4(6):e386-94.

53. Mirabel M, Bacquelin R, Tafflet M, Robillard C, Huon B, Corsenac P, et al. Screening for rheumatic heart disease: evaluation of a focused cardiac ultrasound approach. Circ Cardiovasc Imaging. 2015;8(1):e002324.

54. Sims Sanyahumbi A, Sable CA, Karlsten M, Hosseinipour MC, Kazembe PN, Minard CG, et al. Task shifting to clinical officer-led echocardiography screening for detecting rheumatic heart disease in Malawi, Africa. Cardiol Young. 2017;27(6):1133-9.

55. Engelman D, Okello E, Beaton A, Selnow G, Remenyi B, Watson C, et al. Evaluation of computer-based training for health workers in echocardiography for RHD. Glob Heart. 2017;12(1):17-23.e8.

56. Engelman D, Watson C, Remenyi B, Steer A. (2014). Echo-cardiographic Diagnosis of Rheumatic Heart Disease: Nurse Training Modules 2014. [online] Available from http://www.wiredhealthresources.net/EchoProject/ [Last accessed August, 2022].

57. Lopes EL, Beaton AZ, Nascimento BR, Tompsett A, Dos Santos JP, Perlman L, et al. Telehealth solutions to enable global collaboration in rheumatic heart disease screening. J Telemed Telecare. 2018;24(2):101-9.

58. Nascimento BR, Beaton AZ, Nunes MC, Diamantino AC, Carmo GA, Oliveira KK, et al. Echocardiographic prevalence of rheumatic heart disease in Brazilian schoolchildren: Data from the PROVAR study. Int J Cardiol. 2016;219:439-45.

59. Perelini F, Blair N, Wilson N, Farrell A, Aitken A. Family acceptability of school-based echocardiographic screening for rheumatic heart disease in a high-risk population in New Zealand. J Paediatr Child Health. 2015;51(7):682-8.

60. Ploutz M, Aliku T, Bradley-Hewitt T, Dantin A, Lemley B, Gillespie CW, et al. Child and teacher acceptability of school-based echocardiographic screening for rheumatic heart disease in Uganda. Cardiol Young. 2017;27(1):82-9.

61. Gurney J, Chong A, Culliford-Semmens N, Tilton F, Wilson NJ, Sarfati D. The benefits and harms of rheumatic heart disease screening from the perspective of the screened population. Int J Cardiol. 2016;221:734-40.

62. Bradley-Hewitt T, Dantin A, Ploutz M, Aliku T, Lwabi P, Sable C, et al. The Impact of Echocardiographic Screening for Rheumatic Heart Disease on Patient Quality of Life. J Pediatr. 2016;175:123-9.

63. Wark EK, Hodder YC, Woods CE, Maguire GP. Patient and health-care impact of a pilot rheumatic heart disease screening program. J Paediatr Child Health. 2013;49(4):297-302.

Prevention and Vaccine for Rheumatic Fever: How Far are We?

IB Vijayalakshmi, Monica Kher

> *"Superior doctors prevent disease. Mediocre doctors treat the disease before it is evident. Inferior doctors treat the full-blown disease."*
>
> **—Chinese proverb, Huang Dee Nai-Chang**

INTRODUCTION

Rheumatic fever (RF) and rheumatic heart disease (RHD) were widely prevalent throughout the world at the beginning of the second half of the 20th century. However, during the ensuing decades, the disease's major impact has been centered in developing countries, which constitute a majority of the world's population. As with so many other health problems, these are countries which can least afford the economic and social costs for the management of RF and RHD. Particularly frustrating has been the fact that RF and RHD are theoretically preventable. In patients who develop RF, therapy is directed toward eliminating the group A streptococcal pharyngitis [group A β-hemolytic streptococci (GABHS)] if still present, suppressing inflammation from the autoimmune response and providing supportive treatment for congestive heart failure. If GABHS infections of the upper respiratory tract are prevented or are effectively treated, neither initial nor recurrent attacks of RF occur and that is the goal of prevention.

The medical and public health issues are further complicated by the fact that group A streptococcal infections are universally endemic. As there is no available vaccine for group A streptococcal infections, preventive measures remain dependent upon accurate clinical diagnosis and appropriate antibiotic treatment. RF prevention programs utilizing recommended clinical and laboratory techniques for diagnosis and antibiotic treatment of GABHS infections are cost effective. It is important to know the currently accepted and effective methods of prevention of RF and role of vaccine in RF control program.

PREVENTION

"Prevention is better than cure" is very apt for RF. There are four aspects to the prevention of acute rheumatic fever (ARF) and its sequelae.

1. Primordial prevention
2. Prevention of ARF by accurate and prompt recognition and treatment of streptococcal pharyngitis (Primary prevention)
3. Prevention of recurrent ARF through compulsive ongoing prophylaxis against streptococcal infection (Secondary prevention)
4. Prevention of bacterial endocarditis in individuals with chronic rheumatic cardiac valve disease

Algorithm of prevention of ARF and RHD is given in **Flowchart 1**.

Primordial prevention requires preventing the development of "risk factors" in the community to prevent the disease in the population and thus protect individuals.

Measures for primordial prevention in relation to ARF and RHD consist of:

- Improvement in socioeconomic status
- Prevention of overcrowding

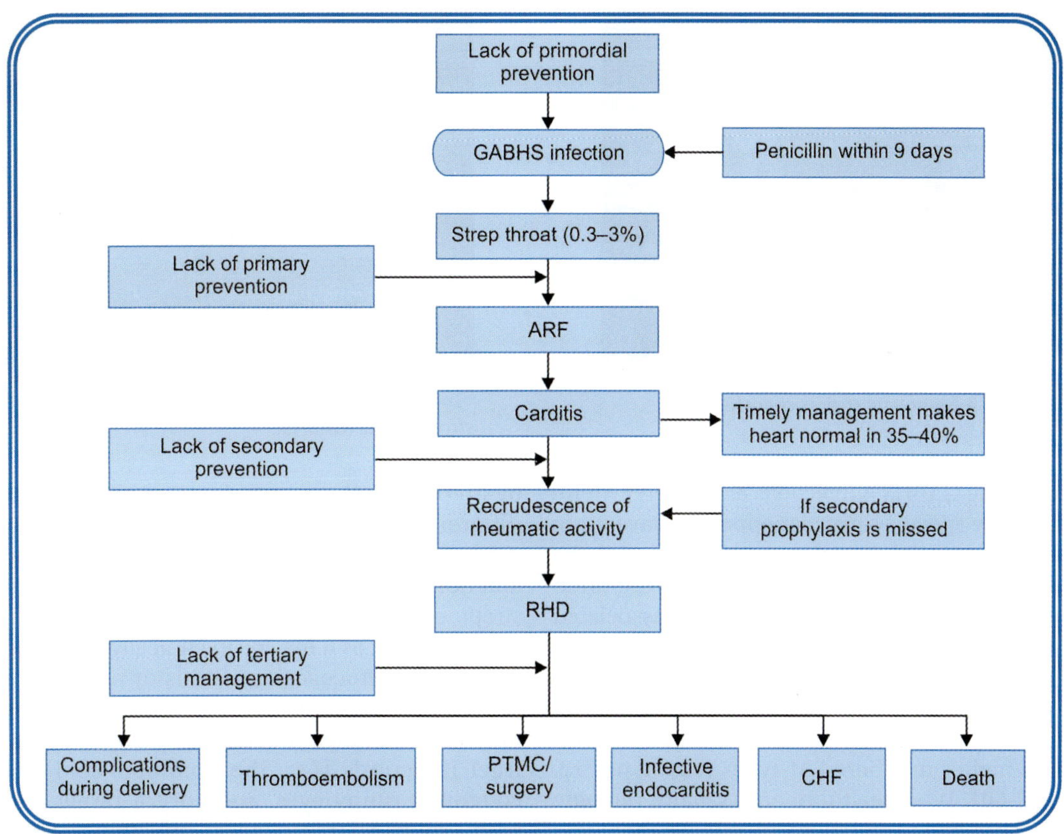

FLOWCHART 1: Algorithm of prevention of ARF and RHD.

(ARF: acute rheumatic fever; CHF: congestive heart failure; GABHS: group A β-hemolytic streptococci; PTMC: percutaneous transvenous mitral commissurotomy; RHD: rheumatic heart disease)

- Prevention of undernutrition and malnutrition
- Availability of prompt medical care
- Public education regarding the risk of ARF from sore throat especially below the age of 15 years.

The last one, i.e., public education is the most important component for primordial prevention. Basically "Primordial prevention" involves measures to prevent the occurrence of a GABHS sore throat. Clean and healthy environment is an important measure.

Mass chemoprophylaxis can work in some high-risk situations. Vaccines are in experimental phase and not feasible in all situations.

Primary prevention involves effective recognition and treatment of GABHS sore throat and, in turn, prevent the development of ARF and appropriate detection and treatment of streptococcal pharyngitis.

EPIDEMIOLOGY OF GROUP A STREPTOCOCCAL UPPER RESPIRATORY TRACT INFECTIONS[1]

There is an incontrovertible relationship between group A β-hemolytic streptococcal upper respiratory infections and development of RF. The only significant reservoir of these organisms is the human body. For incompletely defined reasons, the infection has a predilection for children between the ages of 5 and 15 years, but adults are also susceptible. Although capable of causing epidemics in newborn nurseries and infection in younger children, the majority of streptococcal infections occur in school-age children. Adult infections have been most frequently observed in unique epidemiologic situations such as schools, military bases, and residential institutional facilities.

Group A β-hemolytic streptococci infections appear to be quite frequent and, therefore, result in a high incidence of RF in socially and economically disadvantaged populations, especially where overcrowding is frequent. GABHS upper respiratory tract infection is spread by droplets, thus accounting for its high transmissibility in such situations. Most outbreaks are associated with respiratory tract transmission, but food-borne outbreaks (often associated with dairy products and eggs) have been documented. In contrast to other infectious agents with only single strain (e.g., type b *Haemophilus influenzae*), there are approximately 100 recognized serotypes of group A streptococci. Therefore, although infection with a given serotype is thought to confer long-lasting type specific immunity, the abundance of serotypes makes the threat of a new infection continuous. The result of endemic and epidemic infections is a continuous worldwide public health problem.

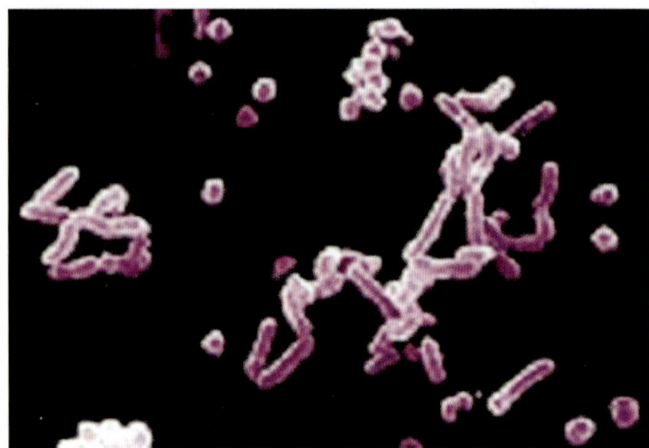

FIG. 1: Group A β-hemolytic streptococci (GABHS).

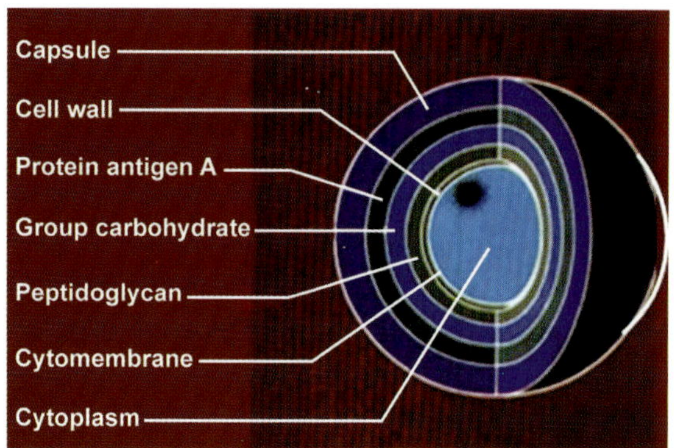

FIG. 2: Diagrammatic structure of group A β-hemolytic streptococci (GABHS).

Complicating the GABHS A infections associated with RF is the fact that some specific serotypes appear to have more "rheumatogenic" potential than do others. Epidemiologic observations suggest that these serotypes are more often associated with the development of RF. Serotypes associated with RF (e.g., M-types 1, 3, 5, 6, 14, 18, and 24) are most often found to infect the upper respiratory tract **(Fig. 1)**. In contrast, serotypes which most frequently cause superficial skin infection (pyoderma) and are not associated with RF are among the higher numbered M-types (e.g., types 12, 49, 55, 57, and 60). Whether there are actually biologic differences in these latter serotypes which make them less of a threat to cause RF remains incompletely understood. These epidemiologic observations may also be responsible for the belief that RF follows only upper respiratory tract infection and not skin infection. This is in contrast to acute poststreptococcal glomerulonephritis, which may follow either upper respiratory tract or skin infection. The understanding of differences between skin and throat infections remains incomplete. Antigen of outer protein cell wall of GABHS induces antibody response in victim which results in autoimmune damage to heart valves, subcutaneous tissue, tendons, joints, and basal ganglia of brain **(Fig. 2)**.

MANAGEMENT OF GROUP A STREPTOCOCCAL UPPER RESPIRATORY TRACT INFECTION

Diagnosis

Young children, school-age children, and adults may present with significantly different clinical findings. An accurate clinical diagnosis of group A streptococcal upper respiratory tract infection can be very difficult emphasizing the advantage of laboratory confirmation of the infection whenever possible. The patient presents with: (1) sore throat with high fever (often >38°C), (2) painful deglutition, (3) headache, abdominal pain, nausea, and vomiting. These classical signs and symptoms are frequently not present, especially in endemic situations. Likewise, in very young children (those below 3 years of age), the presentation of streptococcal upper respiratory tract infection is often different. These children initially present with a low-grade fever, irritability, and a serous discharge from the anterior nares. This latter syndrome has been referred to as streptococcosis.

As difficult as it may be to clinically establish a diagnosis of acute streptococcal tonsillitis or pharyngitis, the signs and symptoms of this bacterial infection typically are quite different from those associated with viral upper respiratory tract infections (i.e., the common cold). Hoarseness, coughing, runny eyes, and coryza rarely are associated with group A streptococcal infections. Although many children have palpable anterior cervical lymph nodes (lymphadenopathy), the characteristic finding of true group A streptococcal upper respiratory tract infections is that of tender anterior cervical lymph nodes (lymphadenitis).

This lack of precision in confirming a clinical diagnosis has reinforced the need, whenever possible, of the diagnostic microbiology or immunology laboratory. The throat culture continues to be the "gold standard" for determining the presence of group A streptococci in the upper respiratory tract. However, failure to properly sample the posterior pharynx, tonsils or tonsillar fossae may result in false negative cultures. Similarly, prior administration of antibiotics may also result in a false negative culture. Rapid antigen detection tests are available which allow the detection of group A streptococcal antigens from the throat swab. Generally, rapid tests have acceptable specificity but their sensitivity has been reported to be unacceptably low in some studies. This has led to the recommendation that if a rapid antigen test is "negative" in a patient suspected of having a streptococcal infection, throat culture is advisable. Rapid antigen tests are not widely available in many countries and when they are, their cost tends to exceed that of a throat culture. Group A streptococcal antibody tests such as antistreptolysin O (ASLO) and antideoxyribonuclease B (anti-DNase B) are very useful supporting evidence in the diagnosis of RF or acute glomerulonephritis. However, they are neither useful nor are they indicated for the routine management of patients with acute group A streptococcal pharyngitis. At the time of presentation with acute pharyngitis, there will have been insufficient time to mount a rise in antibody titer.

Group A β-hemolytic streptococci pharyngitis is an acute infection of the oropharynx or nasopharynx that is caused by *Streptococcus pyogenes*. Accurate diagnosis and optimal treatment of this infection are important to:

- Prevent ARF
- Prevent suppurative complications (e.g., mastoiditis, peritonsillar abscess, and cervical lymphadenitis)
- Improve clinical signs and symptoms
- Reduce transmission to close contacts of patients
- Minimize potential adverse effects of inappropriate antibiotic therapy

ANTIMICROBIAL TREATMENT OF GROUP A STREPTOCOCCAL PHARYNGITIS

Prevention of Initial Attacks (Primary Prevention)

Group A β-hemolytic streptococci infections of the pharynx are the precipitating cause of RF. Primary prevention is the treatment of acute streptococcal pharyngitis in order to prevent the initial attack of RF. During epidemics over a half century ago, as many as 3% of untreated acute streptococcal sore throats were followed by RF and in endemic infections, the incidence of RF is substantially less.[2] Appropriate antibiotic treatment of streptococcal pharyngitis prevents ARF in most cases.[3] Unfortunately, at least one-third of episodes of ARF results from inapparent streptococcal infections.[4] In addition, some symptomatic patients do not seek medical care. In these instances, RF is not preventable. In general, once the diagnosis has been made, prevention of RF requires adequate antibiotic therapy for GABHS pharyngitis.

In selecting a regimen for the treatment of GABHS pharyngitis, physicians should consider various factors, including bacteriologic and clinical efficacy, ease of adherence to the recommended regimen (frequency of daily administration, duration of therapy, and palatability), cost, spectrum of activity of the selected agent, and potential side effects. No regimen eradicates GABHS from the pharynx in 100% of treated patients, even though 100% of GABHS demonstrate in vitro susceptibility to all #-lactam agents (penicillins and cephalosporins) **(Table 1)**.

Penicillins

Penicillin remains the recommended antimicrobial drug and the treatment of choice for GABHS upper respiratory tract infections, except in individuals with histories of penicillin allergy. Pencillin is available as intramuscular benzathine penicillin G and oral penicillin V. In fact, penicillin is the only antibiotic that has ever been evaluated in controlled studies which clearly demonstrate that RF can be prevented by antibiotic therapy. The only currently recommended antimicrobial therapy that has been investigated in controlled

TABLE 1: Primary prevention of rheumatic fever (treatment of streptococcal tonsillopharyngitis).			
Agent	**Dose**	**Mode**	**Duration**
Penicillins			
Penicillin V (phenoxymethyl penicillin)	Children: 250 mg 2–3 times daily for <27 kg (60 lb); Children > 27 kg (60 lb), adolescents, and adults: 500 mg 2–3 times daily	Oral	10 days
Or			
Amoxicillin	50 mg/kg once daily (maximum 1 g)	Oral	10 days
Or			
Benzathine penicillin G	6,00,000 U for patients < 27 kg (60 lb); 12,00,000 U for patients > 27 kg (60 lb)	Intramuscular	Once
For individuals allergic to penicillin			
Narrow spectrum cephalosporin[†] (cephalexin and cefadroxil)	Variable	Oral	10 days
Or			
Clindamycin	20 mg/kg/day divided in 3 doses (maximum 1.8 g/day)	Oral	10 days
Or			
Azithromycin	12 mg/kg once daily (maximum 500 mg)	Oral	5 days
Or			
Clarithromycin	15 mg/kg/day divided into BID (maximum 250 mg BID)	Oral	10 days

[†]To be avoided in those with immediate (type I) hypersensitivity to a penicillin.

(BID: twice per day. The following are not acceptable: sulfonamides, trimethoprim, tetracyclines, and fluoroquinolones)

studies and demonstrated to prevent initial attacks of ARF is intramuscular repository penicillin therapy.[3,5]

These studies were performed with procaine penicillin G in oil containing aluminum monostearate, a preparation that subsequently has been replaced by benzathine penicillin G.

Penicillin has a narrow spectrum of activity, long-standing proven efficacy, and is an inexpensive regimen. GABHS resistant to penicillin has never been documented. Penicillin may be administered intramuscularly or orally depending on the physician's assessment of the patient's likely adherence to an oral regimen and the risks of RF in a particular population. Even when started as long as 9 days after the onset of acute illness, penicillin effectively prevents primary attacks of RF.[6] Therefore, a 24–48 hours delay to process the throat culture before antibiotic therapy is started does not increase the risk of RF. However, early diagnosis (e.g., by rapid antigen test) and therapy may reduce the period of infectivity and morbidity, which would allow the patient to return to normal activity sooner. Patients are considered no longer contagious after 24 hours of antibiotic therapy.[7]

Oral Penicillins

The oral antibiotics of choice are penicillin V and amoxicillin **(Table 1)**. Comparative clinical trials used penicillin V dosages of 40 mg/kg (not to exceed 750 mg for those weighing < 27 kg)/24 hours, given in three equally divided doses.

Generally, 250 mg two times daily is recommended for most children.[8,9] Little information is available about comparable penicillin doses in adults. A dose of 500 mg two to three times daily is recommended for adolescents and adults. All patients should continue to take penicillin regularly for an entire 10-day period, even though they will be asymptomatic after the first few days. Penicillin V is preferred to penicillin G because it is more resistant to gastric acid. An oral and time-released formulation of amoxicillin has been approved in the US for once daily therapy of GABHS pharyngitis in those 12 years of age and older. In comparative clinical trials, once daily amoxicillin (50 mg/kg, maximum 1,000 mg) for 10 days has been shown to be effective for GABHS pharyngitis.[10-13] This somewhat broader spectrum agent has the advantage of once daily dosing, which may enhance adherence, and is relatively inexpensive and amoxicillin suspension is considerably more palatable than penicillin V suspension. However, as 10 days of oral therapy has been the recommended duration, adherence remains a problem for patients taking an oral antibiotic. Reduced adherence to prescribed oral medications for the purpose of RF prevention is common. Educational efforts by healthcare professionals to promote adherence can significantly enhance efficacy.

Intramuscular Benzathine Penicillin G

A single injection of intramuscular benzathine benzyl-penicillin, a long-acting repository form of the antibiotic, is the most effective treatment in eradicating group A streptococci, probably due to its long duration of action. It can also be used for mass prophylaxis. Benzathine penicillin G should be considered particularly for patients who are unlikely to complete a 10-day course of oral therapy and for patients with personal or family histories of RF or RHD or environmental factors (such as crowded living conditions or low socioeconomic status) that place them at enhanced risk for RF.[14-17] Benzathine penicillin G should be given as a single injection in a large muscle mass. This formulation is painful and injections that contain procaine penicillin in addition to benzathine penicillin G are less painful. Less discomfort is associated with intramuscular benzathine penicillin G if the medication is warmed to room temperature before administration.

The recommended dosage of benzathine penicillin G is 600,000 U IM for patients who weigh 27 kg (60 lb) or less and 1,200,000 U for patients who weigh > 27 kg. The combination of 900,000 U of benzathine penicillin G and 300,000 U of procaine penicillin G is satisfactory therapy for most of smaller children.[18] The efficacy of this combination for heavier patients such as large teenagers or adults requires further study.

Allergic reactions to penicillin are more common in adults than in children. Reactions occur in only a small percentage of patients are more frequent after injection and include urticaria and angioneurotic edema. A serum sickness like reaction characterized by fever and joint pain may be mistaken for ARF. Anaphylaxis is rare, especially in children. A careful history regarding allergic reactions to penicillin should be obtained.

Other Antimicrobial Agents

Oral Cephalosporins

A 10-day course of a narrow spectrum oral cephalosporin is recommended for most penicillin allergic individuals. Several reports indicate that a 10-day course with an oral cephalosporin is superior to 10 days of oral penicillin in eradicating GABHS from the pharynx.[19-22] Analysis of these data suggests that the difference in eradication is due mainly to a higher rate of eradication of carriers included unintentionally in these clinical trials. Narrow spectrum cephalosporins, such as cefadroxil or cephalexin, are much preferred to broad spectrum cephalosporins such as cefaclor, cefuroxime, cefixime, cefdinir, and cefpodoxime. Some penicillin allergic persons (up to 10%) are also allergic to cephalosporins and these agents should not be used in patients with immediate (anaphylactic type) hypersensitivity to penicillin.[23]

Most oral broad spectrum cephalosporins are considerably more expensive than penicillin or amoxicillin and the former agents are more likely to select for antibiotic resistant flora. Other reports suggest that a 5-day course with selected oral broad spectrum cephalosporins is comparable to a 10-day course of oral penicillin in eradicating GABHS from the pharynx.[24-27]

Oral Clindamycin

Clindamycin resistance among GABHS isolates in the United States is 1%, and this is a reasonable agent for treating penicillin allergic patients.

Macrolides

The use of an oral macrolide (erythromycin or clarithromycin) or azalide (azithromycin) is reasonable for patients allergic to penicillins. 10 days of therapy is indicated, except for azithromycin, which is given for 5 days **(Table 1)**. Macrolides (erythromycin and clarithromycin) and to a much lesser extent azalides (azithromycin) can cause prolongation of the QT interval in a dose-dependent manner. Because macrolides are metabolized extensively by cytochrome P-450 3A, they should not be taken concurrently with inhibitors of cytochrome P-450 3A such as azole antifungal agents, HIV protease inhibitors, and some selective serotonin reuptake inhibitor antidepressants.[28,29] Erythromycin might be considered but is associated with substantially higher rates of gastrointestinal side effects than the other agents. Strains of GABHS resistant to these agents have been highly prevalent in some areas of the world, which has resulted in treatment failures.[30] In recent years, macrolide resistance rates among pharyngeal isolates in most areas of the United States have been approximately 5–8%.[31]

Other Considerations

Studies suggesting that β-lactamase producing upper respiratory tract flora may interfere with penicillin in the treatment of GABHS pharyngitis have not been confirmed.[32] Antibiotic therapy directed against these organisms remains controversial and is not indicated in patients with acute pharyngitis.

Certain antimicrobials are not recommended for treatment of group A streptococcal upper respiratory tract infections. Tetracyclines should not be used because of the high prevalence of resistant strains. Sulfonamides and trimethoprim sultamethoxazole do not eradicate GABHS in patients with pharyngitis and should not be used to treat active infections.[33] Older fluoroquinolones (e.g., ciprofloxacin) have limited activity against GABHS and should not be used to treat GABHS pharyngitis.[34] Newer fluoroquinolones (e.g., levofloxacin and moxifloxacin) are active in vitro against GABHS but are expensive and have an unnecessarily broad spectrum of activity and, therefore, they are not recommended for routine treatment of GABHS pharyngitis.[35]

Other Treatment Recommendations

Follow-up Throat Cultures

The majority of patients with GABHS pharyngitis respond clinically to antimicrobial therapy, and GABHS are eradicated from the pharynx.[36] Post-treatment throat cultures 2–7 days after completion of therapy are indicated only in the relatively few patients who remain symptomatic, whose symptoms recur or who have had RF and are therefore at unusually high risk for recurrence.

Treatment Failures

Failure to eradicate GABHS from the throat occurs more frequently after the administration of oral penicillin than after the administration of intramuscular benzathine penicillin G.[37] Repeated courses of antibiotic therapy are rarely indicated in asymptomatic patients who continue to harbor GABHS after appropriate therapy. Many patients in whom treatment fails are chronic carriers who have prolonged periods of GABHS colonization.[38] A second course of therapy in asymptomatic individuals should be considered only for those with previous RF themselves or in members of their families. Symptomatic individuals who continue to harbor GABHS in their pharynx after completion of a course of therapy can be retreated with the same antimicrobial agent, given an alternative oral agent or given an intramuscular dose of benzathine penicillin G, especially if poor adherence to oral therapy is likely. However, expert opinions differ about the most appropriate therapy in this situation. Agents such as a narrow spectrum cephalosporin, clindamycin, or amoxicillin clavulanic acid, or the combination of penicillin with rifampin are reasonable in the treatment of patients with GABHS pharyngitis in whom initial penicillin treatment has failed.

It is often difficult to diagnose streptococcal sore throat, even for experienced clinicians, because no single element of history taking, or physical examination is accurate enough to exclude or diagnose streptococcal throat infection. The inability to utilize primary prevention at the community level is due to the large number of sore throats required to be treated to prevent ARF. Community level management requires a sledgehammer approach, i.e., treating each sore throat. Bacteriological facilities required to diagnose streptococcal sore throat at the community level for the whole country, at present, do not exist and are not likely in the near future, hence, each sore throat will need to be treated. Recent data suggests that almost 90% of those who get ARF develop RHD. Hence, if 10,000 sore throats are treated by the sledgehammer approach, anywhere between 300 and 2,000 streptococcal sore throats would be required to be treated (assuming that 3–20% of these are streptococcal), this would result in preventing ARF in one to six children (0.3% streptococcal sore throats cause RF) and RHD in five or six children. Thus, community level primary prevention is not feasible, although it may be possible for select individual patients. Another problem with sledgehammer approach is the identification of sore throat and its treatment, this is logistically not feasible for the whole country. Anywhere from 3 to 20% of sore throats can be streptococcal, the rest being viral infections which do not require treatment antibiotic therapy of group A streptococcal pharyngitis.

Prompt and effective antibiotic therapy eradicates group A streptococci from upper respiratory infection and can prevent ARF if therapy is started within 9 days after the onset of symptoms, but the patients do not reach unless a sore throat is symptomatic. Hence, if not treated this can result in ARF and this makes primary prevention, based on the diagnosis of streptococcal sore throat and use of oral penicillin, inadequate to reduce the burden of RHD in the country. Rapid antigen detection tests are not available universally. ASLO and anti-DNase B have little or no use in diagnosing acute group A streptococcal pharyngitis or tonsillitis, since they can be accurately interpreted only in retrospect. But, this should not detract from their importance in assisting with the diagnosis of acute RF, which requires evidence of a preceding group A streptococcal infection.

An overall protective effect for the use of penicillin against ARF of 80% with a numbers needed to treat (NNT) of 60 children per year to prevent even one episode of RF.

Management of Household Contacts

Household contacts may harbor group A streptococci in their upper respiratory tract but have no symptoms. It is usually not necessary to test these asymptomatic contacts or to treat them if test results are positive. When posttreatment testing of a patient is necessary, it is recommended to do cultures for asymptomatic family contacts with treatment given to those who have positive results. Close contacts of patients with invasive group A streptococcal infections (e.g., necrotizing fasciitis and toxic shock syndrome) should be treated.

Carriers

Chronic streptococcal carriers (defined as individuals with positive throat cultures for GABHS without clinical findings or immunologic response to GABHS antigens) usually do not need to be identified or treated with antibiotics.[39] Streptococcal carriage may persist for many months and a difficult diagnostic problem arises when symptomatic upper respiratory tract viral infections develop in carriers. Because it is impossible in that setting to distinguish carriers from infected individuals, a single course of appropriate antibiotic therapy should be administered to any patient with acute pharyngitis and evidence of GABHS by a throat swab culture or an antigen detection test. Streptococcal carriers appear to be at little risk for development of RF. In general, chronic carriers are thought not to be important in the spread of GABHS to individuals who live and work around them.[39]

Non-GABHS Pharyngitis

Both group C and group G β-hemolytic streptococci can cause acute pharyngitis with clinical features similar to those of GABHS pharyngitis. Group C streptococci are a relatively common cause of acute pharyngitis among college students and among adults who go to an emergency department for treatment.[40,41] ARF has not been described as a complication of either group C or group G streptococcal pharyngitis. Therefore, the primary reason to identify either group C

or group G *Streptococcus* as the cause of acute pharyngitis is to initiate antimicrobial therapy that may mitigate the clinical course of the infection. However, there is currently no convincing evidence from controlled studies of clinical response to antimicrobial therapy in patients with acute pharyngitis and either group C or group G *Streptococcus* isolated from their pharynx.

PREVENTION OF RECURRENT ATTACKS OF RHEUMATIC FEVER (SECONDARY PREVENTION)

General Considerations

An individual with a previous attack of RF in whom GABHS pharyngitis develops is at high risk for a recurrent attack of RF. A recurrent attack can be associated with worsening of the severity of RHD that developed after a first attack or less frequently with the new onset of RHD in individuals who did not develop cardiac manifestations during the first attack. Prevention of recurrent episodes of GABHS pharyngitis is the most effective method to prevent the development of severe RHD. Secondary prophylaxis has been documented to reduce significantly the risk of recurrent attacks with their attendant morbidity and mortality. A GABHS infection need not be symptomatic to trigger a recurrence. For these reasons, prevention of recurrent RF (secondary prophylaxis) requires continuous antimicrobial prophylaxis rather than recognition and treatment of acute episodes of streptococcal pharyngitis. Continuous prophylaxis is recommended for patients with well-documented histories of RF (including cases manifested solely by Sydenham's chorea) and those with definite evidence of RHD. Such prophylaxis should be initiated as soon as ARF or RHD is diagnosed. A full therapeutic course of penicillin (as outlined in **Table 1**) should be given to patients with ARF to eradicate residual GABHS, even if a throat culture is negative at that time. Streptococcal infections that occur in family members of patients with current or previous RF should be treated promptly.

Duration of Prophylaxis

Continuous antimicrobial prophylaxis provides the most effective protection from RF recurrences. In 1955, Stollerman formulated the general principles of prophylaxis with an antibiotic for at least 5 years after the initial bout of RF, preferably penicillin, in monthly injections because it eliminated the difficulties of multiple daily dosing.[42] The recommendation extended even to children who did not suffer carditis as a major manifestation of RF, out of concern that a second or third bout might attack the heart.[43] Risk of recurrence depends on several factors. The age of the patient and the risk posed by the environment are likely to affect the recurrences of RF. Risk increases with multiple previous attacks, whereas the risk decreases as the interval since the most recent attack lengthens.[44-46] In addition, the likelihood of acquiring a GABHS upper respiratory tract infection is an important consideration. Individuals with increased exposure to streptococcal infections include children and adolescents, parents of young children, teachers, physicians, nurses, and allied health personnel in contact with children, military recruits, and others living in crowded situations (e.g., college dormitories). A higher risk of recurrences in economically disadvantaged populations has been demonstrated.[14,47]

Just how long to continue prophylaxis was a debated point. Clearly the risk of recurrence declined with time, especially after 20 years of age, but it never went away.[48] Physicians must consider each individual situation when determining the appropriate duration of prophylaxis. In addition to the risk factors for recurrence described above, the presence of RHD also needs to be taken into consideration. The American Heart Association (AHA) recommendations are given in **Table 2**. The duration of prophylaxis depends on whether residual heart damage (valvular disease) is present or absent. Patients who have had rheumatic carditis, with or without valvular disease, are at a relatively high risk for recurrences of carditis and are likely to sustain increasingly severe cardiac involvement with each recurrence.[49,50] Therefore, patients who have had rheumatic carditis should receive long-term antibiotic prophylaxis well into adulthood and perhaps for life.

For patients with persistent valvular disease, the committee recommends prophylaxis for 10 years after the last episode of ARF or until 40 years of age (whichever is longer). After that time, the severity of the valvular disease and the potential for exposure to GABHS should be discussed and continued prophylaxis (potentially lifelong) should be considered for high-risk patients. Prophylaxis should continue even after valve surgery, including prosthetic valve replacement. For patients without persistent valvular disease, prophylaxis should continue for 10 years or until the patient is 21 years of age, whichever is longer.

Patients who have had RF without rheumatic carditis are also at risk for cardiac involvement with recurrences, although the risk is lower. In general, prophylaxis should continue in these patients until the patient reaches 21 years of age or until 5 years has elapsed since the last RF attack, whichever is longer. In all situations, the decision to discontinue prophylaxis or to reinstate it should be made after discussion with the patient of the potential risks and benefits and careful consideration of the epidemiological risk factors enumerated above.

The World Health Organization[1] recommends secondary rheumatic prophylaxis as lifelong in patients with severe valvular disease and after valve surgery. In patients with mild carditis (mild mitral regurgitation or healed carditis), the duration is for 10 years after the last attack or at least up to the age of 25 years whichever is longer. In patients with RF but no carditis, secondary prophylaxis is recommended for 5 years after the last attack or at least up to the age of 18 years (whichever is longer).

Despite prophylaxis, rheumatic recurrence, in terms of 100-patient years, has been shown to be 0.45% for parenteral penicillin, 5.5% for oral penicillin, 2.8% for sulfa drugs, and 15% in controls.[51]

Choice of Regimen for Prevention of Recurrent Rheumatic Fever

Intramuscular Benzathine Penicillin G

An injection of 1,200,000 U of this long-acting penicillin preparation every 4 weeks is the recommended regimen for secondary prevention of RF **(Table 3)**. After intramuscular injection, peak plasma concentrations are usually reached within 12–24 hours and are usually detectable for 1–4 weeks. In populations in which the incidence of RF is particularly high, the administration of benzathine penicillin G every 3 weeks is justified and recommended, because serum drug levels may fall below a protective level before the 4th week after administration of this dose of penicillin.[52,53] The administration of benzathine penicillin G every 3 weeks is recommended only for those who have recurrent ARF despite adherence to each and every 4-week regimen. Long-acting penicillin is of particular value in patients with a high risk of RF recurrence, especially those with RHD, in whom the consequences of recurrence may be serious. The advantages of benzathine penicillin G must be weighed against the inconvenience to the patient and the pain of injection, which causes some individuals to discontinue prophylaxis.

Although there has been concern about the risk of serious allergic reactions in patients receiving long-term intramuscular benzathine penicillin G prophylaxis for RF, a large, international, and prospective study determined that life-threatening allergic reactions are rare in these patients.[54] It has been demonstrated that the long-term benefits of such prophylaxis far outweigh the risk of serious allergic reactions.

Hypersensitivity reactions reported with penicillin ranging from skin rashes to immediate anaphylaxis which may be fatal. The overall incidence of hypersensitivity reactions is from 2 to 5%. Anaphylaxis is very rare and occurs in about 1/10,000 injections. Death has been reported

TABLE 2: Duration of secondary rheumatic fever prophylaxis.[39]

Category	Duration after last attack
Rheumatic fever with carditis and residual heart disease (persistent valvular disease*)	10 years or until 40 years of age (whichever is longer), sometimes lifelong prophylaxis
Rheumatic fever with carditis but no residual heart disease (no valvular disease*)	10 years or until 21 years of age (whichever is longer)
Rheumatic fever without carditis	5 years or until 21 years of age (whichever is longer)
*Clinical or echocardiographic evidence	

in about 1/30–50,000 injections. There is no evidence of teratogenicity with benzathine penicillin. It can be used during pregnancy.[1]

Several technical factors related to the benzathine penicillin injection can affect its bioavailability. For this reason it is recommended that healthcare workers responsible for administering the injection are trained in the technique of giving injections. The injection should be deep into the gluteus maximus muscle as recommended. More superficial injections allow the benzathine penicillin to remain in the subcutaneous tissue leading to decreased absorption and lower serum levels. Care should be taken, particularly in adults, that the whole content of the vial is fully removed and injected. The vial is diluted in sterile water to allow for a homogeneous suspension to be obtained to avoid obstruction of the injecting needle. A needle gauge of size 19 or 20 is preferred. Smaller bore needles have been noted to be more easily obstructed.

Although the activity of benzathine penicillin remains stable in the vial for several years if adequately stored, the activity may be affected by the presence of preservatives, metal ions, or bicarbonate in the vial. The physical properties of the solution, if not optimum, may also affect its degree of solubility and hence its absorption from the injection site. All of the above affect the biological activity of benzathine penicillin. Since different brands are produced in the market, continuous quality assurance is important to optimize not only its chemical activity but also its biological activity. This is needed to reduce variations between different brands and to assure effective serum penicillin levels.

Oral Agents

For patients for whom the regular and repeated injections of benzathine benzylpenicillin are not given, an alternative but lesser effective method is the use of daily oral phenoxymethylpenicillin. The potential problems with successful oral prophylaxis depends primarily on patient's compliance to prescribed regimens. Patients need careful and repeated instructions about the importance of continuing prophylaxis. Most failures of prophylaxis occur in nonadherent patients. Even with optimal patient adherence, the risk of recurrence is higher in individuals receiving oral prophylaxis than in those receiving intramuscular benzathine penicillin G.[37] Oral agents are more appropriate for patients at lower risk for RF recurrence. Accordingly, some physicians may consider switching patients to oral prophylaxis when they have reached late adolescence or young adulthood and have remained free of rheumatic attacks for at least 5 years.

Penicillin V

The recommended oral agent is penicillin V. The dosage for children and adults is 250 mg twice daily **(Table 3)**. There are no published data about the use of other penicillins, macrolides, azalides, or cephalosporins for the secondary prevention of RF.

TABLE 3: Secondary prevention of rheumatic fever (prevention of recurrent attacks).[39]

Agent	Dose	Mode
Benzathine penicillin G	600,000 U for children ≤27 kg (60 lb), 1,200,000 U for those >27 kg (60 lb) every 4 weeks*	Intramuscular
Penicillin V	250 mg twice daily	Oral
Sulfadiazine	0.5 g once daily for patients ≤27 kg (60 lb), 1.0 g once daily for patients >27 kg (60 lb)	Oral
For individuals allergic to penicillin and sulfadiazine		
Macrolide or azalide	Variable	Oral

*In high-risk situation, administration of every 3 weeks is justified and recommended.

In Indian subcontinent, as ARF is endemic, penicillin prophylaxis, once in 3 weeks is preferable.

Sulfadiazine

For patients allergic to penicillin, sulfadiazine is recommended. Although sulfonamides are not effective in the eradication of GABHS, they do prevent infection. The recommended dose of sulfadiazine is 0.5 g once per day for patients weighing 27 kg (60 lb) or less and 1 g once per day for patients weighing >27 kg. Sulfadiazine and sulfisoxazole appear to be equivalent; therefore, the use of sulfisoxazole is acceptable on the basis of extrapolation from data demonstrating that sulfadiazine has proven effectiveness in secondary prophylaxis. The recommended dose of sulfisoxazole is the same as that for sulfadiazine. Sulfonamide prophylaxis is contraindicated in late pregnancy because of transplacental passage of the drugs and potential competition with bilirubin for albumin-binding sites.

Macrolides

For the patient who is allergic to both penicillin and sulfisoxazole, an oral macrolide (erythromycin or clarithromycin) or azalide (azithromycin) is recommended. Macrolides (erythromycin and clarithromycin) and to a much lesser extent azalides (azithromycin) can cause prolongation of the QT interval in a dose-dependent manner. Because macrolides are metabolized extensively by cytochrome P-450 3A, they should not be taken concurrently with inhibitors of cytochrome P-450 3A such as azole antifungal agents, HIV protease inhibitors, and some selective serotonin reuptake inhibitor antidepressants.[28,29]

Bacterial Endocarditis Prophylaxis

The AHA has recently published updated recommendations regarding the use of prophylactic antibiotics to prevent infective endocarditis.[55] Because of the lack of published evidence indicating that the principle of prophylaxis is definitively valid, as it has been applied to infective endocarditis prevention, the value of infective endocarditis prophylaxis has been called into question by the AHA, as well as by other international scientific bodies.[56] However, the AHA and others continue to recognize that certain conditions, such as patients with prosthetic valves, those with previous endocarditis, cardiac transplant recipients who develop cardiac valvulopathy and specific forms of congenital heart disease, are associated with the highest risk of adverse outcome from endocarditis and given that documented high-risk prophylaxis remains indicated. Notably, the current AHA recommendations no longer suggest prophylaxis for patients with RHD, which may not be right in the developing countries where RF is endemic. Any damaged valve like the one in RHD definitely requires endocarditis prophylaxis, apart from the maintenance of optimal oral healthcare which is important. For the patients with RHD infective endocarditis prophylaxis is recommended, along with those with prosthetic valves or prosthetic material used in valve repair. The current AHA recommendations may not be adequate in poor developing countries where most of the children live in poor hygienic conditions.[57] These recommendations advise the use of an agent other than a penicillin to prevent infective endocarditis in those receiving penicillin prophylaxis for RF, because oral β-hemolytic streptococci are likely to have developed resistance to penicillin.

VACCINE FOR RHEUMATIC FEVER AND RHEUMATIC HEART DISEASE

Introduction

Development of a vaccine for RHD started in the early 1960s with crude cell wall to purified M proteins.[58] It is estimated that 95% of RF and RHD occur in the developing countries and most commonly found in the regions of Australia, Pacific Islands, India, Middle East, and sub-Saharan Africa.[5] GAS pharyngitis is considered to be the primary cause for RHD; however, genetic polymorphism among certain molecules such as human leukocyte antigen (HLA) class II, tumor necrosis factor-alpha (TNF-α), interleukin (IL)-10, IL-6, and IL-1Ra, angiotensin I-converting enzyme (ACE) showed an increased risk of RF/RHD.[59-61] Various autoimmune mechanisms based on cross-reactivity between streptococcal proteins and human cardiac proteins were proposed to explain the pathogenesis of RHD.[59,62-64] Recently, there is an alternative hypothesis proposed based on the binding of certain rheumatogenic M serotypes such as M3 and M18 to human collagen IV results in autoantibody response to collagen which have a potential to cause ARF.[65] Further, it was reported that the autoantibody formed against collagen is not cross-reactive with M proteins and no molecular mimicry occurs,[66] unlike

other reports around the autoimmune hypothesis of RHD. Similar anticollagen antibodies were also observed in the sera of RF patients, implying clinical significance of collagen binding to M proteins in the pathogenesis of RHD.[65,67] WHO in its publication state that "In light of the current lack of a clear strategy for primary prevention of GABHS infections, there is definitely a place for a safe, effective, affordable, and practical GABHS vaccine".[57]

Historical Perspective

Vaccine designing for RHD has been continuing over several decades, nevertheless, there is no protective vaccine available yet to prevent GAS infection. This might be due to several factors such as: (i) widespread diversity of *Streptococcus pyogenes* strains [>250 *emm* (gene encoding M protein) types], (ii) cross-reactivity between streptococcal and host proteins, and (iii) lack of relevant animal model for studying the pathogenesis of RHD.[68-70] Since the extraction of M protein by Rebecca Lancefield,[71] its further purification by Beachey and colleagues in Memphis, Tennessee, and Fischetti at Rockefeller University, New York has led to its molecular definition.[72,73] It was observed that opsonic antibodies to M protein protected animals from lethal challenge.[74] These antibodies persisted for up to 30 years after natural infection in humans[75] and appeared to be the basis of acquired type specific immunity.

Recently, the proteomic approach combined with two other technologies protein array and FACS (Fluorescence-Activated Cell Sorting) helps to identify well expressed, highly conserved cell surface/secreted proteins which are considered to be important characteristics of protective antigens.[76] The availability of genome sequences for most of the pathogens has led to the development of a new vaccine design method known as reverse vaccinology. Using this approach, researchers look at the entire genome of the pathogen to identify a novel protective antigen, instead of studying known virulent factors of the pathogen as a vaccine target.

Vaccine Targets

Vaccine targets for *Streptococcus pyogenes* can be classified into three major types **(Fig. 3)**: (i) vaccines based on cell surface proteins, (ii) vaccines based on secreted proteins, and (iii) vaccines based on carbohydrates.

VACCINES BASED ON CELL SURFACE PROTEINS

M Protein Vaccines

Among the cell surface proteins, M protein of *S. pyogenes* has been studied extensively. Especially, the hypervariable amino-terminal and the highly conserved carboxyl regions have long been the target for vaccine development against

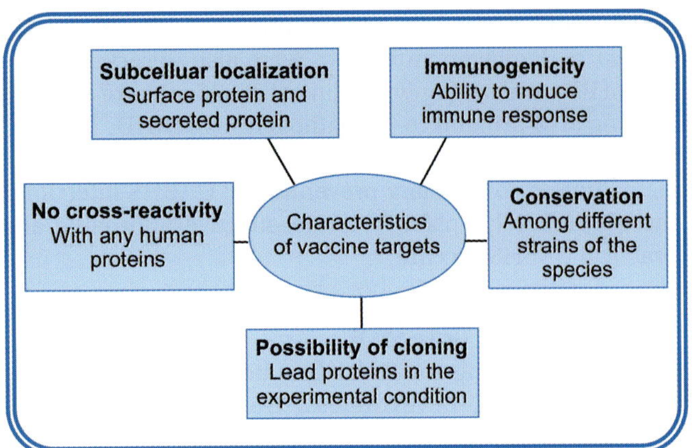

FIG. 3: Common characteristics of a potential vaccine candidate.

RHD due to its immunogenicity and no cross-reactivity properties.[69]

Recently, Dale and colleagues[77] constructed a new 30-valent M protein-based vaccine. This vaccine construct consists of N-terminal fragments (first 50 residues) of M proteins from 30 different M serotypes that are predominant in North America and Europe and further they shown to be immunogenic in rabbits. Interestingly, they have further found that this multivalent vaccine is protective against another 24 nonvaccine M serotypes, which are not included in the 30 valent vaccine constructs. The reason for this crossprotection may be due to the amino-acid sequence similarity present in the N-terminal or high-sequence similarity across the whole M protein found within the same emm cluster.[78]

Although some studies suggested that the level of bactericidal antibodies produced by C-terminal region of M protein may not be adequate to give complete protection against group A streptococcal (GAS) infection,[79] vaccine candidates such as StreptInCor and 14 peptide and J14 peptide which are derived from the C-terminal of M protein shown to be protective in animal models against RHD.

C5a Peptidase

SCPA (C5a peptidase of GAS) is another important cell surface molecule, which is highly conserved in all GAS serotypes and has not been associated with crossreactivity.[80] These features make it a possible vaccine candidate for GAS infection. As it is an endopeptidase, it can cleave the leukocyte binding site of the complement-derived chemotaxin C5a,[81] resulting in the inhibition of the recruitment of phagocytic cells to the site of infection, thereby helping *S. pyogenes* escape from the host immune response. A study by O'Connor et al. started to use C5a peptidase as a vaccine component in which they showed that measurable levels of IgA and IgG anti-SCPA antibodies are present in most of the healthy adults, but in much lower levels in uninfected children.[82]

One advantage of using C5a peptidase as a vaccine target is that, since it shares amino-acid sequence similarity with group B, C, and G *Streptococcus*, it could be used to prevent the infection caused by other groups of *Streptococcus*.

Fibronectin-binding Proteins

S. pyogenes has 11 fibronectin (Fn)-binding proteins, which are classified into two major types based on the presence of their binding repeats. It is found to be present in type I Fn-binding proteins, but not in type II Fn-binding proteins. Type I includes protein F1 (PrtF1)/SfbI, protein F2 (PrtF2)/PFBP, FbaA (formerly Fba), FbaB, SfbII/serum opacity factor (SOF), SfbX, and Fbp54. Proteins such as M1 protein, GAPDH/Plr, Shr, and Scl1 fall under type II Fn-binding proteins. Among these Fn-binding proteins, studies were available for FBP54,[83] FbaA,[84] PrtF1/SfbI,[85] serum opacity factor,[79] and Shr[86] for eliciting good immune response against GAS infection.[87]

Serum Opacity Factor

Serum opacity factor (SOF) is an Fn-binding protein expressed at the cell surface of *S. pyogenes*. Interestingly, it was found that the antibodies produced against opacity factor are type-specific, which can be used to determine the M serotype of GAS by using opacity factor inhibition test.[88] Courtney et al. showed that SOF is able to elicit a protective immune response against SOF-positive serotypes of *S. pyogenes*.[79] Studies suggested that combining SOF with other protective antigens such as Fn-binding protein I (SfbI) would stimulate strong systemic and mucosal immune responses which are required to prevent the disease.

Streptococcal Hemoprotein Receptor

Streptococcal hemoprotein receptor (Shr) is another highly conserved surface protein of GAS, which binds to hemoproteins and mediates heme acquisition.[89]

Streptococcus Pyogenes Cell Envelope Protein

Streptococcus pyogenes cell envelope protein (SpyCEP) is a highly conserved, subtilin-like protease known to cleave and inactivate IL-8.[90] A study by Turner et al. shows that the immunization of mice with recombinant SpyCEP protects against bacterial dissemination from both intramuscular soft-tissue infection and intranasal upper respiratory infection caused by M81 strain.[91]

R28

R28 is a highly repetitive streptococcal surface protein closely related to three different Group B *Streptococcus* surface proteins, α, β, and Rib, which are known to be protective determinants.[92-94]

Streptococcus Protective Antigen

A study by Dale et al. demonstrated that *antistreptococcus protective antigen* (Spa) antibodies opsonize some heterologous serotypes of group A streptococci (M3 and M28) in addition to the parent strain (M18), which confirms the presence of cross-protective epitopes which could aid in the development of broad spectrum vaccines against GAS infection.[95] Another study by McLellan et al. proves that Spa is required for the virulence of type 18 streptococci along with M protein and further evidence suggests that patients with ARF contained antibodies against Spa proteins, which clearly shows that the Spa protein is highly immunogenic in humans.[96]

Streptococcal Immunoglobulin-binding Protein

Streptococcal immunoglobulin-binding protein (Sib35) is an immunoglobulin-binding protein that binds to immunoglobulin (Ig)G, IgA, and IgM antibodies.[97] Immunization of mice with Sib35 induces high IgG antibody titer, which is shown to be protective when challenging mice with GAS strains.[97]

■ VACCINES BASED ON SECRETED PROTEINS

Secreted proteins of *S. pyogenes* include at least 11 pyrogenic exotoxins such as SPEA, SPEC, SPEG, SPEH, SPEI, SPEJ, SPEK, SPEL, SPEM, streptococcal mitogenic exotoxin Z (SMEZ), and streptococcal superantigen A (SSA).[98] Vaccines based on most of the secreted proteins of GAS are shown to be the most effective for systemic and invasive diseases, but have not been tested extensively for RHD.[99-103]

■ VACCINES BASED ON CARBOHYDRATES

Vaccines based on group A *Streptococcus* carbohydrate (GAS-CHO) are of less interest because of the cross-reactive autoantibodies that recognize these molecules and cardiac myosin. Nevertheless, a study by Sabharwal et al. shows that the active and passive immunization of GAS-CHO, conjugated to tetanus toxoid, protects mice against lethal challenges with live GAS strains.[104]

Cunningham[105] revealed that human monoclonal antibodies (mAbs) derived from RHD and Sydenham chorea share a common epitope, N-acetyl-β-D-glucosamine (GlcNAc) of group A carbohydrate, which recognize cross-reactive structures on the heart valve and on the neuronal cells in the brain, which may lead to RHD and Sydenham chorea respectively.

■ IN SILICO APPROACHES FOR VACCINE DESIGNING AGAINST RHD (FIG. 4)

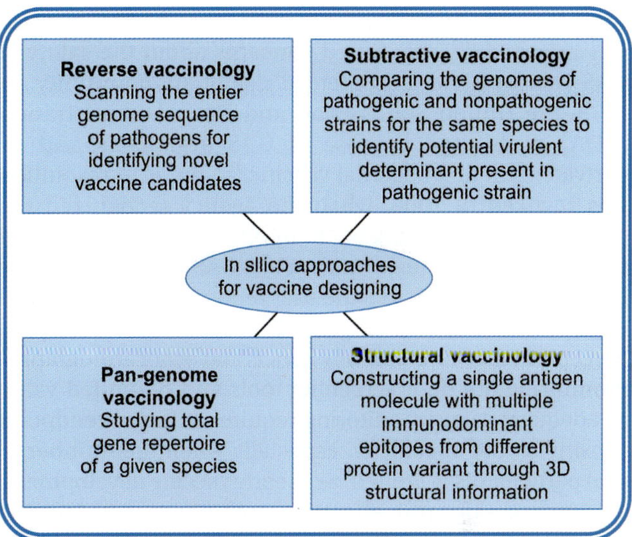

FIG. 4: Different types of in silico approaches for identifying potential targets for vaccine development.

■ HUMAN TRIALS/SAFETY CONSIDERATIONS

Vaccine Pipeline

Only two candidate vaccines are actively under evaluation in human trials. A phase I clinical trial of the MJ8VAX vaccine candidate developed by the Queensland Institute of Medical Research, Australia, was recently reported. The vaccine antigen is a 29-amino acid long peptide (J8) from the conserved carboxyl terminus region of the M protein[106] conjugated with diphtheria toxoid and adsorbed onto aluminum hydroxide. The 30-valent StreptAnova, developed at the University of Tennessee, USA and Dalhousie University, Canada, is an M-protein-based vaccine with four recombinant subunits, each containing seven or eight N-terminal fragments of 30 different emm types linked in tandem.[77] The N-terminal fragment of the Spa antigen is also included in the construct.[77] A phase I clinical trial of the vaccine adjuvanted with alum was recently completed. This program builds on favorable safety and immunogenicity evaluation of previous related constructs including a lower number of emm-type sequences.[77] In preclinical development, the StreptIncor vaccine candidate construct developed by the University of São Paulo, Brazil, is based on the conserved region of the M5 protein, which comprises a 55-amino acid polypeptide containing conserved B- and T-cell epitopes.

Safety Considerations

Safety concerns have constituted an important impediment to past vaccine development efforts. In 1969, the occurrence of ARF following streptococcal vaccination in three out of 21 volunteers vaccinated with a partially purified M3 protein was reported.[107] This raised concerns about the safety of GAS vaccines and a theoretical risk of autoimmunity. In 1979, the United States Food and Drug Administration (FDA) prohibited the use of GAS organisms and its derivatives in any bacterial vaccine.[108] The FDA resolution was revoked in 2006, when the agency recognized the previous understanding as "both obsolete and a perceived impediment to the development of a GAS vaccine".[108] There had not been a GAS vaccine trial reported during a period of 25 years. While due diligence is needed, there is a strong perception that autoantibody panels and echocardiographic monitoring are poor screening tools and of limited value as adequate safety monitoring requires sufficient endpoint sensitivity and specificity, especially when the number of trial participants is limited, as in early vaccine development.

Once a safe and effective streptococcal vaccine is available, there are many practical issues that need to be addressed. The highest rates of ARF tend to occur in areas with limited resources and public health infrastructure and ways of delivering a vaccine under these conditions need to be examined. Other issues, such as cost, route of administration, number and frequency of required doses, potential side effects, stability of the material under field conditions, and durability of immunity, would all influence the usefulness of any vaccine. In India, information on prevailing strains of streptococci based on *emm* typing is available from two Indian reference laboratories located in North (PGI, Chandigarh) and South India (CMC, Vellore).[109] A large number of GABHS emm-subtypes have been identified in them and there are relatively few strains common to both centers. A significant number of novel strains have been identified in both centers. Thus, it would be challenging to develop a polyvalent vaccine that would cover all M protein serotypes in India.

A global vaccine that covers other regions of the world, especially low-income countries, would be extremely helpful to eradicate RHD completely. With the recent computational advancements in the field of vaccinology, we hope that a protective vaccine against RHD is within reach, either through identification of novel antigens or through structure-based design of known antigens of GAS.

CONCLUSION

Acute rheumatic fever and RHD can be prevented by sustainable control strategies including:

- Trained healthcare staff who diagnose and manage disease effectively
- Secondary prophylaxis to prevent further ARF and the development or worsening of RHD
- Community education and awareness
- Screening for unknown RHD in the community Control strategies should focus on:
  - Prompt identification and treatment of GABHS infections
  - Identifying people who have had ARF once and preventing further ARF and the development of RHD

The persistence of ARF in many developing countries of the world, the apparent increase in life-threatening invasive group A *Streptococcus* infections in North America and Europe and the revolution in molecular biology have all spurred attempts to achieve a safe and effective vaccine against group A streptococci. The most promising approaches are M protein-based, including those using multivalent type specific vaccines, and those directed at non-type specific, highly conserved portions of the molecule. Success in developing vaccines may be achieved in the next 5–10 years, but this success would have to contend with important question about the safest, most economical and most efficacious way in which to employ them, as well as their cost effectiveness in a variety of epidemiologic and socioeconomic conditions.

ACKNOWLEDGMENT

Our grateful thanks to AHA for the kind permission to material from their article. Reproduced with permission Circulation. 2009;119:1542-51@ 2009 American Heart Association. Inc.

REFERENCES

1. World Health Organization. WHO Model Prescribing Information: Drugs Used in the Treatment of Streptococcal Pharyngitis and Prevention of Rheumatic Fever. 1999.

2. Siegel AC, Johnson EE, Stollerman GH. Controlled studies of streptococcal pharyngitis in a pediatric population, 1: Factors related to the attack rate of rheumatic fever. N Engl J Med. 1961;265:559-65.

3. Denny FW, Wannamaker LW, Brink WR, Rammelkamp CH Jr, Custer EA. Prevention of rheumatic fever: Treatment of the preceding streptococcal infection. JAMA. 1950;143:151-3.

4. Dajani AS. Current status of nonsuppurative complications of group A streptococci. Pediatr Infect Dis J. 1991;10(suppl): S25-7.

5. Wannamaker LW, Rammelkamp CH Jr, Denny FW, Brink WR, Houser HB, Hahn EO, et al. Prophylaxis of acute rheumatic fever by treatment of preceding streptococcal infection with various amounts of depot penicillin. Am J Med. 1951;10:673-95.

6. Catanzaro FJ, Stetson CA, Morris AJ, Chamovitz R, Rammelkamp CH Jr, Stolzer BL, et al. The role of the *Streptococcus* in the pathogenesis of rheumatic fever. Am J Med. 1954;17:749-56.

7. Snellman LW, Stang HJ, Stang JM, Johnson DR, Kaplan EL. Duration of positive throat cultures for group A streptococci after initiation of antibiotic therapy. Pediatrics. 1993;91: 1166-70.

8. Gerber MA, Spadaccini LJ, Wright LL, Deutsch L, Kaplan EL. Twice-daily penicillin in the treatment of streptococcal pharyngitis. Am J Dis Child. 1985;139:1145-8.

9. Bass JW, Person DA, Chan DS. Twice-daily oral penicillin for treatment of streptococcal pharyngitis: Less is best. Pediatrics. 2000;105:423-4.

10. Shvartzman P, Tabenkin H, Rosentzwaig A, Dolginov F. Treatment of streptococcal pharyngitis with amoxicillin once a day. BMJ. 1993;306:1170-2.

11. Feder HM Jr, Gerber MA, Randolph MF, Stelmach PS, Kaplan EL. Once-daily therapy for streptococcal pharyngitis with amoxicillin. Pediatrics. 1999;103:47-51.

12. Clegg HW, Ryan AG, Dallas SD, Kaplan EL, Johnson DR, Norton HI, et al. Treatment of streptococcal pharyngitis with once-daily compared with twice-daily amoxicillin: A noninferiority trial. Pediatr Infect Dis J. 2006;25:761-7.

13. Lennon DR, Farrell E, Martin DR, Stewart JM. Once-daily amoxicillin versus twice-daily penicillin V in group A beta-hemolytic streptococcal pharyngitis. Arch Dis Child. 2008;93:474-8.

14. Griffiths SP, Gersony WM. Acute rheumatic fever in New York City (1969 to 1988): a comparative study of two decades. J Pediatr. 1990;116:882-7.

15. Gordis L, Lilienfeld A, Rodriguez R. Studies in the epidemiology and preventability of rheumatic fever, II: socioeconomic factors and the incidence of acute attacks. J Chronic Dis. 1969;21: 655-66.

16. Ferguson GW, Shultz JM, Bisno AL. Epidemiology of acute rheumatic fever in a multiethnic, multiracial urban community: The Miami-Dade County experience. J Infect Dis. 1991;164: 720-5.

17. Chun LT, Reddy DV, Yamamoto LG. Rheumatic fever in children and adolescents in Hawaii. Pediatrics. 1987;79:549-52.

18. Bass JW, Crast FW, Knowles CR, Onufer CN. Streptococcal pharyngitis in children: A comparison of four treatment schedules with intramuscular penicillin G benzathine. JAMA. 1976;235:1112-6.

19. Pichichero ME, Margolis PA. A comparison of cephalosporins and penicillin in the treatment of group A beta-hemolytic streptococcal pharyngitis: a meta-analysis supporting the concept of microbial copathogenicity. Pediatr Infect Dis J. 1991;10:275-81.

20. Block SL, Hedrick JA, Tyler RD. Comparative study of the effectiveness of cefixime and penicillin V for the treatment of streptococcal pharyngitis in children and adolescents. Pediatr Infect Dis J. 1992;11:919-25.

21. WM III, Gooch SE, McLinn GH, Aronovitz ME, Pichichero A, Kumar EL, et al. Efficacy of cefuroxime axetil suspension compared with that of penicillin V suspension in children with group A streptococcal pharyngitis. Antimicrob Agents Chemother. 1993;37:159-63.

22. Dajani AS, Kessler SL, Mendelson R, Uden DL, Todd WM. Cefpodoxime proxetil vs penicillin V in pediatric streptococcal pharyngitis tonsillitis. Pediatr Infect Dis J. 1993;12:275-9.

23. Pichichero ME. A review of evidence supporting the American Academy of Pediatrics recommendation for prescribing cephalosporin antibiotics for penicillin-allergic patients. Pediatrics. 2005;115:1048-57.

24. Tack KJ, Hedrick JA, Rothstein E, Nemeth MA, Keyserling C, Pichichero ME. Cefdinir Pediatric Pharyngitis Study Group. A study of 5-day cefdinir treatment for streptococcal pharyngitis in children. Arch Pediatr Adolesc Med. 1997;151:45-9.

25. Pichichero ME, Gooch WM, Rodriguez W, Blumer JL, Aronoff SC, Jacobs RF, et al. Effective short-course treatment of acute group A beta-hemolytic streptococcal tonsillopharyngitis: Ten days of penicillin V vs 5 days or 10 days of cefpodoxime therapy in children. Arch Pediatr Adolesc Med. 1994;148:1053-60.

26. Aujard Y, Boucot I, Brahimi N, Chiche D, Bingen E. Comparative efficacy and safety of four-day cefuroxime axetil and ten-day penicillin treatment of group A beta-hemolytic streptococcal pharyngitis in children. Pediatr Infect Dis J. 1995;14:295-300.

27. Dajani AS. Pharyngitis/tonsillitis: European and United States experience with cefpodoxime proxetil. Pediatr Infect Dis J. 1995;14(4 Suppl):S7-11.

28. Ray WA, Murray KT, Meredith S, Narasimhulu SS, Hall K, Stein CM. Oral erythromycin and the risk of sudden death from cardiac causes. N Engl J Med. 2004;351:1089-6.

29. Huang BH, Wu CH, Hsia Chen CP, Yin C. Azithromycin-induced torsade de pointes. Pacing Clin Electrophysiol. 2007;30:1579-82.

30. Seppälä H, Nissinen A, Järvinen H, Huovinen S, Henriksson T, Herva E, et al. Resistance to erythromycin in group A streptococci. N Engl J Med. 1992;326:292-7.

31. Tanz RR, Shulman ST, Shortridge VD, Kabat W, Kabat K, Cederlund E, et al. North American Streptococcal Pharyngitis Surveillance Group. Community-based surveillance in the United States of macrolide-resistant pediatric pharyngeal group A streptococci during 3 respiratory disease seasons. Clin Infect Dis. 2004;39:1794-801.

32. Gerber MA. Antibiotic resistance: Relationship to persistence of group A streptococci in the upper respiratory tract. Pediatrics. 1996;97(pt 2):971-5.

33. Gerber MA. Antibiotic resistance in group A streptococci. Pediatr Clin North Am. 1995;42:539-51.

34. Coonan KM, Kaplan EL. In vitro susceptibility of recent North American group A streptococcal isolates to eleven oral antibiotics. Pediatr Infect Dis J. 1994;13:630-5.

35. Wickman PA, Black JA, Moland ES, Thomson KS. In vitro activities of DX-619 and other comparison quinolones against Gram-positive cocci. Antimicrob Agents Chemother. 2006;50:2255-7.

36. Gerber MA. Treatment failures and carriers: Perception or problems? Pediatr Infect Dis J. 1994;13:576-9.

37. Feinstein AR, Wood HF, Epstein JA, Taranta A, Simpson R, Tursky E. A controlled study of three methods of prophylaxis against streptococcal infection in a population of rheumatic children, II: Results of the first three years of the study, including methods for evaluating the maintenance of oral prophylaxis. N Engl J Med. 1959;260:697-702.

38. Markowitz M, Gerber MA, Kaplan EL. Treatment of streptococcal pharyngotonsillitis: Reports of penicillin's demise are premature. J Pediatr. 1993;123:679-85.

39. Gerber AM, Baltimore RS, Eaton CB, Gewitz M, Anne H, Shulman ST. Prevention of rheumatic fever and diagnosis and treatment of Acute Streptococcal Pharyngitis: A Scientific Statement From the American Heart Association Rheumatic Fever, Endocarditis, and Kawasaki Disease Committee. Circulation. 2009;119; 1541-51.

40. Meier FA, Centor RM, Graham L Jr, Dalton HP. Clinical and microbiological evidence for endemic pharyngitis among adults due to group C streptococci. Arch Intern Med. 1990;150: 825-9.

41. Turner JC, Hayden FG, Lobo MC, Ramirez CE, Murren D. Epidemiologic evidence for Lancefield group C beta-hemolytic streptococci as a cause of exudative pharyngitis in college students. J Clin Microbiol. 1997;35:1-4.

42. Stollerman GH. The Prevention of Rheumatic Fever by the Use of Antibiotics. Bull N Y Acad Med. 1955;31:165-80.

43. Kuttner AG, Mayer FE. Carditis during Second Attacks of Rheumatic Fever: Its Incidence in Patients without Clinical Evidence of Cardiac Involvement in Their Initial Rheumatic Episode. N Engl J Med. 1963;268:1259-61.

44. Bland EF, Duckett JT. Rheumatic fever and rheumatic heart disease: a twenty year report on 1000 patients followed since childhood. Circulation. 1951;4:836-43.

45. Taranta A, Kleinberg E, Feinstein AR, Wood HF, Tursky E, Simpson R. Rheumatic fever in children and adolescents: a long term epidemiologic study of subsequent prophylaxis, streptococcal infections, and clinical sequelae, V: relation of the rheumatic fever recurrence rate per streptococcal infection to pre-existing clinical features of the patients. Ann Intern Med. 1964;60(suppl 5):58-67.

46. Wilson MG, Lubschez R. Recurrence rates in rheumatic fever: Evaluation of etiologic concepts and consequent preventive therapy. JAMA. 1944;126:477-80.

47. Gordis L, Lilienfeld A, Rodriguez R. Studies in the epidemiology and preventability of rheumatic fever, I: Demographic factors and the incidence of acute attacks. J Chronic Dis. 1969;21: 645-54.

48. Johnson EE, Stollerman GH, Grossman BJ. Rheumatic Recurrences in Patients Not Receiving Continuous Prophylaxis. J Am Med Assoc. 1964;190:407-13.

49. Majeed HA, Yousof AM, Khuffash FA, Yusuf AR, Farwana S, Khan N. The natural history of acute rheumatic fever in Kuwait: A prospective six year follow-up report. J Chronic Dis. 1986;39: 361-9.

50. Lee GM, Wessels MR. Changing epidemiology of acute rheumatic fever in the United States. Clin Infect Dis. 2006;42:448-50.

51. Garvin JB, Tursky E, Albam B, Feinstein AR. Rheumatic fever in children and adolescents: a long term epidemiologic study of subsequent prophylaxis, streptococcal infections and clinical sequelae. II. Maintenance and preservation of the population. Ann Intern Med. 1964;60(suppl 5):18-30.

52. Lue HC, Wu MH, Hsieh KH, Lin GJ, Hsieh RP, Chiou JF. Rheumatic fever recurrences: Controlled study of a 3-week versus 4-week benzathine penicillin prevention programs. J Pediatr. 1986;108:299-304.

53. Lue HC, Wu MH, Wang JK, Wu FF, Wu YN. Long-term outcome of patients with rheumatic fever receiving benzathine penicillin G prophylaxis every three weeks versus every four weeks. J Pediatr. 1994;125(Pt 1):812-6.

54. International Rheumatic Fever Study Group. Allergic reactions to long-term benzathine penicillin prophylaxis for rheumatic fever. Lancet. 1991;337:1308-10.

55. Wilson W, Taubert KA, Gewitz M, Lockhart PB, Baddour LM, Levison M, et al. Prevention of infective endocarditis: Guidelines from the American Heart Association: A guideline from the American Heart Association Rheumatic Fever, Endocarditis, and Kawasaki Disease Committee, Council on Cardiovascular Disease in the Young, and the Council on Clinical Cardiology, Council on Cardiovascular Surgery and Anesthesia, and the Quality of Care and Outcomes Research Interdisciplinary Working Group. Circulation. 2007;116:1736-54.

56. Gould FK, Elliott TS, Foweraker J, Fulford M, Perry JD, Roberts GJ, et al. Working Party of the British Society for Antimicrobial Chemotherapy. Guidelines for the prevention of endocarditis: Report of the Working Party of the British Society for Antimicrobial Chemotherapy. J Antimicrob Chemother. 2006;57:1035-42.

57. World Health Organization. Group A streptococcal vaccine development: Current status and issues of relevance to less developed countries. Group A streptococcal disease. Discussion papers on child health. Geneva: WHO; 2005.

58. Cunningham MW. Pathogenesis of group A streptococcal infections. Clin Microbiol Rev. 2000;13(3):470-511.

59. Chang C. Cutting edge issues in rheumatic fever. Clin Rev Allergy Immunol. 2012;42(2):213-37.

60. Bryant PA, Robins-Browne R, Carapetis JR, Curtis N. Some of the people, some of the time: Susceptibility to acute rheumatic fever. Circulation. 2009;119(5):742-53.

61. Tian Y, Ge Z, Xing Y, Sun Y, Ying J. Correlation of angiotensin I-converting enzyme gene insertion/deletion polymorphism with rheumatic heart disease: A meta-analysis. Biosci Rep. 2016;36(6):e00412.

62. Carapetis JR, McDonald M, Wilson NJ. Acute rheumatic fever. Lancet. 2005;366(9480):155-68.

63. Ellis NM, Li Y, Hildebrand W, Fischetti VA, Cunningham MW. T cell mimicry and epitope specificity of cross-reactive T cell clones from rheumatic heart disease. J Immunol. 2005;175(8):5448-56.

64. Root-Bernstein R. Rethinking molecular mimicry in rheumatic heart disease and autoimmune myocarditis: Laminin, Collagen IV, CAR, and B1AR as initial targets of disease. Front Pediatr. 2014;2:129.

65. Dinkla K, Nitsche-Schmitz DP, Barroso V, Reissmann S, Johansson HM, Frick IM, et al. Identification of a streptococcal octapeptide motif involved in acute rheumatic fever. J Biol Chem. 2007;282(26):18686-93.

66. Tandon R, Sharma M, Chandrashekhar Y, Kotb M, Yacoub MH, Narula J. Revisiting the pathogenesis of rheumatic fever and carditis. Nat Rev Cardiol. 2013;10(3):171-7.

67. Dinkla K, Rohde M, Jansen WT, Kaplan EL, Chhatwal GS, Talay SR. Rheumatic fever-associated Streptococcus pyogenes isolates aggregate collagen. J Clin Invest. 2003;111(12):1905-12.

68. Smeesters PR, McMillan DJ, Sriprakash KS. The streptococcal M protein: A highly versatile molecule. Trends Microbiol. 2010;18(6):275-82.

69. Pandey M, Batzloff MR, Good MF. Vaccination against rheumatic heart disease: A review of current research strategies and challenges. Curr Infect Dis Rep. 2012;14(4):381-90

70. Zabriskie JB. Rheumatic fever: The interplay between host, genetics, and microbe. Lewis A. Conner memorial lecture. Circulation. 1985;71(6):1077-86.

71. Lancefield RC. Specific relationship of cell composition to biological activity of hemolytic streptococci. Harvey Lect. 1941(1940-1941);35:251.

72. Beachey EH, Stollerman GH, Johnson RH, Ofek I, Bisno AL. Human immune response to immunization with a structurally defined polypeptide fragment of streptococcal M protein. J Exper Med. 1979;150:862-77.

73. Fischetti VA, Jones KF, Hollingshead SK, Scott JR. Structure, function and genetics of streptococcal M protein. Rev Infect Dis. 1988;10:(Suppl 2):S356-9.

74. Lancefield RC. Current knowledge of type-specific M antigens of group A streptococci. J Immunol. 1962;89:307-13.

75. Lancefield RC. Persistence of type-specific antibodies in man following infection with group A streptococci. J Experiment Med. 1959;110:271-92.

76. Bensi G, Mora M, Tuscano G, Biagini M, Chiarot E, Bombaci M, et al. Multi high-throughput approach for highly selective identification of vaccine candidates: The Group A *Streptococcus* case. Mol Cell Proteomics. 2012;11(6):M111 015693.

77. Dale JB, Penfound TA, Chiang EY, Walton WJ. New 30-valent M protein-based vaccine evokes cross-opsonic antibodies against non-vaccine serotypes of group A streptococci. Vaccine. 2011;29(46):8175-8.

78. Sanderson-Smith M, Oliveira DM, Guglielmini J, McMillan DJ, Vu T, Holien JK, et al. A systematic and functional classification of *Streptococcus pyogenes* that serves as a new tool for molecular typing and vaccine development. J Infect Dis. 2014.

79. Courtney HS, Hasty DL, Dale JB. Serum opacity factor (SOF) of *Streptococcus pyogenes* evokes antibodies that opsonize homologous and heterologous SOF-positive serotypes of group A streptococci. Infect Immun. 2003;71(9):5097-103.

80. Park HS, Cleary PP. Active and passive intranasal immunizations with streptococcal surface protein C5a peptidase prevent infection of murine nasal mucosa-associated lymphoid tissue, a functional homologue of human tonsils. Infect Immun. 2005;73(12):7878-86.

81. Wexler DE, Chenoweth DE, Cleary PP. Mechanism of action of the group A streptococcal C5a inactivator. Proc Natl Acad Sci U S A. 1985;82(23):8144-8.

82. O'Connor SP, Darip D, Fraley K, Nelson CM, Kaplan EL, Cleary PP. The human antibody response to streptococcal C5a peptidase. J Infect Dis. 1991;163(1):109-16.

83. Kawabata S, Kunitomo E, Terao Y, Nakagawa I, Kikuchi K, Totsuka K, et al. Systemic and mucosal immunizations with fibronectin-binding protein FBP54 induce protective immune responses against *Streptococcus pyogenes* challenge in mice. Infect Immun. 2001;69(2):924-30.

84. Terao Y, Okamoto S, Kataoka K, Hamada S, Kawabata S. Protective immunity against *Streptococcus pyogenes* challenge in mice after immunization with fibronectin-binding protein. J Infect Dis. 2005;192(12):2081-91.

85. Olive C, Schulze K, Sun HK, Ebensen T, Horvath A, Toth I, et al. Enhanced protection against *Streptococcus pyogenes* infection by intranasal vaccination with a dual antigen component M protein/SfbI lipid core peptide vaccine formulation. Vaccine. 2007;25(10):1789-97.

86. Huang YS, Fisher M, Nasrawi Z, Eichenbaum Z. Defense from the Group A *Streptococcus* by active and passive vaccination with the streptococcal hemoprotein receptor. J Infect Dis. 2011;203(11):1595-601.

87. Yamaguchi M, Terao Y, Kawabata S. Pleiotropic virulence factor—*Streptococcus pyogenes* fibronectinbinding proteins. Cell Microbiol. 2012.

88. Beall B, Gherardi G, Lovgren M, Facklam RR, Forwick BA, Tyrrell GJ. emm and sof gene sequence variation in relation to serological typing of opacity-factor-positive group A streptococci. Microbiology. 2000;146(Pt 5):1195-209.

89. Bates CS, Montanez GE, Woods CR, Vincent RM, Eichenbaum Z. Identification and characterization of a *Streptococcus pyogenes* operon involved in binding of hemoproteins and acquisition of iron. Infect Immun. 2003;71(3):1042-55.

90. Edwards RJ, Taylor GW, Ferguson M, Murray S, Rendell N, Wrigley A, et al. Specific C-terminal cleavage and inactivation of interleukin-8 by invasive disease isolates of *Streptococcus pyogenes*. J Infect Dis. 2005;192(5):783-90.

91. Turner CE, Kurupati P, Wiles S, Edwards RJ, Sriskandan S. Impact of immunization against SpyCEP during invasive disease with two streptococcal species: *Streptococcus pyogenes* and *Streptococcus equi*. Vaccine. 2009;27(36):4923-29.

92. Bevanger L, Naess AI. Mouse-protective antibodies against the Ibc proteins of group B streptococci. Acta Pathol Microbiol Immunol Scand B. 1985;93(2):121-4.

93. Michel JL, Madoff LC, Kling DE, Kasper DL, Ausubel FM. Cloned alpha and beta C-protein antigens of group B streptococci elicit protective immunity. Infect Immun. 1991;59(6):2023-8.

94. Stalhammar-Carlemalm M, Stenberg L, Lindahl G. Protein rib: A novel group B streptococcal cell surface protein that confers protective immunity and is expressed by most strains causing invasive infections. J Exp Med. 1993;177(6):1593-603.

95. Dale JB, Chiang EY, Liu S, Courtney HS, Hasty DL. New protective antigen of group A streptococci. J Clin Invest. 1999;103(9):1261-8.

96. McLellan DG, Chiang EY, Courtney HS, Hasty DL, Wei SC, Hu MC, et al. Spa contributes to the virulence of type 18 group A streptococci. Infect Immun. 2001;69(5):2943–9.

97. Okamoto S, Tamura Y, Terao Y, Hamada S, Kawabata S. Systemic immunization with streptococcal immunoglobulin-binding protein Sib 35 induces protective immunity against group: A *Streptococcus* challenge in mice. Vaccine. 2005;23(40):4852-9.

98. Commons R, Rogers S, Gooding T, Danchin M, Carapetis J, Robins-Browne R, et al. Superantigen genes in group A streptococcal isolates and their relationship with emm types. J Med Microbiol. 2008;57(Pt 10):1238-46.

99. Roggiani M, Stoehr JA, Olmsted SB, Matsuka YV, Pillai S, Ohlendorf DH, et al. Toxoids of streptococcal pyrogenic exotoxin A are protective in rabbit models of streptococcal toxic shock syndrome. Infect Immun. 2000;68(9):5011-7.

100. McCormick JK, Tripp TJ, Olmsted SB, Matsuka YV, Gahr PJ, Ohlendorf DH, et al. Development of streptococcal pyrogenic exotoxin C vaccine toxolds that are protective in the rabbit model of toxic shock syndrome. J Immunol. 2000;165(4):2306-12.

101. Kapur V, Maffei JT, Greer RS, Li LL, Adams GJ, Musser JM. Vaccination with streptococcal extracellular cysteine protease (interleukin-1 beta convertase) protects mice against challenge with heterologous group A streptococci. Microb Pathog. 1994;16(6):443-50

102. Chiarot E, Faralla C, Chiappini N, Tuscano G, Falugi F, Gambellini G, et al. Targeted amino acid substitutions impair streptolysin O toxicity and group A *Streptococcus virulence*. mBio. 2013;4(1):e00387-12.

103. Liu M, Zhu H, Zhang J, Lei B. Active and passive immunizations with the streptococcal esterase Sse protect mice against subcutaneous infection with group A streptococci. Infect Immun. 2007;75(7):3651-7.

104. Sabharwal H, Michon F, Nelson D, Dong W, Fuchs K, Manjarrez RC, et al. Group A *Streptococcus* (GAS) carbohydrate as an immunogen for protection against GAS infection. J Infect Dis. 2006;193(1):129-35.

105. Cunningham MW. *Streptococcus* and rheumatic fever. Curr Opin Rheumatol. 2012;24(4):408-16.

106. Sekuloski S, Batzloff MR, Griffin P, Parsonage W, Elliott S, Hartas J, et al. Evaluation of safety and immunogenicity of a group A

Streptococcus vaccine candidate (MJ8VAX) in a randomized clinical trial. PLoS One. 2018;13:e0198658.

107. Massell BF, Honikman LH, Amezcua J. Rheumatic Fever Following Streptococcal Vaccination. Report of three cases. JAMA. 1969;207:1115-9.

108. GoVInfo. (1996). Centre for Disease Control. 21 CFR 610.19—Status of specific products; Group A *Streptococcus*. Code of Federal Regulations. [online] Available from https://www.govinfo.gov/app/details/CFR-1996-title21-vol7/CFR-1996-title21-vol7-sec610-19 [Last accessed Sept., 2022].

109. Dey N, McMillan DJ, Yarwood PJ, Joshi RM, Kumar R, Good MF, et al. High diversity of group A Streptococcal emm types in an Indian community: The need to tailor multivalent vaccines. Clin Infect Dis. 2005;40:46-51.

18

Natural History of Rheumatic Fever and Rheumatic Heart Disease

IB Vijayalakshmi, Asha Moorthy, Jain T Kallarakkal

"Diseases are but parts of a course of natural history."

—**Sir William Withey Gull** (1816–1890)
British Physician, Guy's Hospital
London British Medical Journal (1874)

INTRODUCTION

In many developing countries, acute rheumatic fever (ARF) and its sequelae "rheumatic heart disease" (RHD) are a major cardiovascular health problem in children, adolescents, and young adults. Though, traditionally considered as the disease of poor and driven by poor sanitation, overcrowding, malnutrition, and limited access to health care, it continues to afflict the middle class who have access to medical care in many countries. The natural history of ARF and RHD has changed dramatically, thanks to the improved living conditions, advent of antibiotics, balloon interventions, and improved surgical techniques like repair or replacement of the valves. Unfortunately, the disease exists in its native form in many places in underdeveloped countries like Africa, some urban slums of developing countries like India and in certain pockets of remote areas of developed countries like Australia and New Zealand. In 2015, RHD affected 33.4 million people globally and caused 319,400 deaths.[1] Hence, it is very important to know the natural history so that the patients can be cautioned, coaxed, and impressed upon for the newer methods of management.

NATURAL HISTORY OF ACUTE RHEUMATIC FEVER

In 1928, a study organized the experience recorded in 3,000 children and adolescents who had received protracted hospital care for rheumatic fever at the House of the Good Samaritan in Boston. About 1,000 patients were followed up for the next 20 years in special clinics, at the interval of 6–12 months and the natural history was published by Bland and Duckett Jones.[2] Nearly 30% of patients with ARF had uneventful life and 34% presented with signs and symptoms of heart failure. Atrial fibrillation occurred in 9.4% of patients. Almost one-third of the patients died in two decades and of these more than a third succumbed in the first 5 years of their disease. When postmortem examination was conducted, the cause of death was due to greatly enlarged heart and congestive heart failure (CHF), in nearly 81% of them. Pericarditis was observed in 63% of patients. The least mortality of 12% was seen in patients with chorea. The rate of death at the end of 10 years and 20 years is given in **Table 1**.

In this study, they noticed that those who began their rheumatic career with considerable cardiac enlargement did poorly and it is unusual for patients who survive adolescence with greatly enlarged hearts to attain the age of 30 years. On the other hand, little or no cardiac enlargement early in the disease speaks for a higher degree of natural resistance, relative freedom from serious recurrences and a longer life. The degree of disability and ultimate longevity are further influenced by the frequency, duration, and severity of recurrences. The severity of recurrence of rheumatic activity is by far the most significant factor.

In patients with polyarthritis, if untreated, the inflammatory findings last from 1 to 5 days in each joint, reach the higher intensity in the first 2 days, with the entire process subsiding over 2–4 weeks.[3] Subcutaneous nodules persist from days to weeks and rarely last longer than 1 month. In erythema marginatum, the manifestation is transient, may last a few minutes and more usually for days. It may last intermittently for months. Mild form of chorea may subside in few weeks, but most frequently the recovery takes up to 6 months. In severe cases, the manifestation may persist for >2 years.[4] Chorea characteristically was associated with a benign form of the disease (12% mortality) with much overlapping of this symptomatology.[5] Fever, which is usually low grade, is mainly present in the early stage of the disease and can persist for 2–3 weeks.[6]

The algorithm of natural history of ARF and RHD is given in **Flowchart 1**.

Carditis is predominantly responsible for the morbidity and mortality associated with ARF.[7] Carditis occurs in 0.3% of ARF cases in epidemic areas and 3% of cases in endemic areas. Carditis is an early manifestation of ARF and nearly 80% of patients develop carditis within 2 weeks of onset of ARF.[8,9] Out of these carditis patients, nearly 50% go undetected clinically and later present as chronic RHD after many years. Carditis can present in a number of ways including subclinical, indolent, subacute, fulminant with congestive heart failure or mitral/or aortic regurgitation

TABLE 1: Rate of mortality at the end of 10 and 20 years.[1]		
Onset (No. of cases)	*10 years (fatalities)*	*20 years (fatalities)*
Greatly enlarged heart (70)	56 (80%)	57 (81%)
Congestive failure (207)	148 (71%)	152 (80%)
Pericarditis (130)	73 (56%)	77 (63%)
Nodules (88)	34 (38%)	37 (43%)
Arthritis (410)	91 (22%)	109 (27%)
Chorea (518)	49 (9.4%)	63 (12%)

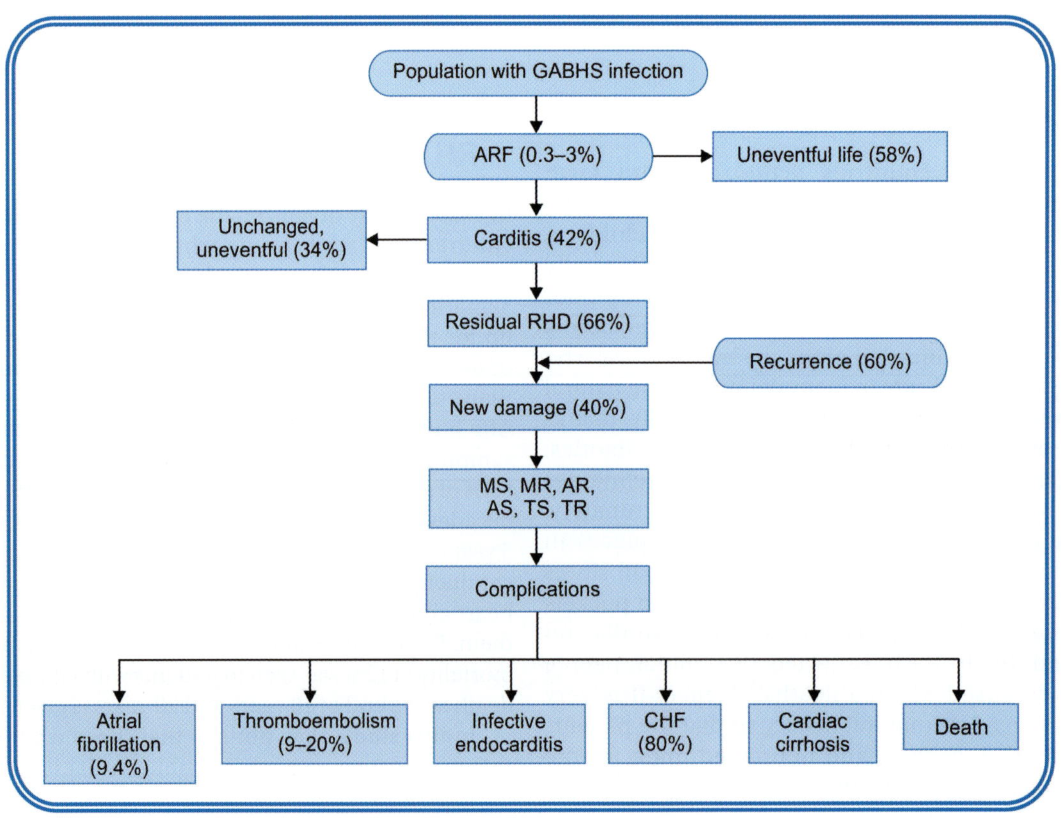

FLOWCHART 1: Algorithm showing natural history of rheumatic fever and rheumatic heart disease

(AR: aortic regurgitation; ARF: acute rheumatic fever; AS: aortic stenosis; CHF: congestive heart failure; MR: mitral regurgitation; MS: mitral stenosis; RHD: rheumatic heart disease; TR: tricuspid regurgitation; TS: tricuspid stenosis)

(AR) of varying severity. The younger patients often present with insidious onset of carditis, whereas joint involvement is common in older patients.[10]

The patients who have significant arthritis less commonly have severe carditis.[8,11] The joint discomfort often forces patients to seek medical attention sooner and more often than patients with carditis, which is often asymptomatic or mildly symptomatic initially. This is unfortunate because arthritis invariably recovers completely without any residual defect, whereas carditis which goes on to develop RHD in future goes untreated. Hence, with every recurrence of rheumatic activity, the heart valves get further damaged. Ultimately, when patient develops enlarged heart and becomes highly symptomatic, the patient is brought to the hospital in a very moribund state.

Among the valves, mitral valve (MV) is the most commonly affected in 80% and the aortic valve is second in frequency and affects 48% of the patients. The tricuspid valve is deformed in only 12% of patients and is almost always associated with mitral and aortic lesions. The involvement of pulmonary valve is extremely rare and affects 5%,[12] and occurs especially among the people living at high altitude. The most accepted reason for affection of the valves in this order is the degree of stress and strain these inflamed leaflets of rheumatic carditis bear during each cardiac cycle rather than any intrinsic factor within the leaflets. The relative frequency with which each valve is affected is proportional to pressure load against which each normally functions. Thus, the load against which the mitral, aortic, tricuspid, and pulmonary valves have to work is in the proportion of about 100, 60, 15, and 6 mm Hg, respectively.[12] The proof for this explanation also comes from the fact that the incidence of rheumatic involvement of the pulmonary valve which is extremely rare, increases at high altitude, where pulmonary hypertension is common. Severe valve insufficiency, during the acute phase may result in CHF and even death (1% of patients). Whether myocardial dysfunction during ARF is primarily related to myocarditis or is secondary to CHF from severe valve insufficiency is not known. Pericarditis, when present, rarely affects cardiac function and does not result in constrictive pericarditis.

While the first attack of carditis may be severe and fatal in some, the majority of the subjects survived subsequent recurrent active carditis. The average age of death was 12.6 years and the highest incidence was in the age group of 12–16 years. The type of rheumatic manifestation, exclusive of active carditis, did not appear to be of prognostic significance.

The incidence of heart disease was comparable, whether patients exhibited joint pains alone or chorea or polyarthritis, with or without joint pains. All of the subjects, presented evidence of cardiac involvement, only in 39%, symptoms of carditis were above the clinical horizon and capable of recognition. Those patients with the symptoms of active carditis had multiple valvular lesions and marked cardiac enlargement and higher mortality. During the course of

the disease, physical signs of valvular involvement may disappear, may be inconstant or uncharacteristic, leading to the erroneous opinion that the heart is left unscathed. The presence of considerable cardiac enlargement, established by adequate radiographic examination in a large series, which were under continuous careful observation, indicates the limitations of a diagnosis of the absence of cardiac involvement in rheumatic individuals based on physical examination alone.

The natural history of individuals who have had documented ARF varies considerably from patient to patient. Thompkins et al. demonstrated that if secondary prophylaxis is reliably followed, 70% of individuals developing the murmur of MR, at the time of acute attack lose that murmur over the next 5 years.[13] Hence, continuous secondary prophylaxis is very important.

The delayed appearance of RHD can occur as sequelae to ARF. The counterpart of the above group is represented by those who recovered unscarred from their original ARF, but whom in later years, insidiously and often without further recognizable rheumatic activity, developed signs of valvular damage, most often "pure" mitral stenosis (MS). The valvular heart disease developed after 10 years in 24% and at the end of 20 years in 44%.[2] In some part of the world like Indian subcontinent; however, an entity known as juvenile or malignant MS occurs.[14] Chronic manifestations due to residual and progressive valve deformity occur in 9–39% of adults with previous RHD. Fusion of the valve apparatus resulting in stenosis or a combination of stenosis and insufficiency develops 2–10 years after an episode of ARF and recurrent episodes may cause progressive damage to the valves. Fusion occurs at the level of the valve commissures, cusps, chordal attachments, or any combination of these. RHD is responsible for 99% of mitral valve stenosis in adults. Associated atrial fibrillation or left atrial thrombus formation **(Fig. 1)** from chronic mitral valve involvement and atrial enlargement may be observed.

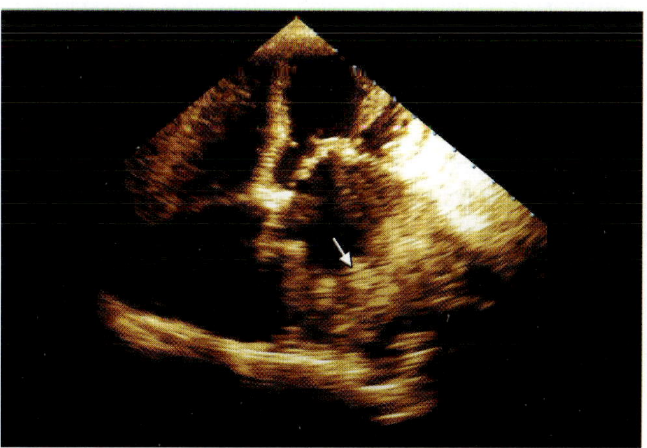

FIG. 1: Apical four-chamber view in a 40-year-old man with severe mitral stenosis (MS) with atrial fibrillation shows enlarged left atrium with large body thrombus (arrow).

In Wood's series,[12] the latency period from ARF (average age – 12 years) until the onset of cardiac symptoms due to MS (average age – 31 years) was 19 years. Selzer and Cohn[15] suggested that the initial valvulitis (at the time of rheumatic carditis) causes an abnormal flow pattern across the valve leaflets that eventually lead to thickening, fibrosis, and possible calcification of the valve cusps.

■ NATURAL HISTORY OF MITRAL STENOSIS

The natural history of rheumatic MS is characterized by an asymptomatic latent period, following the initial rheumatic fever.[16] The most common cause of MS is rheumatic fever and approximately 40% of patients with RHD have isolated MS.[17] Conversely, rheumatic involvement is present in 99% of stenotic mitral valves, excised at the time of mitral valve replacement. In rheumatic MS, the valve leaflets are diffusely thickened by fibrous tissue and/or calcific deposits. The mitral commissures fuse and the chordae tendinae shorten, the valvular cusps become rigid and these changes, in turn, lead to the narrowing at the apex of the funnel-shaped (normal valve is fish mouth). Although, the initial insult to the valve is rheumatic, the later changes may be nonspecific process resulting from trauma to the valve caused by the altered flow patterns due to the initial deformity. Calcification of the stenotic valve immobilizes the leaflets and narrows the orifice further.[18] Left ventricular end-diastolic pressure and cardiac output are usually normal in the person with isolated MS. As the severity of stenosis increases, the cardiac output becomes subnormal at rest and fails to increase during exercise. Approximately one-third of patients with rheumatic MS have depressed left ventricular systolic function as a result of chronic rheumatic myocarditis and underfilling. The presence of concomitant mitral regurgitation (MR), systemic hypertension, aortic stenosis (AS) and/or AR can also adversely affect left ventricular function and cardiac output. The natural history of MS is typically progressive with a slow and stable course early on followed by progressive acceleration in the later years.[19]

When MS is symptomatic, the anatomic features consist of thickened mitral cusps with or without calcific deposits, fusion of the valve commissures along with shortening and fusion of the chordae tendinae.[20] The prime symptoms of MS are caused by pulmonary venous hypertension leading to dyspnea, orthopnea, and paroxysmal nocturnal dyspnea. If pulmonary capillary pressure exceeds by 25 mm Hg and if the lymphatics are unable to decompress the resultant transudate, acute pulmonary edema develops. Usually symptoms generally develop in the fourth and fifth decade. Approximately 50% of patients develop symptoms gradually, while the others experience a precipitation of symptoms from complications such as atrial fibrillation,[15] thromboembolism, and superadded respiratory infection.

TABLE 2: 10 years survival, in patients with mitral stenosis without any surgery/PTMC.	
NYHA class	*Survival in percentage*
I	85
II	55
III	20
IV	None (at end of 5 years)

(NYHA: the New York Heart Association; PTMC: percutaneous transseptal mitral commissurotomy)

One of the most common complications of MS, atrial fibrillation occurs as paroxysmal episodes or as a sustained arrhythmia. In most series of patients with MS, the incidence of atrial fibrillation is about 40–80%. However, the incidence is clearly related to age, according to Deverall et al.[21] It is observed particularly in those in over the age of 40 years. The most important impact of atrial fibrillation on the patient with MS is that it greatly increases the probability of systemic embolism and the incidence ranges from 9 to 20%.[22] The chances of survival dwindle as the years pass and the functional class increases **(Table 2)**.

Commissurotomy improves the outcome of patients with the New York Heart Association (NYHA) class III to 10 years survival of 80%. Even the patients in NYHA class IV, who usually do not survive, can improve and survive (65%) after percutaneous transseptal mitral commissurotomy (PTMC)/closed mitral valvotomy (CMV). In Rapaport series, of randomly selected patients, 80% of MS were alive at end of 5 years and 6% at 10 years.[23] The average age at the time of death in patients with MS is 48 years.[24]

Although mitral valve is frequently affected by infective endocarditis, endocarditis is relatively uncommon in isolated MS and is frequent when MS is associated with MR or AR.

■ NATURAL HISTORY OF MITRAL REGURGITATION

The initial mild MR has been noted to disappear over periods ranging from 2 months to 9 years, while new lesions such as MS or stenosis combined with regurgitation, appeared over a period of up to 12 years.[25] Patients with MR are far more likely to have suffered a more severe acute episode than those with MS.[26] Significant insufficiency may progress rapidly leading on to CHF. In contrast, a systolic murmur of moderate valvular incompetence may well persist throughout the lifetime of the patient without any symptoms or further complications. In general, mild-to-moderate MR is better tolerated than similar degrees of MS.

Rheumatic MR is often associated with some degree of stenosis and fusion of the commissures, but in approximately 10% of rheumatic mitral valve disease, it is pure without associated stenosis.[27] A 10-years study showed 60% and survival rate.[23] The predictors of poor survival in patients medically treated are: severe symptoms (NYHA class III), pulmonary hypertension, markedly increased LV end-diastolic and systolic volume, and reduced ejection fraction (EF).[1] Sudden death should be considered in cases of delayed surgery, even in patients with normal EF. The comparison of prognosis in medically and surgically treated patients shows a trend in favor of surgically treated patients, especially early surgery.[28] A greatly enlarged heart or congestive failure, early in the disease exacted the highest toll, with an 80% mortality in 20 years, mostly in the first decade.[1] Prognosis of patients with MR depends on LV function. The left atrial enlargement leads to atrial fibrillation and embolism. But, the incidence of embolism is lesser than in MS patients. MR patients are susceptible for infective endocarditis. 80% of MR patients live at 5 years and 60% at 10 years.

NATURAL HISTORY OF AORTIC VALVE DISEASE

The usual natural history of rheumatic AS and AR is a long asymptomatic period in which mild-to-moderate regurgitation is well tolerated during the compensated phase. In adults, a rate of <6% per year is estimated for the progression to symptoms and/or systolic dysfunction. Asymptomatic patients with left ventricular dysfunction develop cardiac symptoms at a rate >25% per year and the rate of death for symptomatic patients surpasses 20% annually.[19,29] Patients who have recurrent rheumatic episodes may have a more rapid progression.

In developing countries, as with mitral valvular disease, severe aortic incompetence may become established within 1 to 2 years of the initial episode. Those with associated mitral valvular disease, especially mitral incompetence, have a more rapid downhill course. The progression of disease and natural history of AR is given in **Table 3**. Patients who have undergone mitral valve interventions with insignificant aortic valve disease seldom require aortic valve interventions in long-term follow-up.

NATURAL HISTORY OF TRICUSPID VALVE DISEASE

Isolated tricuspid regurgitation (TR) or stenosis is rare in RHD (10%). Tricuspid valvar regurgitation is frequently a functional lesion, though occasionally it can be organic. There is right ventricular over load and dilation occurring as a result of the severe pulmonary hypertension. Functional TR generally coexists with severe significant aortic and mitral valvular diseases and progressing pulmonary hypertension. Such pulmonary hypertension occurs in almost half of children and adolescents and four-fifths of patients older than 8 years.[30]

Tricuspid stenosis (TS) is most frequently associated with MS **(Fig. 2)**, followed by MS and regurgitation, although it does also occur in combination with mitral and aortic valvar disease. RHD is the most common cause of TS and on autopsy 15–30% of patients diagnosed to have RHD have tricuspid valve involvement. The cusps are thickened and the commissures fused so that the valve area becomes small and the valve leaflets dome toward the right ventricle in diastole, similar to rheumatic mitral valve leaflets. In contrast to mitral valve disease, the subvalvar apparatus is not usually involved[31-33] but the annulus may dilate. As the disease progresses, the right atrium dilates and becomes congested. This is always associated with some degree of TR. Severe TR has been increasingly recognized after mitral valve replacement for rheumatic disease, in the absence of significant left-sided disease or pulmonary hypertension. Recent evidence suggests an organic rheumatic cusp involvement and ring dilatation in this condition.[34] It was always thought that rheumatic tricuspid disease was under reported due to unclear echocardiographic criteria to differentiate organic from functional tricuspid involvement.

TABLE 3: Natural history of aortic regurgitation.[19]	
Asymptomatic patients with normal LV systolic function	
Progression to symptoms and/ or LV dysfunction	<6% per year
Progression to asymptomatic LV dysfunction	<3.5% per year
Sudden death	<0.2% per year
Asymptomatic patients with LV dysfunction	
Progression to cardiac symptoms	>25% per year
Symptomatic patients	
Mortality rate	>10% per year

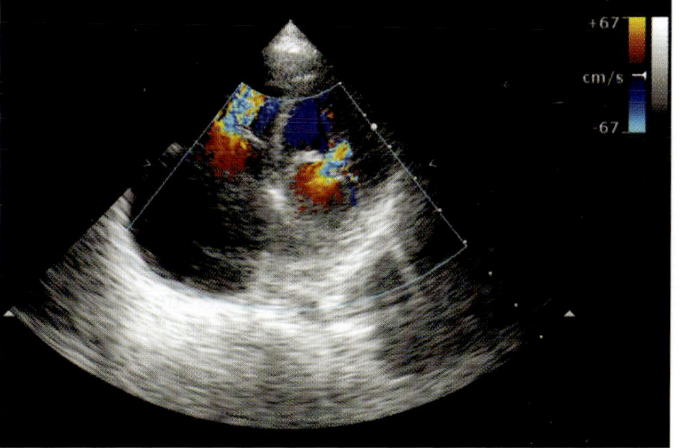

FIG. 2: Combined mitral stenosis and tricuspid stenosis in a 2 years and 3 months old child.

■ SUBACUTE BACTERIAL ENDOCARDITIS

Subacute bacterial endocarditis (SBE) in the damaged valves is a major problem in RHD patients. Infective endocarditis (IE) is a potential complication of valves afflicted by chronic rheumatic lesions because of the disturbed pattern of flow of blood and also the irregular endocardial surface. The incidence of IE continues to raise with a yearly incidence of 15,000–20,000 new cases. Thus, IE now represents the fourth leading cause of life-threatening infectious disease syndromes (after urosepsis, pneumonia, and intra-abdominal sepsis). Advances in antimicrobial therapy and the development of better diagnostic and surgical techniques have reduced the morbidity and mortality.[35] Studies from India, Turkey, and Lebanon, all found that RHD was the most common underlying factor in endocarditis (range 33–66%),[36-39] whereas studies from Hong Kong and Thailand found RHD in 18% and 12% of cases, respectively[40,41] and a study from Singapore found RHD in only 4% of endocarditis cases.[42]

Even though the valvular lesions are mild initially, once the SBE occurs, patients deteriorate very fast and the valve gets damaged beyond repair. There is no evidence that the incidence of SBE is declining in patients with RHD.[43] Although, it is known that penicillin resistant organisms can colonize in the individuals receiving penicillin,[44] there is no evidence that rheumatic individuals on secondary prophylaxis are at increased risk of SBE with penicillin resistant organisms.[45] Prophylaxis for SBE is often confused with that of ARF. It should be emphasized that doses used for ARF prophylaxis are very much inadequate as far as prophylaxis for SBE is concerned. Further gram-negative bacteria may need coverage in a number of instances and this is not achieved with drugs used for ARF. Hence, the end for the RHD patients could be due to SBE, as operating on them is extremely difficult and carries high mortality.

Complications and Outcome of Infective Endocarditis

In the absence of appropriate therapy, IE typically progresses to the development of various intra- and extracardiac complications. Cardiac complications are overwhelmingly common and affect up to 50% of patients.[46] Heart failure or pulmonary edema is probably the most common complication, occurring in about one-third to one-half of patients with IE, as well as the deadliest complication and the most frequent indication for urgent surgery. Heart failure occurs as a result of valvular destruction and ensuing insufficiency or in rare cases of large vegetations, as a result of valvular stenosis. Heart failure may result in the setting of moderate, rather than severe, regurgitation, particularly involving the aortic valve,[47] since the left ventricle is unable to compensate for the acute increase in preload and afterload in this condition. Heart failure is found to complicate aortic valve IE more frequently than mitral or tricuspid endocarditis.

Embolic complications may arise in any patient with IE but particularly in those with larger lesions. Even in the absence of prior embolization, vegetations > 10 mm seem to have high predictive validity for embolic events.[48] The location of the primary vegetation also may be a factor. In adults, mitral lesions have been associated with higher rates of embolization than aortic vegetations (25% vs. 10%, respectively) with the highest rate of embolization (37%) occurring when vegetations are attached to the anterior rather than the posterior mitral leaflet.[49] This may be related to the fact that the mitral valve (as compared with the aortic valve) undergoes two excursions per cardiac cycle. Staphylococcal and fungal infections carry a high risk of embolism regardless of vegetation size or location. Although embolization can occur before diagnosis, during therapy, or even after therapy is completed, most embolic episodes occur within the first 2–4 weeks after the therapy is instituted.[50] Although persistent vegetations are not predictive of adverse events,[51] an increase in vegetation size during the fourth to the eighth week of therapy is predictive of embolic events and abscess formation. Systemic embolization occurs in 22–50% of cases of IE.[52-55] Emboli often involve major arterial beds, including lungs, coronary arteries, spleen, bowel, and extremities **(Figs. 3A and B)**. Up to 65% of embolic events involve the central nervous system and 90% of central nervous system emboli lodge in the distribution of the middle cerebral artery.

These latter emboli are associated with a high mortality rate.[56] The highest incidence of embolic complications is seen with aortic and mitral valve infections **(Fig. 4)** and in IE due to *Staphylococcus aureus* and *Candida* and HACEK and *Abiotrophia* organisms. Among such patients, the predictive accuracy for embolism with large mitral vegetation was nearly 100%.[48] Of note, the rate of embolic events drops dramatically during the first 2 weeks of successful antibiotic therapy, from 13 to <1.2 embolic events per 1,000 patient days.[57] Mortality in medically treated IE patients with concomitant RHD can be as high at 35% and reports have even reported mortality rate as high as 68%.[58-60] This is not necessarily due to poor medical management or inadequate antimicrobial coverage but mortality may be secondary to a severely compromised physical or hemodynamic condition before the onset of IE aggravated by a sudden hemodynamic deterioration.

■ CARDIAC CIRRHOSIS

Cardiac cirrhosis is the end stage of RHD. In cardiac cirrhosis, the liver shows centrilobular hepatic necrosis due to CHF. After repeated attacks of failure or after years of persistent distention, cirrhotic changes may occur. These patients are usually in a moribund, cachectic state, and in CHF **(Fig. 5)**. They have associated hydrothorax, due to biventricular failure, ascites and jaundice. The underlying heart disease is usually the cause of death in cardiac cirrhosis.

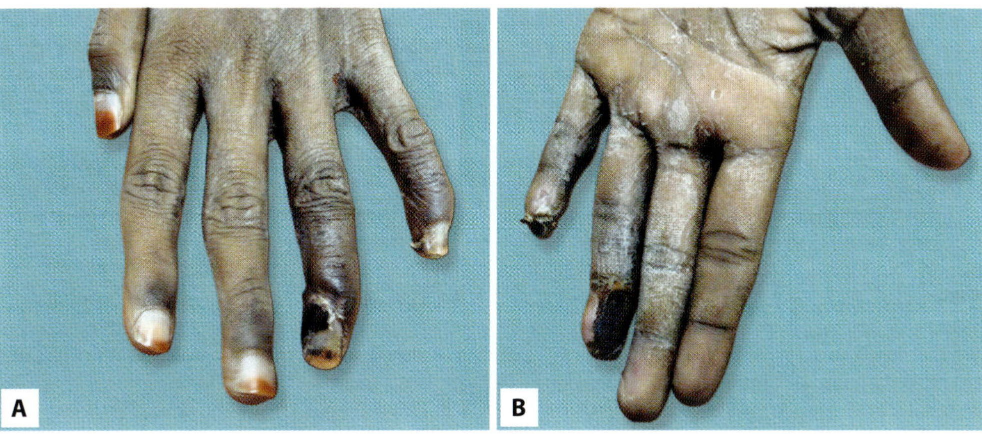

FIGS. 3A AND B: Peripheral embolization of infective endocarditis (IE) of the mitral valve leading to gangrene of index and little finger.

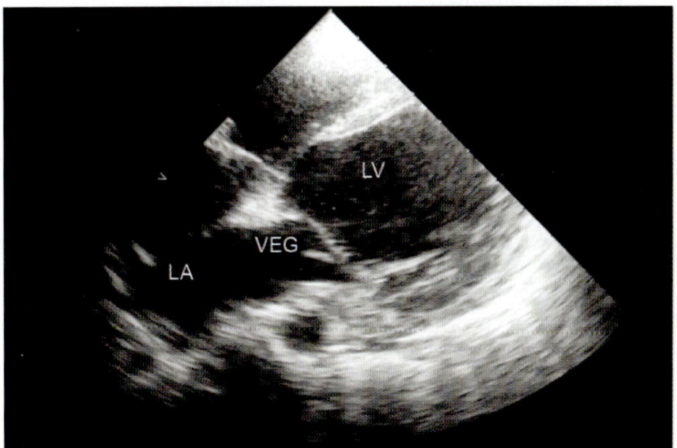

FIG. 4: Freely mobile vegetation on mitral valve.
(LA: left atrium; LV: left ventricle)

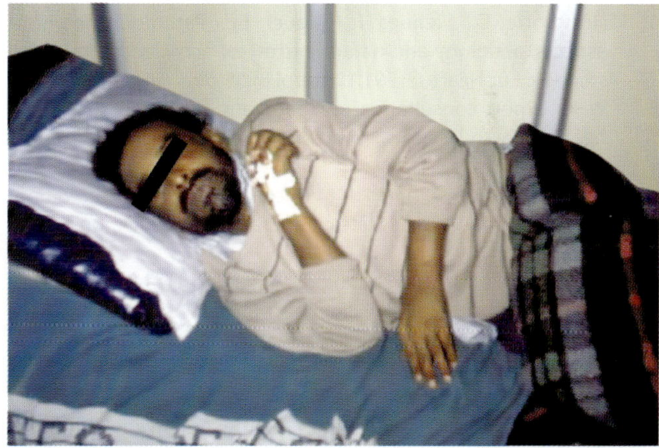

FIG. 5: A 42-year-old man with multivalvular disease in congestive heart failure (CHF).

CONCLUSION

The natural history of ARF and RHD is very important because the clinical manifestations are complex maze of events that are diagnostically difficult but significant for the patient's well-being, as the end is devastating for these patients. IE continues to remain a potentially life-threatening disease. The rising incidence of IE, its significant morbidity and mortality rates, its substantial prognostic, and financial implications for the patients are enormous.

REFERENCES

1. GBD 2015 Mortality and Causes of Death Collaborators. Global, regional, and national life expectancy, all-cause mortality, and cause-specific mortality for 249 causes of death, 1980–2015: a systematic analysis for the Global Burden of Disease Study 2015. Lancet. 2016;388:1459-544 .

2. Bland EF, Jones D. Rheumatic Fever and Rheumatic Heart Disease: A Twenty Years Report on 1000 Patients Followed Since Childhood. Circulation. 1951;4:836-43.

3. Markowitz M, Kuttner AG, Gordis L. Rheumatic Fever: Diagnosis, Management and Prevention. Philadelphia: WB Saunders; 1965. p. 242.

4. World Health Organization. Rheumatic Fever and Rheumatic Heart Disease: Report of a WHO Expert Consultation. Geneva, 29 October–1 November 2001. WHO technical report series No. 923. Geneva: WHO; 2004.

5. Martino D, Tanner A, Defazio G, Church AJ, Bhatia KP, Giovannoni G, et al. Tracing Sydenham's chorea: historical documents from a British Paediatric hospital. Arch Dis Child. 2005;90:507-11.

6. Homer C, Shulman ST. Clinical aspects of acute rheumatic fever. J Rheumatol. 1991;18:2-13.

7. Padmavati S. Rheumatic fever and rheumatic heart disease in developing countries. Bull WHO. 1978;56:543-50.

8.   Feinstein AR, Stern EK, Spagnuolo M. The prognosis of acute rheumatic fever. Am Heart J. 1964;68:817-34.

9.   Massell BF, Fyler DC, Roy SB. The clinical picture of rheumatic fever. Diagnosis, immediate prognosis, course and therapeutic implications. Am J Cardiol. 1958;1:436-49.

10.   Massell BF, Narula J. Rheumatic fever and rheumatic heart carditis. In: Braunwald E (Ed). The Atlas of Heart Diseases. Philadelphia: Current Medicine Inc.; 1994. p. 10.

11.   Feinstein AR, Spagnuolo M. The clinical pattern of acute rheumatic fever, a reappraisal. Medicine (Baltimore). 1962;41: 279-305.

12.   Wood P. An appreciation of mitral stenosis. Part I. Clinical features. Br Med J. 1954;8(1):1051-63.

13.   Thompkins DG, Boxerbaum B, Liebman J. Long term prognosis of rheumatic fever patients receiving regular intramuscular benzathine penicillin. Circulation. 1972;45:543-51.

14.   Ilyas M, Haidry JG. Juvenile mitral stenosis: A pathogenic puzzle. J Pakistan Med Assoc. 1980;30:254-6.

15.   Selzer A, Cohn KE. Natural history of mitral stenosis: a review. Circulation. 1972;45:878-90.

16.   Horstkotte D, Niehues R, Strauer BE. Pathomorphological aspects, aetiology and natural history of acquired mitral valve stenosis. Eur Heart J. 1991;12(suppl B):55-60.

17.   WHO Expert consultation on rheumatic fever and rheumatic heart disease. Geneva, Switzerland: WHO technical report series; 2001. p. 923.

18.   Fauci A. Harrisons Principles of Internal Medicine, 17th edition, Chapter 230. United States: McGraw Hill Education; 2008. pp. 1465-9.

19.   American College of Cardiology/American Heart Association Task Force on Practice Guidelines; Society of Cardiovascular Anesthesiologists; Society for Cardiovascular Angiography and Interventions; Bonow RO, Carabello BA, Kanu C, et al. ACC/AHA 2006 guidelines for the management of patients with valvular heart disease: a report of the American College of Cardiology/American Heart Association Task Force on Practice Guidelines (writing committee to revise the 1998 Guidelines for the Management of Patients with Valvular Heart Disease): developed in collaboration with the Society of Cardiovascular Anesthesiologists: endorsed by the Society for Cardiovascular Angiography and Interventions and the Society of Thoracic Surgeons. Circulation. 2006;114:e84-231.

20.   Roberts WC, Perloff JK. Mitral valvular disease. A clinico-pathologic survey of the conditions causing the mitral valve to function abnormally. Ann Intern Med. 1972;77:939-75.

21.   Devarall PB, Olley PM, Smith DR, Watson DA, Whitaker W. Incidence of systemic embolism before and after mitral valvotomy. Thorax. 1968;23:530-6.

22.   Abernathy WS, Willis PW 3rd. Thromboembolic complications of rheumatic heart disease. Cardiovasc Clin. 1973;5(2):131-75.

23.   Rapaport E. Natural history of aortic and mitral valve disease. Am J Cardiol. 1975;35:221-7.

24.   Olesen KH. Natural history of 271 patients with mitral stenosis under medical treatment. Br Heart J. 1962;24:349-57.

25.   Ravisha MS, Tullu MS, Kamat JR. Rheumatic fever and rheumatic heart disease: Clinical profile of 550 cases in India. Arch Med Res. 2003;34:382-7.

26.   Kouchoukos NT, Blackstone EH, Doty EH. Acquired valvar heart disease. In: Kouchoukos NT, Blackstone EH, Doty EH (Eds). Kirklin/Barratt-Boyes Cardiac Surgery: Morphology, Diagnostic Criteria, Natural History, Techniques, Results and Indications, 3rd edition. Philadelphia: Churchill Livingstone; 2003. pp. 483-714.

27.   Selzer A, Katayama F. Mitral regurgitation: Clinical patterns, pathophysiology and natural history. Medicine (Baltimore). 1972;51:337-6.

28.   Hochreiter C, Niles N, Devereux RB, Kligfield P, Borer JS. Mitral Regurgitation—Relationship of noninvasive descriptors of right and left ventricular performance to clinical and haemodynamic findings and to prognosis in medically and surgically treated patients. Circulation. 1986;73:900-12.

29.   Bonow RO, Rosing DR, McIntosh CL, Jones M, Maron BJ, Lan KK, et al. The natural history of asymptomatic patients with aortic regurgitation and normal left ventricular function. Circulation. 1983;68:509-17.

30.   Chockalingam A, Gnanavelu G, Elangovan S, Chockalingam V. Clinical spectrum of chronic rheumatic heart disease in India. J Heart Valve Dis. 2003;12:577-81.

31.   Daniels SJ, Mintz GS, Kotler MN. Rheumatic tricuspid valve disease: two-dimensional echocardiographic, hemodynamic and angiographic correlations. Am J Cardiol. 1983;51:492-6.

32.   Guyer DE, Gillam LD, Foale RA, Clark MC, Dinsmore R, Palacios I, et al. Comparison of the echocardiographic and hemodynamic diagnosis of rheumatic tricuspid stenosis. J Am Coll Cardiol. 1984;3:1135-44.

33.   Shimada R, Takeshita A, Nakamura M, Tokunaga K, Hirata T. Diagnosis of tricuspid stenosis by M-mode and two-dimensional echocardiography. Am J Cardiol. 1984;53:164-8.

34.   Henein MY, O'Sullivan CA, Li W, Sheppard M, Ho Y, Pepper J, et al. Evidence for rheumatic valve disease in patients with severe tricuspid regurgitation long after mitral valve surgery: role of 3D reconstruction. J Heart Valve Dis. 2003;12:566-72.

35.   Bayer AS, Bolger AF, Taubert KA, Wilson W, Steckelberg J, Karchmer AW, et al. Diagnosis and Management of Infective Endocarditis and its Complications. Circulation. 1998;98:2936-48.

36.   Kanafani ZA, Mahfouz TH, Kanj SS. Infective endocarditis at a tertiary care centre in Lebanon: predominance of streptococcal infection. J Infect. 2002;45:152-9.

37.   Garg N, Kandpal B, Tewari S, Kapoor A, Goel P, Sinha N. Characteristics of infective endocarditis in a developing country: clinical profile and outcome in 192 Indian patients, 1992–2001. Int J Cardiol. 2005;98:253-60.

38.   Heper G, Yorukoglu Y. Clinical, bacteriologic and echo-cardiographic evaluation of infective endocarditis in Ankara, Turkey. Angiology. 2002;53:191-7.

39.   Khanal B, Harish BN, Sethuraman KR, Srinivasan S. Infective endocarditis: report of a prospective study in an Indian hospital. Trop Doct. 2002;32:83-5.

40.   Lertsapcharoen P, Khongphatthanayothin A, Chotivittayatarakorn P, Thisyakorn C, Pathmanand C, Sueblinvong V. Infective endocarditis in pediatric patients: an eighteen-year experience from King Chulalongkorn Memorial Hospital. J Med Assoc Thai. 2005;88(suppl 4):S12-6.

41.   Yiu KH, Siu CW, Lee KL, Fong YT, Chan HW, Lee SW, et al. Emerging trends of community acquired infective endocarditis. Int J Cardiol. 2007;121:119-22.

42.   Liew WK, Tan TH, Wong KY. Infective endocarditis in childhood: a seven-year experience. Singapore Med J. 2004;45:525-9.

43.   WHO Study Group. Rheumatic fever and rheumatic heart disease. WHO Technical Report Series No. 764. Geneva: World Health Organization; 1988.

44. Naiman RA, Barrow JG. Penicillin resistant bacteria in the mouths and throats of children receiving continuous prophylaxis against rheumatic fever. Ann Intern Med. 1963;58:768-72.

45. Doyle EF, Spagnuolo M, Taranta A, Kuttner AG, Markowitz M. The risk of bacterial endocarditis during antirheumatic prophylaxis. JAMA. 1967;201:807-12.

46. Mansur AJ, Grinberg M, da Luz PL, Bellotti G. The complications of infective endocarditis. A reappraisal in the 1980s. Arch Intern Med. 1992;152:2428-32.

47. Sexton DJ, Spelman D. Current best practices and guidelines. Assessment and management of complications in infective endocarditis. Cardiol Clin. 2003;21(2):273-82.

48. Mügge A, Daniel WG, Frank G, Lichtlen PR. Echocardiography in infective endocarditis: reassessment of prognostic implications of vegetation size determined by the transthoracic and the transesophageal approach. J Am Coll Cardiol. 1989;14:631-8.

49. Rohmann S, Erbel R, Darius H, Görge G, Makowski T, Zotz R, et al. Prediction of rapid versus prolonged healing of infective endocarditis by monitoring vegetation size. J Am Soc Echocardiogr. 1991;4:465-74.

50. Garvey GJ, Neu HC. Infective endocarditis: an evolving discussion. A review of endocarditis at the Columbia-Presbyterian Medical Center, 1968-1973. Medicine (Baltimore). 1978;57:105-27.

51. Vuille C, Nidorf M, Weyman AE, Picard MH. Natural history of vegetations during successful medical treatment of endocarditis. Am Heart J. 1994;128:1200-9.

52. Roy P, Tajik AJ, Guiliani ER, Schattenberg TT, Gau GT, Frye RL. Spectrum of echocardiographic findings in bacterial endocarditis. Circulation. 1976;53:474-82.

53. Pelletier LL Jr, Petersdorf RG. Infective endocarditis: a review of 125 cases from the University of Washington Hospitals, 1963–1972. Medicine. 1977;56:287-313.

54. Lutas EM, Roberts RB, Devereux RB, Prieto LM. Relation between the presence of echocardiographic vegetations and the complication rate in infective endocarditis. Am Heart J. 1986;112:107-13.

55. De Castro S, Magni G, Beni S, Cartoni D, Fiorelli M, Venditti M, et al. Role of transthoracic and transesophageal echocardiography in predicting embolic events in patients with active infective endocarditis involving native cardiac valves. Am J Cardiol. 1997;80:1030-4.

56. Pruitt AA, Rubin RH, Karchmer AW, Duncan GW. Neurologic complications of bacterial endocarditis. Medicine. 1978;57:329-43.

57. Steckelberg JM, Murphy JG, Ballard D, Bailey K, Tajik AJ, Taliercio CP, et al. Emboli in infective endocarditis: the prognostic value of echocardiography. Ann Intern Med. 1991;114:635-40.

58. Frankl W, Bret A. Endocarditis: recognition, management and prophylaxis. Valvular Heart Dis: Comprehen Evaluat Treat. 1993;139-73.

59. Saccente M, Cobbs CG. Clinical approach to infective endocarditis. Cardiol Clin. 1996;14(3):351-63.

60. Ma Sylvia TD, Adrian CP. Outcome of Infective Endocarditis Complicating Rheumatic Heart Disease: The Philippine Heart Center Experience. Phil J Microbiol Infect Dis. 1999;28:139-46.

19

Nonsurgical Management of Rheumatic Heart Disease

Ramesh Arora, Poonam Malhotra Kapoor

> *"Formerly, when religion was strong and science weak, men mistook magic for medicine; now, when science is strong and religion weak, men mistake medicine for magic."*
>
> **—Thaomas Szasz**

INTRODUCTION

Rheumatic heart disease (RHD) is still one of the most common cardiovascular ailments in India and many other developing countries. This remains a significant health problem. Mitral valve is afflicted in almost all cases of RHD and mitral stenosis (MS) is the most common lesion followed by multivalvular lesions.[1] Following the introduction of nonsurgical balloon dilatation of pulmonary valve in 1982, there is an ever-increasing trend worldwide of percutaneous valvuloplasty as the initial and the only therapeutic modality for stenotic lesions.[2]

MITRAL STENOSIS

Attempts to open the mitral valve are the story of >100 years when in 1898, it was recognized that opening the mitral valve will help the patients. It took nearly 50 years for three surgeons—Bailey, Harken, and Block to perform the successful closed mitral commissurotomy (CMC).[3] This was the preferred method of treatment for more than three decades because of satisfactory immediate and long-term results (excellent symptomatic improvement in 80% at the end of 15 years) as well as being more economical and available at many cardiovascular centers.[4] Based on the same mechanism, i.e., mechanical dilatation without visualization, balloon dilatation by percutaneous technique was introduced by Inoue in 1984[5] and Lock et al. in 1985[6] by using two different types of balloons. Subsequent progress has been at a frenetic pace as scores of operators adopted this simple and effective means of treatment. Al Zaibag in 1986 introduced the technique of double-balloon mitral valvuloplasty.[7] Similarly, Stefanadis (1990) reported the technique of retrograde left atrial catheterization via the ventricle.[8] Finally, Cribier introduced a percutaneous metallic valvulotomy device, which was basically similar to Tubb's dilator used by surgeons for CMC.[9] After various modifications in the procedural techniques and experience, when the immediate and long-term results of percutaneous transluminal mitral commissurotomy (PTMC) were found to be similar to CMC, it became the preferred form of therapy for relief of MS.

Management and Prevention of Rheumatic Heart Disease

Patients with rheumatic valve disease should undergo periodic clinical and echocardiographic evaluation with frequency based upon the severity of disease. The authors also suggested to not treating carditis with glucocorticoids or intravenous immune globulin (Grade 2C). The available limited-quality evidence has not demonstrated an improvement in cardiac outcomes with these agents. The duration of prophylactic antibiotic administration for secondary prevention of ARF is adjusted depending upon the severity of RHD as outlined in **Table 1**.[10]

Among children and adolescents 5–17 years of age with latent RHD, secondary antibiotic prophylaxis reduced

TABLE 1: Secondary prophylaxis for rheumatic fever—duration of therapy.	
Category	*Duration after last attack*
Rheumatic fever with carditis and residual heart disease **(persistent valvular disease)**	10 years or until 40 years of age (whichever is longer)
	Sometimes lifelong prophylaxis
Rheumatic fever with carditis but no residual heart disease **(no valvular disease)**	10 years or until 21 years of age (whichever is longer)
Rheumatic fever without carditis	5 years or until 21 years of age (whichever is longer)

the risk of disease progression at 2 years. In the GOAL trial, secondary antibiotic prophylaxis reduced the risk of progression of latent RHD in children and adolescents. Population-based screening and initiation of prophylaxis may eventually prove to be integral components of the National Rheumatic Heart Disease Action Plans envisioned by the World Health Assembly in 2017 in a resolution on RHD.[11]

Selection of Patients

Percutaneous transluminal mitral commissurotomy is indicated for all symptomatic patients [New York Heart Association (NYHA) Class > II] who have moderate and severe MS (MVOA ≤ 1.5 cm^2). The procedure is not without risk and should not be routinely indicated in asymptomatic patients. Exceptions to the rule are those with severe MS who require other major noncardiac surgery, young women in the reproductive period and patients at high risk of thromboembolism [history of thrombotic phenomenon, dense spontaneous contrast in left atrium (LA), and recurring atrial fibrillation].[12]

Patient selection is fundamental in predicting immediate and follow-up results. This requires a detailed 2D echocardiography, Doppler and color flow imaging (CFI) for assessment of morphologic characteristics of mitral valve apparatus, hemodynamic significance of the stenosis and regurgitation, other associated valvular lesions, and pulmonary artery pressure estimation. The significance of prevalvuloplasty echocardiography emerged from CMC experience showing that the success depends on valve morphology. Wilkins et al. described ECHO score that graded morphologic changes of the mitral valve, i.e., leaflet motility, leaflet thickening, valve calcification, and involvement of subvalvular apparatus and each of them classified in 0–4 scale.[13] Palacious et al. have established that among its components, the only one that correlates with an absolute change in MVOA after valvuloplasty is thickening of the valve.[14] This score does not take into account other factors that are important in predicting results such as asymmetry of fused commissures and their degree of calcification and it fails to predict severe mitral regurgitation (MR).[12] As the principle mechanism by which valvuloplasty helps

in increasing MVOA is by splitting of the commissures, bilateral commissural calcification is the predictor of suboptimal results and should be taken as relative contraindication of valvuloplasty. On the other hand, in presence of extensive subvalvular fusion, graded dilatation should be done starting with 2–4 mm less than the predicted diameter and after each dilatation, 2D ECHO should be done to assess the extent of commissural split. There may be persistence of significant gradient across the mitral valve in spite of split commissures, as fibrosis of subvalvular apparatus may be as much responsible for stenosis of inflow into the left ventricle as valvular stenosis itself. In the presence of mild or moderate MR on color flow Doppler, PTMC can be done while the presence of severe MR is conventionally considered a contraindication. But in the younger population (Juvenile MS) when it is not possible to deploy prosthetic mitral valve of proper size, PTMC needs to be attempted in spite of presence of severe central MR.[15] Another important aspect assessed by echocardiography in the presence of thrombus is the LA or left atrial appendage (LAA). While the mobile thrombus on the interatrial septum (IAS) and in LA cavity is absolute contraindication for transseptal puncture, there are reports of the procedure being performed with caution after anticoagulation with clots localized in LAA **(Figs. 1A to D)**.[16,17]

Techniques of PTMC

The different techniques by which PTMC can be performed are:

- *Transfemoral transvenous antegrade approach*: The most commonly practiced needs transseptal left heart catheterization and the use of antegrade transfemoral venous approach. In this, septal approach from inferior vena cava (IVC) to fossa ovalis is direct but not easy for balloon catheter to traverse the mitral valve—almost bends by 180°. Moreover, the balloon catheter has to traverse anteriorly and simultaneously confirm to the distorted atrial anatomy. Various complex maneuvers are required to cross the mitral valve.[13] PTMC can be accomplished by using single Inoue balloon, double-balloon (Mansfield) technique, bifoil or trifoil balloon, Joseph balloon, multitrack technique or metallic valvulotome **(Figs. 2A to D)**. In adults, the Inoue balloon size is determined according to the height of the patient—height in cm to be divided by 10 and then add 10. In children <12 years of age, use an initial balloon size 2–4 mm less than what is recommended on adult nomogram. Similarly, the success of the procedure should be defined as final MVOA >1 cm^2/m^2 and/or percentage in MVOA ≥50% of baseline. For double-balloon technique, balloon diameter in adults should be 100–110% of mitral valve annulus diameter and in children 21-22 mm/m^2.[15] PTMC during pregnancy is performed preferably by using Inoue balloon as not only it takes less time but also has rapid inflation and deflation. However less, PTMC under fluoroscopy does expose the fetus to the risk of radiation-

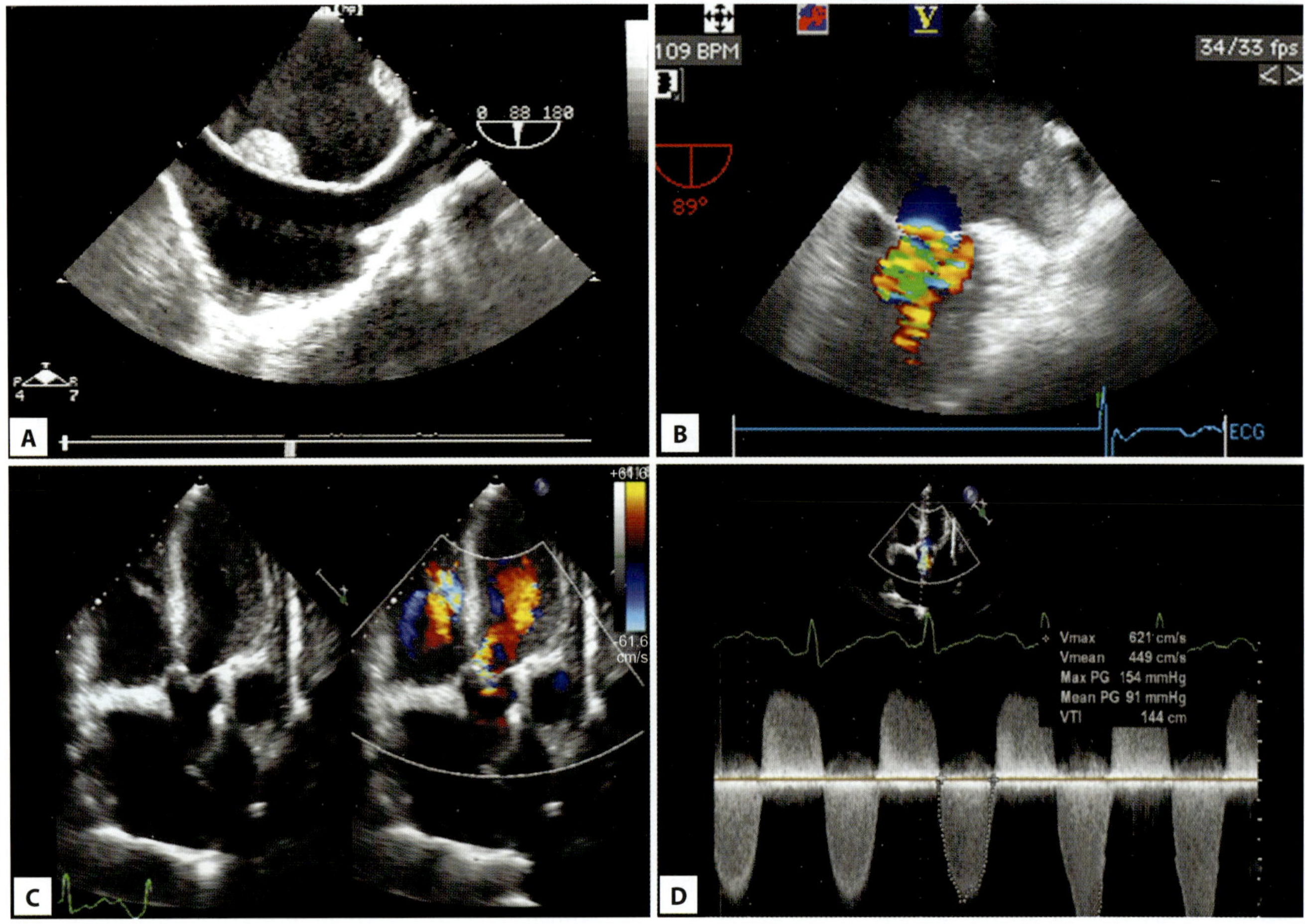

FIGS. 1A TO D: Transesophageal echocardiography (TEE) showing thrombus: (A) on interatrial septum; (B) in left atrial appendage; (C) apical five-chamber view with color Doppler showing severe aortic regurgitation; (D) continuous flow Doppler showed an aortic valve gradient of 154/91 suggestive of severe aortic stenosis.

induced teratogenicity, to avoid that the procedure can be attempted under echocardiography guidance **(Figs. 3A to C)**. In recent times, the role of both transthoracic and transesophageal echocardiography has revealed that could be quadrivalvular involvement of PHD in patients, where all four thickened and calcified systemic valves, where echocardiography diagnosis plays a significant role.[18]

- *Transjugular transvenous antegrade approach*: It finds indication in thrombosed femoral veins, presence of IVC webs or filters, azygous continuation of IVC, distorted atrial anatomy, and operator's preference.[19] The limitations are—approach to IAS is difficult, long and unwieldy conventional Brockenbrough needle, and the operator gets more radiation. But the relative advantages are—direct route to mitral valve, less likely dislodgment of LAA clot, and less radiation to pregnant patient. Inoue, bifoil, and Joseph balloon can all be used by this route.

Retrograde nontransseptal aortic approach (femoral or brachial artery): It also finds application in IVC obstruction or anomalies and when there is inability to perform transseptal puncture (thickened IAS or chest deformity) but

is contraindicated in severe aortic stenosis, prosthetic aortic valve, and peripheral arterial disease.[8] Stefanadis designed a catheter that enters the LA easily but catheter requires 8–9F sheath for its introduction. Although success rate is >90%, but the requirement of large sheath and arterial damages makes this technique less attractive, especially in juvenile MS.

Comparison of PTMC, CMC, and Open Mitral Commissurotomy

Several studies compared the immediate and early follow-up results of PTMC versus CMC in optimal patients. The results have shown either superior outcome from PTMC or no significant difference between both groups.[20] Long-term follow-up results shown by Ben Farhat et al.[21] were similar for PTMC and open mitral commissurotomy (OMC) and significantly superior to CMC. Though the results of PTMC and OMC were quite comparable, the need for cardiopulmonary bypass, thoracotomy, higher cost, longer length of hospital stay, and longer period of convalescence make PTMC the procedure of choice. Since mitral commissurotomy is a

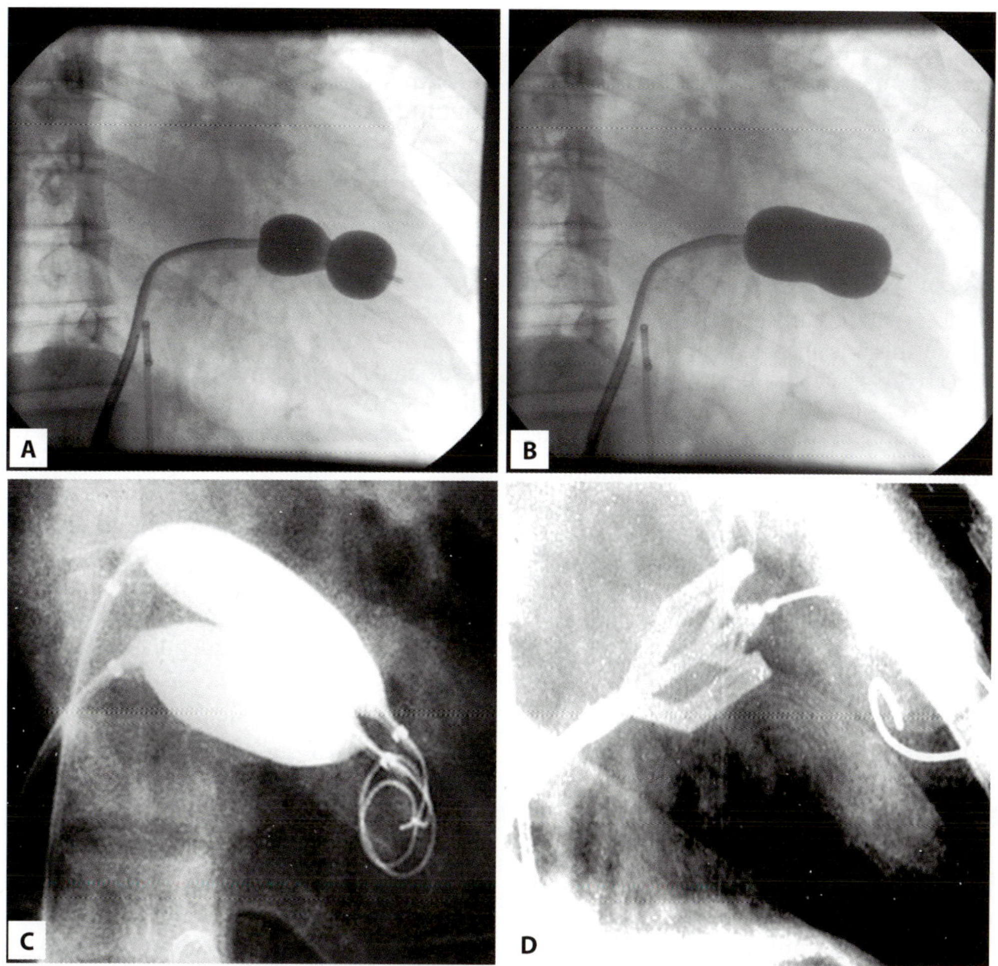

FIGS. 2A TO D: Percutaneous transvenous mitral commissurotomy (PTMC) techniques: (A) Inoue balloon across stenosed mitral valve (MV); (B) fully inflated Inoue balloon at MV; (C) double balloon (Mansfield); (D) metallic valvulotome.

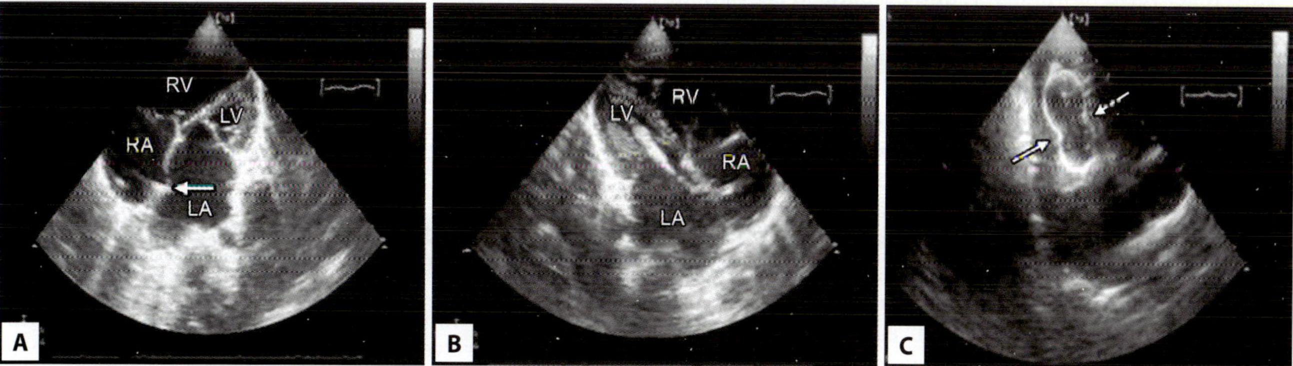

FIGS. 3 A TO C: PTMC under TTE guidance: (A) arrow showing tenting of fossa ovalis by septal puncture needle within Mullin's dilator; (B) balloon across MV into LV; (C) inflated balloon at MV with arrow heads showing constriction by fused commissures.

(LA: left atrium; RA: right atrium; RV: right ventricle; LV: left ventricle; PTMC: percutaneous transvenous mitral commissurotomy; TTE: transthoracic echocardiogram; MV: mitral valve) palliative procedure, the likelihood that thoracotomy will be needed at some point later in the course of the disease, the complications of repeat thoracotomy can thus be prevented.

Comparison of Double Balloon and Inoue Balloon

The double-balloon technique resulted in superior immediate outcome as reflected in a large MVOA (2.1 ± 0.7 vs. 1.8 ± 0.6 cm², p = 0.004) and a lower incidence of 3 + MR (5.4% vs. 10.6%) in the early experience of 113 cases of Inoue technique.[14] This was observed only in the group of patients with ECHO score ≤8. On the other hand, post PTMC MVOA (1.9 ± 0.6 vs. 1.7 ± 0.6 cm², p = 0.008) and success rate were significantly higher in the late experience Inoue group as well as there was a trend toward lower incidence of severe MR ≥3+ (6.8% vs. 12%, p = 0.16).[14] Despite the differences in the immediate outcome, there were no significant differences in the event-free survival at long-term follow-up between the two techniques, left to right shunt, cardiac tamponade, thromboembolic event, and in-hospital mortality.[22] Moreover, the use of double-balloon technique is limited by the fact that the procedure is more complex. In comparison, the Inoue balloon is more user friendly, requiring less procedure and fluoroscopy time. This has important implications particularly in high-risk and pregnant patients.

Therapeutic Results

Excellent acute hemodynamic results have consistently been reported in numerous clinical studies involving a large number of patients.[23,24] In author's series of 4,838 cases, successful valvuloplasty was achieved in 99.8%, while optimal results were obtained in 91% only (defined as MVOA ≥1.5 cm², MVEDG <5 mm Hg, and ≤2 + MR). Among the various factors analyzed for determining the success of PTMC (age, valve morphology, and baseline MVOA), none predicted the outcome in these patients.[24] In patients with calcified versus noncalcified valves and mitral restenosis after previous commissurotomy (CMC, OMC, or PTMC) versus native valve, there was less increase in MVOA but not statistically significant. The overall complications were low hemopericardium in 2%, severe MR requiring mitral valve replacement (MVR) in 1.4%, systemic arterial embolization and infective endocarditis in 0.1%, persistent left to right shunt in 0.02% and mortality in 0.15%. At a follow-up of 12–166 months, >90% of cases were in functional class I or II, restenosis resulted in 4.8% and elective MVR was required in 1% due to symptomatic functional deterioration of severity of MR.

Newer Applications

Percutaneous transluminal mitral commissurotomy has found newer applications including for restenosis after surgical commissurotomy, the treatment of choice during

pregnancy, juvenile cases of MS with severe MR, nonpliable and calcified valves, few select cases with documented left atrial thrombus, associated moderate regurgitation, multivalvular stenosis, coexistent coronary artery disease, and as an emergency life-saving procedure in acute pulmonary edema with hypoxia/hypotension.[24,25]

Role of Surgery in MS

At present, CMC is only recommended in technically unsuccessful PTMC or if this facility is not available. Direct vision OMC is the procedure of choice only in patients with associated left atrial thrombus especially mobile and close to the IAS. MVR is reserved for adult patients with severe MR, acute severe MR, symptomatic patients with suboptimal balloon valvuloplasty having densely calcified valve, and restenosis of a bioprosthesis. Surgery is also indicated in the presence of associated conditions mandating cardiac surgical intervention, e.g., organic tricuspid regurgitation, severe calcified aortic stenosis or failed balloon aortic valvuloplasty, aortic regurgitation with left ventricular volume overload or dysfunction, and coronary artery bypass surgery.

■ AORTIC STENOSIS

Aortic stenosis due to rheumatic pathology never occurs as an isolated lesion and is almost always associated with mitral valve disease. Very rarely associated tricuspid and pulmonary valve may be of hemodynamic significance. Conventionally like surgical procedure, aortic valve should be opened prior to mitral valve. After transseptal puncture, Inoue balloon is positioned in the LA. Balloon dilatation of aortic valve (ABV) is done by retrograde approach using Mansfield balloon. Post-ABV, in the absence of grade-3 AR, PTMC is performed. The procedure has been successful in 25 patients of Santhosh et al. with fall in mean aortic peak gradient from 89 to 38 mm Hg and increase in MVOA from 0.8 to 1.8 cm², while none required urgent surgical valve replacement.[26]

■ TRICUSPID STENOSIS

Tricuspid stenosis (TS) is an uncommon disease, almost of rheumatic origin and virtually never occurs as an isolated lesion. Its incidence may be underestimated because it is commonly overlooked, particularly when associated with MS. Tricuspid valve (TV) pathology is present at autopsy in about 15% of patients with RHD and is of clinical significance in only about 5% of cases.[27] The clinical diagnosis of TS is usually difficult and there is no perfect diagnostic method. The characteristic clinical features are of low cardiac output, fatigue, edematous feet, hepatomegaly, ascites, and anasarca out of proportion to the degree of dyspnea. The absence of symptoms due to pulmonary congestion (hemoptysis, paroxysmal nocturnal dyspnea, and acute pulmonary edema) in a patient with obvious MS should suggest the possibility of TS. Like other valvular lesions, echocardiography provides an accurate noninvasive tool and compares very well to catheterization in the quantification of TS.

After balloon valvuloplasty emerged as an alternative procedure for pulmonic, aortic, or MS, an attempt was made to dilate the TV concomitantly to obviate surgery and the improvement in valve area and symptoms were found to be similar to surgical commissurotomy.[28]

Selection of Patients

Those with clinical features of intractable edematous feet, ascites and hepatomegaly out of proportion to the degree of dyspnea on optimal diuretic therapy as well as those with other valvular stenotic lesions who are being considered for intervention should be carefully screened for TS by detailed echocardiography (2D, Doppler, and color flow imaging). Apical four-chamber and parasternal long-axis inlet views are the most useful as all three leaflets can be visualized by taking these two views.[29] Patients taken up for valvuloplasty are those with: (a) an echocardiographic mean TV diastolic gradient of 2 mm or more and a TV area (TVA) $\leq$2 cm^2, (b) in the presence of a grade I-II/III tricuspid regurgitation mean TV diastolic gradient of 5 mm or more and TVA of $\leq$2 cm^2.

Techniques of Tricuspid Valve Dilatation: Tricuspid Balloon Valvuloplasty

It can be performed by percutaneous transvenous femoral or transjugular route by using double balloon or Inoue balloon:

- *Double-balloon technique*: From the two right femoral vein hemostatic sheaths 7F, tip hole balloon catheters are placed, one in the right atrium and other in the right ventricle. The TV gradient is measured by simultaneously recording of right ventricle and right atrial pressures. Both catheters are then advanced into the distal pulmonary artery and 0.035" × 260 cm guidewires are then positioned through them into the pulmonary artery. Two Mansfield balloons 15–20 mm in diameter with effective balloon diameter of 90–110% of annulus size are then advanced and positioned across the TV. Both balloons are inflated simultaneously to a maximum of four atmospheres. After withdrawal of balloon catheters, tiphole catheters are placed one in the right atrium and the other in the right ventricle for recording the trans TV gradient.[30]
- *Inoue balloon over the wire*: A 0.025" exchange guidewire is positioned into the left lobe pulmonary artery branch or right ventricle through the Swan–Ganz catheter. The Inoue balloon, nearly 100% of the size of the annulus diameter, is inserted with the stretching tube through the right groin over the 0.025" guidewire. After reaching the right atrium, the stretching steel tube is then withdrawn so as to direct the balloon catheter tip toward the tricuspid orifice. Then, withdrawal of golden stylet up to

the 2-inch mark helps in negotiating the balloon catheter over the wire into the right ventricle. The distal portion of the balloon is then inflated in the right ventricle and the catheter shaft is withdrawn until it straddles against the TV. Rapid inflation and deflation of the balloon are done until the waist disappears. Hemodynamic measurements are repeated.
- *Inoue balloon floatation technique*: A simple algorithm for negotiating the TV is:
  - *Step 1*: Simply float the Inoue balloon into the right ventricle such as Swan–Ganz catheter.
  - *Step 2*: If step 1 fails, use the J-stylet with clockwise rotation
  - *Step 3*: If step 2 fails, use the J-stylet and utilize the Swan–Ganz property of the Inoue balloon to enter the right ventricle.
  - *Step 4*: If step 3 fails, use over the wire technique or a special loop in the right atrium for distorted right atrial anatomy.

Combined Lesions with TS

In patients with combined mitral and TS, the mitral valve is usually dilated first. This is especially relevant to patients with pre-existing tricuspid regurgitation as dilating the mitral valve first provides the opportunity to confirm a satisfactory split of the mitral valve and a fall in pulmonary artery pressures before dilating the TV. Because of the high right atrial pressures, a close watch should be kept for hypoxemia developing due to right to left shunt across the IAS.[31] In such an event, TV has to be dilated as quickly as possible. If attempted before the mitral valve, to prevent right to left shunt and clinical compromise, there is a possibility of worsening the pulmonary congestion due to the increase in blood flow, given the extremely high left atrial pressures and transmitral gradient. If there is associated aortic or pulmonary valve stenosis, dilatation of these valves is attempted before tricuspid stenotic valve. When two stenotic lesions exist in tandem, the manifestations of the more proximal of the two tend to mask those produced by the distal lesion. This is particularly true if the proximal lesion is more severe than the distal one.

Complications of Tricuspid Balloon Valvuloplasty

Because of the proximity of the atrioventricular conduction system to the tricuspid annulus, balloon dilatation of the TV may be associated with transient heart block due to barotrauma.[28]

Therapeutic Results of Tricuspid Balloon Valvuloplasty

Following tricuspid balloon valvuloplasty (TBV), satisfactory immediate hemodynamic results have been consistently reported in various cases and small serious reports.[28,31]

Most of the cases of TBV apart from bioprosthesis have been performed concomitantly with mitral, aortic, and pulmonary balloon dilatation. No separate criteria for optimal valvuloplasty have been defined and are being considered the same as for mitral valve, i.e., a valve area of >1.5 cm^2 and <3+ degree of regurgitation.[24] Sharma et al. combined PTMC and TBV in 10 patients using Mansfield double-balloon technique in six and Inoue balloon in four patients. Hemodynamic parameters revealed an increase in TVA from 1.11 + 0.41 to 2.52 + 0.6 cm^2 ($p < 0.005$), a fall in the mean valve gradient from 11.80 ± 4.70 to 4.14 ± 3.40 mm Hg along with an increase in cardiac index. There was continuous relief of stenosis after 3–24 months in four patients.

Multivalvular heart disease is not well tolerated during pregnancy and TBV has been successfully performed in symptomatic patients along with mitral and aortic valve.[32] The specific impact of TS on pregnancy is not known. Gamra et al. found recurrent miscarriages in a patient with TS and that patient had a normal pregnancy after successful dilatations.[33] The mechanism by which TS could be the cause of miscarriages has been ascribed to low cardiac output, resulting in an impairment of uterine blood flow. In addition, elevated venous pressure may have some adverse effects on venous drainage of the uterus/placenta and thus reduce both placental and fetal viability.

Tricuspid Transcathether Intervention

The scenarios for the percutaneous treatment of TV is rapidly expanding **(Fig. 4)**.[34] These newer percutaneous device such as the PASCAL device **(Figs. 5A to D)** has low complication rates, especially for edge-to-edge technique, provied they are used on a case-based individual scenario as shown by a signifiant reduction in right atrial volume, right ventricular end-diastolic pressure (RVEDP) was achieved.[35]

Transcatheter Aortic Valve

Intervention: For elderly, comorbid patients, needing treatment of severe aortic stenosis, needs a good catheter laboratory patients workup with a coronary angiogram and a right heart catheter with PAP, with aortogram and iliofemoral and transesophageal echocardiography (TEE) **(Boxes 1 and 2 and Figs. 6 to 10)** angiogram with both transfemoral or transapical approach.

BOX 1	**Procedure and hardware of TAVR.**

BAV → Valve implantation

Balloon aortic valvotomy:

- Prepping and draping → Anesthesia → Diagnostic arterial access: C/L FA access with 6F sheath → pigtail catheter for C/L iliofemoral angiography, location of puncture marked
- *Femoral vein access*: To diagnostic access with 7F sheath, for RHC and pacing leads
- *Therapeutic arterial access*: Percutaneous puncture/surgical preparation → standard diagnostic J 0.035 guidewire +14F long (24 cm) sheath, heparin
- *Valve crossing*: Amplatzer length 1 catheter (AL1) into ascending aorta → exchanged with straight tip 0.035 guidewire to cross AV → AL1 into LV and wire exchanged with Amplatz extra stiff 0.035, 260 cm length guidewire

(BAV: balloon aortic valvotomy; RHC: right heart catheterization; TAVR: transcatheter aortic valve replacement)

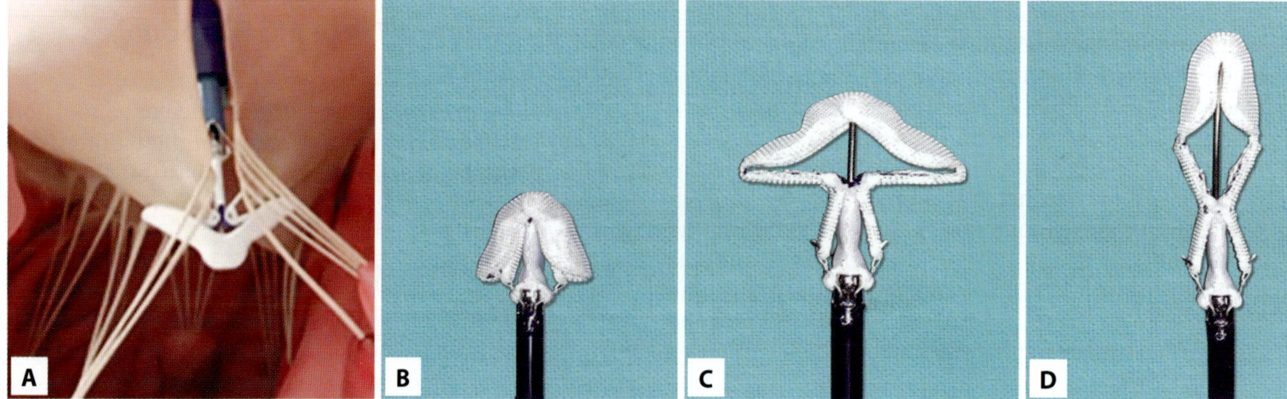

FIG. 4: Transcatheter tricuspid valve interventions with different percutaneous device.

FIGS. 5A TO D: (A) The PASCAL device for tricuspid transcatheter implantation in situ. (B and C) the PASCAL original and PASCAL ace implant. (D) This device is percutaneously implanted and is most suitable for tricuspid valve.

<table>
<tr><td>

BOX 2   **Cardiac catheterization.**

- Coronary angiogram
- RH catheterization with PAP
- *Aortogram (PA or LAO):* 30 mL @ 15 mL/s
- *Iliofemoral angiogram:* 30 mL @ 6 mL/s
- No angioseal!

(LAO: left anterior oblique; PAP: pulmonary artery pressure; RH: right heart)

</td></tr>
</table>

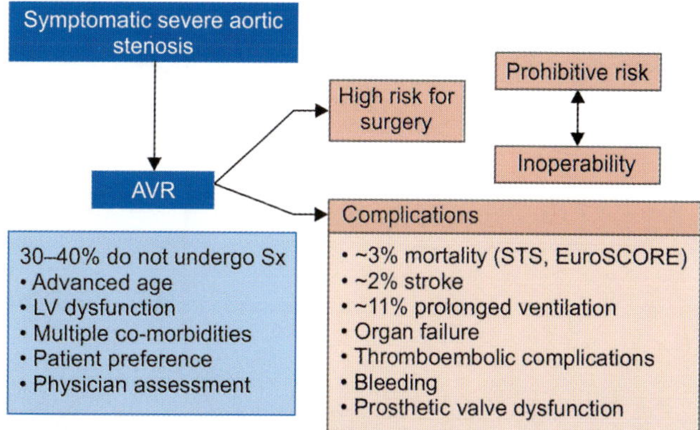

FIG. 6: Indications for transcatheter aortic valve replacement.

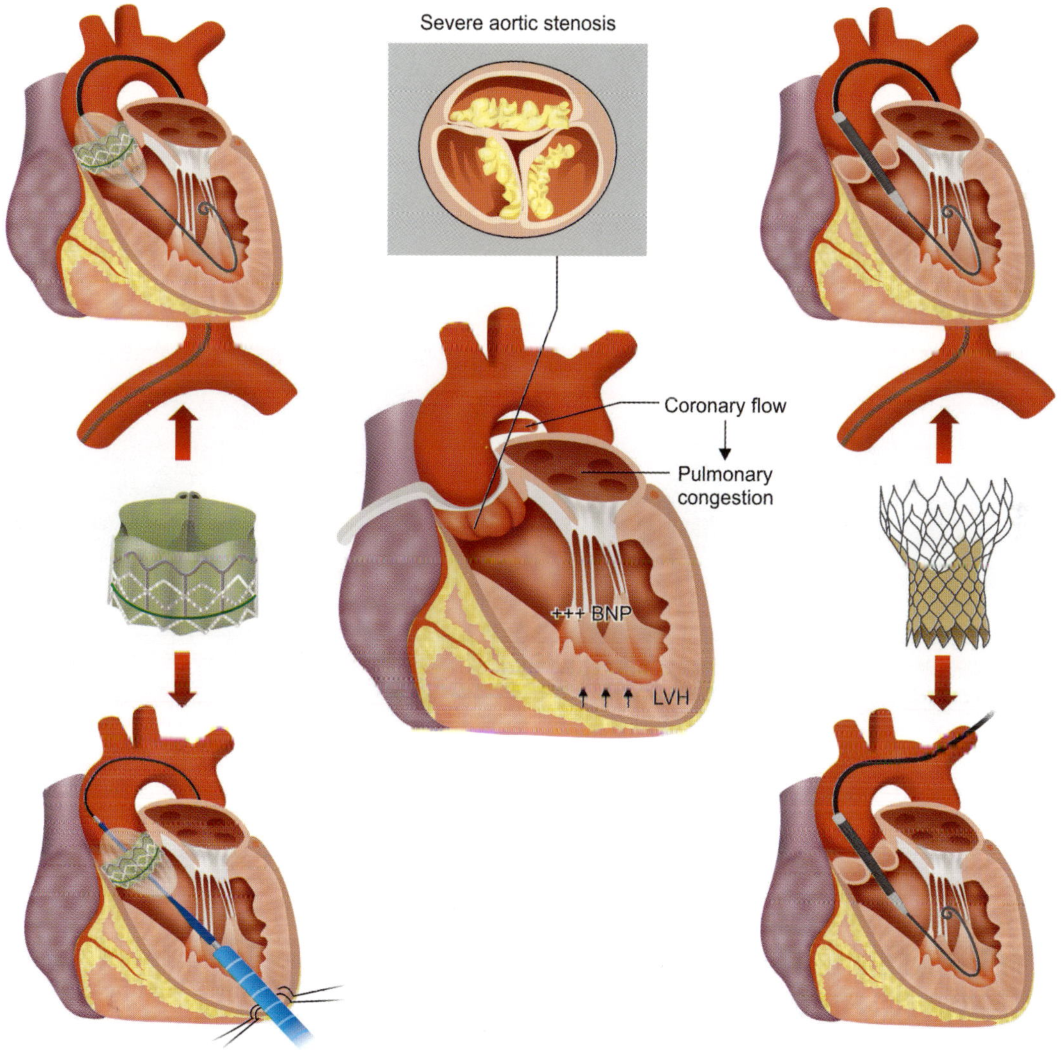

FIG. 7: Transcatheter aortic valve implantation.
(BNP: B-type natriuretic peptide; LVH: left ventricular hypertrophy)

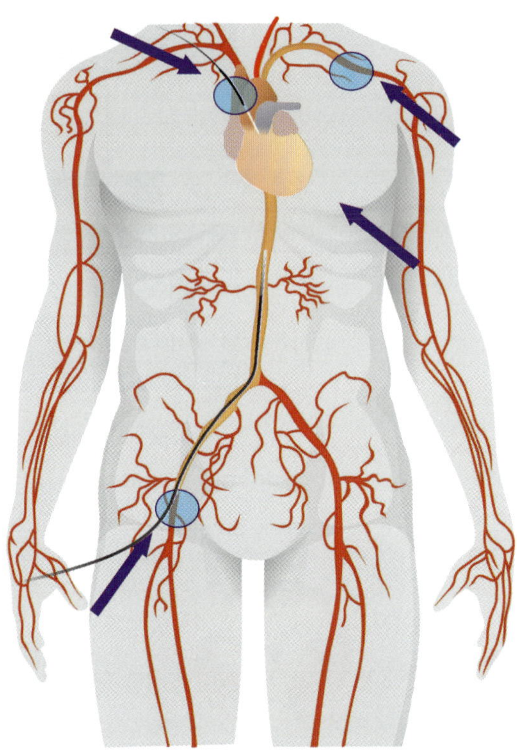

FIG. 8: Procedure and hardware of transcatheter aortic valve replacement.

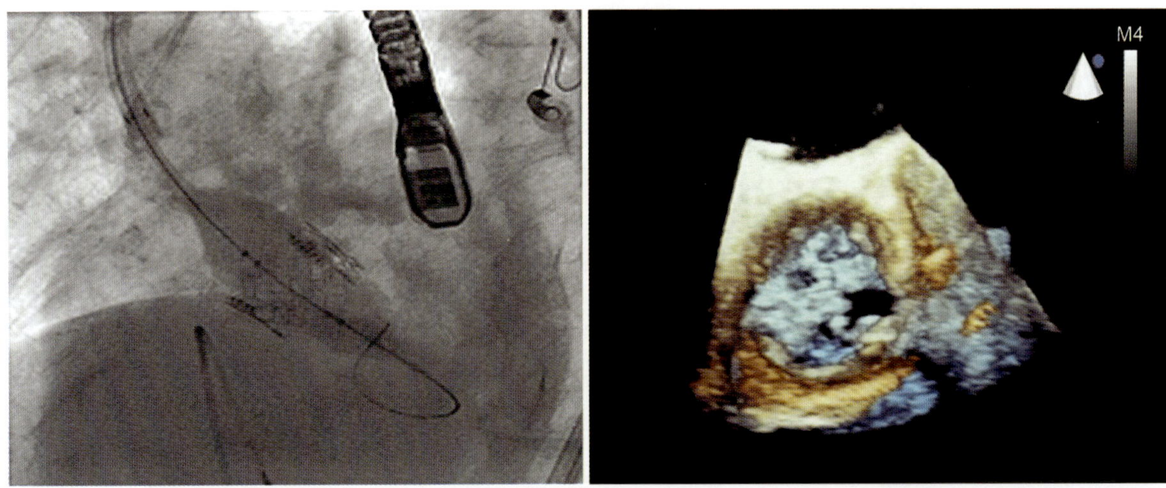

FIG. 9: Transfemoral (TF) valve deployment and stenosed native aortic valve.

CATHETER-BASED INTERVENTIONS FOR RHEUMATIC HEART DISEASE MANAGEMENT

In 1997, Cribier et al., in a robust publication, reiterated that percutaneous transvenous mitral commissurotomy using a mitral commissurotome with a definitive ease of resterilization and unchanged physical properties made this device popular as a good alternative to balloon valvotomy and was economical as well.[36] In 2021, when the profile of rheumatic MS was significantly changing over time, Ofir Koren et al.[37] opined that over the decades, as the demographic and echocardiographic profile of RHD patients changed, PTMC could be successfully carried out in more number of patients with multiple comorbidities, more complex and calcified valvular structures, with a Wilkin's score of >8, postprocedural MR $\geq$1.5 cm^2 being independent predictors for the time for surgery and heart failure hospitalization.

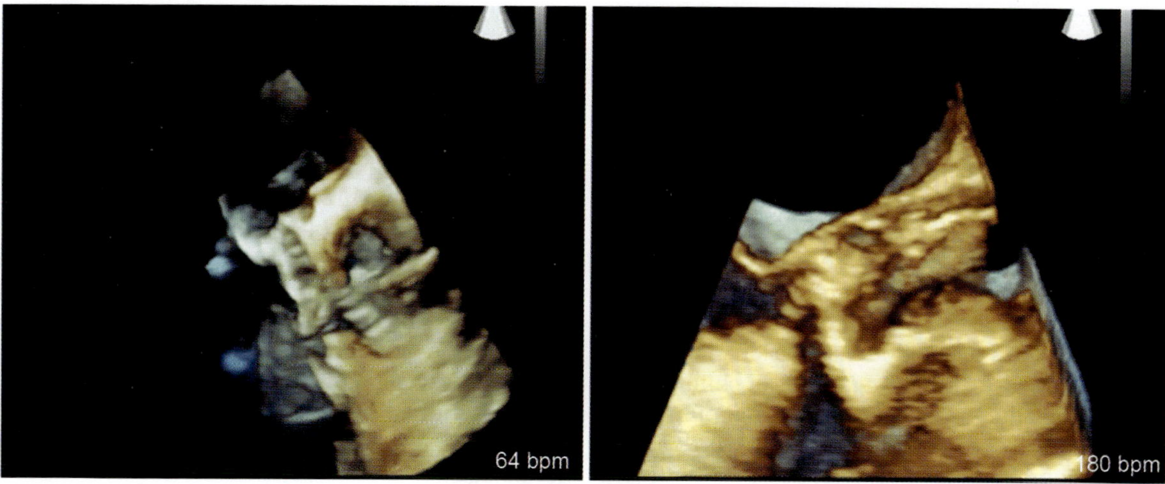

FIG. 10: Guidewire across native aortic valve and valve deployment.

The American Heart Scientific Association, in their statement in 2020, has also confirmed to (Ref T is AHP) palliative care is essential first especially in resource-poor setting[13] for management of RHD. The World Heart Federation (WHF) has also called for 25% reduction in the burden of RHD by 2015. Early diagnosis with echocardiography added to clinical diagnosis, with screening, can avoid the need for intervention. Balloon mitral valvotomy (BMV) is often the preferred option in younger patients who have an absolute or relative contraindication to anticoagulation, severe MS that manifests during pregnancy, and selected patients with restenosis after surgical valvotomy. It can be repeated for those who develop restenosis after previous BMV. Almost 80% of symptomatic patients with severe RHD MS are candidates for BMV, leaving only 20% to undergo surgery because of unfavorable anatomy and high Wilkins score.

Given the fact that BMV is much less resource intensive than surgery, it is necessary to develop a sustainable, low-cost model for BMV in environments that need it the most. A BMV center that performs the Inoue technique with conscious sedation, transthoracic echocardiography guidance, and the possibility of resterilization and reuse of the balloon can make it relatively affordable. Percutaneous valve implantation holds promise, especially if this work can be expanded to the mitral valve as a treatment for severe MR or mixed mitral disease. However, the application of these technologies in young rheumatic patients appears less probable in the foreseeable future, primarily because current techniques and devices are less appropriate for rheumatic MR that requires valves with annulus sizes well over 3 cm.

In doing a PTMC, an appropriate balloon diameter is most essential.[38] Selection of the appropriate balloon diameter is crucial for the success of the procedure. The formula using patient's height is a simple and effective way to determine the optimal size of balloon to use [balloon diameter (mm) = height (cm)/10+10].[39] Studies in the past decade have considered percutaneous mitral commissurotomy (PMC) success as an increase in mitral valve area (MVA) (>50% or MVA $\geq$1.5 cm^2), without a significant increase in MR. The main echocardiographic predictors of immediate procedural results are related to MV anatomy including baseline MVA, subvalvular thickening, and valve calcification, especially at the commissural level.[40]

■ CONCLUSION

The goals of therapy for RHD are to prevent progression and optimize cardiac function. Secondary antibiotic prophylaxis can reduce the long-term severity of RHD.

Patients with RHD, including those receiving benzathine benzylpenicillin G prophylaxis, should receive amoxicillin prophylaxis before undergoing high-risk dental or surgical procedures. If they have recently been treated with a course of penicillin or amoxicillin, or have immediate penicillin hypersensitivity, clindamycin is recommended.[41]

With improvement in cardiac imaging and balloon technology, nonsurgical catheter dilatation has revolutionized the approach to management of rheumatic valvular heart disease. During the last three decades, the number and types of procedures have increased dramatically. For rheumatic MS, PTMC has now become the standard treatment modality in most centers replacing surgical commissurotomy with excellent improvement in clinical and hemodynamic parameters. This has also obviated the need for MVR in the elderly patients with nonpliable valves as well as in the selected cases of pediatric age group with severe MR, when it is not possible to deploy prosthetic valve of proper size, thus avoiding the second open-heart surgery and its complications.

Psychologically, there is more acceptability for nonsurgical procedure as there is no thoracotomy scar, no general anesthesia, no regular use of blood transfusion, less hospital stay, as well as possibility of repeat balloon valvotomy, if required. A subset of patients undergoing balloon mitral valvuloplasty have associated stenosis of aortic, tricuspid, or pulmonary valves. Moreover, multivalvular interventions in RHD are a safe treatment resulting in significant improvement in hemodynamics and functional class. Above all, the prerequisite of availability for closed and open-heart surgery should be kept in mind even with experienced operators and in centers performing balloon valvuloplasty on a routine basis.

Rheumatic heart disease remains the major acquired valvular heart disease among children and young adults. Patients with chronic RHD often presented with complications of the disease or with reactivation of RHD. Mitral valve lesion was the predominant lesion, particularly in a dual-valve disease, presenting as MR in children and stenosis in young adults. Tricuspid, aortic, and pulmonary valve involvements were commonly seen with various patterns and combinations. Multivalve lesions indicated an advanced stage of disease. Poor compliance and limited access to secondary prophylaxis remain significant challenges to rheumatic fever (RF)/RHD control programs, especially in rural areas.[42]

Percutaneous mitral balloon commissurotomy (PMBC) is the most fruitful percutaneous intervention in RHD and remains the treatment of choice in MS patients with a suitable valve. PBMC is accomplished by splitting the commissures by inflating a balloon placed transseptally across the mitral valve. Isolated rheumatic TS can also be successfully treated by balloon tricuspid valvuloplasty. The role of percutaneous interventions remains less well established for other rheumatic valvular lesions such as rheumatic MR and aortic stenosis. The skill set for invasive hemodynamic evaluation and PMBC continues to be essential for an interventional cardiologist.

■ REFERENCES

1. Padmavati S. Present status of rheumatic fever and rheumatic heart disease in India. Ind Heart J. 1995;47:395-8.

2. Kan JS, White RI, Mitchell SE, Gardner TJ. Percutaneous balloon valvuloplasty: A new method for treating congenital pulmonary valve stenosis. N Eng J Med. 1982;307:540-2.

3. Bailey CP. The surgical treatment of mitral stenosis. Dis Chest. 1949;15:377.

4. John S, Bashi W, Jairaj PS, Muralidharan S, Ravikumar E, Rajarajeswari T, et al. Close mitral valvotomy: Early results and long-term follow-up of 3724 consecutive patients. Circulation. 1983;68:891-6.

5. Inoue K, Owaki T, Nakamura T, Kitamura F, Miyamoto N. Clinical application of transvenous mitral commissurotomy by a new balloon catheter. J Thorac Cardiovasc Surg. 1984;87:394-402.

6. Lock JE, Khalilullah M, Shrivastava S, Bahl V, Keane JF. Percutaneous catheter commissurotomy in rheumatic mitral stenosis. N Eng J Med. 1985;313:1515-8.

7. AlZaibag M, Ribiero PA, Alkasab S, Alfagih MR. Percutaneous double balloon mitral valvotomy for rheumatic mitral valve stenosis. Lancet. 1986;1:757-61.

8. Stefanadis C, Kourouklis C, Strates C, Pitsavos C, Tentolouris C, Toutouzas P. Percutaneous balloon mitral valvuloplasty by retrograde left atrial catheterisation. Am J Cardiol. 1990;65:650-4.

9. Cribier A, Eltchanioff H, Koning R, Rath PC, Arora R, Imam A, et al. Percutaneous mechanical mitral commissurotomy with a newly designed metallic valvulotome. Immediate results of the initial experience in 153 patients. Circulation. 1999;99:793-9.

10. Zühlke L, Cupido B; UpToDate. (2022). Management and prevention of rheumatic heart disease. [online] Available from https://www.uptodate.com/contents/management-and-prevention-of-rheumatic-heart-disease. [Last accessed November, 2022]

11. Beaton A, Okello E, Rwebembera J, Grobler A, Engelman D, Alepere J, et al. Secondary antibiotic prophylaxis for latent rheumatic heart disease. N Engl J Med. 2022;386:230-40.

12. Arora R, Kalra GS, Murty GS, Trehan V, Jolly N, Mohan JC, et al. Percutaneous transatrial mitral commissurotomy. Immediate and intermediate results. J Am Coll Cardiol. 1994;23:1327-32.

13. Wilkins GT, Weyman AE, Abascal VM, Block PC, Palacious IF. Percutaneous balloon dilatation of the mitral valve: An analysis of echocardiographic variables related to outcome and mechanism of dilatation. Br Heart J. 1988;60:299-308.

14. Palacious IF. Chapter 17: Percutaneous mitral balloon valvuloplasty. In: Sievert H, Qureshi SA, Wilson N, Hijazi ZM (Eds). Percutaneous Interventions for Congenital Heart Disease. Boca Raton, Florida, United States: CRC Press; 2007. pp. 177-84.

15. Arora R, Mukhopadhyay S, Yusuf J, Trehan V. Transcatheter treatment of rheumatic mitral stenosis in children: Technique, immediate and follow-up results. Cardiol Young. 2007;17(1): 3-11.

16. Chen WJ, Chen MS, Liau CS, Wu CC, Lee YT. Safety of percutaneous transvenous mitral commissurotomy in patients with mitral stenosis and thrombus in left atrial appendage. Am J Cardiol. 1992;70:117-9.

17. Satvic CM, Chaudhury AG, Devegowda L, Bhat P, Manjunath CN. Quadrivalvular involvement in rheumatic heart disease: A rare case report. J Indian Acad Echocardiogr Cardiovasc Imaging. 2022;6:56-8.

18. Arora R, Lal P. Valvular heart disease in pregnancy: Problems and practice. Cardiology Today. 2008;12: 207-14.

19. Joseph G, Baruah DK, Kuruttukulam SV, Chandy ST, Krishnaswami S. Transjugular approach to transseptal balloon mitral valvuloplasty. Cathet Cardiovasc Diagn. 1997;42: 219-26.

20. Arora R, Nair M, Kalra GS, Nigam M, Khalilullah M. Immediate and long term results of balloon and surgical closed mitral valvotomy: A randomized comparative study. Am Heart J. 1993;125:1091-4.

21. Farhat BM, Ayari M, Maatouk F, Betbout F, Gamra H, Jarra M, et al. Percutaneous balloon versus surgical closed and open mitral commissurotomy: Seven-year follow-up results of a randomized trial. Circulation. 1998;97:245-50.

22. Leon MN, Harell LC, Simosa HF, Mahdi NA, Pathan AZ, Lopez-Cuellar J, et al. Comparison of immediate and long-term results of mitral balloon valvotomy with the double balloon versus Inoue techniques. Am J Cardiol. 1999;83:1356-63.

23. Chen CR, Cheng TO. Percutaneous balloon mitral valvuloplasty by the Inoue technique: A multicentre study of 4832 patients in China. Am Heart J. 1995;129:1197-203.

24. Arora R, Kalra GS, Singh S, Mukhopadhyay S, Kumar A, Mohan JC, et al. Percutaneous transvenous mitral commissurotomy. Immediate and long-term follow-up results. Cathet Cardiovasc Intervent. 2002;55:450-6.

25. Palacious IF. Farewell to surgical mitral commissurotomy for many patients. Circulation. 1998;97:223-6.

26. Satheesh S, Gobu P, Binaya BB, Karthikeyan B, Arunprasath P, Ajith A, et al. Percutaneous balloon valvuloplasty for concurrent mitral, aortic and tricuspid rheumatic stenosis. Indian Heart J. 2009;61(208):555.

27. Kitchin A, Turner R. Diagnosis and treatment of tricuspid stenosis. Br Heart J. 1964;26:354-79.

28. Khalilullah M, Tyagi S, Yadav BS, Jain P, Choudhry A, Lochan R. Double balloon valvuloplasty of tricuspid stenosis. Am Heart J. 1987;114:1232-3.

29. Arora R. Chapter 20: Tricuspid valve stenosis. In: Sievert H, Qureshi SA, Wilson Nand Hijazi ZM (Eds). Percutaneous Interventions for Congenital Heart Disease. Boca Raton, Florida, United States: CRC Press; 2007. pp. 201-6.

30. Patel TM, Dani SI, Shah SC, Patel TK. Tricuspid balloon valvuloplasty: A more simplified approach using Inoue balloon. Cathet Cardiovasc Diagn. 1996;37:86-8.

31. Sharma S, Loya YS, Desai DM, Pinto RJ. Percutaneous double valve balloon valvotomy for multivalve stenosis. Immediate results and intermediate-term follow-up. Am Heart J. 1997;133:64-70.

32. Savas V, Grines CL, O'Neill WW. Percutaneous tricuspid valve balloon valvuloplasty in a pregnant woman. Cathet Cardiovasc Diagn. 1991;24:288-94.

33. Gamra H, Betbout F, Ayari M, Addad F, Jarrar M, Maatouk F, et al. Recurrent miscarriages as an indication for percutaneous tricuspid valvuloplasty during pregnancy. Cathet Cardiovasc Diagn. 1997;40:283-6.

34. Alperi A, Almendárez M, Álvarez R, Moris C, Leon V, Silva I, et al. Transcatheter tricuspid valve interventions: Current status and future perspectives. Front Cardiovasc Med. 2022; 9:994502.

35. Aurich M, Volz MJ, Mereles D, Geis NA, Frey N, Konstandin MH, et al. Initial experience with the PASCAL ace implant system for treatment of severe tricuspid regurgitation. Circ Cardiovasc Interv. 2021;14(9):e010770.

36. Harikrishnan S, Bhat A, Tharakan J, Titus T, Kumar A, Sivasankaran S, et al. Percutaneous transvenous mitral commissurotomy using metallic commissurotome: long-term follow-up results. J Invasive Cardiol. 2006;18(2):54-8.

37. Koren O, Israeli A, Rozner E, Darawshy N, Turgeman Y. Clinical and echocardiographic trends in percutaneous balloon mitral valvuloplasty. J Cardiothorac Surg. 2021;16(1):68.

38. Nunes MCP, Nascimento BR, Lodi-Junqueira L, Tan TC, Athayde GR, Hung J. Update on percutaneous mitral commissurotomy. Heart. 2016;102:500-7.

39. Lau KW, Hung JS. A simple balloon-sizing method in Inoue-balloon percutaneous transvenous mitral commissurotomy. Cathet Cardiovas Diagn. 1994;33:120-9; discussion 30–1.

40. Korkmaz S, Demirkan B, Guray Y, Yılmaz MB, Aksu T, Saşmaz H. Acute and long-term follow-up results of percutaneous mitral balloon valvuloplasty: a single-center study. Anadolu Kardiyol Derg. 2011;11:515-20.

41. Ralph AP, Currie BJ. Therapeutics for rheumatic fever and rheumatic heart disease. Aust Prescr. 2022;45:104-12.

42. Lilyasari O, Prakoso R, Kurniawati Y, Roebiono PS, Rahajoe AU, Sakidjan I, et al. Clinical Profile and Management of Rheumatic Heart Disease in Children and Young Adults at a Tertiary Cardiac Center in Indonesia. Front Surg. 2020;7:47.

Transcatheter Treatment of Rheumatic Mitral Stenosis in Pediatric Age Group

Ramesh Arora, IB Vijayalakshmi,
Sivasubramanian Ramakrishnan

> *"Children may be victims of fate; let them not be victims of our negligence."*
>
> **—John F Kennedy**

INTRODUCTION

The prevalence of rheumatic fever (RF) has declined significantly in most of the developed world. It continues, nonetheless, to be the most common cause of acquired heart disease in children and adolescent population of most developing countries.[1] Awareness regarding the early onset of rheumatic mitral stenosis in India was provided by Roy et al. who coined the term "juvenile" mitral stenosis for patients presenting with mitral stenosis below the age of 20 years.[2] The disease in these patients results in severe pulmonary artery hypertension, with the early appearance of symptoms and congestive heart failure at a very young age.[3]

Until the early 1980s, the only option for symptomatic patients with mitral stenosis uncontrollable by medical therapy was surgery. Surgical procedures included closed or open mitral commissurotomy [closed mitral valvotomy (CMV) or open mitral valvotomy (OMV)] and replacement of the mitral valve. A major breakthrough in the treatment of stenotic valves came in 1982, when Kan et al. performed the first nonsurgical dilatation of the pulmonary valve, using a balloon introduced percutaneously.[4] The technique soon developed to such an extent that dilatation of the mitral valve was attempted initially using single balloon[5] and then by two balloons positioned side by side within the valve, the so-called double balloon technique.[6] At the same time, Inoue et al. used a single rubber nylon balloon for open mitral commissurotomy under direct vision and following

that in 1984 reported successful percutaneous transvenous mitral commissurotomy (PTMC).[7] Subsequently, the use of the Inoue balloon gained widespread acceptance and at present is the preferred technique for treating symptomatic patients of rheumatic mitral stenosis, which is applicable to patients of all age groups.[8]

SELECTION OF PATIENTS

All symptomatic patients of mitral stenosis with significant stenosis [mitral valve orifice area (MVOA ≤ 1.5 cm^2)] should be considered for PTMC. Prior to the procedure, a detailed clinical and echocardiographic examination should be undertaken. On clinical examination, it is important to document the staging with the functional classification of the New York Heart Association (NYHA), any history of systemic embolism or hemoptysis and any continuing features of rheumatic activity. Another important aspect to be established is the presence of any severe cardiothoracic deformity, which may make fluoroscopic-guided transseptal puncture difficult and in such cases, septal puncture can be performed under echocardiographic guidance.[9]

Indeed, two-dimensional and Doppler echocardiographic techniques are essential noninvasive tools for assessing the structure of the mitral valvular apparatus, along with the hemodynamic significance of the stenosis **(Figs. 1A and B)**. The assessment of valvular and subvalvular anatomy

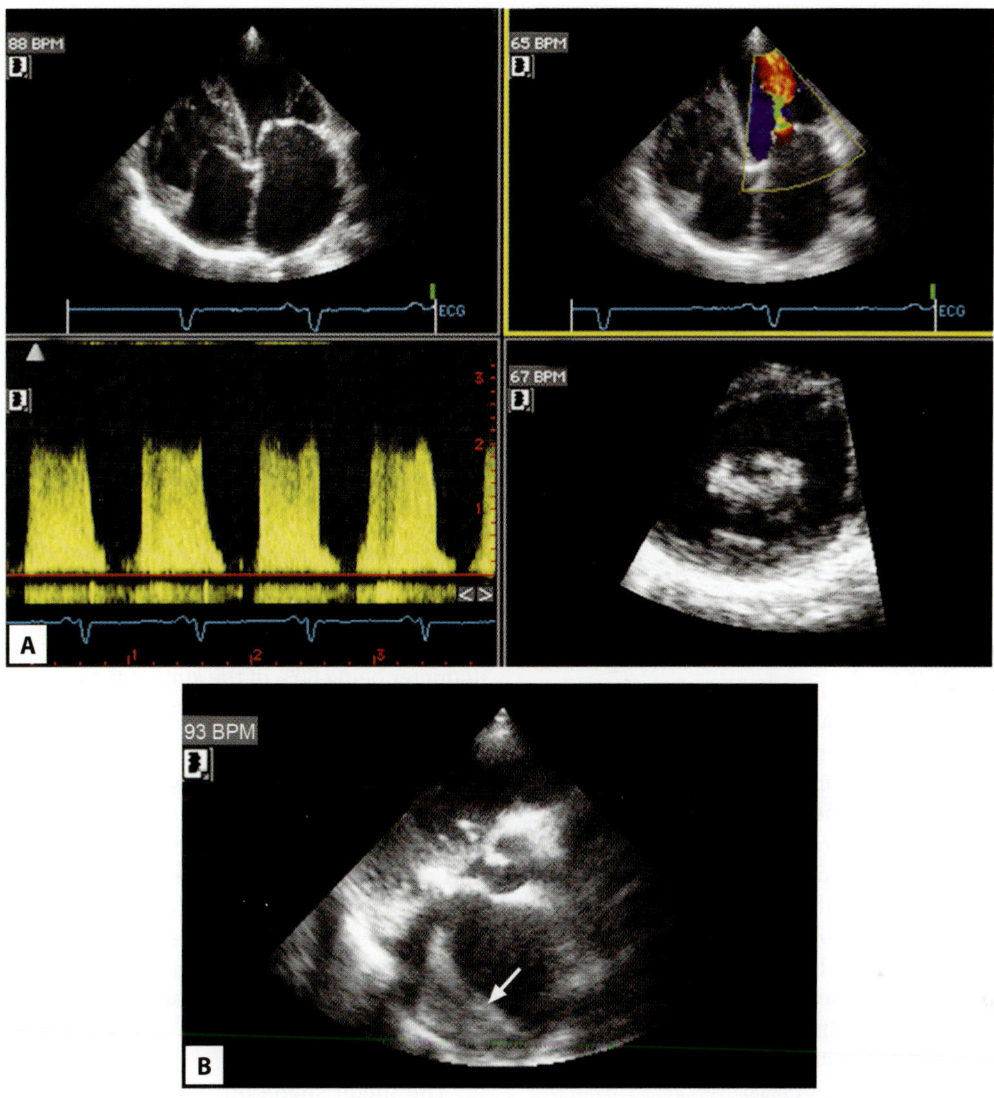

FIGS. 1A AND B: Cross-sectional echocardiographic, Doppler and Color flow imaging showing (A) the evaluation of the mitral valvular area and the degree of MR and (B) a large left atrial clot (arrow).

is frequently expressed as Wilkin's score with higher scores indicating more severe pathological deformities.[10] No doubt, the echocardiographic score gives an indication of the severity of the deformity but the predictive accuracy of the score in defining the likely success of the procedure[11] or the chance of development of complications like severe mitral regurgitation (MR) is limited.[12] But in the presence of high (>8) Wilkin's score, it is possible to proceed by graded dilatation, starting with a balloon measuring 2–4 mm less than the predicted diameter based on height and after each dilation intraprocedural echocardiography should be done to assess the extent of commissural split. Apart from assessing the structure of the valvular apparatus, color Doppler interrogation is used to assess the presence and severity of associated MR **(Fig. 1A)**.

While patients with mild or moderate MR can be suitable candidates for PTMC, the presence of severe MR is conventionally considered a contraindication. However, in younger population, when it is not always possible to deploy prosthetic mitral valve of adequate size, percutaneous dilatation may need to be attempted in spite of the presence of severe central jet of MR.[13] Another important aspect assessed by echocardiography is the presence of thrombus in the left atrium (LA) or left atrial appendage **(Fig. 1B)**. The presence of mobile thrombus on the interatrial septum and in LA cavity is absolute contraindication for transseptal puncture. There are reports of the procedure being performed with caution in severely symptomatic patients with clots localized in the left atrial appendage.[14]

TECHNICAL ASPECTS OF PERCUTANEOUS TRANSVENOUS MITRAL COMMISSUROTOMY

The various techniques by which PTMC can be performed are: transfemoral transvenous antegrade approach, transjugular venous approach, or retrograde femoral/brachial arterial approach.

Transfemoral Transvenous Antegrade Approach

The technique does not differ in children from that used in adults, except that the hemostatic sheath used for femoral arterial access is smaller, usually 4 French so as to minimize the local complication of arterial occlusion. PTMC is usually performed under local anesthesia. Transseptal puncture is done via the right femoral vein, monitoring arterial pressure by placing a pigtail catheter at the aortic root through the right femoral artery. After accessing the femoral vein, a pediatric Mullins dilator is passed over an exchange length guidewire of 0.025 diameter into the superior vena cava and also pediatric Brockenbrough needle is used. Although the septal approach from inferior vena cava (IVC) to fossa ovalis is direct, it is not easy for balloon catheter to traverse the mitral valve, as it has to bend by almost 180°. Various complex maneuvers are required for LV entry and the most important in children is by using the reverse loop technique **(Figs. 2A and B)**. PTMC is usually done by using single Inoue balloon. Nowadays double balloon or single Mansfield balloon dilatations are not done. The formula used for calculation of the size of Inoue balloon in adults cannot be used for children. This is because while using this formula, a high incidence of MR and restenosis was reported in a small series of children aged 12 years or less.[15]

Kothari et al. therefore, recommended a principle of staged balloon dilatation, starting with a balloon of 2–4 mm less than the recommended diameter and using progressive dilatation with increments of 1–2 mm until the endpoint is reached,[11] which should be any of the following:

- Mitral valve orifice area > 1 cm^2/m^2 and it is important to estimate the extent of splitting of the zone of apposition by using cross-sectional echocardiography in the short-axis view. If both ends of the zone of apposition are sufficiently split to a point near the annulus, further dilatation will cause significant MR. Similarly, if only one end is adequately split, further dilatation requires extra care because of risk of excessive avulsion of that area to the mitral annulus, resulting in severe MR.
- Mean gradient across mitral valve of <5 mm Hg **(Figs. 3A and B)**.
- Development of severe MR or an increase in severity of MR by one grade in patients with preexisting mild to moderate MR.

With Mansfield technique, for optimal dilatation, balloon diameter should be 21 or 22 mm/m². After transseptal puncture, the site of puncture is dilated with a balloon of 6–8 mm. Two balloons of appropriate size with their effective diameter being 80% of the sum of the required diameter are positioned across the mitral valve and inflated until the waist disappears.

Multitrack system utilizes two separate balloon catheters positioned on a single guidewire. The first catheter, with only a distal guidewire lumen, is introduced into the vein and then advanced into the mitral orifice. Subsequently, a rapid exchange balloon catheter running on the same guidewire is inserted and lined up with the first catheter so the two are positioned side by side. Both balloons are then inflated simultaneously. The sum of the diameters of the two balloons chosen is around 90–100% of the measured mitral valvular annulus.[16]

The metal shafts on both balloon catheters allow for very precise and stable manipulations on the balloons. The multitrack approach combines user friendliness, short

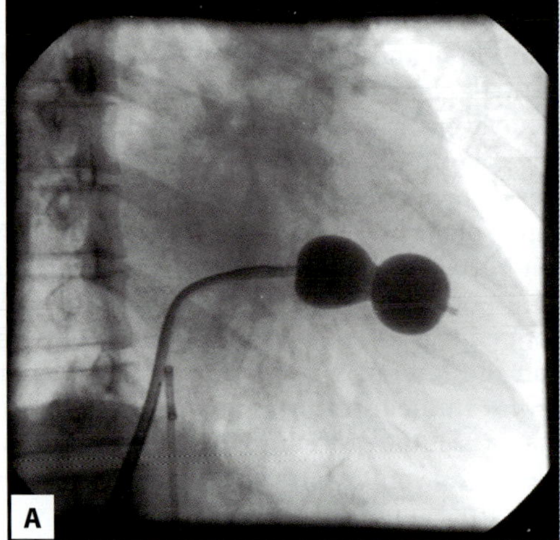

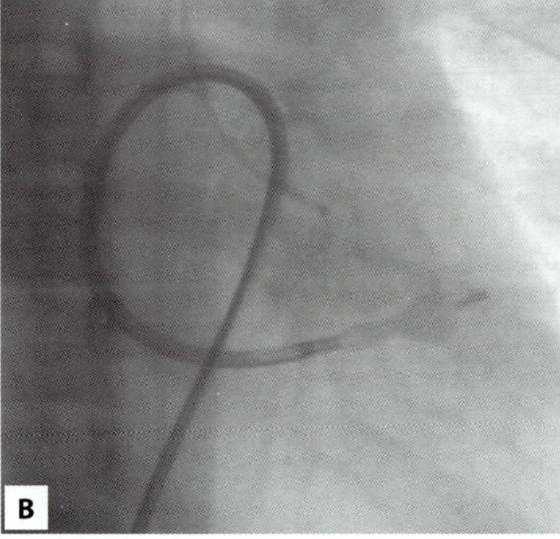

FIGS. 2A AND B: Entry of the Inoue balloon from the left atrium to the left ventricle by the (A) direct method; (B) reverse loop method.

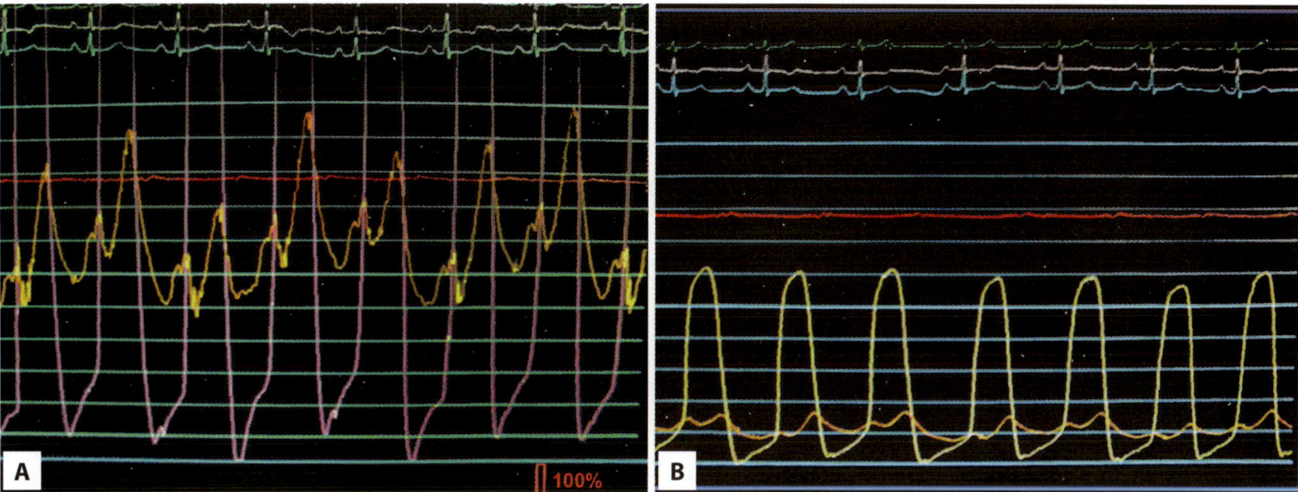

FIGS. 3A AND B: Simultaneous pressure tracings taken in the left atrium and left ventricle, showing a gradient across the mitral valve (A) predilatation and (B) postdilatation.

procedural time, and cost effectiveness along with the advantages of the double-balloon technique.

Transjugular Transvenous Approach

It is feasible and advantageous in certain cases of mitral stenosis with webs, interruption, obliteration or thrombosis of IVC or iliofemoral vein. The right internal jugular vein serves as a safe conduit for use of large balloon catheters in children.[17] This approach also provides a more direct route to the mitral valve, without catheters having to bend backward to cross the mitral valve, as occurs when using the femoral transvenous approach. Further, in patients with huge LA and distorted septal anatomy, the outcome of success of the procedure, particularly crossing of the mitral valve, is critically dependent, when using the transfemoral route. When using the jugular approach, as long as the superior part of the septum is punctured about 2 cm below the roof of the LA, midway between the aorta and the anterior border of the spine, the crossing of the mitral valve is then consistently simple and quick.[17] For transseptal puncture through the jugular vein, an Endrys pediatric transseptal set (Cook, Bloomington, IN) should be used. This transseptal set consisting of an outer metal tube and an inner stylet is more suitable since its extra curvature, which can be increased easily, allows a more perpendicular orientation of the needle tip to the atrial septum, while its short length makes the assembly easy to handle.

Retrograde Nontransseptal Aortic Approach

Catheter is big and requires a large sheath 8 or 9 French which makes it less attractive in children due to risk of injury to the femoral artery.[18]

ACUTE AND LONG-TERM RESULTS

Percutaneous transvenous mitral commissurotomy has become an established method of treatment for mitral stenosis in adults, with several series reporting the intermediate and long-term results.[19-21] There is paucity of information, however, regarding the long-term efficacy of the procedure in young children. While the majority of the reports available on the procedure as used for juvenile mitral stenosis include patients of adolescent age, from 12 to 18 years and in whom the results are quite comparable to adults.[22-24] Studies describing the efficacy of the procedure in children aged <15 years are limited.[11,13,15,25]

While Essop et al.[25] first reported its feasibility and success exclusively in children aged <12 years, it was Krishnamoorthy et al.[15] who undertook a study to determine whether the definition of mitral stenosis and the recommendation for using Inoue balloon as in adults based on height, is applicable for children and also to assess the effects of age and body surface area on the immediate outcome of the procedure. In their study, success was defined as achieving MVOA > 1.5 cm^2 with less than grade 2 MR, with these criteria being similar to those used in adults. A stepwise dilatation was carried out at 1 mm increments, commencing with a balloon sized at 2 mm less than that calculated using the height-based nomogram and going up to 2 mm above that obtained by the formula. Though the procedure was successful in over nine-tenths of the series, two children (15%) developed moderate MR, this being higher than by the one-tenth incidence of this complication reported in the Inoue balloon registry obtained for adult patients.[26] The authors attributed this problem to use of a height-based nomogram in selecting the size of the balloon and also in targeting a valvular area >1.5 cm^2 to define the procedure as successful. Similarly, while using the criteria of MVOA < 1.5 cm^2 on follow-up as the definition of restenosis, as is the case in adults, a restenosis rate of almost 40% was reported on follow-up of 20 months, though none of the patients were symptomatic. Subsequently, Kothari et al.[11] addressed the issues of success and restenosis with respect to body surface area. They modified procedural success as achieving a MVOA > 1 cm^2/m^2 in the absence of complications such as death, tamponade, systemic embolism or severe MR. They considered restenosis as a decrease in the MVOA < 0.8 cm^2/m^2 or greater than or equal to half the loss in the initial gain.[11] The initial size of the balloon chosen was 2–4 mm less than the size as if calculated on the basis of height. The procedure was successful in 97 out of 100 patients and maximum size of the balloon used was less than or equal to the recommended size. With this policy, the incidence of severe MR was 4% and restenosis rate of 12%, well within the acceptable limits. The result of this study in children <12 years of age, with intermediate term follow-up at a mean of 34 months, reported echocardiographic restenosis in one-sixth of patients, which is comparable to that reported by Arora et al.[13] in one-eighth of children aged <15 years followed for over 96 months and much less than reported by Krishnamoorthy et al.[15] albeit that the latter group did not define restenosis on the basis of body surface area. Kothari et al.[11] have also reported event free survival at 100 months of 75% compared to 56% at similar duration of follow-up in a large Western series in adults.[27] Moreover in authors' series of 17 patients of severe MR, there was regression of MR in 16 by 1 grade or more and only one required MVR.[13]

Juvenile mitral stenosis is called "malignant mitral stenosis"; however, PTMC significantly reduces the morbidity and mortality in the otherwise undernourished children and helps in avoiding or postpones surgery.[28]

In series of Vijayalakshmi et al.[28] a total of 14,560 cases of MS underwent PTMC with Inoue/Accura balloon, from April 1994 to August 2010, at Sri Jayadeva Institute of Cardiovascular Sciences and Research, out of which 6,550 cases were below the age of 20 years, youngest patient was 6 years old (73 cm height), mean age was 14.39 years and female:male ratio was 2:1 (female: 4,377 cases and male: 2,183 cases). The smallest mitral MVOA was 0.2 cm^2 **(Fig. 4)**. Compared to adults, MVOA was smaller, both before and after PTMC. One exceptional girl who had CMV at the age of 6 years underwent PTMC twice and OMV later at the age of 18 years as she had LA thrombus. Post PTMC, MR could be due to over splitting of commissure or chordal tear as the balloon can be trapped in the chordae **(Fig. 5)**. If the balloon is deformed then it is likely that it is caught in the chordae **(Fig. 6)** and such a balloon should not be inflated. None had severe MR **(Fig. 7A)**. 1965 cases (30%) had mild MR. 106 children came for recrudescence of rheumatic activity and 32 had restenosis. None had significant atrial septal defect (ASD) **(Fig. 7B)**. Most of them had significant residual gradient because of severe submitral fusion and very thick valve with reduced mobility, especially immobile PML **(Figs. 8A and B)**. **Table 1** gives the comparison of PTMC in adult with children. Comparable results of

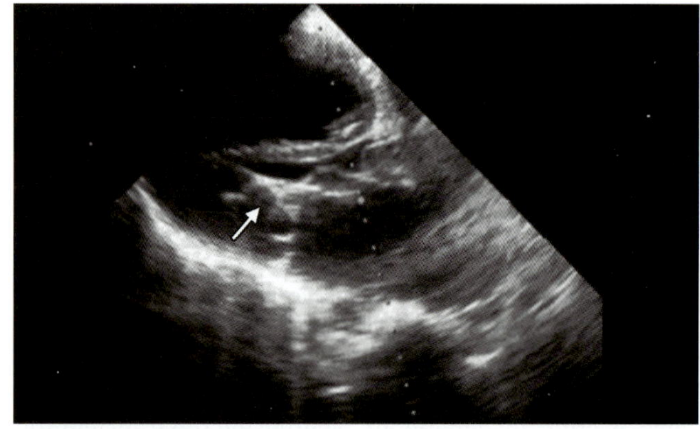

FIG. 5: Parasternal long-axis shows Inoue balloon caught in submitral structure (arrow).

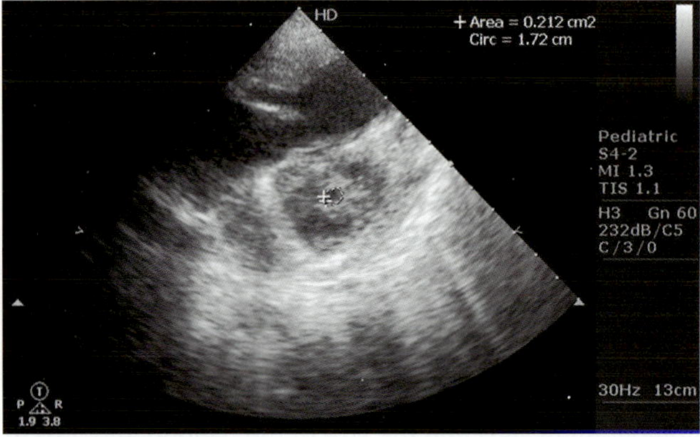

FIG. 4: Parasternal short-axis shows 0.2 cm^2 MVOA in an 8-year-old child with critical MS.

(MS: mitral stenosis; MVOA: mitral valve orifice area)

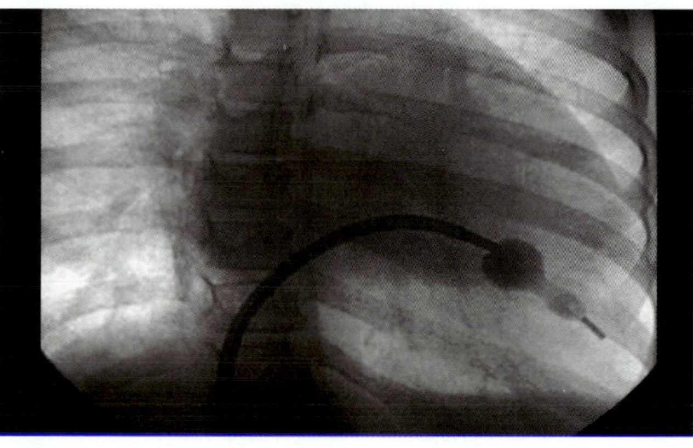

FIG. 6: Cine picture of deformed Inoue balloon caught in the chordae.

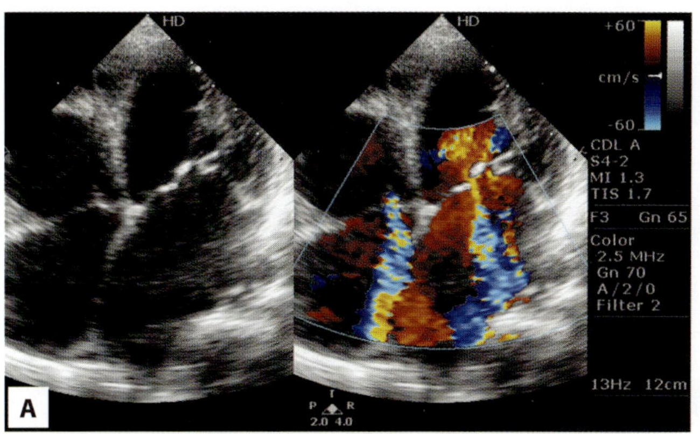
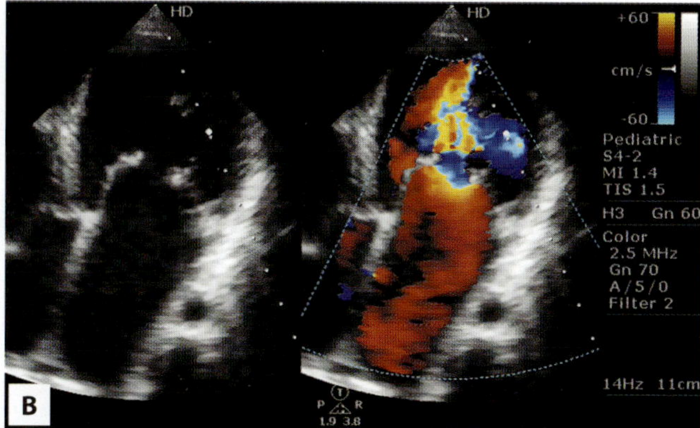

FIGS. 7A AND B: (A) Apical four chamber view in a 10-year-old boy with MS before PTMC. (B) Apical two chamber view after PTMC. No significant ASD.

(ASD: atrial septal defect; PTMC: percutaneous transvenous mitral commissurotomy; MS: mitral stenosis)

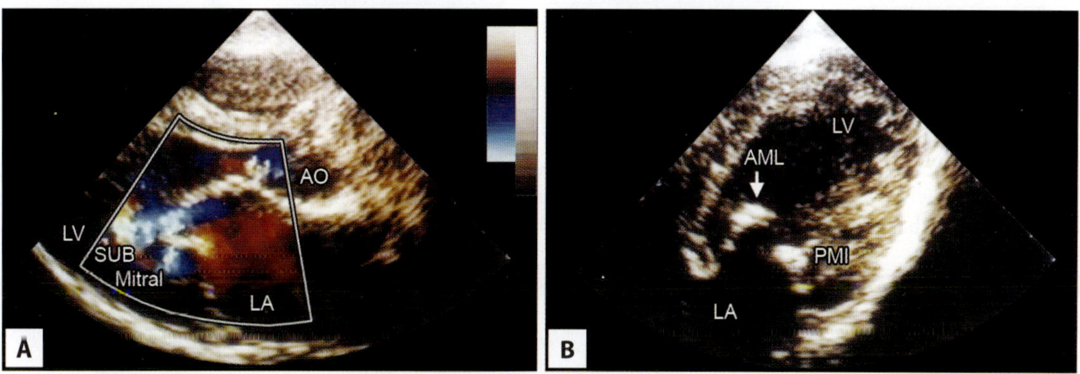

FIGS. 8A AND B: (A) Parasternal long axis with color Doppler shows submitral stenosis; (B) Shows thickened deformed AML and PML.

(AML: anterior mitral leaflet; LA: left atrium; LV: left ventricle PML: posterior mitral leaflet; AO: Aorta)

TABLE 1: Ten years data of PTMC in adult MS and JMS at Sri Jayadeva Institute of Cardiovascular Sciences and Research, Bengaluru.

	Mean age (Year)	MVOA cm²		PASP (mm Hg)		Peak MV Gradient (mm Hg)	
		Pre	Post	Pre	Post	Pre	Post
Adult MS 19,478	32.7	0.8 + 0.18	2.3 + 0.25	54.8 ± 20.16	30.6 ± 10.6	18.5 ± 6.12	3.0 ± 3.1
JMS 6,550	14.39	0.73 ± 0.164	1.85 ± 0.32	72.38 ± 23.03	42.95 ± 14.54	28.46 ± 7.18	11.47 ± 4.04

(MS: mitral stenosis; MVOA: mitral valve orifice area; PTMC: percutaneous transvenous mitral commissurotomy)

PTMC in children are published from other major Indian institutes and from Nepal.[29,30] All the studies in children and adolescents across the globe are reviewed in detail by Saxena A in 2015.[31]

Percutaneous transvenous mitral commissurotomy may also be performed in rare children who present with refractory symptoms of heart failure and an episode of recurrence of RF. In a small study, the acute results were comparable in children presenting with acute activity; however, the restenosis rate was higher.[32]

MITRAL STENOSIS WITH ASSOCIATED CONGENITAL HEART DISEASE

Rarely rheumatic mitral stenosis can be associated with congenital heart diseases (CHDs) like:

- ASD called as Lutembacher's syndrome; where we can do both balloon mitral valvotomy (BMV) and device closure of ASD.
- Coarctation of aorta (COA) in which case we must dilate the COA first and then do the BMV **(Figs. 9A to E)**.

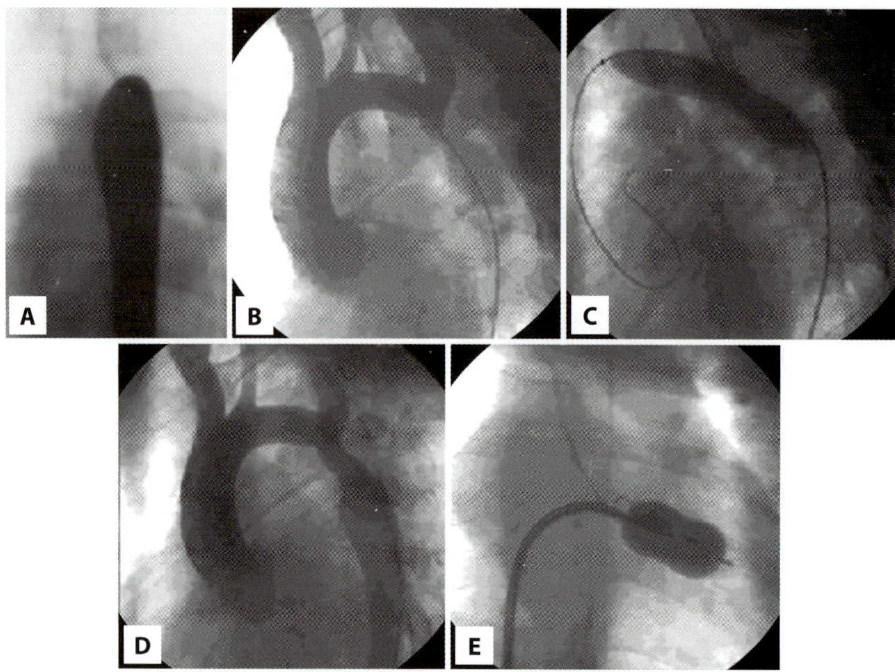

FIGS. 9A TO E: (A) The descending aortic angiogram in AP view shows severe COA; (B) After crossing the COA the ascending aortic angiogram in left lateral view shows severe COA; (C) Inflated balloon in situ; (D) Check angio shows good dilatation of coarcted segment with no dissection; (E) Inoue balloon dilatation of MS in a patient oh rheumatic heart disease with atrial fibrillation with pulmonary edema in a 14 years old boy.

(AP: anteroposterior; COA: coarctation of aorta; MS: mitral stenosis)

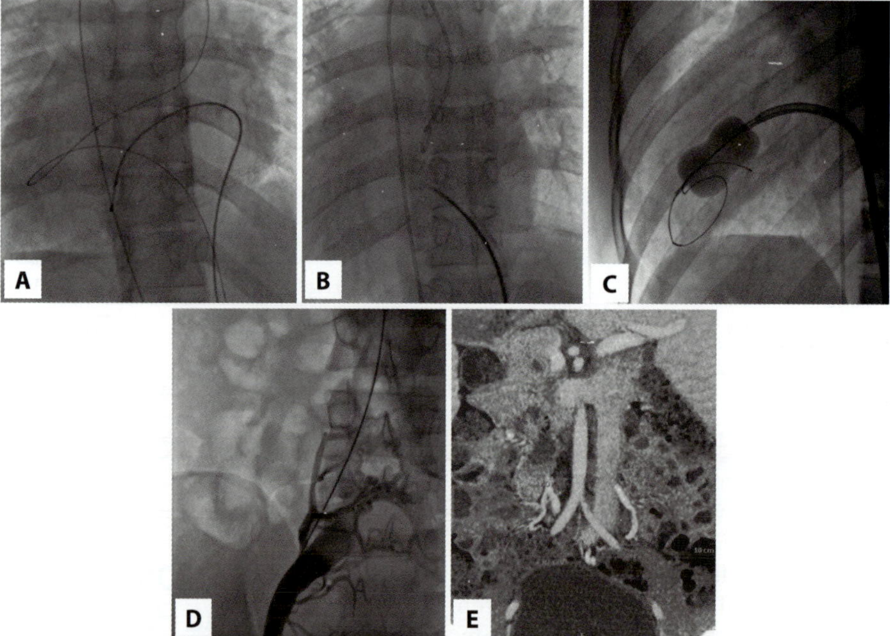

FIGS. 10A TO E: (A) Fluoroscopy shows a good AV loop in LV, 12 × 40 mm Tyshak II balloon was inflated across the aortic orifice and the pacing lead seen is used to pace at a rate of 220/min; (B) The puncture of the IAS was done from left femoral vein approach keeping the arrow of Brockenbrough needle between 7 and 8 o'clock position instead of 4 o'clock position; (C) Over the guidewire balloon was negotiated through IAS into LV directly, without using the usual 'U' guidewire and the inflation was done with 24 mm accura BMV balloon; (D) The pacemaker lead was not going through right femoral vein, hand injection into the sheath showed stasis of dye and partial obstruction of right common iliac vein; (E) CTA showing compression of right common iliac vein by left common iliac artery (reverse of May–Thurner syndrome) in a 16 years old boy who presented with chest pain and echo showed dextrocardia, situs inversus, severe MS (gradient 63/34 mm Hg), with bicuspid aortic valve with severe AS (200/122 mm Hg).

(AV: arteriovenous; BMV: balloon mitral valvotomy; CTA: computed tomography angiography; IAS: interatrial septum; LV: left ventricle; MS: mitral stenosis)

- Bicuspid aortic stenosis (AS) in such cases dilate the AS first and then do BMV **(Figs. 10A to E)**.

CONCLUSIONS AND FUTURE DIRECTIONS

Though there are few guidelines about the optimal size of Inoue balloon to be used in children undergoing PTMC, it seems appropriate to follow the strategy of using an Inoue balloon sized at 2–4 mm less than the size recommended on the basis of height or a Mansfield balloon sized at 21–22 mm/m^2. Procedural success should also be defined as achieving a MVOA > 1 cm/m^2 and restenosis as ≤0.8 cm/m^2. Nonetheless, it should be remembered that surgical procedures nowadays also carry a low mortality, almost similar to that achieved using percutaneous balloon dilatation but in juvenile mitral stenosis, repeated restenosis, necessitating redilatation makes PTMC as the preferred choice of therapy.

ACKNOWLEDGMENT

Our grateful thanks to Dr Jamal Yusuf his kind assistance.

REFERENCES

1. Rheumatic fever and rheumatic heart disease. World Health Organ Tech Rep Ser. 2004;923:1-122.
2. Roy SB, Bhatia ML, Lazaro EJ, Ramalingaswami V. Juvenile mitral stenosis in India. Lancet. 1963;2:1193-6.
3. Srivastava S, Tandon R. Severity of mitral stenosis in children. Int J Cardiol. 1991;30:163-7.
4. Kan JS, White RI, Mitchell SE, Gardner TJ. Percutaneous balloon valvuloplasty: A new method for treating congenital pulmonary valve stenosis. N Engl J Med. 1982;307:540-2.
5. Lock JE, Khalilullah M, Srivastava S, Bahl V, Keane JF. Percutaneous catheter commissurotomy in rheumatic mitral stenosis. N Engl J Med. 1985;313:1515-8.
6. Al Zaibag M, Ribiero PA, Alkasab S, Alfagih MR. Percutaneous double balloon mitral valvotomy for rheumatic mitral valve stenosis. Lancet. 1986;1:757-61.
7. Inoue K, Owaki T, Nakamura T, Kitamura F, Miyamoto N. Clinical application of transvenous mitral commissurotomy by a new balloon catheter. J Thorac Cardiovasc Surg. 1984;87:394-402.
8. Cheng TO. Percutaneous balloon mitral valvuloplasty with Inoue balloon is applicable to all age groups. Cathet Cardiovasc Diagn. 1998;43:412.
9. Trehan V, Mukhopadhyay S, Nigam A, Yusuf J, Mehta V, Gupta MD, et al. Mitral valvuloplasty by Inoue balloon under transthoracic echocardiographic guidance. J Am Soc Echocardiogr. 2005;18:964-9.
10. Wilkins GT, Weyman AE, Abascal VM, Block PC, Palacious IF. Percutaneous balloon dilatation of the mitral valve: An analysis of echocardiographic variables related to outcome and mechanism of dilatation. Br Heart J. 1998;60:299-308.
11. Kothari SS, Ramakrishnan S, Kumar CK, Juneja R, Yadav R. Intermediate term results of percutaneous transvenous mitral commissurotomy in children less than 12 years of age. Cathet Cardiovasc Interv. 2005;64:487-90.
12. Arora R, Kalra GS, Murty GS, Trehan V, Jolly N, Mohan JC, et al. Percutaneous transatrial mitral commissurotomy: Immediate and intermediate results. J Am Coll Cardiol. 1994;23:1327-32.
13. Arora R, Trehan V, Thakur AK, et al. Percutaneous transvenous mitral commissurotomy in the pediatric age group. Indian Heart J. 2003;55(442):575.
14. Chen WJ, Chen MF, Liau CS, Wu CC, Lee YT. Safety of percutaneous transvenous mitral commissurotomy in patients with mitral stenosis and thrombus in left atrial appendage. Am J Cardiol. 1992;70:117-9.
15. Krishnamoorthy KM, Tharakan JA. Balloon mitral valvotomy in children aged less than or equal to 12 years. J Heart Valve Dis. 2003;12:461-8.
16. Bonhoeffer P, Esteves C, Casal U, Tortoledo F, Yonga G, Patel T, et al. Percutaneous mitral valve dilatation with the multitrack system. Cathet Cardiovasc Intervent. 1999;48:178-83.
17. Joseph G, Baruah DK, Kuruttukulam SV, Chandy ST, Krishnaswami S. Transjugular approach to transseptal balloon mitral valvuloplasty. Cathet Cardiovasc Diagn. 1997;42:219-26.
18. Stefanadis C, Stratos C, Pitsavos C, Kallikazaros I, Triposkiadis F, Trikas A, et al. Retrograde nontransseptal balloon mitral valvuloplasty: immediate results and long term follow up. Circulation. 1992;85:1760-7.
19. Chen CR, Cheng TO. Percutaneous balloon mitral valvuloplasty by the Inoue technique: A multicentre study of 4832 patients in China. Am Heart J. 1995;129:1197-203.
20. Arora R, Kalra GS, Singh S, Mukhopadhyay S, Kumar A, Mohan JC, et al. Percutaneous transvenous mitral commissurotomy: immediate and long-term follow-up results. Cathet Cardiovasc Intervent. 2002;55:450-556.
21. Palacious IF. Percutaneous mitral balloon valvuloplasty. In: Sievert H, Qureshi SA, Wilson N, Hijazi ZM (Eds). Book of Percutaneous Interventions for Congenital Heart Disease. London, United Kingdom: Informa Health Care; 2007. pp. 177-84.
22. Fawzy ME, Mimish L, Awad M, Galal O, el-Deeb F, Khan B. Mitral balloon valvotomy in children with Inoue balloon technique immediate and intermediate term results. Am Heart J. 1994;127:1559-62.
23. Srivastava S, Chandra YV, Krishnamoorthy KM, Radhakrishnan S. Mitral valvotomy with Inoue balloon in juvenile rheumatic mitral stenosis. Am J Cardiol. 1995;76:404-6.
24. Joseph PK, Bhat A, Francis B, Sivasankaran S, Kumar A, Pillai VR, et al. Percutaneous transvenous mitral commissurotomy using an Inoue balloon in children with rheumatic mitral stenosis. Int J Cardiol. 1997;62:19-22.
25. Essop MR, Govendrageloo K, Du Plessis J, van Dyk M, Sareli P. Balloon mitral valvotomy for rheumatic mitral stenosis in children aged < 12 years. Am J Cardiol. 1993;72:850-1.
26. Harrison JK, Wilson JS, Hearne SE, Bashore TM. Complications related to percutaneous transvenous mitral commissurotomy. Cathet Cardiovasc Diagn. 1994;Suppl 2:52-60.
27. Iung B, Garbarz E, Michaud P, Helou S, Farah B, Berdah P, et al. Late results of percutaneous mitral commissurotomy in a

series of 1024 patients. analysis of late clinical deterioration–frequency, anatomic findings and predictive factors. Circulation. 1999;99:3272-8.

28. Vijayalakshmi IB, et al. Percutaneous Transvenous Mitral commissurotomy in Juvenile Rheumatic Mitral Stenosis vs Adult. Cathet Cardiovasc Intervent. 2002:57(1):120.

29. Patnaik AN, Srinivas B, Seshagiri Rao D. Percutaneous transvenous mitral commissurotomy in rheumatic mitral stenosis in children: NIMS experience. Clin Proc NIMS. 2008; 19:9-11.

30. Shrestha M, Adhikari CM, Shakya U, Khanal A, Shrestha S, Rajbhandari R. Percutaneous Transluminal Mitral Commissurotomy in Nepalese children with Rheumatic Mitral Stenosis. Nepalese Heart J. 2013;10:23-6.

31. Saxena A. Catheter Interventions for Mitral Stenosis in Children: Results and Perspectives. World J Pediatr Congen Heart Surg. 2015;6(2):250-6.

32. Kothari SS, Ramakrishnan S, Juneja R, Yadav R. Percutaneous Transvenous Mitral Commissurotomy in Patients with Severe Mitral Stenosis and Acute Rheumatic Fever. Pediatr Cardiol. 2006;27(3):347-50.

21

Surgical Management of Rheumatic Heart Disease

Prasanna Simha Mohan Rao

> *"Speed in operating should be the achievement, Not the aim, of every surgeon."*
>
> —**Russel John Howard** (1875–1942)
> British Surgeon, Royal London Hospital, London

INTRODUCTION

Historically, attempts to relieve rheumatic mitral stenosis were one of the first attempts at intracardiac surgery. Sir Lauder Brunton was one of the first persons to propose surgical correction of mitral stenosis. Elliot Cutler made initial experimental and human attempts to relieve mitral stenosis. Souttar was the first person to successfully dilate a stenotic mitral valve and this was later popularized by Bailey, Smithy, Harken, and Brock. Closed mitral valvotomy became popular with the introduction of the graded dilator by Oswald Tubbs. Many attempts were made to correct mitral insufficiency by closed methods using obturators and plugs which were not successful. The first attempt at reconstruction was by Lillehei and later with the introduction of the Starr Edwards valve consistent replacement became possible. Aortic valve replacement was first done in the orthotopic subcoronary position by Harken.

Repair techniques were championed by Carpentier and Duran who also demonstrated the clinical benefits of repairing the mitral valve.

PATHOLOGY

Rheumatic Mitral Disease

Mitral stenosis: There is initial valvular inflammation, lymphocytic infiltration and neovascularization. The characteristic pathological finding is the Aschoff nodule which is found in the ventricular and atrial tissue. Inflammation subsides with fibrosis. The commissural damage promotes fibrin deposition and adhesion of the leaflets to a varying degree causing mitral stenosis. Leaflet fibrosis causes a decrease in the surface area of the leaflet and varying degree of tethering. Progression of this stenosis is due to a combination of recurrent carditis and local turbulence, fibrin deposition, and organization with fibrous tissue deposition. In chronic cases, there is calcification in the fibrotic areas and this can be in the leaflet, commissures, and annulus. Fusion of the commissures and leaflet thickening causes the mitral annulus to become more planar, a fixed orifice develops giving the classical "fish mouth" appearance of the mitral valve (**Fig. 1**). Fibrotic nodules may form in the leaflet and commissure. Chordal inflammation causes the chordae to initially have a fibrinous exudative cover which organizes giving rise to chordal thickening and shortening. This progresses to fusion of the chordal apparatus, shortening of the chordae, and fusion of papillary muscle heads. In extreme cases, the whole chordal apparatus may form a fused sheet which can significantly cause subvalvular obstruction. The posterior leaflet and its chordal apparatus may become plastered to the posterior left ventricular (LV) wall in extreme cases.

Mitral regurgitation: In the acute phase of carditis, there can be annular dilatation secondary to myocarditis and this gives rise to acute mitral regurgitation giving rise to the classical Carey Coombs murmur. This acute regurgitation due to myocarditis can be significant and can contribute

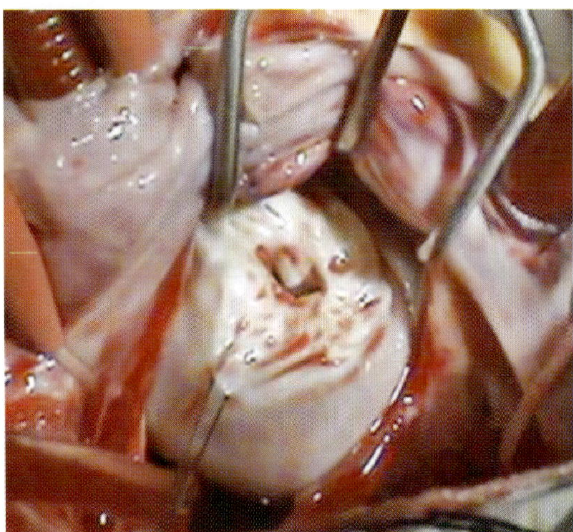

FIG. 1: The classical "fish mouth" appearance of mitral valve.

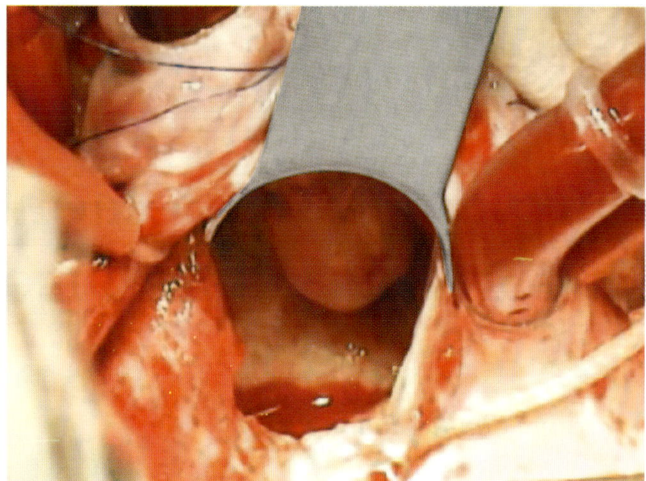

FIG. 2: Anterior leaflet prolapse, posterior leaflet retraction, and commissural fusion.

to severe cardiac failure in addition to myocarditis per se. With resolution of carditis there is resolution of this regurgitation. At times there can be dramatic resolution of severe mitral regurgitation with resolution of carditis, so it is unwise to consider patients with active carditis for surgery unless there is severe hemodynamic compromise such that survival till resolution of carditis is possible. In most cases, medical stabilization with aggressive medical management is possible in these cases.

Following resolution of rheumatic carditis, there is progressive fibrosis of the leaflets with varying degrees of fusion giving rise to specific entities that need to be addressed during repair of rheumatic mitral regurgitation.

Annular dilatation is a progressive occurrence and regurgitation begets dilatation which begets regurgitation. The annulus may not dilate in cases with significant mitral stenosis and in cases with significant annular fibrosis. Patients who do not have significant annular dilatation (typical above 10 cm) usually have deficiency of leaflet tissue due to extensive fibrosis and these patients may need leaflet augmentation procedures to achieve competence. Significant annular dilatation is to the surgeon's advantage when repairing a valve as this indicates that subsequent annular reduction will allow greater tissue coaptation increasing the chances of a successful repair.

Leaflet fusion is seen to a variable extent in rheumatic mitral disease and when present, it is pathognomonic. The fusion may be minimal or it may be extensive resulting in a fixed orifice mitral regurgitation. Release of this fusion is mandatory as it will cause a "hinge point restriction" during repair which will preclude a good result.

Leaflet fibrosis causes leaflet retraction, shortening, and nodularity. Retraction is seen maximally in the P3 region of the mitral valve and is the Achilles heel of mitral valve repair.[1] Leaflet retraction causes the posterior mitral leaflet (PML) height to be reduced and thus systolic anterior motion of the mitral valve, post repair, is extremely rare after rheumatic

mitral valve repairs.[2,3] The anterior mitral leaflet (AML) may be significantly fibrosed and retracted. These patients are poor candidates for repair and may need extensive patching with pericardium to achieve mitral competence. Focal fibrotic nodules may affect leaflet motion and may require excision to allow leaflet pliability and motion.

Leaflet prolapse–very commonly the anterior leaflet in rheumatic mitral regurgitation is prolapsed. There is chordal elongation and the leaflet may have varying degrees of fibrosis. The margin of the leaflet may have focal areas of dilatation which represent a sinuous leaflet margin with areas of focal increased prolapse and these areas can lead to significant regurgitation post repair if not identified and attended **(Fig. 2)**.

Calcification occurs at the annulus, leaflet, and chordal apparatus. Calcified valves are usually extremely distorted and are poor candidates for repair and are not usually repairable. Selected cases with focal calcium can be debrided and focal nodules may be excised and the area patched. Commissural calcium and calcium on the leaflets extending down to the subvalvular apparatus usually precludes repair.

Rheumatic Aortic Disease

Rheumatic aortic valve disease is characterized by an initial inflammation and neovascularization followed later by varying degrees of fibrosis and commissural fusion. There is fibrosis and rolling up and shortening of the leaflets so there is often a combination of stenosis and regurgitation. With progressive disease there is finally calcification and often a fixed orifice which is stenotic and regurgitant **(Fig. 3)**.

Rheumatic tricuspid valve disease can be primary and secondary. Tricuspid regurgitation (TR) is very common in patients with severe pulmonary hypertension due to mitral valve disease due to annular dilatation. This secondary TR was considered to resolve with correction of the mitral disease but it is increasingly being understood that even moderate degrees of TR and patients with an annulus > 27 mm/m^2 are

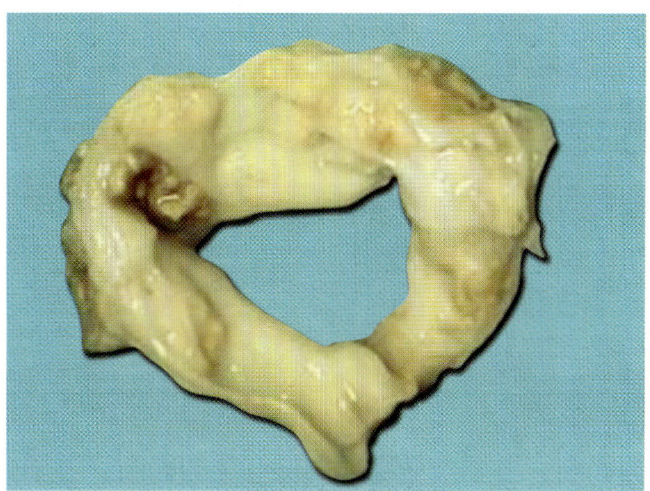

FIG. 3: Excised valve of a case of calcific rheumatic aortic stenosis with regurgitation.

at risk for progression of regurgitation and while temporary resolution of symptoms may occur TR recurs in a few years in these patients. Organic tricuspid disease is a combination of varying degrees of tricuspid stenosis and retraction and fibrosis of leaflets that cause significant regurgitation and stenosis. Some patients may have pure tricuspid stenosis.

INDICATIONS FOR SURGERY

Mitral Stenosis

Intervention is indicated in patients with mitral stenosis who are symptomatic. Patients with asymptomatic disease and a pulmonary artery (PA) pressure of >50 mm Hg at rest or 60 mm Hg with exercise, mean transmitral gradient of above 15 mm Hg or a PA wedge pressure >25 mm Hg require intervention. Usually patients with a valve area > 1 cm/m^2 require intervention. Percutaneous balloon mitral valvotomy is the procedure of choice, if there are no contraindications and if it is available. When not available closed mitral valvotomy is an alternative which is being used infrequently. Open mitral valvotomy, mitral valve repair, or mitral valve replacement may be indicated in patients who have a contraindication for balloon mitral valvotomy.

Closed mitral valvotomy is currently only indicated in patients who are suitable for balloon mitral valvotomy but are not balloonable for various technical reasons like access problems or inability to cross the interatrial septum (IAS). With increasing skill this has become a relatively rare event in areas where balloon mitral valvotomy is done in high volumes.

Open mitral valvotomy is done in patients who are not candidates for balloon mitral valvotomy. The usual reason is a left atrial appendage clot that is protruding into the body that precludes balloon mitral valvotomy. The valvotomy is combined with left atrial thrombectomy and an additional Maze surgery can be done. Concomitant tricuspid problems are addressable. Patients undergoing concomitant aortic valve surgery also can have their mitral stenosis addressed at the same time with open valvotomy. Patients with Lutembacher's syndrome are often subjected to surgery as the large interatrial septal defect poses a problem in stable anchorage of the balloon during balloon mitral valvotomy. It has also been a personal observation that these patients often have severe subvalvular disease which tends to make the results of balloon dilatation less than optimal or can result in severe mitral regurgitation in many cases.

Mitral valve replacement is indicated in patients who have valves which are not suitable for balloon or open mitral valvotomy. Typically, these are calcified valves or having severe valvular and subvalvular fibrosis and fusion with nonpliable valves.

Mitral Regurgitation

Surgery for mitral regurgitation is indicated in patients with the New York Heart Association (NYHA) Class III or IV symptoms.

Patients with asymptomatic mitral regurgitation and progressive LV dysfunction as evidenced by an ejection fraction (EF) < 60% and end-systolic diameter left ventricular internal dimensions in systole (LVIDS) > 40 mm. Patients with low EF (<30% or LVIDS > 55 mm) should still be offered surgery albeit with a higher risk if repair is possible or replacement with chordal preservation or neochord construction is to be done. Dimensions have to be indexed to body surface area in children and left atrial dimension of >45 mm, pulmonary artery hypertension, and new onset atrial fibrillation are additional indications for intervention especially if referring to a surgeon who has a high repair rate and experience in repairing rheumatic valves.

Combined lesions of rheumatic heart disease often presents as a combination of mitral stenosis with regurgitation. This presents a peculiar problem where regurgitation increases left atrial volume whereas the stenosis causes obstruction to the normal flow and the added regurgitant volume. Patients with combined lesions are symptomatic earlier and also have one of the largest left atria and increased propensity for atrial fibrillation. Valve areas of 1.5 cm^2 and less can become significantly stenotic in the presence of significant regurgitation (II+). Pulmonary hypertension and increasing left atrial and LV dimensions should guide earlier intervention before atrial fibrillation and left atrial thrombi form. These lesions are amenable to repair with good results if the leaflets are pliable. They are more difficult to repair and are best done by experienced surgeons. Mitral valve replacement in these patients is done if the lesion is not repairable.

Aortic Valve Disease

The approach to rheumatic aortic valve disease has to be tempered by the fact that repair is not consistently possible and long-term durability has not been consistently achieved with repair. The Ross procedure in these patients is not a very good option in patients <35 years as recurrent carditis can affect the neoaortic valve and damage it. Bioprosthetic valve implantation has its own set of problems and when implanted in the typically young patient group has a sobering incidence of rapid valve degeneration. Mechanical valves are also not an ideal substitute but are commonly implanted for socioeconomic reasons. Unfortunately, thrombohemorrhagic episodes and obstructive pannus are a real problem. Also when implanted in growing teens rapid increase in weight during the teenage growth spurt poses challenges in maintaining therapeutic anticoagulation levels.

Aortic Stenosis

Symptomatic aortic stenosis is an indication for surgery. Patients undergoing concomitant surgery and with moderate or severe aortic stenosis also should undergo aortic valve replacement. Patients with moderate aortic stenosis have a fairly rapid progression of disease, so if the patient is undergoing any other cardiac surgery it is better to intervene. Patients with severe aortic stenosis and LV dysfunction and an EF of <50% can also undergo aortic valve replacement. Patients with an abnormal response to stress testing should also undergo aortic valve replacement. Rheumatic aortic stenosis is rarely an isolated disease and is usually combined with regurgitation and mitral valve disease. Aortic valve repair is not consistently possible with rheumatic aortic disease and replacement is needed.

Aortic Regurgitation

Aortic valve replacement is indicated in patients with symptomatic severe aortic regurgitation or when undergoing concomitant procedures of the mitral valve. Asymptomatic patients should undergo AVR when there is evidence of declining LV function and increasing ventricular dimensions. It is important to index the dimensions and volumes to body surface area as patients with rheumatic heart disease are often malnourished and have growth retardation.

Tricuspid Valve Disease

Severe medically nonresponsive tricuspid regurgitation has been the traditional indication for tricuspid valve repair/replacement. It has been increasingly recognized that the concept that "correcting the left sided lesion" will restore tricuspid competence in hypertensive TR is fallacious and while temporary resolution of right heart symptoms may come down immediately after left-sided intervention, TR will recur in the short or medium term and will require attention. Prophylactic tricuspid repair is done in our practice when the tricuspid annulus is >27 mm/m^2 even in the absence of regurgitation as it is a risk factor for developing regurgitation in the near future. We prefer to stabilize the tricuspid annulus in any patient with a history of right heart failure and wavering

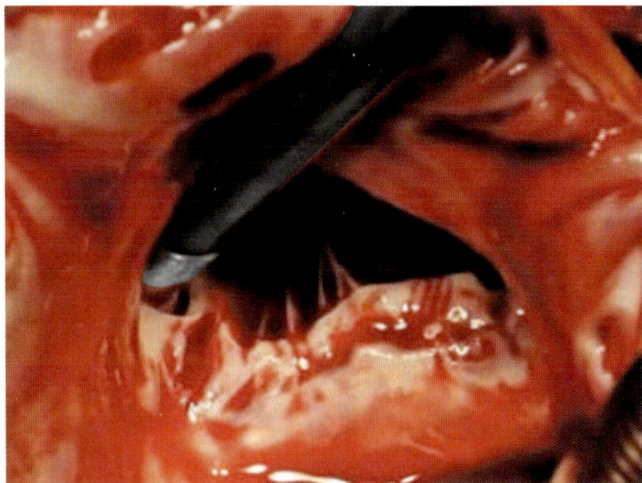

FIG. 4: Tricuspid stenosis with regurgitation–the anteroseptal commissure is partly fused.

TR. Patients with normotensive TR, organic tricuspid valve disease, and associated with tricuspid stenosis need to have their valve repaired. Most valves can be repaired and in case of leaflet area deficiency liberal augmentation of the AML with autologous pericardium may be required. Patients who cannot be repaired should undergo tricuspid valve replacement preferably with a bioprosthetic valve.

Patients with organic tricuspid stenosis and right heart failure should undergo tricuspid valvotomy at the time of their surgery **(Fig. 4)**. Isolated tricuspid stenosis should undergo balloon valvotomy, if feasible.

Open Mitral Valvotomy

Open mitral valvotomy is indicated in patients who are not candidates for balloon (or closed mitral valvotomy). These include patients who have a left atrium (LA) body clot, patients undergoing concomitant procedures like an aortic valve replacement, and in patients where there is a technical hindrance to balloon valvotomy or in cases where there is a complication of balloon valvotomy where the mitral valve cannot be opened and requires cardiopulmonary bypass (CPB).

Patients are placed on standard CPB with bicaval cannulation. The mitral valve can be exposed through a standard left atriotomy or via an interatrial septal approach. Any loose LA clot is removed with a Russian forceps and after this lamellated white thrombus is removed by first dissecting a plane between the yellow organized clot and bluish white left atrial endocardium. This plane is developed and the whole organized clot can be delamellated. It is particularly adherent toward the atrial appendage and it helps to intussuscept the atrial appendage to remove the clot in the left atrial appendage. A whole cast of the LA can be removed at times as shown in **Figure 5**.

After removing the clot, a thorough wash is given using an asepto syringe and any loose fragments are picked up. A wet

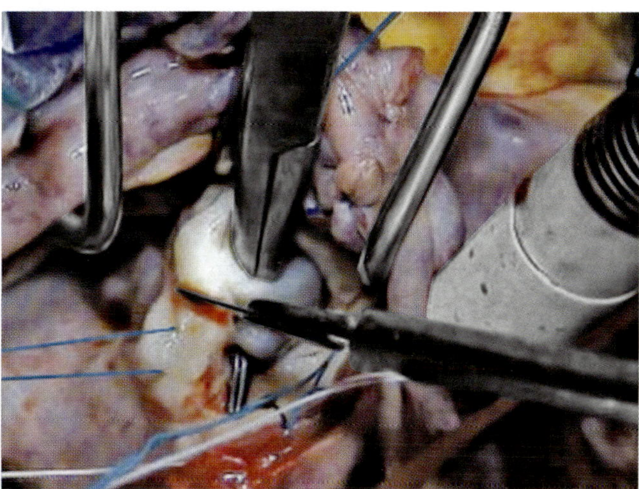

FIG. 5: Valvotomy in progress.

single layer gauze is swept repeatedly over the endocardium to pick up loose fibrin strands and the process is repeated till no strands or clots are seen sticking to the gauze. Subsequently, individual pulmonary veins are checked for clots and the anesthesiologist inflates the lungs while strong suction is applied to the pulmonary veins to pick up any clots.

After this the mitral valve is exposed by placing a tethering stitch at 6 o'clock position and the valve is inspected for feasibility of valvotomy. Commissural calcification will usually preclude commissurotomy. Two stay sutures are placed on the anterior and PML at the proposed site of valvotomy and are pulled across. This creates a furrow which marks the commissure. A stab incision is placed 3–4 mm from the annulus at the proposed extreme of the commissure which marks the limit of the valvotomy. Extending beyond this point will lead to commissural regurgitation and is to be avoided. Now the subvalvular apparatus is hooked with a Mixter forceps and inspected. Commissurotomy is now done by sharp incision of the furrow which indicates the line of fusion **(Fig. 5)**.

After the leaflet is divided further division of the subvalvular apparatus is done by splitting the fused chordae or sharing chordae between the anterior and posterior leaflet such that the chordae provide support. The fused papillary muscle chordal complex is divided down to the papillary muscle using a Potts scissor following which splitting of the papillary muscle is done by incising the papillary endocardium and the papillary muscle is teased to divide it. The same process is repeated at the posterolateral commissure. After this posterobasal chordae are divided. Fused chordae which form a wall of subvalvular tissue benefit from fenestration which is essentially cutting a triangular wedge of fused subvalvular tissue that frees up the posterior leaflet. After this saline insufflation is done using an asepto syringe and compression over the LV is done with a forceps to check for competence of the valve. Mild central leak in

the flaccid state is acceptable. Apical saline insufflation via a stab in the LV apex after opening the aortic root vent is an alternate technique. If perfect competence is not achieved repair techniques as described in mitral valve repair are carried out to ensure competence. The atrial appendage is either ligated externally or closed with a running suture from within ensuring that the circumflex artery which runs between the appendage and the mitral valve is not ensnared by a suture (by taking relatively superficial bites and close to the appendage in that area). A Maze procedure as described by us is conveniently done during rewarming, the atriotomy is closed, and the heart is deaired and the cross clamp is removed. After a period of rest, the heart is weaned off CPB. A post CPB transesophageal or epicardial echocardiogram is done to check the valve area, transmitral gradients, and presence of significant mitral regurgitation. These patients can be typically fast tracked and discharged. Patients who are in atrial fibrillation are anticoagulated. Rheumatic prophylaxis is mandatory for all patients as per the World Health Organization (WHO) guidelines.

Mitral Valve Repair

This is the procedure of choice in patients with repairable valves. Unfortunately, repair is considered difficult or impossible in mitral valve disease and with proper selection of cases especially in endemic areas, where the disease afflicts young adults; a large proportion of patients can undergo conservative surgery with good results.

Selection of cases with pliant noncalcified valves lend themselves to repair. Valve analysis has to be done preoperatively by the surgeon in conjunction with an echocardiographer. We do our "planning echocardiography" preoperatively by transthoracic echocardiography and intraoperative, transesophageal echocardiography (TEE) can be used to further delineate the anatomy. In many parts of the world, TEE access intraoperatively may be a problem and epicardial echocardiography can represent a good alternative. We have been able to find a good correlation between careful surgeon-guided preoperative transthoracic echocardiography for evaluating suitability of repair. It is very essential to have some echocardiographic control, be it transesophageal or epicardial intraoperatively.

The first step in assessment for repairing rheumatic valves is to evaluate the amount of tethering and plastering of the posterior leaflet and the amount of anterior leaflet available for repair. Significant leaflet tethering precludes or complicates the repair and we have described an infraposterior leaflet triangle (infra-PML triangle) and have found that patients who have an area <1 cm^2 are usually not repairable and are at risk for poor long-term results **(Fig. 6)**. Such patients very often require leaflet augmentation to allow repair to be done.

We then estimate the amount of prolapse and retraction of the leaflets. Interrogation in the parasternal long-axis (PLAX) echocardiogram view gives an estimate of the amount of noncoaptation. Relative noncoaptation above

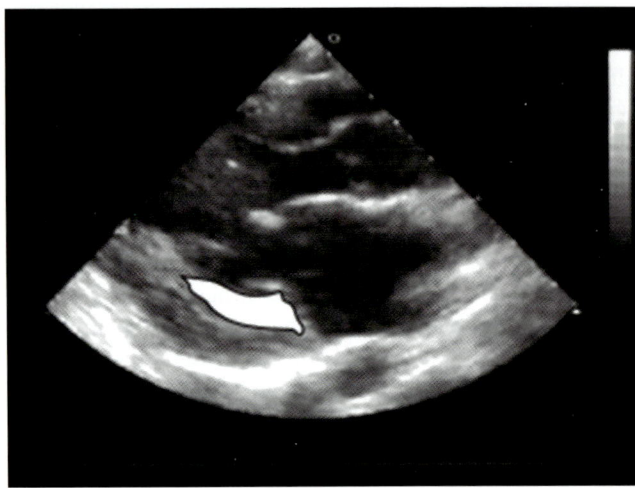

FIG. 6: The infraposterior mitral leaflet triangle.

5 mm in the PLAX view usually necessitates a chordal shortening procedure.

Absolute anterior leaflet length has been used by Sampath Kumar et al. for estimating operability. A height of the AML of <16 mm precludes repair or requires extensive AML patching.

Patients with rheumatic valves and calcification are poor candidates for repair. Only those cases which have focal deposits of excisable/debridable calcium are repairable. Caution has to be exercised in patients who have thick nonpliant leaflets where a repair may be achieved but with such severe dismobility that functional mitral stenosis occurs on dynamic testing post repair. Such patients may also have a "hinge problem", i.e., failure of leaflet folding and unfolding due to nonpliant leaflets that can result in mitral regurgitation.

Measurement of the annular circumference is another important indicator of operability. Patients with dilated annuli >10 cm (typically >15 cm) (or according to body surface area in very small children) usually lend themselves to repair as subsequent annuloplasty helps in achieving better leaflet apposition provided good leaflet level matching is achieved. Patients with a small annulus and significant mitral regurgitation in the absence of significant mitral stenosis usually have retracted and deficient leaflet tissue and thus a lesser tissue substrate for repairing. These patients may need extensive leaflet augmentation and often have very nonpliant valves that do not lend themselves to repair.

SURGERY

Surgery is done on conventional CPB with antegrade and retrograde cardioplegia. We use a modified St Thomas solution which is added to blood and we also use adenosine and esmolol as additives. Most surgeries are done at 28°C unless the patient has significant hepatorenal dysfunction when we perform the surgeries at 32°C. We use a pump flow index between 2.8 and 3.4 L/m^2. These cases may require long cross-clamp and CPB times so efficient myocardial protection and good whole body perfusion is mandatory to get good outcomes. We typically withdraw all angiotensin-converting enzyme inhibitors (ACEIs) and long-acting calcium-channel blockers and keep patients on oral nitrates/short-acting calcium-channel blockers and vasodilators. This prevents postoperative vasoplegia which can be particularly troublesome in patients who are taking these drugs. This becomes particularly important in patients with hepatic dysfunction where the use of perioperative vasoconstrictors to counteract vasoplegia may cause progressive hepatic dysfunction, fulminant hepatic failure, hepatorenal syndrome and death despite an anatomically successful repair. We prefer not to operate cases with active carditis as significant regurgitation may disappear with resolution of carditis. Repairing valves in patients with active carditis can also result in mitral regurgitation during the postoperative period due to ongoing carditis with the valve being damaged during the resolution of carditis.

A variety of approaches to the mitral valve have been described and we used to use the traditional standard left atriotomy after dissecting the Sondergaard's groove. This provides excellent exposure in most cases. With our policy of aggressive tricuspid repair and increased referral of smaller and smaller children with small atria as well as increased use of lower hemisternotomy we have shifted to a transseptal approach by means of a vertical atriotomy in the interatrial septal tissue without any extension to the roof of the LA. This avoids conduction problems that are associated with Guiradon's incision and is easy to close. Placement of everything stay sutures on the incision on the septum everts the anterior lip and provides excellent exposure. The key to better exposure is not to introduce large retractors and usually fine ventricular septal defect (VSD) retractors are all that is required.

After atriotomy exposure and good visualization of the mitral valve is of paramount importance. We usually tape the superior vena cava (SVC) and inferior vena cava (IVC) and hitch the snares up to bring up the IAS and mitral valve up. A suture placed at the 6 o'clock position brings up the mitral valve, though with an interatrial approach not much retraction is required.

Inspection of the mitral valve is done. The jet lesion due to the regurgitant jet is noted and gives an idea of the affected area (the leaflet opposite the jet). Commissural fusion and any calcification are noted. Graduated valve hooks are used to pick up the leaflets and areas of prolapse and retraction are noted. A good commissurotomy with splitting of the subvalvular apparatus is the first step and the aim is to convert mixed mitral disease into pure regurgitant disease **(Fig. 7)**. It is also required to release the hinge points of the mitral leaflets to allow good leaflet mobility.

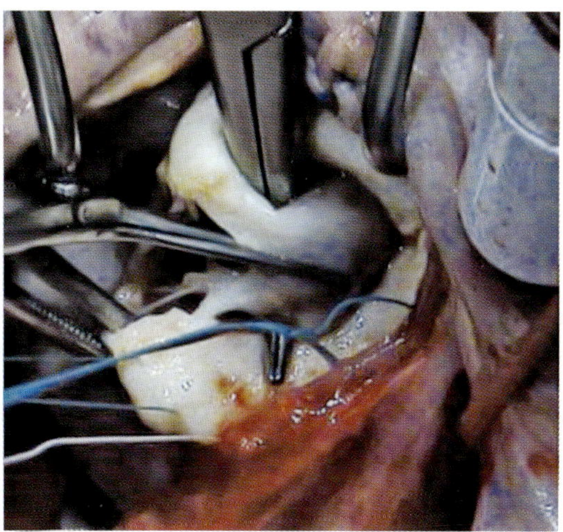

FIG. 7: Splitting of the fused subvalvular apparatus in progress.

After commissurotomy each segment of the mitral valve is lifted up and usually the noninvolved segment (area P1) is examined and compared with the immediately adjacent area. In rheumatic mitral valves, different segments may have different pathologies and it is critical to examine each segment (A123 and P123) and the plan of repair is drawn up and compared to the preoperative findings.

After evaluation of the segment after commissurotomy, the next step is to release and divide all the posterobasal chordae to release and increase the mobility of the posterior leaflet as posterior leaflet retraction is the most common pathology encountered. A fine nerve hook is used to pick up the posterobasal chordae which are identified by the fact that they are secondary chordae not attached to the free margin and are not commissural fan chordae. Division of these chordae causes increased leaflet mobility and if the relative noncoaptation between the AML and PML is <5 mm this usually allows sufficient PML mobility such that an additional annuloplasty allows good coaptation, after release of the posterobasal chordae. Valve hooks are now used to determine the amount of release and compare it with the AML to mark the degree of AML prolapse. After this, Goretex neochordae are placed in the AML. We use a method which we describe as combined chordoplasty where we do an initial trenchless chordal shortening using Goretex suture **(Fig. 8A)** and this shortens a whole bunch of chordae and the use of the same arms of the Goretex suture to create neochordae **(Fig. 8B)**. The neochordae act as a shock absorber and prevent elongation of the shortened chordae and we use a trenchless shortening of the chordae to prevent suture abrasion injury of the native chordae, both problems that are associated with the Carpentier trenched chordal shortening method. We have followed up patients for over a decade with this method with gratifying and stable results.

Reassessment at this stage is done using saline insufflations to check the level of coaptation. Usually we

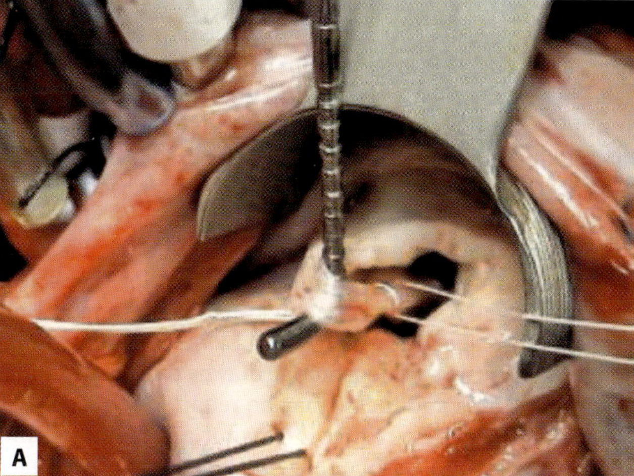

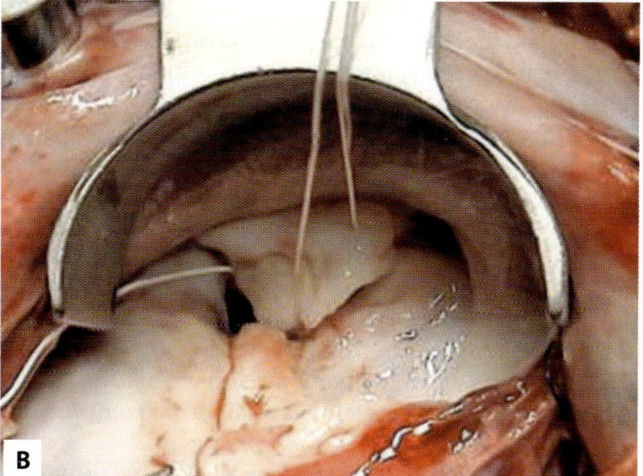

FIGS. 8A AND B: Goretex neochordae being implanted.

hold the posterior annulus and move it to one or another side creating a functional annuloplasty to give an assessment of the repair.

The AML is now sized and an annuloplasty is done. We have used a wide variety of methods. Patients coming with rheumatic disease are often poor and cannot afford commercial rings. We have used a variety of annuloplasty techniques like fashion ring started with a modified De Vega–Panneth Burr type of annuloplasty. We used epicardial pacing wires to give additional annular stability. We used Goretex and pericardial strips with success. We found that while these worked and allowed a large percentage of patients to be repaired, these nonrigid annuloplasty methods did not allow remodeling of the annulus and thus some patients could not be repaired as there would be buckling of the annulus creating a distorted "V" shape if the posterior leaflet was rigid and thus causing unacceptable regurgitation. In our quest for making a cheap indigenous ring, we fabricated annuloplasty rings using No. 5 sternal steel wires which are threaded into a 7-Fr double lumen central neck line and fashioned rings on formers/sizers which we cut out of a sheet of thick acrylic. The two ends of the wire neckline ring are sutured together after forming. We prepare various sizes and ETO to sterilize them for use. The former/sizers are used to size the ring by estimating the size of the AML. The annuloplasty sutures are placed around the annulus using interrupted 4/0 polyester sutures and passed through the ring and tied down. We have also used commercial rings and the indigenous rings work as well as the commercial rings.

After placing the annuloplasty ring reassessment is done of the repair using saline insufflations—either transvalve or transapically till saline comes out of the aortic root vent. Additional compression of the LV may be done. Final adjustment of Goretex neochordae may be done at this time. Additional "nips and tucks" may be required to lie closure of leaking pseudoclefts that form after annuloplasty and application of the Carpentiers magic stitch to eliminate commissural leaks. If the line of coaptation is parallel to the annulus and there is no leak or trivial central leak the repair is considered acceptable subject to reconfirmation by post-CPB echocardiography.

We then do concomitant procedures like Maze (we use an ordinary monopolar cautery Maze) and always exclude the left atrial appendage by either external ligation or internal suture. We usually ligate the appendage externally as soon as we go on CPB if there is no appendage clot as the prolapsing inverted appendage can be a troublesome distraction. If there is a left atrial appendage clot we evacuate it and suture the mouth of the left atrial appendage close. In large floppy atria we do a Kawazoe type of atrial placation to reduce bronchial, lung, and posterobasal left atrial compression **(Fig. 9)**.

It is very important to delamellate all left atrial thrombus including the white adherent clot when doing a left atrial thrombectomy especially if there is a left atrial body clot **(Figs. 10 and 11)**.

A thorough wash is given and the IAS is closed with care taken to see that the extreme ends are closed well with

pledgeted sutures as they are the sites of external bleeding if closed hastily. I usually do the tricuspid procedure on a beating heart prior to the mitral procedure along with the right-sided Maze lesions but if it has not been done then it can be conveniently done now.[4] Retrograde warm "hotshot" cardioplegia followed by normokalemic perfusion is done and by the time the right atrium is closed, the heart is usually beating in sinus rhythm. The heart is deaired and the cross clamp is removed. After adequate rest, the patient is weaned off CPB. Despite long cross clamp times, it is very necessary to have an efficient myocardial protection system so that the patients can be weaned off CPB with minimal inotropes. My usual rule is that if we cannot wean off CPB with >3 µg/kg/min of dopamine and dobutamine along with sodium nitroprusside in patients who were not in preoperative cardiogenic shock and not predisposed to vasoplegia then assiduous examination of the mitral valve

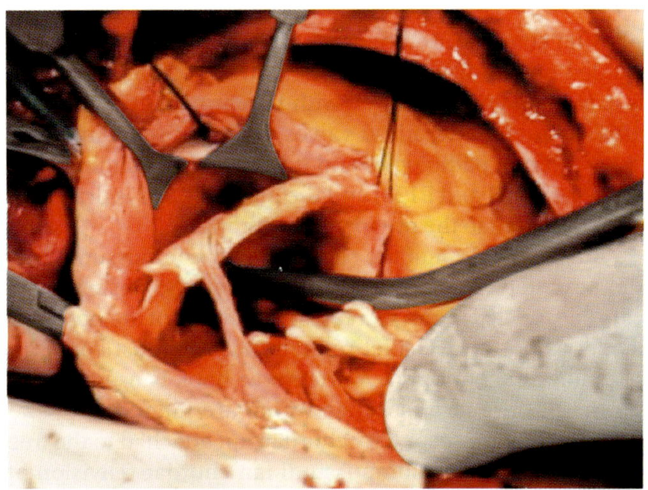

FIG. 10: Left atrial organized thrombus being delamellated.

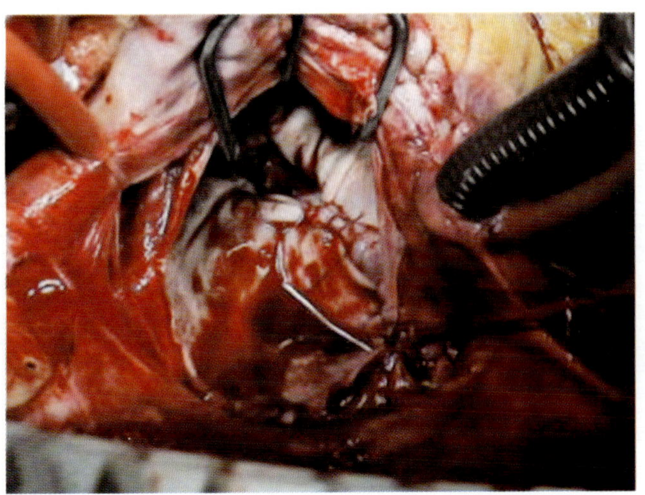

FIG. 9: Kawazoe placation of the left atrium in progress.

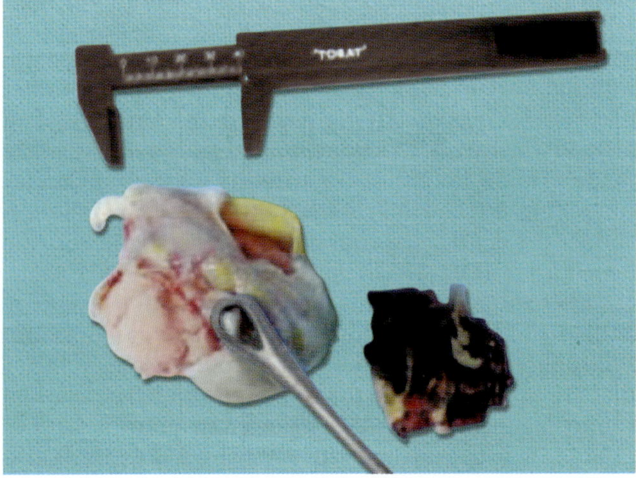

FIG. 11: Left atrial whole body clot being removed forming a left atrial cast.

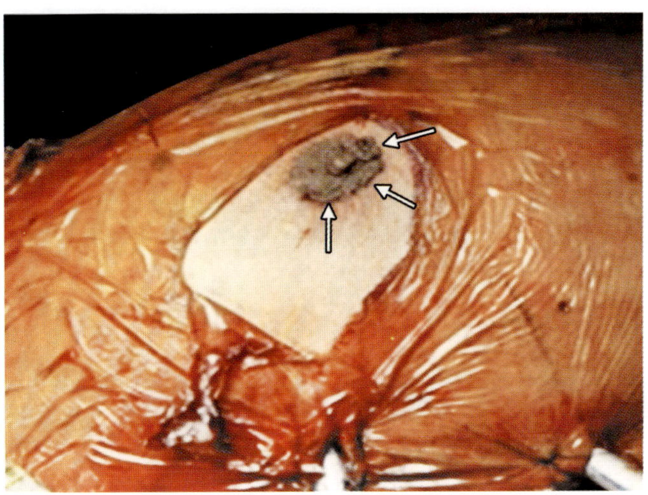

FIG. 12: Nonrobotic totally endoscopic mitral valve repair.

for unrecognized regurgitation must be done. Inappropriate tachycardia is also a warning sign of regurgitation.

In selected children and adults, various minimally invasive access methods ranging from hemisternotomy, minithoracotomy, totally endoscopic (nonrobotic or robotic) can be used **(Fig. 12)**. These offer a cosmetically appealing incision but as the incision becomes smaller the learning curve is sharper and technically becomes more complex with additional skill sets need to be employed.

The postweaning transesophageal or epicardial echocardiogram must be done after adequate preload augmentation and with a good pressure. If there is any doubt quantification may be done after increasing the afterload with boluses of phenylephrine or placing a partial clamp on the aorta to simulate increased afterload. Load independent indices like jet vena contracta and examination with appropriate hemodynamics are important to evaluate the regurgitation. Any significant regurgitation must be analyzed and if considered significant the patient must be put back on CPB and the valve must be repaired or replaced.

Patients are usually fast tracked and are extubated when hemodynamically stable and there is no bleeding. Patients usually are able to be discharged within the third or fifth day, if they have not had significant hepatorenal impairment. We usually start them on ACEIs and β-blockers and a diuretic. Patients who have had a Maze are put on amiodarone for 3 months. All patients need to be on antirheumatic prophylaxis and based on anecdotal observation of inadequate blood levels in the 3rd week we recommend all repairs to be on 2 weekly weight adjusted long-acting penicillin rather than 3 weekly penicillin as any bout of carditis will damage the repaired valve. We usually continue ACEI and β-blockers till the LV regresses and then withdraw the drug and re-evaluate for persistent LV regression. All patients get echocardiograms after 3 months of discharge and then 6 monthly evaluations to rule out carditis check the repair and also to ensure compliance of antirheumatic

prophylaxis, antibacterial endocarditis prophylaxis, and to reinforce the importance of continued evaluation.

Results

We initially had a repair rate of 70% in our initial 50 cases but with experience and case selection we are now able to repair 96% of our cases. Till October 2019, we have done 1,686 repairs of which 1,348 are rheumatic repairs. Till May 2010, we have done 896 repairs of which 712 are rheumatic repairs. The median follow-up at that time was 8.2 years. We have had eight deaths within 30 days in the whole cohort and these deaths were in patients who had preoperative hepatorenal dysfunction which progressed. We have gratifying results with combined chordoplasty and we studied 104 patients who received repairs with this method with a median follow-up of 8.9 years. In 104 cases, 92 were rheumatic in pathology and the remaining 12 were myxomatous valves. One patient died due to fungal endocarditis, four patients were reoperated (all rheumatic) and intraoperatively the recurrence was found to be due to progression of rheumatic activity with posterior leaflet retraction. The combined chordoplasty was intact and there was no recurrent anterior leaflet prolapse. Four cases have had progression of mitral regurgitation due to recurrent rheumatic activity and ECHOES have shown further PML scarring to be the etiology with no AML prolapse. None of the myxomatous valves had recurrent MR.

The most common pathology encountered is anterior leaflet prolapse (Carpentier type II + Posterior leaflet retraction (Carpentier type IIIa) with most cases having annular dilatation (Carpentier type I) as the pathology in over 90% of cases. Pure annular dilatation is seen in <1% of cases.

Stability of repair over time is an issue and on a follow-up of a median of 8.2 years (2010 data). It is expected that patients will come back for redo-surgery as previous reports show a 10-year freedom from resurgery of 70% at 10 years.

We have reoperated now 32 patients who have had rheumatic repair after the initial 30 days postsurgery. In all these cases, the finding on table has been progression of rheumatic disease with retraction of P3 segment which I call the area of sorrow of rheumatic mitral disease. The median time of resurgery has been 4.8 years. 10 out of 12 patients had recurrent carditis and two patients had moderate mitral regurgitation at the post discharge ECHO but it was accepted as both were small children. Most patients with recurrent mitral regurgitation had their valves replaced with a mechanical valve. Selected patients have undergone re-repair. Depending on the quality of the leaflets **(Fig. 13)**.

Patients with irreparable mitral valve disease can undergo mitral valve replacement with a bioprosthetic or mechanical valve after due discussion with the patient. We have done five cases of autopericardial implantation for calcific mitral valve disease as described by Deac et al. **(Fig. 14)**.

Mechanical valve replacement poses a unique problem in young rheumatics as they are growing children and young

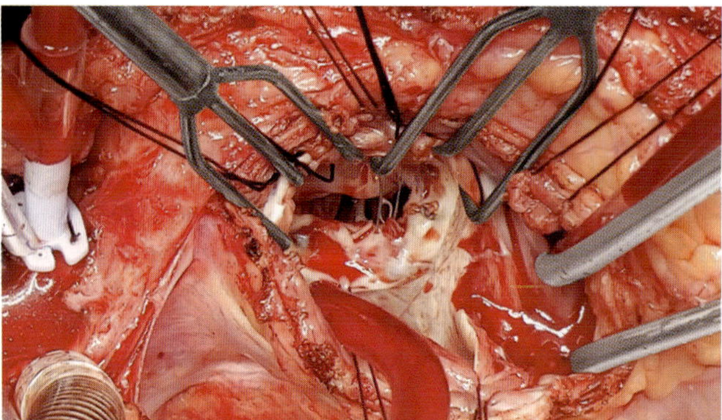

FIG. 13: Redo mitral valve surgery for a patient who had mitral valve repair done 18 years ago and now requiring replacement. Not the shrunken anterior mitral valve leaflet and retracted P3 segment of the mitral valve rendering the valve irreparable a second time.

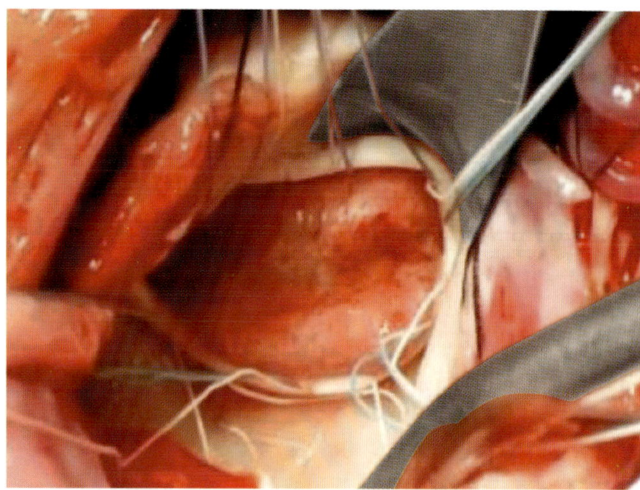

FIG. 14: Autopericardial valve with an indigenous ring.

adults and females in the child-bearing age. Rapid calcium turnover causes dismal longevity of bioprosthetic valves. Implantation of a valve in a small child can be especially problematic and at times an aortic valve in reverse position may have to be used. Standard methods of implantation are used and we try to do total chordal preservation or neochordal placement in all patients. We use a standard everting horizontal mattress suture technique and we bivalve the AML and PML and suture them to the annulus. If the leaflets are bulky we trim them down to essential chords and if that is not possible we place polybutylate ester (Ticron/Ethibond) neochords which function very well. Careful debridement of calcium is very important to prevent paravalvular leaks. It is better to place sutures and carefully around residual chunks of calcium rather than through them to prevent fracturing of the calcium leading to paravalvular leaks.

Tricuspid Valve Disease

We have now been very aggressive in managing tricuspid valve disease and in adult patients do not hesitate to place a ring in patients with secondary tricuspid vale disease if the annulus is dilated above 27 mm/m^2. Patients who have concomitant tricuspid stenosis require a valvotomy followed by ring implantation. Patients with organic tricuspid disease with a small annulus may require augmentation of the anterior mitral valve leaflet with autologous pericardium. Truly destroyed valves may require tricuspid valve replacement. These procedures are usually done on CPB on beating heart either initially (our preference) along with the right-sided Maze procedure as they commonly have atrial fibrillation) or conveniently after cross clamp removal and during rewarming.

Care should be taken while implanting rings to avoid the atrioventricular node and bundle of His during implantation of rings/valves. This can be avoided by taking sutures on the septal leaflet of the tricuspid valve during ring implantation.

In children who are growing, a Kay's annuloplasty can be placed if a ring equivalent to a 26 size Carpentier Edwards ring cannot be implanted. This allows annular growth and avoids early repeat surgery for changing a ring as the child grows.

Aortic Valve Surgery

Repairs in aortic valves have not been reproducible consistently with good long-term results. Only a small percentage lends themselves to repair and we have used cuspal thinning, cuspal extension with pericardium, and aortic valve repair in 22 patients. Three patients developed fungal endocarditis after 9 months to 2 years after surgery and all related to a bout of diarrhea were IV fluid administration was given. Probable fungal contamination of IV fluid source may be a possibility. All three patients died. Of the remaining we have had to replace three patients at a median of 5 years for recurrent regurgitation. We currently attempt repair in the aortic valve only in small children with a favorable anatomy to delay valve replacement so that a larger valve can be placed later with somatic growth.

Aortic valve replacement is done with standard techniques. Careful debridement of the annulus and suprannular placement of a mechanical or bioprosthetic valve is to be done. Supra-annular placement with nonpledgeted mattress sutures taken from ventricle to aortic side allows placement of a larger prosthesis. Careful and complete leaflet excision is required to prevent leaflet impingement of any tissue in the LV outflow tract.

The Ross operation is not a good option in young rheumatics as they develop recurrent carditis and damage of the neoaortic valve.

We are increasingly using autopericardial reconstruction based on the tenets elucidated by Ozaki et al. from 2016.[5,6] We had noted favorable hemodynamics in the initial cases compared to mechanical valve replacement and subsequently have used this as an attractive option. Out of 95

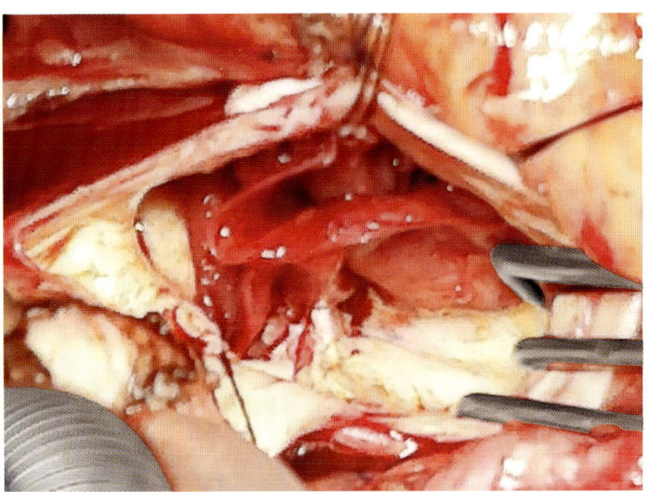

FIG. 15: Autopericardial aortic valve reconstruction.

patients done till November 2020 we have done 54 rheumatic cases of which 50 had concomitant mitral valve repair done **(Fig. 15)**. The long-term durability of this operation in younger rheumatic cohort is yet to be determined but so far appear promising. We have noted that patients with a preoperative Z value of LVIDd or LVIDs above +7 are to be avoided as they were associated with 100% mortality either perioperatively or within the first year and should be considered for mechanical assist or transplant pathway.

Patients with mechanical valve replacement need to be on regular follow-up for anticoagulation and this can be also troublesome as in the mitral valve with a thrombo-hemorrhagic rate of around 2% in patients with good international normalized ratio (INR)/prothrombin time (PT) monitoring and can practically go up to 20% when patients have irregular monitoring.

Anticoagulation after Mechanical Valve Replacement

Anticoagulation after mechanical valve replacement is mandatory. Patients may be anticoagulated after bioprosthetic valves for 6 weeks to 3 months but many surgeons do not anticoagulate and prefer to keep the patient on aspirin with or without clopidogrel in patients in sinus rhythm with equally good results. We do not anticoagulate patients with bioprosthetic valves in sinus rhythm and administer antiplatelet drugs.

Patients with mechanical valves need to have regular monitoring of the prothrombin time standardized against a standard thromboplastin, the INR. We usually ask patients to get monthly INRs. The highest thrombohemorrhagic events occur in the first year. Patients with aortic valves and mitral valves with sinus rhythm, newer generation prostheses and mitral valve replacements with no spontaneous echogenic contrast (SEC) in the LA can be anticoagulated with an INR between 2.2 and 3.5 and patients with older generation mitral prostheses, atrial fibrillation and SEC on echocardiography, and previous valve thrombosis should require a higher level anticoagulation with an INR maintained between 3.5 and 4.5. Antiplatelet therapy may be added selectively. There have been attempts to use antiplatelets exclusively with disastrous results though reports of exclusive antiplatelet therapy with only aspirin with the On-X valve seem to be promising.

Patients have to be warned about signs of thrombohemorrhagic complications. They need to be warned about potential drug interactions especially with respect to over the counter drugs like nonsteroidal anti-inflammatory drugs (NSAIDs), contraceptive drugs, antiepileptic drugs, and antituberculosis medications. Patients have to also be explained about importance of regular drug therapy, keeping adequate stock of anticoagulant drugs at home and regular follow-up. A common misconception and erroneous advice is regarding eating green leafy vegetables and tomatoes. It needs over 500 g of green leafy vegetables/tomatoes to alter the INR so moderate consumption of these food items can be allowed and prevents development of unintended anemia and malnutrition.

Bacterial endocarditis prophylaxis has to be given to all patients who have undergone valve repair and valve replacement who are undergoing any procedure breaking the integrity of the skin and mucosal barrier as per the latest WHO guidelines.

Rheumatic heart disease is an unfortunate affliction which attacks the poorest patients who can least afford advanced medical therapies and till the root cause of social deprivation and poverty is eliminated such cases are wedded to the physician. Patients with these diseases have a less than normal lifespan and are committed to multiple interventions and surgeries in their lifetime.

CONCLUSION

Rheumatic heart disease is an avoidable affliction that unfortunately causes significant morbidity and mortality in young and poor population. Aggressive prevention programs should be applied to prevent this scourge. Efficient medical management and appropriate surgery can significantly alleviate the suffering of these patients. Unfortunately once afflicted by rheumatic disease the patients need life long monitoring and multiple procedures that need to be timed appropriately to extend life and improve the quality of life.

REFERENCES

1. Duran CM, Gometza B, Saad E. Valve repair in rheumatic mitral disease: An unsolved problem. J Card Surg. 1994;9(Suppl 2): 282-5.

2. Sampath AK, Dhareshwar J. Mitral Valve repair in RHD. J Card Sur. 2004;19(4):30-7.

3. Chauvaud S, Fuzellier JF, Berrebi A, Deloche A, Fabiani JN, Carpentier A. Long-term (29 years) results of reconstructive surgery in rheumatic mitral valve insufficiency. Circulation. 2001;104(suppl 1):I12-5.

4. Simha P, Bhat PS, Prabhudeva N. The Electrocautery Maze—How I Do It. Heart Surg Forum. 2001;4(4):340-5; discussion 344-5.

5. Vijayan J, Lachma RN, Rao PSM, Bhat AS. Autologous pericardial aortic valve reconstruction: early results and comparison with mechanical valve replacement. Indian J Thorac Cardiovasc Surg. 2020;36(3):186-92.

6. Ozaki S, Kawase I, Yamashita H, Uchida S, Nozawa Y, Takatoh M, et al. A total of 404 cases of aortic valve reconstruction with glutaraldehyde-treated autologous pericardium. J Thorac Cardiovasc Surg. 2014;147:301-6.

22

Rheumatic Fever, Rheumatic Heart Disease Registry, and Control Program

IB Vijayalakshmi

> *"Education never ends, Watson. It is a series of lessons with the greatest for the last."*
>
> **—Arthur Conan Doyle** (1856–1930)
> (British Crime Novelist)

INTRODUCTION

It is estimated that 15.6 million people are affected worldwide by acute rheumatic fever (ARF) and 3 lakhs out of 5 lakhs individuals that acquire ARF every year go on to develop rheumatic heart disease (RHD). ARF follows 0.3–3% of cases of group A β-hemolytic streptococcal (GABHS) pharyngitis. As many as 39% of persons with ARF may develop varying degrees of pancarditis associated with valve insufficiency, heart failure, and even death. 3 million people have chronic heart failure requiring repeated hospitalization.[1,2] A large proportion would have valvular heart disease requiring cardiac surgery in the next 5–10 years. The majority of the affected populations are children in the school-aged group in low and middle socioeconomic groups.[3] There are estimated 330,000 deaths annually and many survivors are left with disabilities with no access to the required medical and surgical care.[4-6] According to the World Health Organization (WHO) bulletin of 1981, >50% of ARF/RHD detected in surveys and health check-up camps are unaware of their disease and >70% do not receive secondary prophylaxis regularly.[7]

BACKGROUND OF THE PROBLEM AND ITS PUBLIC HEALTH IMPORTANCE

In developing countries, rheumatic fever is endemic and remains one of the major causes of cardiovascular disease, accounting for nearly 25–45% of the cases. It is a major cause of mortality among subjects under 50 years of age and has been identified as one of the major problems in large cities of the third world countries by the WHO. The annual incidence of rheumatic fever is 100–200 times greater than that observed in developed countries and fluctuates between 100 and 200 per 100,000 children of school age (from 5 years to 17 or 18 years depending on the study). The prevalence of RHD per 1,000 children has been reported as follows: Egypt—10, Thailand—1.2–2.1, India—6–12, Pakistan—1.8–11, Sri Lanka—100–150 with a very high prevalence in China, Taiwan, French and American Polynesia, South Africa, and among the Maori population in New Zealand.

India is in the phase of "epidemiological transition". On one hand, there is a substantial burden due to RHD, on the other hand resources are scarce to treat and prevent the disease. More than 20,382 cases of RHD (10% of total admission) were admitted at Sri Jayadeva Institute of Cardiovascular Sciences and Research in Bengaluru (1998–2010). The approximate cost of treatment was more than ₹100 million ($2,272,727) in the last 12 years. In cardiology department from April 1994 to August 2010, more than 14,560 cases percutaneous transluminar balloon commissurotomy (PTMC) were done, out of which 6,550 cases were below the age of 20 years and the youngest patient was 6 years old. Despite the subsidized rates the cost for management of mitral stenosis has been ₹30,250,000 ($6,875,000) and valve replacement has cost ₹80 million ($1,818,181) over the last few years in our hospital alone. Not only the cost of treatment is phenomenal, the morbidity and mortality is also enormous.

The reasons for ARF and RHD remaining a burning problem are confusion in diagnosis, confusion in management, poor socioeconomic conditions, lack of hygiene and awareness, lack of prophylaxis, not utilizing the modern tool like echocardiography, lack of vaccine and most importantly there is no "National Rheumatic Fever Control Program" in our country.

The incidence and prevalence of RHD has declined when primary and secondary prevention programs have been implemented.[8,9] Hence, it is high time we have a registry of rheumatic fever and RHD and secondary prevention program in our country. Secondary prevention is the mainstay to the prevention of ARF and RHD in most developing countries. In spite of the problems of compliance encountered with regular long-term antibiotic prophylaxis, secondary prevention programs have been feasible, relatively inexpensive, and cost effective in developing countries.[8-11] Moreover, they can be implemented through the existing healthcare services without major additional costs.[12,13]

The prevention program should employ strategies for secondary prevention of ARF and RHD through existing primary healthcare structures (Health and Family Welfare Department) with the participation of the Indian Council of Medical Research (ICMR) and medical colleges throughout the country.

The strategies include:
- Health education targeted to parents, children, and teachers as well as medical and nonmedical healthcare providers with the aim of increasing awareness and knowledge of the disease.
- Baseline survey and community screening of the selected regions to map the extent of the problem by primary healthcare units (PHU), primary healthcare centers (PHC), and district hospitals.
- Facilitating the incorporation of strategies for implementing secondary prophylaxis into existing healthcare systems by the director of health services.
- Establishing a workable surveillance system for ARF/RHD in each district and medical colleges.

Program Planning

The program planned should be implemented in three phases in selected regions. The first phase should include a prevalence survey in urban and rural demonstration areas of selected regions by the medical students and the house surgeons of medical colleges and start the ARF and RHD registry. This is in addition to the establishment of simple clinic registers to facilitate follow-up and secondary prophylaxis. The proven strategies in the control of ARF should be adapted to wider regions in the second phase. Finally, a national spread of the program must be done for the third phase as the "National ARF and RHD control program".

Socioeconomic Implications

Environmental and socioeconomic factors linked to low income, poverty, overcrowding, poor housing conditions, poor nutritional states, and inadequate health services have a very important influence in its occurrence and severity. Furthermore, medical treatment is not curative and usually PTMC or surgical care of RHD becomes necessary. In India, it is difficult to estimate the cost of care for one RHD patient because either they get treatment in government hospitals, where the treatment is free, or go to corporate hospitals with some hope and pay through the nose by selling their meager property and land up in a hopeless state. Hence, along with the national poverty elevation programs, maintaining the hygiene, especially oral hygiene in poor should be included and implemented.

Constraints to Prevention Programs at Country Level

Lack of information and training of health personnel, low level of health education among patients, parents, population at risk (school age children who are not normally included in most child health projects). The dangers of droplet infection should be taught. The importance of covering the nose and mouth while sneezing and coughing and the repeated hand wash should be explained to the poor and illiterates. Though these are very simple measures they will surely have a great impact in preventing the spread of sore throat. Teaching the healthy habits does not cost but it requires the will on the part of health personnel.

Objectives of ARF and RHD Secondary Prevention Program

Overall objective is to reduce the number of recurrent attacks of ARF, decrease the incidence and the severity of heart valve damage, reduce the number of young people requiring PTMC and surgery, so that there is reduction in the healthcare expenditure for RHD and ultimately to reduce number of deaths.
- *Phase I objective*: To estimate the prevalence of the disease in a defined population in an urban and rural setting.
- *Phase II objective*: To plan and develop the ARF and RHD secondary prevention pilot program in defined areas.
- *Phase III objective*: To extend the program in other defined areas or nationwide as a national policy.

▉ PROGRAM STRATEGIES

The programs start in a demonstration area and is later extended depending on the availability of resources with due consideration of issues of sustainability.

The main activities of the program should consist of the following:

- Program planning (coordination and contact meeting with key responsible persons)
- Survey to estimate prevalence in urban and rural area
- Capacity assessment of the health facilities within the program area with respect to management of ARF.
- Integration of ARF/RHD secondary prevention activities integrated into the existing health and school system including:
  - Personnel training (primary care physicians, nurses, community healthworkers, and teachers)
  - Case detection—active and passive recruitment
  - Supply of benzathine penicillin (or alternative oral drugs for patients with penicillin allergy) for the pilot project
  - Administration of benzathine penicillin once in 2–3 weeks
  - Follow-up of patients with ARF/RHD regularly
- Epidemiological surveillance through maintenance of ARF and RHD registries
- Health education including school-based health education, development of health education material, and mass media input in local languages.
- Patient's self-care education (for children 5–15-year-old) and parents' education

Phase I

Objective: To estimate the prevalence of the disease in a defined population in an urban and rural setting. Planning and survey should be completed in 12 weeks' time.

The following activity should be conducted in phase I:

- Preprogram planning
- *Coordination*: Meeting with national central officials and focal person. Meeting at local level with project personnel, country managers, community heads, opinion of leaders and community associations, recruitment of a program manager for each model.
- *Resource and logistic design.*
- Training of project personnel through seminars, CMEs, and satellite teaching programs wherever connectivity is available.
- Field work should include survey, validation of screening by medical team, capacity assessment of the PHC where the pilot project will be implemented.
- Data management activities and project evaluation
- Presentation and dissemination of the results at the central office

Field work: Timeline—8 weeks.

Household Survey

The survey should be performed in the urban and rural settings to estimate the prevalence of ARF and RHD in different areas of the same country. The sample size, based upon estimated prevalence of approximately 5 and 10 per 1,000 in rural and urban areas respectively and considering a confidence interval of 95%, will be 4,000 children for the rural setting and 2,000 children for the suburban setting. The household survey, based on interview and quick cardiac auscultation, should be conducted by community healthworkers after interview and auscultation training.

Sampling procedures: Clusters of households methodology should be used and all children in the family must be interviewed.

Interview procedures: Children must be interviewed in a friendly way in the presence of a parent or relative.

Follow-up action: Children with a positive answer for the history of sore throat, joint pain, chest pain, palpitation, breathlessness and/or any murmur should be referred to the higher medical center for confirmation of diagnosis. The child should be given a form reporting the date and center to visit for the medical examination, probably linked with *Suvarna Aarogya Chetana* school program in which crores of school-going children are screened.

(Annexure I: Rheumatic Fever/Rheumatic Heart Disease Community Survey Questionnaire)

Medical Examination

The medical examination should validate the survey results and confirm the diagnosis of ARF/RHD. It should be performed by a qualified medical practitioner. The medical examination should consist of detailed history, clinical examination including cardiac auscultation, laboratory investigation, and detailed echocardiography should be done for each child to evaluate the condition completely. Protocol proforma containing all the detailed information should be completed.

The ARF/RHD register collecting the standardized registration forms for all patients detected through the community screening will be started at the health center directly after confirmation of diagnosis by medical examination.

Data Management Activities

- *Data entry*: Depending upon setting characteristic, the record officer or record assistant at the local government health department can perform it. Alternatively, all questionnaires from the community survey and the medical examination forms can be directly sent to headquarters (HQ).
- *Data analysis*: At headquarters.

Advocacy and Community Participation

The survey data will provide prevalence figure of ARF and RHD in suburban and rural areas. A meeting will be held after completion of the study to present the result of the survey and advocate the program.

The following stakeholders should be invited:
- Representative from the Ministry of Health
- Representative from the Ministry of Education
- District medical representatives
- Teacher representatives
- Community representatives (National Women Association and Sports Association)
- Religious leaders
- Opinion leaders
- Media representative

Human Resources Assessment

- Number of staff by category
- Type of service (inpatient/outpatient)
- *For outpatient clinic*: Types of clinics and day
- Staff training activities (refer to the local government health department)
- Health education activities

Drugs

- Benzathine and phenoxymethyl penicillin availability (stock, expiration date, and last replenishment date)
- Penicillin average use per month (injections tablets)
- Disposable syringe availability
- Penicillin procurement procedure
- Penicillin storage
- Sulfadiazine, amoxicillin, and cephalosporin availability
- Erythromycin availability

Additional Services

- Availability of emergency trolley with appropriate drugs to treat anaphylaxis
- Knowledge and competence of staff to treat anaphylaxis

Record System

- Presence of outpatients attendance record
- Number of people attending the PHC in the last 3 months
- Number of children in the 5–15 years age group
- Number of children with ARF/RHD in the last year
- Number of children performing ARF/RHD secondary prophylaxis

Follow-up Procedures

Procedures/Process available for follow-up of patients diagnosed as having ARF/RHD.

Evaluation

- *Training evaluation*: Pre- and post-training evaluation
- Testing and validation of screening instruments chi square (χ^2 test at 95% CI) matching analysis of field diagnosis matched with doctor diagnosis of the cases sent to the clinic.
- *Response rate*: Percentage of patients attending clinic when referred by field workers.

- *Procedural evaluation*: Identification of anticipated problems.

Phase II: Pilot Project

Objective: Demonstration of project in a defined area to develop and test locally appropriate methods and procedure for the implementation of the program. According to the prevalence data obtained from the survey, a pilot project should start incorporating rural and urban areas. The project should be implemented in a local primary healthcare center. A similar primary healthcare center where prevention of rheumatic fever should continue according to the local standards should serve as control. The primary healthcare center selected should fix a day to receive patients for secondary prophylaxis.

Case Finding Identification of Active and Inactive Cases of ARF/RHD

- Positive cases resulting from the household survey and medical examination
- Screening in school through teachers
- Hospital retrospective case surveys in the hospital in the project area
- Continuing detection of any ARF/RHD patients from the local hospital, polyclinic or any other sources available, to be referred to the central/local register or referral center
- Advertisement of the program with district doctors and district health centers
- Advocacy of the program at the local community level
- Advocacy of the program in schools

Registration

All patients detected through passive recruitment will be entered in the ARF and RHD register started in phase I. A central register should be started in a main hospital collecting all active and passive recruitment cases.

Logistics

The pilot project should be implemented in the primary health centers assessed during phase I. The children with RF and RHD resulting from the community screening and passive recruitment should be directly enrolled in the secondary prophylaxis program. Facilities for secondary prevention should be distributed in such a way that accessibility will not be a problem.

The nurse should start collecting the standardized forms to send at central RF and RHD register. She/He will need to follow-up and provide the register with the requested information. A follow-up and reminder card should be given to the patient. The specifically trained nurse at a selected close health center should then continue the program. The children who underwent the first injection of penicillin should then be transferred to this center to continue secondary prophylaxis.

Drug procurement: Penicillin will be provided for the pilot program. The syringe should be either provided by the center or brought personally by the patient. Only disposable syringe should be used. Sulfadiazine or erythromycin should be provided only for patients allergic to penicillin.

Dropouts management: School teachers should be informed about the children undergoing secondary prophylaxis and shall have a calendar with injections schedule. They should follow up with the children. The nurse or the community health worker should visit the family of children missing more than two appointments.

Monitoring

The program should be monthly monitored by the program manager. Each participating center should complete a monitoring proforma each month which shall be submitted monthly to the program manager. A quarterly summary shall then be sent to HQ. A final report should be requested for each participating center at the end of the year.

Evaluation

The program will be evaluated by the national program manager and HQ at the end of 1 year. At the end of phase I, chief coordinator should carry out a site visit to the center to evaluate progress, outcomes, and discuss with health authorities, the program manager and the program advisory committee, and to train personnel. During the site visit, the expert shall also evaluate methods of work, relationship between participating units, cost analysis, effectiveness, and available epidemiological trends.

The evaluation will be performed according to the procedure as follows:

Patient-directed Evaluation
- Registered patient rate (all identified cases during the active and passive recruitment)
- Patients enrolled rate (all patients starting secondary prophylaxis)
- Drop out rate (patients stopping secondary prophylaxis)
- Recurrence rates
- Adverse reaction and rate (strictly not related to evaluation but important to know)

Facilities-directed Evaluation
- Failed injection rate
- Drop out tracing indicators
- Drug replenishment procedure
- Drugs storage

It is very important to have facility for adequate monitoring of anticoagulation therapy in patients with atrial fibrillation and/or mechanical prosthetic valves. A single and centralized (preferably computerized) ARF/RHD register for each program should be established. Each patient will receive a smart card which will serve as ID as well as source for medical information collection and dissemination **(Fig. 1)**. All the clinics will receive card reader. The data obtained will be transmitted to a central server as well as any other data base available in the Health Care System. In addition to the trained doctors or healthcare workers, we will also develop a web based 24 × 7 consulting service.

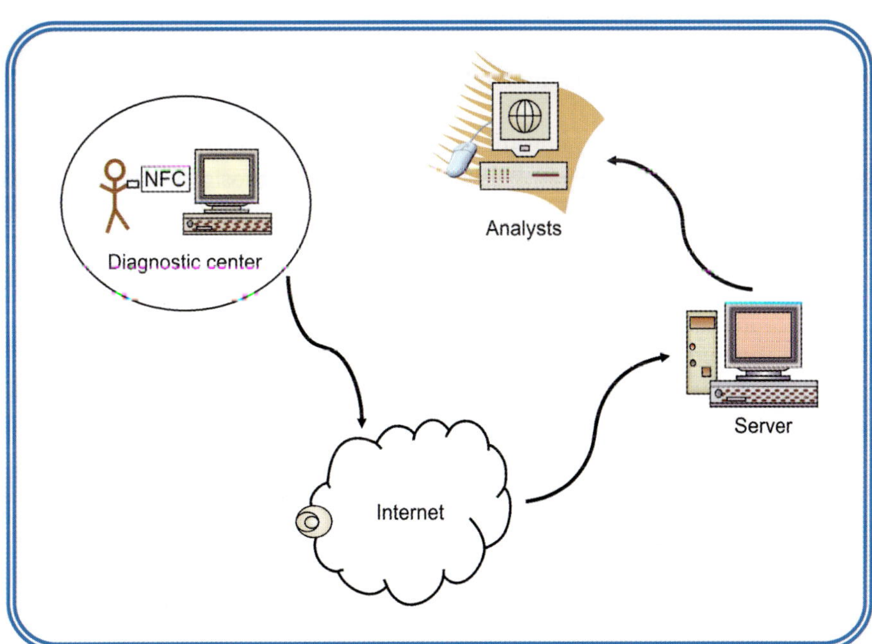

FIG. 1: The working system of smart card and IT-based diagnostic data collection, storage, and retrieval of the same by the analysts.

Phase III: National Program

Timeline: 5 years

Application of Vijaya's Echocardiography Criteria for Changing the Epidemiological Face of Rheumatic Fever and Rheumatic Heart Disease

Among the various manifestations of ARF, carditis is the only one that can cause death during the acute stage of the disease or may lead to long-term morbidity and mortality. It is very pertinent to realize that ECHO can assist in:

- Precise and early diagnosis of ARF and carditis, as timely management can make the heart normal in 35–40% of cases of ARF and in remaining children the secondary prophylaxis can prevent the recrudescence of rheumatic activity.
- Echocardiography can prevent overdiagnosis of carditis by depending on the traditional clinical auscultatory findings, which could be fallacious and lead to unnecessary drugging and psychological impact on the children and their family.
- Regular check-up with noninvasive ECHO can help to evaluate of status of RHD and decide for elective balloon valvuloplasty for mitral stenosis (PTMC) and timely decision for valve repair/replacement, which can reduce the morbidity and mortality before the patient develops congestive cardiac failure.

Despite knowing the importance of echocardiography several authors have raised questions like:

- Can echocardiography reliably differentiate valve regurgitation (physiological) from minor degree of pathological valvular regurgitation?
- Can the detection of echocarditis (subclinical) translate into clinical benefit?
- Would the detection of subclinical carditis alter the management strategy?
- If management is not altered, should the finding of echocardiographic subclinical carditis help in better assessment of prognosis and prophylaxis?
- If echocardiography is not likely to significantly alter either acute management or prognostication, then should it influence the long-term prophylaxis strategy?
- Should echocarditis be accepted as a major manifestation in the Jones criteria in the absence of clinical evidence of carditis?

Background

Adherence to revised Jones criteria may lead to under diagnosis among the Indian children with polyarthralgia and overdiagnosis in clinically diagnosed carditis. To avoid morbidity and mortality and heavy expenditure incurred on sophisticated treatment with balloon or valve replacement by the government and family, an early precise diagnosis of ARF and secondary prophylaxis is very important and ECHO is a very useful investigation in this direction. With this background two prospective pilot studies were conducted.

Phase I study done: 452 children with clinically diagnosed ARF were studied by ECHO for the pilot project, "Role of echocardiography in diagnosing carditis in setting of ARF".[14] This study helped us to evolve the ECHO criteria.

The efficacy of thus evolved Vijaya's criteria was studied in the second study.

Phase II study done: Prospective study of 333 consecutive cases titled, "Efficacy of echocardiographic criteria for diagnosis of carditis in ARF".[15]

Phase III to be done: The proposed project "Application of Vijaya's ECHO criteria for changing the epidemiological face of rheumatic fever and RHD".

The aim of this project is to do ECHO in all the cases of clinically suspected ARF and RHD and conduct free heart check-up camps in endemic areas and other districts, so that ECHO is done at the doorstep of the patients free of cost to the poor patients who fail to reach the hospital in order to assess:

- Role of Vijaya's ECHO criteria in precise and early diagnosis of carditis/valvulitis
- The need to include ECHO criteria in Jones criteria
- The regression or progression of rheumatic carditis, valvulitis, and valvular regurgitation on follow-up
- The evolution of RHD
- Timely detection and need for interventions such as balloon valvuloplasty, valve repair, or replacement

Methods

Every suspected case of ARF and RHD will be thoroughly examined clinically. The laboratory investigations would be done by qualified pediatricians. Those who fit into Jones criteria are taken into Study Group A and those who do not fit into the criteria are taken into the Control Group B. All cases will undergo echocardiographic examination M-mode and 2D echocardiography thoroughly in all views by experienced and qualified sonographers without knowing the clinical details and diagnosis (blinded) and the details of ECHO will be filled in proforma (enclosed as Annexure II).

The ECHO score to be calculated according to Vijaya's criteria as given in **Table 1**. Any patient getting ≥ 6 scores will be taken as ECHO positive.

M-mode for:
- Dimensions of left atrium (LA), aorta (AO), and their ratio (LA:AO)
- Left ventricular (LV) dimension in diastole and systole.

Two-dimensional echocardiography:
- Beaded appearance of valves [especially anterior mitral leaflet (AML)]
- Thickness of the valves (<3 mm: normal; >4 mm: thickened)
- Mitral valve prolapse (MVP)
- Mobility of the valves
- Thickening of submitral structures (increased echo-genicity)

TABLE 1: Echo features and their scores.

Echo features	Score
MV and AV thickness > 4 mm	2
Increased echogenicity of submitral structures	2
Rheumatic nodules (beaded appearance)	2
Mitral valve prolapse (MVP)/AVP/TVP	2
MV regurgitation/AVR/TVR	2
Reduced mobility of valves	2
Chordal tear	2
Pericardial effusion	2
Total score	**16**

(AV: aortic valve; AVP: aortic valve prolapse; AVR: aortic valve regurgitation; MV: mitral valve; TVP: tricuspid valve prolapse; TVR: tricuspid valve regurgitation)

- Chordal tear
- Pericardial effusion
- End-diastolic volume (EDV) and end-systolic volume (ESV) and ejection fraction (EF%)

The echocardiographic features and diagnosis of sonographers are fed back to the pediatricians for proper treatment but not told (blinded) to senior pediatric cardiologist who will go through all the echocardiography recordings individually and record their findings independently (for interoperator variability). The final analysis of this triple blind study will be done at the end of the year. Vijaya's criteria of scoring of 6 or more to make the echocardiographic diagnosis will be strictly applied.

(Annexure III: Protocol for detailed entry at the tertiary center where echocardiography facility with trained sonographer is available)

Significance: Scientific evidence about effectiveness and efficiency of echocardiography in ARF and RHD, possibly making it cost effective, may have tremendous impact on reducing the human suffering in children and young adults in developing countries. The results may help in evolving risk stratification and early intervention, thus reducing morbidity and mortality, unnecessary financial burden on the patient in particular and the government in general. Because the saying, "Prevention is better than cure" is literally true in case of ARF and RHD.

The second phase of the study is to visit the remote endemic areas with mobile heart care unit with diagnostic kit and mobile echocardiography machine. The diagnosis is made on the spot and the treatment shall be started and all the newly diagnosed cases in the free heart check-up camp should be persuaded to visit the institute for follow-up echocardiography. This part of the project is aimed to know the feasibility of extending the benefit of precise early diagnosis of ARF with carditis with echocardiography, at the doorstep, free of cost for the poor patients who fail to reach the hospital in time, so that more number of patients are brought into the net of penicillin prophylaxis and to know the effect in future.

Objective: To extend the program nationwide. The model tested in the pilot project should be customized to the requirements of the region and several model projects should be implemented nationwide and do echocardiographic evaluation of every suspected case of ARF and RHD.

KEY EPIDEMIOLOGICAL OBJECTIVES

The fundamental goal in long-term management of chronic RHD is to avoid or at least delay, valve surgery. Therefore, secondary prophylaxis to prevent recurrent ARF is a crucial strategy in managing patients with chronic RHD. Where adherence to secondary prevention is poor, there is greater need for surgical intervention and long-term surgical outcomes are not good.

CONCLUSION

Although strategies for preventing RHD are proven, simple, cheap, and cost effective, unfortunately they are not adequately implemented. In fact, sometimes these are not implemented at all. In the populations at the highest risk of the disease because there is variability in the management of these diseases, with lack of up-to-date training and experience in the management of ARF and RHD. This occasionally results in inappropriate management and access to healthcare services by population groups experiencing the highest rates of ARF and RHD is limited. The timely echocardiography is the most effective approach in improving and in clinical follow up of patients with RHD. Echocardiography, a modern facility when used as diagnostic criteria, can prevent both over diagnosis and under diagnosis. The Mobile Heart Care units with diagnostic kit and mobile echocardiography machine can bring more patients into the net of secondary prophylaxis. The proper implementation of RHD control programs depends on the health personnel along with a coordinated control, including specialist review. A dedicated coordinator working with the missionary zeal (this is critical to the success of the program); and integration of activities into the established health system to ensure the control program continues to function well despite staffing changes.

REFERENCES

1. World Health Organization. (2000). The World Health Report 2000: Health System: Improving Performance. WHO Geneva 2000. [online] Available from https://apps.who.int/iris/handle/10665/42281 [Last accessed August, 2022].

2. WHO Study Group on Rheumatic Fever and Rheumatic Heart Disease. (1988). Rheumatic fever and rheumatic heart disease. Report of a WHO Study Group. Technical Report Series No. 764, World Health Organization, Geneva 1988. [online] Available from http://whqlibdoc.who.int/trs/WHO_TRS_764.pdf. [Last accessed August, 2022].

3. World Health Organization. (1997). The World Health Report 1997: Conquering suffering. Enriching humanity. WHO Geneva 1997. [online] Available from https://apps.who.int/iris/handle/10665/41900. [Last accessed August, 2022].

4. Murray CJL, Lopez AD. Global Burden of Disease and Injury Series. Global Health Statistics. United States: Harvard University Press; 1996.

5. Murray CJ, Lopez AD. World Health Statistical Annual. Geneva: World Health Organization; 1990-2000.

6. World Health Organization. Joint WHO/ISFC Meeting on RF/RHD Control with emphasis on primary prevention. Geneva 1994. WHO Document WHO/CVD 94.1. Geneva: World Health Organization; 1994.

7. Strasser T, Dondog N, El Kholy A, Gharagozloo R, Kalbian VV, Ogunbi O, et al. The community control of rheumatic fever and rheumatic heart disease: Report of a WHO international cooperative project. Bull World Health Organ. 1981;59(2):285-94.

8. Bach JF, Chalons S, Forier E, Elana G, Jouanelle J, Kayemba S, et al. Ten years educational programme aimed at rheumatic fever in two French Caribbean islands. Lancet. 1996;347:644-6.

9. Neilson G, Streatfield RW, West M, Johnson S, Glavin W, Baird S. Rheumatic fever and chronic rheumatic heart disease in Yarrabah Aboriginal community, North Queensland. Establishment of a prophylactic program. Med J Aust. 1993;158:316-8.

10. Bitar FF, Hayek P, Obeid M, Gharzeddine W, Mikati M, Dbaibo GS. Rheumatic fever in children: A 15-year experience in a developing country. Pediatr Cardiol. 2000;21(2):119-22.

11. Comprehensive programme for prevention. Havana, Cuba 1972-87. Rev Cub Ped. 1989;61(2):228-31.

12. Johannesson M, Weinstein MC. On the decision rules of cost-effectiveness analysis. J Health Econ. 1993;12:459-67.

13. Jaysemy E. Chronic rheumatic heart disease in childhood. Its costs and economic implications. Trop cardiol. 1982;8:55-7.

14. Vijayalakshmi IB, Mithravinda J, Deva AN. The role of echocardiography in diagnosing carditis in the setting of acute rheumatic fever. Cardiol Young. 2005;15:583-8.

15. Vijayalakshmi IB, Vishnuprabhu RO, Chitra N, Rajasri R, Anuradha TV. The efficacy of echocardiographic criterions for the diagnosis of carditis in acute rheumatic fever. Cardiol Young. 2008;18:586-92.

■ ANNEXURE I: RHEUMATIC FEVER/RHEUMATIC HEART DISEASE COMMUNITY SURVEY QUESTIONNAIRE

Name: Village: PHC number: Respondent number:	Location (town/city/village): Suburban ☐ Rural ☐

1. Have you ever had swollen and painful knees, ankles, elbows, wrists with high fever?

☐ Yes

☐ No

2. When you play, have you ever felt tired or had shortness of breath and needed to stop earlier as compared to your friends?

☐ Yes

☐ No

3. Are you undergoing repeated "painful" injection or have you ever had in the past?

☐ Yes

☐ No

4. Have you ever been diagnosed with rheumatic fever or heart disease or heart murmur before?

☐ Yes

☐ No

5. Have you ever had suddon and not controllable movement of your arms, legs, hands and facial muscles?

☐ Yes

☐ No

6. Cardiac auscultation Murmur

☐ Yes

☐ No

ANNEXURE II: PROFORMA FOR ECHO IN ACUTE RHEUMATIC FEVER – 2011

Name	OP No.	Age	Sex	Date	ECHO No.
MV: Thickness-AML	mm, PML	mm, TV	mm, AV	mm	
By tissue harmonics					
Thickness at tip	Base	Throughout			
Submitral structures: Increased echogenicity	Yes	No			
M-mode: Excursion of AML	PML				
Mobility of AML: Normal	Reduced	Increased			
Mobility of PML					
MVP: Clinically	SS	MSM			
ECHO: MVP with-thin valve	Myxomatous valve	Thick valve			
AMLP	PMLP	Both pro	Flial V	TVP	AVP
Beaded appearance: MV	TV	Both			
Mitral regurgitation: Clinically murmur		Absent			
MR grade	Jet central	Eccentric	Jet velocity		
Chordal tear: AML	PML				
AR: Mumur clinically	ECHO grade				
TR: Clinical murmur	ECHO grade	Jet velocity			
Pericardial effusion: Mild	Moderate	Severe			
Pancarditis:	Yes	No	Total ECHO score		
LVIDS EDV First diagnosed on	LVIDs ESV Final diagnosis	RVD EF	Aorta dim	LAD	IVS LVPW
Rh nodules	Chorea	Chest pain	Arthritis/Arthralagia		
ESR	ASLO	CRP	Hb%		
Aspirin: Low dose	High dose	Steroids			
PTMC/CMV	MV repair/ replacement		H/O SBE		

■ ANNEXURE III: PROTOCOL FOR DETAILED ENTRY AT THE TERTIARY CENTER

PROFORMA

Role of echocardiography in precise and early diagnosis of acute rheumatic fever and evolution of rheumatic heart disease

Core proforma for echocardiography in ARF and RHD patients

Registration number:

Name of the patient:

Date of birth:

Age: Sex:

Religion:

Socioeconomic status: Rural ☐ Urban☐

Number of persons in family:

Source of registration:

Hospital:

Diagnostic center:

Consultant:

General practitioner:

Family details	Age	Sex	Relation	Education
1.				
2.				
3.				
4.				
5.				
6.				

Address of the patient

Door No.	Cross	Main	Phase	Block	Locality

Telephone No. ☐☐☐☐☐☐☐☐☐☐ Pin code ☐☐☐☐☐☐☐☐

Diagnosis (Rheumatic fever)

Jones criteria

1. Carditis	☐	Fever	☐	Preceding streptococcal infection	☐
2. Polyarthritis	☐	Arthralgia	☐	H/o Scarlet fever	☐
3. Chorea	☐	Previous H/o RF/RHD	☐	+ve throat culture	☐
4. Rh nodules	☐	C-reactive protein	☐	ASLO titer and other streptococcal antibodies	☐
5. Erythema marginatum	☐	Prolonged P-R interval	☐		☐

Investigations:

1. ESR

2. ECG

3. Echocardiography

SI No.	Types of involvement	Date / /	Date / /	Date / /
1.	Mitral valve thickness 0 for No, 1 for <4 mm, 2 for >4 mm	☐	☐	☐
2.	Mitral regurgitation 0 for No, 1 for Gr 1, 2 for Gr II, 3 for Gr III	☐	☐	☐
3.	Mitral valve prolapse 0 for No. 1 for Gr 1, 2 for Gr II, 3 for Gr III	☐	☐	☐
4.	Aortic regurgitation 0 for No, 1 for Gr 1, 2 for Gr II, 3 for Gr III	☐	☐	☐
5.	Tricuspid regurgitation 0 for No, 1 for Gr 1, 2 for Gr II, 3 for Gr III	☐	☐	☐
6.	Pericardial effusion 0 for No, 1 for Gr 1, 2 for Gr II, 3 for Gr III	☐	☐	☐
7.	Pancarditis 0 for No, 1 for Gr 1, 2 for Gr II, 3 for Gr III	☐	☐	☐
8.	Rheumatic nodules 0 for No, 1 for Yes	☐	☐	☐
9.	Chordal tear 0 for No, 1 for Yes	☐	☐	☐
10.	Reduced mobility and increased echogenicity of the valve and submitral structures 0 for No, 1 for Yes	☐	☐	☐

Progress of disease (Rheumatic heart date)

Valvular disease

	Date	Date	Date
1. MS			
2. MR			
3. AR			
4. AS			
5. TS			
6. TR			
7. PH, CCF			
8. SBE			

Interventional procedure

Cardiac: PTMC ☐

Surgical: CMV ☐   OMV ☐   MVR ☐   AVR ☐   DVR ☐

NYHA class

	At diagnosis	During follow-up	At the end of the study
0			
1			
2			
3			
4			

Disease status as assessed by pediatrician:

Remarks by pediatric cardiologist:

Index

Page numbers followed by *b* refer to box, *f* refer to figure, *fc* refer to flowchart, and *t* refer to table.